Challenges in Pediatric Kidney Transplantation

Katherine E. Twombley
Editor

Challenges in Pediatric Kidney Transplantation

A Practical Guide

Springer

Editor
Katherine E. Twombley
Department of Pediatrics, Division of Pediatric Nephrology
MUSC Shawn Jenkins Children's Hospital/Medical University of South Carolina
Charleston, SC
USA

ISBN 978-3-030-74782-4 ISBN 978-3-030-74783-1 (eBook)
https://doi.org/10.1007/978-3-030-74783-1

This Springer imprint is published by the registered company Springer Nature Switzerland AG
The registered company address is: Gewerbestrasse 11, 6330 Cham, Switzerland

Contents

Contributors

Shumyle Alam, MD Department of Urology, MUSC Shawn Jenkins Children's Hospital/Medical University of South Carolina, Charleston, SC, USA

Kaushalendra Amatya, PhD Children's National Hospital Washington DC, Division of Nephrology, Washington, DC, USA

Isa F. Ashoor, MD Department of Pediatrics, LSU Health and Children's Hospital New Orleans, New Orleans, LA, USA

Sharon M. Bartosh, MD University of Wisconsin, Division of Pediatric Nephrology, Pediatric Kidney Transplantation, Madison, WI, USA

Tom D. Blydt-Hansen, MDCM, FRCPC Department of Pediatrics, University of British Columbia, Vancouver, BC, Canada

Aleah L. Brubaker, MD, PhD Division Abdominal Transplantation, Department of Surgery, Stanford University, Stanford, CA, USA

Alesa Campbell, PharmD Department of Pharmacy, Montefiore Medical Center, Bronx, NY, USA

Rachel M. Engen, MD, MS Department of Pediatrics, Northwestern University Feinberg School of Medicine, Chicago, IL, USA

Rouba Garro, MD Pediatric Nephrology, Emory University School of Medicine Department of Pediatrics, Atlanta, GA, USA

Children's Health Care of Atlanta, Atlanta, GA, USA

Howard M. Gebel, PhD Histocompatibility & Immunogenetics Labs, Emory Medical Laboratory, Emory University School of Medicine, Atlanta, GA, USA

Roshan George, MD, PhD Department of Pediatrics; Division of Pediatric Nephrology, Emory University and Children's Healthcare of Atlanta, Atlanta, GA, USA

Mileka Gilbert, MD, PhD Department of Pediatrics, Division of Pediatric Rheumatology, MUSC Shawn Jenkins Children's Hospital/Medical University of South Carolina, Charleston, SC, USA

Aviva Goldberg, MD Department of Pediatrics and Child Health, Max Rady College of Medicine, University of Manitoba, Winnipeg, MB, Canada

German Lozano Guzman, MD Section of Nephrology St Christopher Hospital, Philadelphia, PA, USA

Lyndsay A. Harshman, MD University of Iowa Organ Transplant Center, Iowa City, IA, USA

James Johnston, MD Department of Pediatrics and Child Health, Max Rady College of Medicine, University of Manitoba, Winnipeg, MB, Canada

Beau Kelly, MD, MBA, FACS DCI Donor Services, West Sacramento, CA, USA

Sarah Kizilbash, MBBS, MS Department of Pediatrics, University of Minnesota, Minneapolis, MN, USA

Samantha Lang, MBBS, BSc Department of Experimental Medicine, University of British Columbia, Vancouver, BC, Canada

Asha Moudgil, MD Children's National Hospital Washington DC, Division of Nephrology, Washington, DC, USA

Satish N. Nadig, MD, PhD Division of Transplant Surgery, Department of Surgery, Medical University of South Carolina, Charleston, SC, USA

Oana Nicoara, MD Department of Pediatrics, Division of Pediatric Nephrology, MUSC Shawn Jenkins Children's Hospital/Medical University of South Carolina, Charleston, SC, USA

Raphael H. Parrado, MD Department of General Surgery, Medical University of South Carolina, Charleston, SC, USA

Maziar Riazy, MD, PhD, FRCPC Department of Pathology and Laboratory Medicine, University of British Columbia, Vancouver, BC, Canada

Sonia I. Savani, MD Department of Medicine and Department of Pediatrics, Medical University of South Carolina, Charleston, SC, USA

Kristen Sgambat, PhD, RD Children's National Hospital Washington DC, Division of Nephrology, Washington, DC, USA

Nida Siddiqi, PharmD Department of Pharmacy, Sidra Medicine, Doha, Qatar

Hailey Silverii, MD Department of Urology, MUSC Shawn Jenkins Children's Hospital/Medical University of South Carolina, Charleston, SC, USA

Jodi M. Smith, MD, MPH Department of Pediatrics, Seattle Children's Hospital/University of Washington, Seattle, WA, USA

Sonia Solomon, DO Department of Pediatric Nephrology, Maria Fareri Children's Hospital/New York Medical College/Westchester Medical Center/Boston Children's Health Physicians, Valhalla, NY, USA

Priya Verghese, MBBS, MPH Department of Pediatrics, Northwestern University Feinberg School of Medicine, Chicago, IL, USA

Pamela D. Winterberg, MD Pediatric Nephrology, Emory University School of Medicine Department of Pediatrics, Atlanta, GA, USA

Children's Health Care of Atlanta, Atlanta, GA, USA

Joshua J. Zaritsky, MD, PhD Division Chief Section of Nephrology St Christopher Hospital, Philadelphia, PA, USA

Part I

Immunologic Challenges

1 Immunologic Challenges Pre-transplant

Roshan George and Howard M. Gebel

Introduction

There are two major antigen systems that play a role in transplantation, namely, the ABO blood group system and the HLA (human leukocyte antigen) complex.

For solid organs, ABO blood group incompatibilities are almost always a contraindication to transplantation (except in emergency liver transplantation or ABO-incompatible infant heart transplantation) and are rarely crossed. While HLA incompatibilities had long been considered to also contraindicate transplantation, more recent data indicate that such incompatibilities can be sufficiently mitigated to allow transplants to proceed. While the ABO system is limited to four distinct blood groups (A, B, AB, and O), the HLA system is far more complex. The current database of HLA alleles cites over 27,000 distinct HLA alleles in the human genome [1].

The importance of the HLA system in transplant outcomes emerged following the first successful kidney transplant between identical twin siblings in 1954. Subsequent studies between non-identical siblings revealed improved graft survival among HLA identical kidney transplant pairs compared with their HLA mismatched counterparts [2].

R. George (✉)
Department of Pediatrics; Division of Pediatric Nephrology, Emory University and Children's Healthcare of Atlanta, Atlanta, GA, USA
e-mail: roshan.punnoose.george@emory.edu

H. M. Gebel
Histocompatibility & Immunogenetics Labs, Emory Medical Laboratory, Emory University School of Medicine, Atlanta, GA, USA
e-mail: hgebel@emory.edu

K. E. Twombley (ed.), *Challenges in Pediatric Kidney Transplantation*,
https://doi.org/10.1007/978-3-030-74783-1_1

What Is Human Leukocyte Antigen (HLA)?

The HLA system is encoded by the human major histocompatibility complex (MHC) located on the short arm of human chromosome 6 (6p21.3) (Fig. 1.1). The MHC is a highly polymorphic region, spanning approximately 3600 kilobases of DNA [3] encoding for proteins that distinguish "self" from "non-self." The gene products encoded by the MHC complex are inherited in Mendelian fashion, such that each child receives a set of HLA genes (known as a haplotype) from each parent. The proteins encoded by these HLA genes are expressed as co-dominant alleles and play an essential role in the immunologic responsiveness and diversity among and between individuals across all races and ethnicities [4].

The human MHC is referred to as the HLA (human leukocyte antigen) system as these antigens were first identified and characterized using alloantibodies that reacted with leukocytes [5].

The human MHC is divided into three regions: class I, class II, and class III (Fig. 1.1).

The function of the HLA system is to continually present antigens (in the form of small peptides) to T cells, helping each individual's immune system develop tolerance to target tissue expressing "self" antigens and promoting the elimination of targets expressing "non-self" antigens. There are three classes of MHC antigens (classes I, II, and III) of which classes I and II are critically important from the perspective of transplant immunology [6]. Class I antigens include the HLA-A, HLA-B, and HLA-C gene clusters, while class II antigens include HLA-DR, HLA-DQ, and HLA-DP gene clusters.

Class I HLA proteins are expressed by virtually all somatic nucleated cells and platelets and occasionally (approximately in 15% of the population) on red cells [7–9]. Class I genes code for the α polypeptide (heavy) chain of the class I

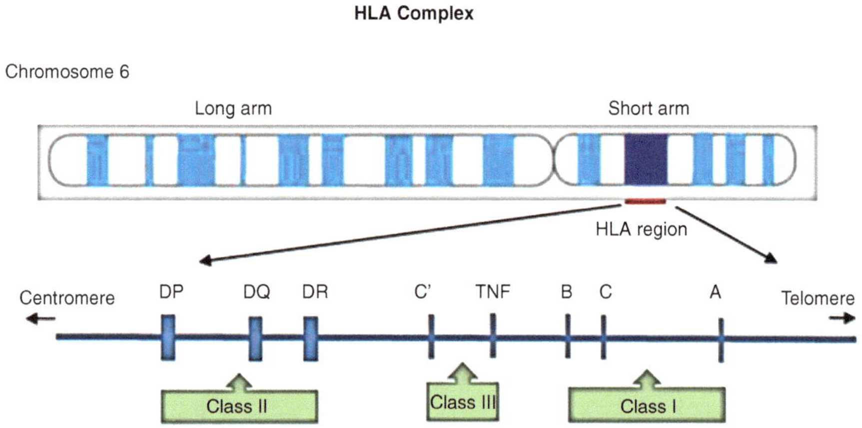

Fig. 1.1 Human major histocompatibility complex (MHC), on the short arm of chromosome 6. Class I, class II, and class III regions represented

molecule. The α chain has five domains: two peptide-binding domains (α1 and α2), one immunoglobulin-like domain (α3), the transmembrane region, and the cytoplasmic tail. The β (light) chain of the class I molecule is encoded by beta2-microglobulin, a gene on chromosome 15. While there are ~20 class I genes in the HLA region, HLA-A, HLA-B, and HLA-C are class Ia genes (the so-called classic genes) and the most clinically relevant class I genes in transplant immunology (Fig. 1.2).

Class II proteins are normally expressed by a subgroup of specialized antigen-presenting cells including B cells, activated T cells, macrophages, dendritic cells, and thymic epithelial cells [7]. Class II genes encode both polypeptide chains (α and β) of class II molecules. In the presence of interferon-γ, such as under conditions of inflammatory stress (e.g., transplant surgery), other types of cells can also express class II HLA molecules [7, 10]. The class II region consists of a series of subregions, each containing *A* and *B* genes encoding α and β chains, respectively [11]. Each of the class II α and β chains has four domains – the peptide-binding domain (α1 or β1), the immunoglobulin-like domain (α2 or β2), the transmembrane region, and the cytoplasmic tail (Fig. 1.2). The *DR* gene family consists of a single *DRA* gene and up to nine *DRB* genes (*DRB1* to *DRB9*).

Under the auspices of the World Health Organization and the International Union of Immunological Societies, a nomenclature committee met in July, 1975, and established an alpha-numeric system of letters and numbers for each antigen that includes a letter designation for the locus, followed by a number unique to each antigen [12].

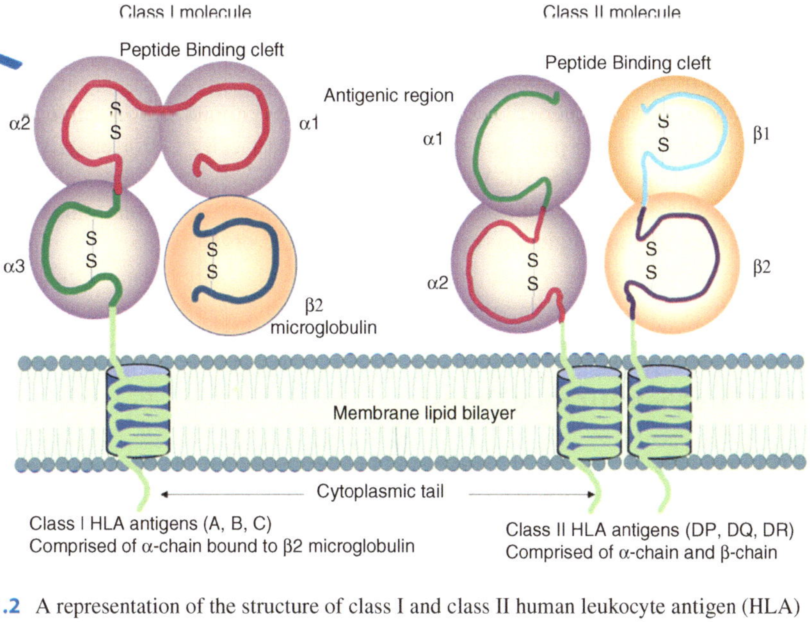

Fig. 1.2 A representation of the structure of class I and class II human leukocyte antigen (HLA)

The designation of the HLA loci on chromosome 6 consists of one or two letters for classes I and II, respectively: for example, for HLA-A and HLA-DR. For class II locus antigens, there are a third letter (A or B) referring to the α or β, respectively, and a number referring to which A or B chain (when there are >1), for example, HLA-DRB3. After the last letter, there is an asterisk (*) which indicates the HLA allele has been identified by molecular methodology. Each individual HLA allele is then identified by a unique number corresponding to up to a total of four sets of digits, each set separated by a colon. In its simplest form, the numbers before the first colon describe the so-called antigen, while the numbers after the colon refer to the allele of that antigen. The set of digits after the second colon refer to changes in nucleotide sequences for the molecule which do not result in a protein change. The numbers after the third colon refer to differences outside the coding region of the HLA molecule. Alleles whose numbers differ in the second set of digits differ in at least one nucleotide substitution that results in an amino acid change (meaning the protein sequence will be different). For example, HLA-DRB1*04:01 and HLA-DRB1*04:02 represent two different subtypes of DR4. Note that while reporting is typically done in alphabetical order, the actual sequence of the loci on chromosome 6 is centromere, D, B, C, and A [13].

The *Class III* region does not encode HLA molecules, but contains genes for complement components (C2, C4, factor B), 21-hydroxylase, tumor necrosis factors (TNFs), and other genes associated with immune responsiveness [3].

HLA class I and class II gene complex are among the most polymorphic loci in the human genome. Polymorphisms (multiple forms of an antigen type each encoded by the same HLA locus) that occur within the peptide-binding regions of an HLA molecule often lead to variations of peptide-binding abilities and specificities, hence playing an important role in an individual's immunological repertoire [14]. Since every individual has two HLA alleles at each HLA locus (A, B, C, DRB1, DRB3/4/5, DQA, DQB, DPA, DPB) [15], the degree of possible genetic diversity is enormous, leading to increased likelihood of species survival.

Both class I and class II molecules function to initiate the adaptive immune response by presenting pathogen-derived peptides to T cells. Unfortunately, in solid organ transplantation, the HLA proteins on donor organs and donor cells are perceived as "foreign" or "non-self" antigen. Without immunosuppression, the recipient will thus immunologically reject the transplanted organ.

Pre-transplant

How Does Sensitization Occur?

HLA sensitization refers to the presence of antibodies to HLA antigens in the potential recipient. If the antibodies are directed against any of the HLA antigens of a specific donor, those antibodies are referred to as DSA (donor-specific antibodies). Those same antibodies would not be considered donor specific if the donor did not possess any of the corresponding HLA antigens. This distinction, while obvious, is nonetheless critically important. Antibodies to HLA antigens can develop if a patient is exposed to non-self HLA and sensitization can occur pre- or post-transplantation. Pre-transplant sensitization is found in ~30% adult kidney transplant candidates; post-transplant, donor-specific sensitization occurs in up to 20% of recipients; de novo donor-specific antibody (DSA) increases based on factors such as donor-recipient mismatch, time since transplant, and compliance with immunosuppressive medication [16–19].

In children, these post-transplant HLA antibodies were even more common [20].

Risk factors for HLA sensitization include prior transplantation, blood product transfusion, pregnancy, and ventricular assist device use [21]. Of these risk factors, the strongest is a history of prior transplantation.

Prior Transplantations In the post-transplant period, over 20% of renal allograft recipients will develop de novo HLA-DSA within 10 years [22]. Re-transplantation recipients displayed stronger antibody production than recipients of a primary transplant transplantation. Re-transplant candidates also had an increased risk of early graft loss compared to their first transplant counterparts [23, 24]. Patients were often broadly sensitized after the removal of the failed renal allograft especially when immunosuppression was halted [25]. This presents a significant challenge in long-term care of pediatric patients as they are more likely to require repeated transplantations in their lifetime.

Pregnancy Sensitization by pregnancy is a significant mechanism by which parous (especially multiparous) women develop HLA class I and class II antibodies. Since a baby inherits its HLA type from each parent, the mother will be exposed to the father's antigens that are expressed in the cells of the developing baby and cross through the placenta into her own system. The HLA antigens from the father which are foreign to the mother will stimulate her immune system to produce anti-HLA antibodies. Interestingly, HLA antibodies made during pregnancy that would be reactive with the baby's cells and tissues do not cross the placenta and harm the baby. This is because the placenta expresses HLA antigens and the antibodies tend to be adsorbed on that tissue before reaching the baby. Antibodies to HLA class I are more frequent than class II [26]. The prevalence of HLA antibodies increases as the number of pregnancies/parities increases [27]. When a wife/mother is in need of a kidney transplant, if they were sensitized and have demonstrable HLA antibodies to their child or the child's biological father, neither the child nor its biological father would be considered suitable donors [28, 29].

While not commonly encountered in pediatric patients, a history of pregnancy should be inquired in all age-appropriate patients during transplant evaluation.

Transfusion Transfusion is a relatively poorly immunogenic stimulus, and multiple transfusions are typically required to induce persistent HLA allosensitization. The use of blood transfusions that matched for HLA-DR antigens was the starting point in transfusion therapy. The use of HLA-matched blood and leukocyte-depleted blood products reduces but does not eliminate the risk of HLA sensitization [30, 31].

Vaccination Prevention of infections through vaccination, in solid organ transplantation, is important and recommended by several clinical guidelines [32–34]; however, there have been concerns about the immune response to vaccination triggering the undesirable development of HLA antibodies [35, 36]. There are limited studies assessing development of de novo DSA and rejection episodes after vaccination in solid organ transplant recipients; however, the overall incidence of post-vaccine de novo DSA and rejection is low and comparable to non-vaccinated patients [37]. It is hence critically important for transplant recipients to get vaccinated as recommended, to be protected from vaccine-preventable infections.

Impact of Sensitization Alloantibodies recognize specific antigenic sequences (epitopes, eplets) displayed by the HLA molecule on the transplanted allograft and contribute to graft damage. There is a clear association between previous exposure to foreign HLA and the occurrence of a high degree of panel reactive antibody (PRA) [38]. The percentage of PRA estimates the likelihood of compatibility or incompatibility with random donors. The higher the PRA (or the more reliable calculated PRA (cPRA)), the lower the likelihood of compatibility with a random donor. Today, cPRA activity is determined using an array of microparticles coated with discrete HLA alleles to determine the antibody specificities a patient possesses. These antibodies are then entered into a web-based cPRA calculator which quickly calculates the percentage of approximately 18,000 HLA-typed deceased donors that react with the antibodies. Historically, when transplants were performed across antibodies that were present pre-transplant, recipients with preformed DSA had a higher likelihood of graft loss [28, 39].

Female patients receiving kidney allografts from their male partners or offspring often experience higher rates of graft rejection [40].

The risk of sensitization increases as there is exposure to more than one sensitizing factor [38].

Collectively, the impact of sensitization in a potential recipient results in longer waiting time for transplantation, post-transplant complications, increased episodes of graft rejection, exposure to more adverse effects of immunosuppressive drugs, and under the worst of circumstances graft loss [41].

The immune system of children is constantly evolving, and their immune maturation is already impacted by their underlying primary disease as well as exposure to pre-transplant immune insults [42]. Approximately 20% of children awaiting transplantation have cPRA >80 percent [43]. Importantly, from 2010 to 2012, only 3% of these children received a kidney transplant [44]. Highly sensitized pediatric patients are hence at a significant disadvantage compared to their unsensitized peers.

Why Is HLA Compatibility Important?

HLA matching between potential donor and recipient pair is determined by comparing their HLA antigens. Accurate typing of HLA is critical to avoid transplanting a donor organ against which the recipient has preformed antibodies and also to determine the degree of HLA mismatch between a donor and recipient. Historically, the degree of mismatch between the donors and recipients only considered mismatches for HLA-A, HLA-B, and HLA-DR antigens. A *six-antigen mismatch* means that two each of the three HLA antigens, namely, HLA-A, HLA-B, and HLA-DR, in the recipient are different from those of the donor's phenotype.

Mismatching for HLA-A, HLA-B, and HLA-DR has been associated with a higher risk of HLA sensitization in both adult and pediatric patients listed for a second kidney transplant. In a study of 2704 pediatric kidney transplant recipients who were relisted after primary graft failure, an increasing number of HLA-DR mismatches at first transplantation were associated with a higher degree of sensitization, and two HLA-DR mismatches at first transplant were associated with a 20 percent lower likelihood of receiving a second transplant [45].

A zero-antigen mismatch is the absence of HLA-A, HLA-B, or HLA-DR antigens in the donor's phenotype different from the recipient's HLA-A, HLA-B, and HLA-DR antigens. Thus, six-antigen HLA matches and zero-antigen HLA mismatches are associated with the best clinical outcomes. Unfortunately, most living-donated allografts for a pediatric recipient are not such identical matches. In fact, allografts for children are commonly from a parent, with whom they share a single haplotype match. In either deceased donor or living-related transplant, superior HLA matching between recipient and donor is associated with improved allograft outcomes in children [46]. Optimal HLA matching is also preferred to minimize sensitization, particularly for young recipients who will need re-transplantations [47, 48].

The number of HLA matches may be a stronger predictor of kidney allograft survival compared to the number of mismatches. In a retrospective study of over 96,000 deceased donor kidney transplants between 1995 and 2012, both HLA matching and mismatching were associated with graft survival when analyzed in individual models. However, when both HLA matching and mismatching were accounted for simultaneously, using a combined model, only the degree of HLA matching was found to be a significant predictor of delayed graft function, 1-year acute rejection, and 10-year graft survival [49].

It is, however, critical to balance HLA matching for long-term outcomes with equitable access to transplantation, since solely using HLA matching for allocation may limit access to transplantation for recipients of minority race and ethnicity, who may have rare HLA antigens not present in a primarily Caucasian donor pool. It is also thus important to advocate for organ donation from a diverse donor pool.

HLA typing was initially performed using serology-based assays, which has since been replaced by the use of DNA-based molecular techniques, leading to high-resolution and more accurate HLA typing. It has also led to typing of all loci

(*HLA-A*, *HLA-B*, *HLA-C*, *HLA-DRB1*, *HLA-DRB3/4/5*, *HLA-DQA*, *HLA-DQB*, and *HLA-DPB*), as opposed to the historic focus on *HLA-A*, *HLA-B*, and *HLA-DR* loci.

In the United States, the United Network for Organ Sharing (UNOS) mandates HLA typing of all loci by molecular methods. Allocation algorithms for deceased donor kidney transplants now take into consideration antibodies against all loci when determining a patient's suitability for transplant from a particular donor.

The specific methodology used for HLA typing in solid organ transplantation differs between HLA laboratories. Currently, the primary method to type deceased donors is referred to as real-time polymerase chain reaction (RT-PCR). High-resolution typing methods (such as sequence-based typing, next-generation sequencing [NGS]) currently take more time to perform and are not yet typically applicable for deceased donor typing. However, this technology-driven and high-resolution typing for deceased donors is likely to be the method of choice in the not too distant future [50]. Interestingly, serologic-based assays are still utilized by numerous laboratories around the world.

Serologic methods: this technique uses a panel of reference sera known to contain antibodies to various HLA antigens. Lymphocytes from the donor or recipient are added to several wells of plates containing different sera and incubated to allow binding between antibody and antigen, following which a complement is added to the wells, and cell lysis is detected using a viability dye. The presence of dead cells is a positive test. Comparison of the serologic specificities of the different sera that reacted allows one to assign the HLA type.

This method had some significant limitations – antisera contained antibodies against more than one specific HLA molecule causing inconclusive reactivity patterns and large number of HLA specificities could not be reliably identified, especially antigens with decreased cell surface expression (such as HLA-C and HLA-DP antigens) was challenging.

In the United States, Canada, and Europe, HLA typing for kidney transplant candidates is performed by intermediate- or high-resolution molecular typing, and serologic equivalents for HLA-A, HLA-B, HLA-C, HLA-Bw4, HLA-Bw6, HLA-DR, HLA-DR51/52/53, and HLA-DQB antigens are reported for organ sharing. HLA-DPB results are reported exclusively at the allele level (no serological equivalents).

Epitope Mismatch

An epitope, also known as antigenic determinant, is the small configuration of amino acids on HLA molecular surfaces, which is recognized by the immune system. It is the specific piece or part of the antigen to which an antibody binds. Epitopes consist of three-dimensional configurations of approximately 15 to 22 amino acid residues, which may be contiguous (linear) in the peptide chain or, more commonly, brought together (conformational) by protein folding.

Immunogenicity and antigenicity of HLA antigens are determined by their stereostructure, amino acid sequence, and physicochemical properties. As initially proposed by Duquesnoy, antigens are composed of multiple subunits referred to as "eplets" [51].

Eplets have been called "functional epitopes" since they include the 2 to 5 amino acids that are recognized by anti-HLA antibodies within the larger 15 to 22 amino acids of an HLA epitope.

Eplets may be unique to a specific HLA antigen, shared among a few HLA antigens, or common to multiple HLA antigens (Fig. 1.3). The restricted number of eplets and their sharing across HLA antigens offer a novel strategy when considering donor- recipient pairs.

The eplet mismatch load is determined by counting the number of eplets that are mismatched between a recipient and the potential donor. The number of donor-recipient eplet mismatches can be determined using an available computer algorithm called the HLAMatchmaker [52, 53].

Several observational studies have shown that a higher number of mismatched eplets are associated with a higher risk of developing DSA post-transplant and a higher risk of graft loss [54–56]. Given the observation that certain HLA allele mismatches are more antigenic than others, studies have looked into the consequences of donor-recipient mismatch at the epitope/eplet level. For example, while two different donor-recipient pairs may each be mismatched for a single HLA antigen, they may be differentially eplet mismatched (e.g., < 5 vs. > 25 eplet mismatches), with a higher load mismatch leading to a greater risk of poor outcomes [54, 57, 58]. Furthermore, the most recent data suggest that not all eplet mismatches carry identical risk. Some (possibly immunodominant mismatches) may be more deleterious than others, and avoiding those mismatches can promote better long-term outcomes. The overall number of donor-recipient eplet mismatches (so-called eplet load) has been linked to the development of de novo DSA

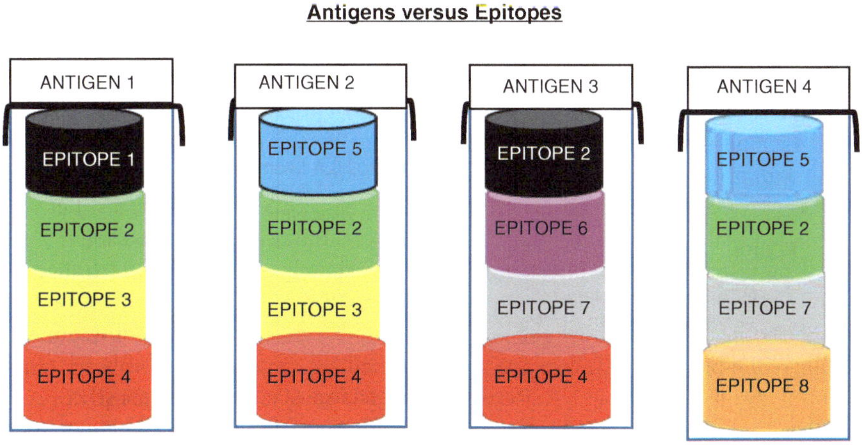

Fig. 1.3 Representing the differences between antigens and epitopes
Four distinct antigens. Each antigen is made up of multiple epitopes. While each antigen is unique, the same epitopes can be shared among different antigens

and immune-mediated allograft injury [55, 59, 60]. Several researchers have sought to identify thresholds of cumulative eplet mismatch loads associated with greater risk of immune-mediated injuries post-transplant at the population level. Recently, it has been suggested or revealed that similar eplet loads may be composed of eplet mismatches with different properties and some eplets may have greater immunogenicity than others [61]. To incorporate eplet matching into organ allocation schemes, it is important to identify which eplets have the greatest adverse impact across the continuum of immune-mediated injuries such as DSA development, reversible and irreversible rejection (e.g., transplant glomerulopathy), and premature graft failure. A recent study by Sapir-Pichhadze et al. reviewed more than 100,000 SRTR kidney transplant records and found a statistically significant relationship between a particular set of eplet mismatches and death-censored graft failure across sensitivity and subgroup analysis [62]. These eplet mismatches were found to be independent predictors of transplant glomerulopathy in a separate Canadian cohort. The relatively small number of these eplets (compared with the comprehensive repertoire of eplets) and their association with transplant outcomes suggest that minimization of mismatches of those particular epitopes is a reasonable, feasible, and clinically justifiable strategy to introduce epitope matching into organ allocation schemes, even for patients who may be deemed unsensitized (Fig. 1.4).

How Are HLA Antibodies Detected and HLA Matching Performed?

To determine pre-transplant HLA sensitization The panel reactive antibody (PRA) score is derived using a panel of HLA-typed cells or microparticles which act

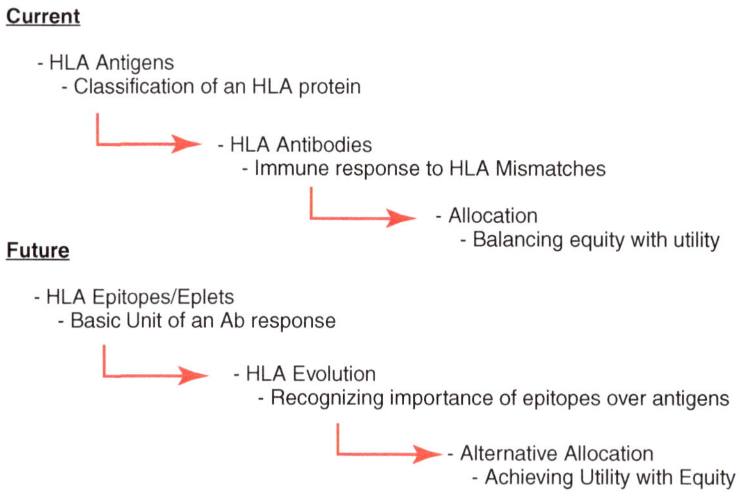

Fig. 1.4 Current and future utilization of our knowledge of HLA antigens and epitopes

as surrogate targets representative of organ donors. PRA is broadly used to determine the degree of HLA sensitization in an individual [63].

As mentioned above, UNOS developed a calculator to determine calculated PRA (cPRA) values. The cPRA is based on the frequency of those HLA specificities deemed unacceptable for an individual sensitized as evaluated with a historic population of HLA-typed deceased donors. Thus, a cPRA represents the percentage of donors who are expected to have unacceptable HLA antigens to which the transplant candidate is sensitized [64].

Antibody Detection

To determine preformed HLA antibodies HLA antibodies are detected through cell-based assays or solid-phase immunoassays. Historically, cell-based assays were developed first and significantly improved transplant outcomes. However, cell-based assays had limited sensitivity and specificity, which led to development of so-called solid-phase assays. The term "solid phase" refers to coating of polystyrene or latex beads with HLA antigens as opposed to cellular targets with membrane-bound HLA molecules [65]. Solid-phase assays are now the most commonly used platform in the HLA laboratories. DSA identified by single-antigen bead (SAB) array are nonetheless questioned for their sensitivity and lack of event prediction after transplantation [66].

Cell-Based Assays

The Complement-Dependent Cytotoxicity Assay (CDC) Patel and Terasaki, in a 1969 study, used CDC to predict humoral hyperacute rejection after they found that 80% of grafts with positive CDC crossmatches failed immediately post-transplant compared to a 4% immediate failure rate among those donor-recipient pairs with a negative crossmatch [67].

In the CDC method, the recipient's serum is mixed with individual donor cells (or panel cells for PRA determination). Following incubation, an exogenous source of complement is added, and viability is then assessed. Dead cells are interpreted as a positive reaction [68]. If HLA antibodies are present in the recipient serum, those bind to HLA proteins on lymphocytes and complement can then bind. This initiates complement-mediated injury, resulting in lymphocyte death [65]. The percent lymphocyte death is assessed by microscopy and expressed as a percentage of panel reactive antibodies (PRA). If the assay is positive, then antigen specificities of HLA antibodies can be determined by follow-up immunoassays.

The major limitations of the CDC method include relatively poor sensitivity and specificity, incomplete identification of HLA antibody specificities, a reliance on cell viability, inability to detect non-complement fixing HLA antibodies, and poor reproducibility and are typically limited to detection of antibodies to class I antigens [69–71].

Solid-phase immunoassays were developed to overcome these challenges.

Solid-Phase Assays

Since 2009, UNOS has mandated the use of solid-phase assays to identify HLA antibodies in potential transplant recipients in the United States. Their technical advantages, which enable automation and rapid turnaround, and their ability to identify both complement- and non-complement-dependent antibodies make them a preferred method. Solid-phase matrix (plates or beads) is coated with single or multiple HLA antigens. Antibodies to these antigens are typically detected by flow cytometry or with a Luminex® instrument [65].

ELISA-Based Detection of HLA Antibodies Patient's serum is incubated with HLA antigens coated on a microtiter plate. The sensitivity of ELISA for HLA antibody detection is higher than CDC (97% versus 78%, respectively) [72], but this method is rarely used now. More sensitive, rapid analyses such as single-antigen bead assays, which utilize flow cytometry and/or laser-based multiplex technology (Luminex®), are now used in place of cell-based assay [65].

Flow Cytometry Detection of HLA Antibodies For HLA antibody detection, patient's serum is incubated with latex beads coated with purified antigens. If antibodies are present, they bind and are detected using fluorescent tags and expressed as number of beads with bound antibodies to the number tested. The beads can be coated with single HLA antigen to increase specificity of the antibodies [72].

Flow cytometry techniques are superior in identifying HLA specificity and to identify antibodies to HLA antigens from a pool of donors and perform a crossmatch [73, 74].

Each center determines their threshold for positivity, and this leads to challenges in standardization. Variability in fluorochromes and flow cytometers and differences in clinical significance of identified antibodies add to these challenges [70].

Luminex®-Based Detection of HLA Antibodies The Luminex® system is a multiplex bead-based platform, where patient's serum is incubated with beads – each coated with a single HLA antigen. Antibodies, if present, bind to the beads and are detected with a fluorescently labeled antibody to human IgG, using a dual laser to identify the bound antibody as well as the HLA antigen-coated bead [75, 76]. The degree of fluorescence exhibited by the presence of the antibody is resulted in terms of its *median fluorescence intensity (MFI).*

Luminex®-based immunoassays allow rapid turnaround time, HLA determination of specific HLA antibodies, distinguishing between class I and II positivity, and enabling virtual crossmatching. However, there is a high degree of technical variation with center-specific thresholds and only semi-quantitative results being available [74].

Is Median Fluorescent Intensity (MFI) Signal a Surrogate Measure of the Level of HLA Antibody?

MFI levels on the beads, using undiluted patient sera, represent a relative amount of antibody that is bound to the antigen on the bead and can vary between individual beads. MFI threshold cutoffs are established by each HLA laboratory (balancing between the sensitivity of the assay and its false-positive rate) and are not standardized.

MFI results are provided as a numerical value and can provide some idea of the amount and strength of alloantibody present. However, the MFI value cannot be used as a quantitative method. MFI values are *not* synonymous with concentration or titer of antibody.

MFI levels can be affected by a number of technical considerations to the assay, including the setup of the flow cytometer or Luminex® instrument, the density of antigen expressed on the beads, and the fluorochrome detection antibody used.

Existing consensus guidelines suggest that quantification of antibody burden is best estimated by titration (serial dilution) studies [70, 77].

Peri-transplant

The Virtual Crossmatch (vXM) in Transplantation

The concept of virtual crossmatching evolved from theoretical to practical, after solid-phase antibody detection assays were implemented [78]. A vXM is based on the specificities of HLA antibodies detected in the transplant recipient compared to the HLA antigen profile of a potential donor. If there are no antibodies in the patient's serum complimentary to the antigens found in the prospective donor, the vXM is considered negative. Presence of donor antibodies at a given MFI threshold (center determined) is considered a positive vXM. Virtual crossmatching enlarges the catchment area for organ procurement and reduces transplant wait times while having similar long-term outcomes as those transplanted using a traditional prospective cell-based physical crossmatch [79, 80].

Unexpected Crossmatch Scenarios

Unexpected/false positive: can occur in the following scenarios:

- High background signal, particularly with B-cell flow cytometry crossmatch. To reduce this background fluorescence and improve the specificity of the test, most labs use pronase (a cocktail of nonspecific proteases) to treat the cells [81, 82] and remove Fc receptors from the target cell surface. However, use of pronase can reduce sensitivity to detect the presence of DSA, reducing HLA expression or causing false-positive crossmatch results by unveiling cryptic or hidden epitopes [83–85].
- The presence of antibodies that react against lymphocyte-specific antigens but are unlikely to cause graft injury as the antibody is not directed against HLA on the allograft tissue.
- The presence of IgM antibodies, often detected in sera of patients with autoimmune disorders [86]. The caveat here is to rule out a newly formed DSA through a recent sensitizing event.
- Humanized monoclonal antibody treatment, such as an anti-CD20 monoclonal antibody (e.g., rituximab), in which scenario T-cell crossmatch results are not impacted but B-cell crossmatches are strongly positive due to binding of the CD20 epitopes by the monoclonal antibody.
- Other causes include donor cell viability and a strict cutoff threshold.

Under- recognition of antibodies Failure to consider shared epitopes can lead to under-recognition of DSA identified by SAB testing. When a number of beads contain a shared epitope, it is possible for the antibody to become "diluted" by combining to multiple beads and all of those beads to register MFI values below the threshold cutoff [87].

Clinical Scenarios and Interpretation of Crossmatch Results in Kidney Transplantation

Clinicians should communicate closely with their own HLA laboratories and lean on their expertise to understand results of the crossmatch and its relevance to their patients.

Various potential clinical scenarios are noted in Table 1.1.

Table 1.1 Clinical scenarios and interpretation of crossmatch results

CDC crossmatch	Flow cytometry crossmatch	DSA by SAB assay/virtual crossmatch	Interpretation	Outcome
Positive	Positive	Positive	Indicates high antibody burden	Contraindication (CI) for Tx as it is associated with hyperacute rejection
Negative	Positive	Positive	Moderate antibody burden	Not necessarily a CI for Tx but intermediate risk for ABMR higher rates of AR and early and late graft loss
Negative	Negative	Positive	May indicate lower thresholds of antibody detection	Conflicting view on clinical significance. The presence of DSA does indicate a prior exposure to the donor-specific HLA antigen, and therefore the patient is at risk for a latent memory response
Negative	Positive	Negative	Likely clinically irrelevant, non-HLA antibody	Does not appear to correlate with graft outcomes (unless in rare cases a false negative SAB result)

CDC complement-dependent cytotoxicity, *DSA* donor-specific antibody, *SAB* single-antigen bead, *Tx* transplantation, *CI* contraindication, *ABMR* antibody-mediated rejection, *AR* acute rejection, *HLA* human leukocyte antigen

Post-transplant Post-transplantation DSA testing at the time of acute graft dysfunction is also crucial as it may support the diagnosis of antibody-mediated rejection and is discussed elsewhere in this book.

Conclusion

Strategies to improve long-term allograft outcomes include more accurate, timely, and actionable information about HLA mismatch, now even to the eplet level. Aligning the results of all HLA testing can provide an immunologic risk assessment between a donor and recipient pair while also considering clinical characteristics such as urgency, access to compatible allograft, and immunosuppressive strategies. Close and constant communication among the HLA and transplant teams is the foundation for successful transplantation. With continued technical advances in HLA, some of the challenges in pediatric transplantation may be overcome in the coming decades, leading to improved quality of life, limited morbidity, and reduced need for re-transplantation in pediatric recipients.

Questions and Answers with Explanation

Question 1. What are the antigens considered traditionally in a six-antigen mismatch when assessing the degree of mismatch between the donors and recipients?

A. HLA-A, HLA-B, HLA-C.
B. HLA-DR, HLA-DP, HLA-DQ.
C. HLA-A, HLA-B, HLA-DR.
D. HLA-A, HLA-B, HLA-DQ.

Answer: C.

Explanation: Historically, only the mismatches of HLA-A, HLA-B, and HLA-DR antigens were considered when assessing the degree of matches between donor and recipients, and if each two of the three HLA antigens in the recipients are different than the donor, then it was considered a six-antigen mismatch. If there was no difference in these (HLA-A, HLA-B, and HLA-DR) in the donor and recipient phenotype, it was considered a zero-antigen mismatch. Currently, the United Network for Organ Sharing (UNOS) mandates HLA typing of all loci by molecular methods.

Question 2. Which of the following statements is accurate?

A. Serology-based HLA typing when compared to molecular techniques provides higher resolution and more accuracy.
B. Calculated panel reactive antibody (cPRA) scores take into account eplet mismatch load.
C. Median fluorescent intensity (MFI) can be used as a quantitative comparison since they are standardized across laboratories and are independent of technical considerations.
D. Solid-phase assays are now most commonly used to determine preformed antibodies in HLA laboratories.

Answer: D.

Explanation: Solid-phase assays such as flow cytometry or Luminex-based detection of antibodies (as opposed to cell-based assays) have improved sensitivity and specificity and are now used most commonly to determine preformed antibodies.

Molecular techniques such as real-time polymerase chain reaction (RT-PCR) provide more accurate HLA typing when compared to serologic methods which have significant limitations. The calculated panel reactive antibody (cPRA) scores determine pre-transplant HLA sensitization and take into account HLA antigens in donors and not the eplet mismatch.

Eplet mismatch load has been shown to be associated with higher risk of developing post-transplant donor-specific antibody and poorer allograft outcomes but is yet to be incorporated into organ allocation schemes. Median fluorescent intensity (MFI) threshold cutoffs are laboratory specific and not standardized currently. MFI is also affected by technical considerations, such as the setup of the instrument and antigen density on the beads, and hence cannot be used as an accurate or reliable quantitative, comparative measure.

Question 3. Virtual crossmatching is now used widely to assess HLA antibodies in a recipient as specifically related to the HLA antigen profile of his/her potential donor. Which one of the following is an effect of virtual crossmatching?

A. Longer wait times for transplant recipients.
B. Greater confidence in accepting offers from import donors.
C. Increased risk of development of de novo donor-specific antibodies.
D. Poorer long-term outcomes as compared to prospective physical crossmatch.

Answer: B.

Explanation: Virtual crossmatching has increased the confidence of transplant centers to accept import offers of deceased donor organs even for highly sensitized patients based on its ability to predict a negative physical crossmatch. Prior to solid-phase antibody detection assays, the technology did not exist to reliably predict a negative physical crossmatch. Instead, transplant centers had to wait for the results of a physical crossmatch before proceeding to transplant. Besides adding cold ischemia time to the imported donor organ, if the crossmatch was positive, the transplant was canceled, and either the organ was offered to a backup recipient (if a waiver from the organ procurement organization or OPO had been obtained), or the organ was shipped back to be sent to another (next in line) transplant center. This, of course, added even more ischemia time. Therefore, and not infrequently, transplant centers would pass on import offers for their highly sensitized patients.

Question 4. A 15-year-old patient with lupus nephritis progressed to end-stage kidney disease after being on various treatments including steroids, monoclonal antibody therapy, and antihypertensive medications. She was just actively listed for a deceased donor kidney transplantation 2 months ago. A deceased donor offer for this patient is received, and on crossmatching, it is found that she has strongly positive B-cell crossmatch. As a clinician taking this call, what would be your next best step?

A. Cancel this transplant since strongly positive B-cell crossmatch is an absolute contraindication to accepting this donor.
B. It is unclear if this is an absolute or relative contraindication so discuss with the family first, describing the potential high risk of accepting this donor offer.
C. Review the patient history, especially the timing of monoclonal antibody (such as rituximab) administration, and discuss with your HLA lab.
D. There is no risk, and the transplant offer should be accepted immediately to prevent any delays.

Answer: C.

Explanation: Anti-CD20 monoclonal antibody treatment can cause strongly positive B-cell crossmatch due to binding of the CD20 epitope; hence, it is critical to review the timing of such medications and have in-depth communication with your HLA laboratory. Patients with autoimmune diseases can also have IgM antibodies in their sera. There may still be a risk in accepting this offer, but the most appropriate next step is to discuss with your HLA laboratory to gather all data and together assess the risk-benefit in this scenario. Once all information is obtained, it is also essential to communicate with the patient and patient family before next steps are decided.

Acknowledgments *Sherine J. Thomas, MD, for assistance with* Figs. 1.1 and 1.2.

References

1. Robinson J, Halliwell JA, Hayhurst JD, Flicek P, Parham P, Marsh SG. The IPD and IMGT/HLA database: allele variant databases. Nucleic Acids Res. 2015;43(Database issue):D423–31. Epub 2014/11/22.
2. Cheigh JS, Chami J, Stenzel KH, Riggio RR, Saal S, Mouradian JA, et al. Renal transplantation between HLA identical siblings. Comparison with transplants from HLA semi-identical related donors. N Engl J Med. 1977;296(18):1030–4. Epub 1977/05/05.
3. Beck S, Trowsdale J. The human major histocompatibility complex: lessons from the DNA sequence. Annu Rev Genomics Hum Genet. 2000;1:117–37. Epub 2001/11/10.
4. Klein J, Sato A. The HLA system. First of two parts. N Engl J Med. 2000;343(10):702–9. Epub 2000/09/07.
5. Terasaki PI. A brief history of HLA. Immunol Res. 2007;38(1–3):139–48. Epub 2007/10/06.
6. Carpenter CB. HLA and renal transplantation. N Engl J Med. 1980;302(15):860–2. Epub 1980/04/10.
7. Klein J. Natural history of the major histocompatibility complex. New York: John Wiley and Sons; 1986.
8. Novotny VM, Doxiadis II, Brand A. The reduction of HLA class I expression on platelets: a potential approach in the management of HLA-alloimmunized refractory patients. Transfus Med Rev. 1999;13(2):95–105. Epub 1999/04/28.
9. de Villartay JP, Rouger P, Muller JY, Salmon C. HLA antigens on peripheral red blood cells: analysis by flow cytofluorometry using monoclonal antibodies. Tissue Antigens. 1985;26(1):12–9. Epub 1985/07/01.
10. Daar AS, Fuggle SV, Fabre JW, Ting A, Morris PJ. The detailed distribution of MHC class II antigens in normal human organs. Transplantation. 1984;38(3):293–8. Epub 1984/09/01.
11. Marsh SG. Nomenclature for factors of the HLA system, update October 2004. Tissue Antigens. 2005;65(2):206–7. Epub 2005/02/17.
12. WHO-IUIS terminology committee nomenclature for factors of the HL-A system. 1976.
13. Carpenter CB. Editorial: the new HLA nomenclature. N Engl J Med. 1976;294(18):1005–6. Epub 1976/04/29.
14. Danzer M, Niklas N, Stabentheiner S, Hofer K, Proll J, Stuckler C, et al. Rapid, scalable and highly automated HLA genotyping using next-generation sequencing: a transition from research to diagnostics. BMC Genomics. 2013;14:221. Epub 2013/04/06.
15. Tshabalala M, Mellet J, Pepper MS. Human leukocyte antigen diversity: a southern African perspective. J Immunol Res. 2015;2015:746151. Epub 2015/09/09.
16. Jordan SC, Tyan D, Stablein D, McIntosh M, Rose S, Vo A, et al. Evaluation of intravenous immunoglobulin as an agent to lower allosensitization and improve transplantation in highly sensitized adult patients with end-stage renal disease: report of the NIH IG02 trial. J Am Soc Nephrol. 2004;15(12):3256–62. Epub 2004/12/08.
17. Terasaki PI, Ozawa M. Predicting kidney graft failure by HLA antibodies: a prospective trial. Am J Transplant. 2004;4(3):438–43. Epub 2004/02/14.
18. Everly MJ, Rebellato LM, Haisch CE, Ozawa M, Parker K, Briley KP, et al. Incidence and impact of de novo donor-specific alloantibody in primary renal allografts. Transplantation. 2013;95(3):410–7. Epub 2013/02/06.
19. Devos JM, Gaber AO, Teeter LD, Graviss EA, Patel SJ, Land GA, et al. Intermediate-term graft loss after renal transplantation is associated with both donor-specific antibody and acute rejection. Transplantation. 2014;97(5):534–40. Epub 2014/03/07.
20. Miettinen J, Perasaari J, Lauronen J, Qvist E, Valta H, Pakarinen M, et al. Donor-specific HLA antibodies and graft function in children after renal transplantation. Pediatr Nephrol. 2012;27(6):1011–9. Epub 2011/10/14.

21. Pirim I, Soyoz M, Ayna TK, Kocyigit AO, Gurbuz BC, Tugmen C, et al. De novo produced anti-human leukocyte antigen antibodies relation to alloimmunity in patients with chronic renal failure. Genet Test Mol Biomarkers. 2015;19(6):335–8. Epub 2015/04/01.
22. Everly MJ. Incidence and hazards of alloantibodies in renal transplantation. Clin Transpl 2013:313–317. Epub 2013/01/01.
23. Hyun J, Park KD, Yoo Y, Lee B, Han BY, Song EY, et al. Effects of different sensitization events on HLA alloimmunization in solid organ transplantation patients. Transplant Proc. 2012;44(1):222–5. Epub 2012/02/09.
24. House AA, Chang PC, Luke PP, Leckie SH, Howson WT, Ball EJ, et al. Re-exposure to mismatched HLA class I is a significant risk factor for graft loss: multivariable analysis of 259 kidney retransplants. Transplantation. 2007;84(6):722–8. Epub 2007/09/26.
25. Scornik JC, Kriesche HU. Human leukocyte antigen sensitization after transplant loss: timing of antibody detection and implications for prevention. Hum Immunol. 2011;72(5):398–401. Epub 2011/03/01.
26. Hickey MJ, Valenzuela NM, Reed EF. Alloantibody generation and effector function following sensitization to human leukocyte antigen. Front Immunol. 2016;7:30. Epub 2016/02/13.
27. Triulzi DJ, Kleinman S, Kakaiya RM, Busch MP, Norris PJ, Steele WR, et al. The effect of previous pregnancy and transfusion on HLA alloimmunization in blood donors: implications for a transfusion-related acute lung injury risk reduction strategy. Transfusion (Paris). 2009;49(9):1825–35. Epub 2009/05/21.
28. Kumbala D, Zhang R. Essential concept of transplant immunology for clinical practice. World J Transplant. 2013;3(4):113–8. Epub 2014/01/07.
29. Akgul SU, Ciftci HS, Temurhan S, Caliskan Y, Bayraktar A, Tefik T, et al. Association between HLA antibodies and different sensitization events in renal transplant candidates. Transplant Proc. 2017;49(3):425–9. Epub 2017/03/28.
30. Scornik JC, Bromberg JS, Norman DJ, Bhanderi M, Gitlin M, Petersen J. An update on the impact of pre-transplant transfusions and allosensitization on time to renal transplant and on allograft survival. BMC Nephrol. 2013;14:217. Epub 2013/10/11.
31. Tambur AR, Campbell P, Chong AS, Feng S, Ford ML, Gebel H, et al. Sensitization in transplantation: assessment of risk (STAR) 2019 working group meeting report. Am J Transplant. 2020;20(10):2652–68. Epub 2020/04/29.
32. Danzinger-Isakov L, Kumar D. Guidelines for vaccination of solid organ transplant candidates and recipients. Am J Transplant. 2009;9(Suppl 4):S258–62. Epub 2010/01/28.
33. Cohn J, Blumberg EA. Immunizations for renal transplant candidates and recipients. Nat Clin Pract Nephrol. 2009;5(1):46–53. Epub 2008/11/26.
34. Danziger-Isakov L, Kumar D. Vaccination of solid organ transplant candidates and recipients: guidelines from the American society of transplantation infectious diseases community of practice. Clin Transpl. 2019;33(9):e13563. Epub 2019/04/20.
35. Katerinis I, Hadaya K, Duquesnoy R, Ferrari-Lacraz S, Meier S, van Delden C, et al. De novo anti-HLA antibody after pandemic H1N1 and seasonal influenza immunization in kidney transplant recipients. Am J Transplant. 2011;11(8):1727–33. Epub 2011/06/16.
36. Danziger-Isakov L, Cherkassky L, Siegel H, McManamon M, Kramer K, Budev M, et al. Effects of influenza immunization on humoral and cellular alloreactivity in humans. Transplantation. 2010;89(7):838–44. Epub 2010/02/25.
37. Mulley WR, Dendle C, Ling JEH, Knight SR. Does vaccination in solid-organ transplant recipients result in adverse immunologic sequelae? A systematic review and meta-analysis. J Heart Lung Transplant. 2018;37(7):844–52. Epub 2018/04/04.
38. Guichard-Romero A, Marino-Vazquez LA, Castelan N, Lopez M, Gonzalez-Tableros N, Arvizu A, et al. Impact of pretransplant exposure to allosensitization factors generating HLA antibodies in the Luminex era. Transpl Immunol. 2016;38:33–9. Epub 2016/08/25.
39. Elgueta S, Fuentes C, Lopez M, Hernandez J, Arenas A, Jimenez M, et al. Effect of implementing anti-HLA antibody detection by Luminex in the kidney transplant program in Chile. Transplant Proc. 2011;43(9):3324–6. Epub 2011/11/22.

40. Higgins R, Lowe D, Hathaway M, Williams C, Lam FT, Kashi H, et al. Human leukocyte antigen antibody-incompatible renal transplantation: excellent medium-term outcomes with negative cytotoxic crossmatch. Transplantation. 2011;92(8):900–6. Epub 2011/10/05.
41. Zachary AA, Kopchaliiska D, Jackson AM, Leffell MS. Immunogenetics and immunology in transplantation. Immunol Res. 2010;47(1–3):232–9. Epub 2010/01/27.
42. George RP, Mehta AK, Perez SD, Winterberg P, Cheeseman J, Johnson B, et al. Premature T cell senescence in pediatric CKD. J Am Soc Nephrol. 2017;28(1):359–67. Epub 2016/07/15.
43. Chaudhuri A, Ozawa M, Everly MJ, Ettenger R, Dharnidharka V, Benfield M, et al. The clinical impact of humoral immunity in pediatric renal transplantation. J Am Soc Nephrol. 2013;24(4):655–64. Epub 2013/03/02.
44. Matas AJ, Smith JM, Skeans MA, Thompson B, Gustafson SK, Schnitzler MA, et al. OPTN/SRTR 2012 annual data report: kidney. Am J Transplant. 2014;14(Suppl 1):11–44. Epub 2014/01/01.
45. Gralla J, Tong S, Wiseman AC. The impact of human leukocyte antigen mismatching on sensitization rates and subsequent retransplantation after first graft failure in pediatric renal transplant recipients. Transplantation. 2013;95(10):1218–24. Epub 2013/03/13.
46. Shi X, Liu R, Xie X, Lv J, Han W, Zhong X, et al. Effect of human leukocyte antigen mismatching on the outcomes of pediatric kidney transplantation: a systematic review and meta-analysis. Nephrol Dial Transplant. 2017;32(11):1939–48. Epub 2017/10/11.
47. Tagliamacco A, Cioni M, Comoli P, Ramondetta M, Brambilla C, Trivelli A, et al. DQ molecules are the principal stimulators of de novo donor-specific antibodies in nonsensitized pediatric recipients receiving a first kidney transplant. Transpl Int. 2014;27(7):667–73. Epub 2014/03/19.
48. Foster BJ, Dahhou M, Zhang X, Platt RW, Hanley JA. Relative importance of HLA mismatch and donor age to graft survival in young kidney transplant recipients. Transplantation. 2013;96(5):469–75. Epub 2013/06/14.
49. Yacoub R, Nadkarni GN, Cravedi P, He JC, Delaney VB, Kent R, et al. Analysis of OPTN/UNOS registry suggests the number of HLA matches and not mismatches is a stronger independent predictor of kidney transplant survival. Kidney Int. 2018;93(2):482–90. Epub 2017/10/03.
50. De Santis D, Truong L, Martinez P, D'Orsogna L. Rapid high-resolution HLA genotyping by MinION Oxford nanopore sequencing for deceased donor organ allocation. Hla. 2020;96(2):141–62. Epub 2020/04/11.
51. Duquesnoy RJ. Are we ready for epitope-based HLA matching in clinical organ transplantation? Transplantation. 2017;101(8):1755–65. Epub 2017/02/17.
52. Duquesnoy RJ, Marrari M. HLAMatchmaker: a molecularly based algorithm for histocompatibility determination. II. Verification of the algorithm and determination of the relative immunogenicity of amino acid triplet-defined epitopes. Hum Immunol. 2002;63(5):353–63. Epub 2002/04/27.
53. Kosmoliaptsis V, Bradley JA, Sharples LD, Chaudhry A, Key T, Goodman RS, et al. Predicting the immunogenicity of human leukocyte antigen class I alloantigens using structural epitope analysis determined by HLAMatchmaker. Transplantation. 2008;85(12):1817–25. Epub 2008/06/27.
54. Wiebe C, Pochinco D, Blydt-Hansen TD, Ho J, Birk PE, Karpinski M, et al. Class II HLA epitope matching-a strategy to minimize de novo donor-specific antibody development and improve outcomes. Am J Transplant. 2013;13(12):3114–22. Epub 2013/10/30.
55. Wiebe C, Nevins TE, Robiner WN, Thomas W, Matas AJ, Nickerson PW. The synergistic effect of class II HLA epitope-mismatch and nonadherence on acute rejection and graft survival. Am J Transplant. 2015;15(8):2197–202. Epub 2015/06/23.
56. Dankers MK, Witvliet MD, Roelen DL, de Lange P, Korfage N, Persijn GG, et al. The number of amino acid triplet differences between patient and donor is predictive for the antibody reactivity against mismatched human leukocyte antigens. Transplantation. 2004;77(8):1236–9. Epub 2004/04/29.

57. Wiebe C, Kosmoliaptsis V, Pochinco D, Gibson IW, Ho J, Birk PE, et al. HLA-DR/DQ molecular mismatch: a prognostic biomarker for primary alloimmunity. Am J Transplant. 2019;19(6):1708–19. Epub 2018/11/11.
58. Sharma A, Lewis JR, Lim WH, Palmer S, Strippoli G, Chapman JR, et al. Renal transplant outcomes and de novo donor-specific anti-human leukocyte antigen antibodies: a systematic review. Nephrol Dial Transplant. 2018;33(8):1472–80. Epub 2018/04/17.
59. Sapir-Pichhadze R, Tinckam K, Quach K, Logan AG, Laupacis A, John R, et al. HLA-DR and -DQ eplet mismatches and transplant glomerulopathy: a nested case-control study. Am J Transplant. 2015;15(1):137–48. Epub 2014/12/19.
60. Wiebe C, Rush DN, Nevins TE, Birk PE, Blydt-Hansen T, Gibson IW, et al. Class II Eplet mismatch modulates tacrolimus trough levels required to prevent donor-specific antibody development. J Am Soc Nephrol. 2017;28(11):3353–62. Epub 2017/07/22.
61. McCaughan JA, Battle RK, Singh SKS, Tikkanen JM, Moayedi Y, Ross HJ, et al. Identification of risk epitope mismatches associated with de novo donor-specific HLA antibody development in cardiothoracic transplantation. Am J Transplant. 2018;18(12):2924–33. Epub 2018/05/31.
62. Sapir-Pichhadze R, Zhang X, Ferradji A, Madbouly A, Tinckam KJ, Gebel HM, et al. Epitopes as characterized by antibody-verified eplet mismatches determine risk of kidney transplant loss. Kidney Int. 2020;97(4):778–85. Epub 2020/02/16.
63. Asante-Korang A, Jacobs JP, Ringewald J, Carapellucci J, Rosenberg K, McKenna D, et al. Management of children undergoing cardiac transplantation with high panel reactive antibodies. Cardiol Young. 2011;21(Suppl 2):124–32. Epub 2011/12/14.
64. Cecka JM, Kucheryavaya AY, Reinsmoen NL, Leffell MS. Calculated PRA: initial results show benefits for sensitized patients and a reduction in positive crossmatches. Am J Transplant. 2011;11(4):719–24. Epub 2010/12/01.
65. Fuggle SV, Martin S. Tools for human leukocyte antigen antibody detection and their application to transplanting sensitized patients. Transplantation. 2008;86(3):384–90. Epub 2008/08/14.
66. Gombos P, Opelz G, Scherer S, Morath C, Zeier M, Schemmer P, et al. Influence of test technique on sensitization status of patients on the kidney transplant waiting list. Am J Transplant. 2013;13(8):2075–82. Epub 2013/07/12.
67. Patel R, Terasaki PI. Significance of the positive crossmatch test in kidney transplantation. N Engl J Med. 1969;280(14):735 9. Epub 1969/04/03.
68. Duquesnoy RJ, Marrari M. Multilaboratory evaluation of serum analysis for HLA antibody and crossmatch reactivity by lymphocytotoxicity methods. Arch Pathol Lab Med. 2003;127(2):149–56. Epub 2003/02/04.
69. Gebel HM, Bray RA. Sensitization and sensitivity: defining the unsensitized patient. Transplantation. 2000;69(7):1370–4. Epub 2000/05/08.
70. Tait BD, Susal C, Gebel HM, Nickerson PW, Zachary AA, Claas FH, et al. Consensus guidelines on the testing and clinical management issues associated with HLA and non-HLA antibodies in transplantation. Transplantation. 2013;95(1):19–47. Epub 2012/12/15.
71. Honger G, Krahenbuhl N, Dimeloe S, Stern M, Schaub S, Hess C. Inter-individual differences in HLA expression can impact the CDC crossmatch. Tissue Antigens. 2015;85(4):260–6. Epub 2015/03/20.
72. Minucci PB, Grimaldi V, Casamassimi A, Cacciatore F, Sommese L, Picascia A, et al. Methodologies for anti-HLA antibody screening in patients awaiting kidney transplant: a comparative study. Exp Clin Transplant. 2011;9(6):381–6. Epub 2011/12/07.
73. Pei R, Lee J, Chen T, Rojo S, Terasaki PI. Flow cytometric detection of HLA antibodies using a spectrum of microbeads. Hum Immunol. 1999;60(12):1293–302. Epub 2000/01/08.
74. Pei R, Lee JH, Shih NJ, Chen M, Terasaki PI. Single human leukocyte antigen flow cytometry beads for accurate identification of human leukocyte antigen antibody specificities. Transplantation. 2003;75(1):43–9. Epub 2003/01/25.
75. Tait BD, Hudson F, Cantwell L, Brewin G, Holdsworth R, Bennett G, et al. Review article: Luminex technology for HLA antibody detection in organ transplantation. Nephrology (Carlton). 2009;14(2):247–54. Epub 2009/02/12.

76. Zachary AA, Vega RM, Lucas DP, Leffell MS. HLA antibody detection and characterization by solid phase immunoassays: methods and pitfalls. Methods Mol Biol. 2012;882:289–308. Epub 2012/06/06.
77. Tambur AR, Herrera ND, Haarberg KM, Cusick MF, Gordon RA, Leventhal JR, et al. Assessing antibody strength: comparison of MFI, C1q, and titer information. Am J Transplant. 2015;15(9):2421–30. Epub 2015/05/02.
78. Bray RA, Nolen JD, Larsen C, Pearson T, Newell KA, Kokko K, et al. Transplanting the highly sensitized patient: the Emory algorithm. Am J Transplant. 2006;6(10):2307–15. Epub 2006/08/31.
79. Yanagida R, Czer LS, Reinsmoen NL, Cao K, Rafiei M, De Robertis MA, et al. Impact of virtual cross match on waiting times for heart transplantation. Ann Thorac Surg. 2011;92(6):2104–10; discussion 11. Epub 2011/11/26.
80. Amico P, Hirt-Minkowski P, Honger G, Gurke L, Mihatsch MJ, Steiger J, et al. Risk stratification by the virtual crossmatch: a prospective study in 233 renal transplantations. Transpl Int. 2011;24(6):560–9. Epub 2011/02/22.
81. Kerman RH, Susskind B, Buyse I, Pryzbylowski P, Ruth J, Warnell S, et al. Flow cytometry-detected IgG is not a contraindication to renal transplantation: IgM may be beneficial to outcome. Transplantation. 1999;68(12):1855–8. Epub 2000/01/11.
82. Lobo PI, Spencer CE, Stevenson WC, McCullough C, Pruett TL. The use of pronase-digested human leukocytes to improve specificity of the flow cytometric crossmatch. Transpl Int. 1995;8(6):472–80. Epub 1995/01/01.
83. Park H, Lim YM, Han BY, Hyun J, Song EY, Park MH. Frequent false-positive reactions in pronase-treated T-cell flow cytometric cross-match tests. Transplant Proc. 2012;44(1):87–90. Epub 2012/02/09.
84. Hetrick SJ, Schillinger KP, Zachary AA, Jackson AM. Impact of pronase on flow cytometric crossmatch outcome. Hum Immunol. 2011;72(4):330–6. Epub 2011/01/26.
85. Apithy MJ, Desoutter J, Gicquel A, Guiheneuf E, Westeel PF, Lesage A, et al. Pronase treatment improves flow cytometry crossmatching results. Hla. 2017;90(3):157–64. Epub 2017/07/01.
86. Przybylowski P, Balogna M, Radovancevic B, Frazier OH, Susskind B, Van Buren C, et al. The role of flow cytometry-detected IgG and IgM anti-donor antibodies in cardiac allograft recipients. Transplantation. 1999;67(2):258–62. Epub 1999/02/12.
87. Gebel HM, Bray RA. HLA antibody detection with solid phase assays: great expectations or expectations too great? Am J Transplant. 2014;14(9):1964–75. Epub 2014/08/05.

Challenges in Post-transplant Immunologic Monitoring

2

Rouba Garro and Pamela D. Winterberg

Challenges in Post-transplant Immunologic Monitoring

Kidney transplant is the preferred modality for renal replacement therapy in children, with better outcomes compared to dialysis [1]. Despite substantial improvement over the last several decades in early acute rejection rates and short-term allograft survival, the long-term outcome of expected half-life of 10 years remains less than optimal [2, 3]. Improving long-term graft survival is especially important in children due to the longer expected remaining years of life post-transplant compared to adults.

Management of pediatric kidney transplant (KT) recipients relies in part on data derived from adult studies because of the low incidence of end-stage renal disease in children and the relatively small size of individual pediatric kidney transplant programs. Post-transplant care of children presents unique challenges compared to adults, and new diagnostics or therapeutics do not necessarily translate easily from adults to children. First, young children with kidney transplants are at higher risk for rejection given the greater immunologic responsiveness of a developing immune system, higher risk for contracting various viral infections, and variations in the metabolism of immunosuppression drugs compared to adults. Second, long-term outcomes in older children are in part compromised by risk-taking behaviors and struggles with adherence to medications and clinical care during adolescence and young adulthood. The propensity for risk-taking behaviors at different stages of psychosocial development highlights the need for more frequent monitoring for

R. Garro (✉) · P. D. Winterberg
Pediatric Nephrology, Emory University School of Medicine Department of Pediatrics, Atlanta, GA, USA

Children's Health Care of Atlanta, Atlanta, GA, USA
e-mail: rgarro@emory.edu; pdwinter@emory.edu

K. E. Twombley (ed.), *Challenges in Pediatric Kidney Transplantation*,
https://doi.org/10.1007/978-3-030-74783-1_2

rejection using validated and non-invasive biomarkers [4]. Considering all the specific challenges in pediatric transplantation, to ultimately improve graft survival, there is a significant need to develop and validate approaches to immunological monitoring post-transplant that predict early rejection and allow safe and effective therapeutic approaches to decrease risk of infection, drug toxicity, and graft injury.

Monitoring pediatric KT recipients is focused on detection of (1) emerging alloimmune response that increases risk for rejection, (2) early signs of graft dysfunction and/or injury, and (3) off-target effects of immunosuppression such as metabolic and infectious complications. In this chapter, we review conventional and emerging biomarkers used for post-transplant monitoring in children with a focus on risk stratification for rejection and/or graft loss. While the assessment for infection or drug toxicity must also be taken into account when determining the risk for rejection or when deciding on a treatment regimen, specifics of monitoring for these complications is beyond the scope of this chapter and is covered elsewhere in this textbook.

Conventional Monitoring Post-Transplant

Serum Creatinine (Graft Function)

Although monitoring kidney function using serum creatinine remains the primary method of detecting graft injury and rejection following kidney transplant, this traditional biomarker has several limitations. First, serum creatinine is an insensitive marker of graft function, as substantial injury and loss of function are required to result in noticeable alterations in serum creatinine, making it an unreliable marker for detecting early or subclinical rejection to facilitate effective intervention. This is further exacerbated in small children receiving large donor kidneys given the mismatch between muscle mass and nephron number [5]. Second, elevations in serum creatinine are not specific for rejection and can be affected by hydration status, certain medications (e.g., trimethoprim-sulfamethoxazole, angiotensin-converting enzyme (ACE) inhibitors, and tacrolimus), urinary obstruction, or bacterial or viral kidney infections. However, creatinine is affordable and readily available in all clinical settings and therefore will likely continue to be utilized as a marker of glomerular filtration rate in conjunction with other more sensitive biomarkers of injury and/or inflammation.

Drug Monitoring and Variability

Therapeutic drug monitoring for calcineurin inhibitors and the mammalian or mechanistic target of rapamycin (mTOR) inhibitors is standard practice post-transplantation to ensure adequate immunosuppressive exposure, with frequent monitoring needed due to narrow therapeutic windows and variation in drug metabolism between individuals [6]. This is especially important in children, who have greater variability in pharmacodynamic and metabolism of medications throughout growth and maturation. Children are also at higher risk for infection at younger ages, and they struggle with medication adherence during adolescence and emerging adulthood, which highlight the need for improved drug monitoring in this population.

Tacrolimus (TAC) remains a primary immunosuppressive medication for maintenance therapy in solid organ transplant, though it has a narrow therapeutic window with significant inter- and intra-patient variability (IPV) [6]. Underexposure might increase the risk for rejection, and higher levels can lead to acute and chronic nephrotoxicity and undesired gastrointestinal and neurologic side effects. Close monitoring of TAC trough level is important to maintain levels within the targeted range, especially since TAC levels and metabolism are affected by multiple factors, particularly early post-transplant, like interaction of concomitant medications and food, CYP3A4/A5 phenotype of the patient, presence of diarrhea, hepatic function, serum albumin level, hematocrit, and inflammation [6–8]. Non-adherence to immunosuppressive medications has been identified as an important factor contributing to intra-patient variability, especially in adolescents and older children >6 months post-transplant [8–10].

When evaluating the effect of drug exposure on outcome or monitoring for non-adherence, it is difficult to make a clinical judgment based on one or two levels, and it is more reasonable to measure the fluctuation of medication levels over a period of time. Early studies evaluated standard deviation (SD) of TAC as a surrogate for drug exposure. More recent studies used coefficient variation (CV), as higher TAC levels can lead to a higher SDs that require manual removal of outliers [11].

Multiple studies found that high IPV in TAC trough levels is associated with worse allograft outcomes in solid organ transplant [7, 10]. Tacrolimus CV of >30% is associated with the development of donor-specific antibodies (DSA), allograft dysfunction, and higher risk of rejection and graft loss in both pediatric [7, 8, 10–14] and adult KT recipients [15–17]. Thus, especially in the adolescent and emerging adult populations, the use of variations in immunosuppressive medication levels, like TAC CV, may provide a promising and practical tool to monitor medication adherence and signal the need for intervention to reduce the risk of rejection [14, 18].

Surveillance Monitoring of Donor-Specific Antibodies

The presence of anti-human leukocyte antigen (HLA) DSA is not uncommon in children following kidney transplant, with reported frequencies of 15–45% by 1–2 years post-transplant [19–22], and has been associated with antibody-mediated rejection (ABMR) and impaired graft survival [22–26]. Serial monitoring for the development of DSA post-transplant has been proposed as a method of detecting emerging humoral alloimmune response. Consensus guidelines published in 2013 recommended screening for de novo DSA (dnDSA) in non-sensitized patients at least every 3–12 months post-transplant and performing a kidney biopsy to evaluate for ABMR when DSA is detected [27]. Reports of this approach detected a significant number of subclinical rejection episodes in patients with dnDSA [28].

Despite existing guidelines, there is variability in the frequency of monitoring and management of DSA post-pediatric KT [29]. Several studies suggested de novo DSA detection can precede and therefore predict the development of antibody-mediated rejection [20], but there are insufficient data to guide clinical management for DSA detected in the absence of histologic injury.

While the advent of single-antigen bead assays to detect anti-HLA antibodies provides increased sensitivity relative to traditional cellular-based assays, there is a debate over the "strength" or threshold to determine clinical relevance of dnDSA post-transplant. There has been progress in developing protocols to reduce variability between centers in multicenter clinical trials [30–32], but the use of median fluorescent intensities (MFI) to quantify the abundance of dnDSA remains in question [33].

The significance and pathogenicity of DSA antibodies for an individual patient is not always straightforward, especially in the absence of graft dysfunction or histological evidence of rejection on biopsy [34]. Not every patient with dnDSA develops acute ABMR or graft loss in these studies, and dnDSA resolve in a few patients [19, 20, 22, 24]. To improve decisions for intervention, in the past decade, there have been several studies aimed at identifying the characteristics of humoral alloimmune responses that are most predictive of pathogenicity. These include evaluation of epitope specificity of the antibody (e.g., HLA class I vs II antigens, native versus denatured antigens), antibody abundance (e.g., median fluorescent intensity (MFI), dilution titrations), and ability to interact with complement as determined by antibody isotype (immunoglobulin (Ig)G subclasses, IgG vs IgM) or via direct testing of ability to fix complement component 1q (C1q) or C3d complement [35]. Of these factors, the ability to interact with complement components appears to be the best predictor of overall graft survival and/or acute antibody-mediated rejection [36–39]. At this time, however, there has not been widespread adoption of these assays because of concerns about variability between centers and about reliability in results due to interfering substances [40].

Another challenge with predicting the pathogenic potential of dnDSA lies in the evolving definitions and clinico-histological subtypes of antibody-mediated rejection (ABMR) that have varying manifestations of graft dysfunction and risk and rapidity for graft loss [23, 41–43]. The use of additional emerging non-invasive biomarkers in combination with DSA may improve prediction and guide therapy. For example, active ABMR on biopsy was associated with elevated donor-derived cell-free DNA levels among adults with detectable dnDSA [44].

Although DSA development is associated with worse graft survival, it is still unclear which interventions prompted by surveillance detection of DSA are effective at reducing the risk for subsequent ABMR and/or prolonging graft survival [34]. There is also a need for improved identification of the most effective approaches to prevent DSA development for individual patients, including the evolving challenges in predicting the risk associated with antigenic mismatch discussed in Chap. 1. Strategies could be developed to personalize the immunosuppressive regimen based on pre-transplant risk stratification for the development of DSA and additional strategies to address "break-through" DSA development. Inadequate immunosuppression – including high variability in tacrolimus levels due to non-adherence and lower antiproliferative drug exposure due to either medication non-adherence, variations in drug metabolism, or medically indicated reduction (e.g., during infections) – are associated with development of dnDSA in several studies [21, 45]. Therefore, as a preventive strategy for dnDSA, some advocate for therapeutic drug monitoring of mycophenolate mofetil (MMF) in addition to tacrolimus and appropriate dose adjustment.

Non-HLA Antibodies

There has been recent recognition of non-HLA antibodies as potential mediators of allograft injury, rejection, and/or worse graft outcome [46–50]. Autoantibodies directed against the angiotensin II type I receptor-antibody (AT1R-Ab), endothelin-1 type A receptor, major histocompatibility complex class 1-related chain a (MICA), perlecan, and collagen V have all been studied as potential mediators of allograft dysfunction [51]. In particular, AT1R-Ab has been the most studied for associations with rejection, vascular injury, and graft injury and loss in adult kidney transplant recipients, with similar reports in pediatric solid organ transplant recipients [47, 50, 52]. AT1R-Ab has also been linked to progressive decline in glomerular filtration rate (GFR), inflammation, and worse graft outcome in pediatric patients [47].

The prevalence of AT1R-Ab pre- and post-transplantation varies among studies, with some suggestion of higher prevalence in children overall and a higher likelihood of developing these antibodies post-transplant [52]. There is also significant uncertainty regarding the direct pathogenicity of AT1R-Ab [53], synergetic effect with HLA antibodies [50], and the role of other factors like ischemic injury contributing to the observed associations [53]. Therefore, there is currently no consensus on monitoring the presence of AT1R-Ab either pre- or post-transplant. However, transplant clinicians should consider evaluating for the presence of non-HLA antibodies in patients with pathologic signs of ABMR on biopsy without detectable anti-HLA antibodies or in the setting of ABMR with severe hypertension.

Surveillance Biopsies (SBs)

While clinical rejection continues to be the most common cause of graft loss in pediatric KT recipients, early diagnosis and treatment of subclinical rejection (SCR) detected on surveillance biopsies in the absence of graft dysfunction is a modifiable risk that can effect long-term graft outcome [54]. Surveillance biopsies have also been used to detect early signs of calcineurin inhibitor (CNI) toxicity, viral infection, and chronic damage like interstitial fibrosis (IF) and tubular atrophy (TA). Early identification of these complications can allow prompt modification of immunosuppressive therapy to prevent further chronic allograft damage and improve long-term outcome.

The utility of performing surveillance biopsies as part of routine post-transplant care in both adult and pediatric centers is debated, with significant variation in adaptation, timing, and the management approach to SCR [55]. According to a 2017 UNOS survey, 17% of responding centers performed surveillance biopsies on all patients, with 3- and 12-month post-transplant biopsies being the most common [56]. An international pediatric survey reported that 34% of the responding pediatric transplant centers performed surveillance biopsies [57].

Multiple recent single-center pediatric studies evaluated the prevalence of different pathological findings, including subclinical rejection, at different time points post-transplant. Pathologic abnormalities were found in 30–50% of surveillance biopsies in pediatric studies, with subclinical rejection described in 11–40% of biopsies [58–60]. Lansberg et al. found that 6-month surveillance biopsy yields the greatest pathologic abnormality (57%), with TCMR diagnosed in 43% of the biopsies, and led to the most modification in immunosuppressive therapy compared to biopsies conducted at 1.5, 3, 12, or 24 months post-transplant [60].

Though there have not been randomized clinical trials in children to determine the effectiveness of treatment for subclinical rejection or borderline rejection on outcome, several pediatric studies have demonstrated renal function and graft survival of treated subclinical rejection comparable to patients with normal SB [61, 62]. This was confirmed in a single-center study by Odum et al., who found that treatment of SCR resulted in resolution or improvement in the SCR in 50% and 18% on follow-up biopsies, respectively [59]. Furthermore, Seifert et al. found that subclinical inflammation was associated with an increased hazard ratio for clinically relevant acute rejection and allograft loss if untreated [63].

Multiple recent pediatric studies examined the safety of surveillance biopsies in children and evaluated complications like infection, bleeding, formation of arteriovenous (AV) fistula, or gross hematuria. Most studies showed very minimal risk associated with these biopsies [57–60, 62]. Although the risk of complications of SBs is minimal, especially when performed at experienced centers, it is not negligible as children require sedation or general anesthesia to perform the procedure, which is not without negative sequelae and is undesired by many families.

Surveillance biopsies are currently the main tool used to monitor for silent immunological events, detect early signs of inflammation, detect drug toxicity, and diagnose SCR, which can be an important short-term end point for graft survival and subsequently affect long-term graft outcome. However, obtaining serial kidney biopsies at a frequency to adjust and individualize immunosuppressive medications based on subclinical injury and to evaluate the effect of treatment is limited by cost, inconvenience, and the potentially serious complications of repeated invasive procedures. Finally, surveillance biopsies can also be limited by sampling and interpretation errors. With all that in mind, there has been substantial work in the transplant community over the last decade to develop non-invasive biomarkers that have sufficient sensitivity and specificity to diagnose early signs of rejection and to discriminate other sources of graft injury (infection, ischemia, drug toxicity) to provide customized interventions and optimize long-term allograft outcome for individual patients [64–67].

Innovative Biomarkers for Immunologic Monitoring Post-transplant

Donor-Derived Cell-Free DNA (dd-cfDNA)

Elevated total cell-free deoxyribonucleic acid (cfDNA) in plasma is thought to be secondary to increased cell turnover of hematopoietic cells in the context of multiple physiologic and pathologic states, including exercise, malignancy, sepsis, myocardial infarction, stroke, and critical illness [68–70]. The level of cfDNA can be correlated with illness severity.

Donor-derived cell-free DNA (dd-cfDNA) detected in the plasma of the organ recipient has been investigated as a possible non-invasive biomarker to diagnose rejection in clinical settings. A key hypothesis in transplantation is that the allograft injury induced by rejection will increase cell apoptosis, leading to increased release of dd-cfDNA into the recipient plasma. Recent studies have developed the use of single nucleotide polymorphisms (SNPs) and computational approaches to determine the donor type and to quantify dd-cfDNA without the need for separate genotyping of the recipient or the donor [71–74].

The validity of dd-cfDNA in diagnosing rejection and graft injury has been studied over the last decade, with some recent data in adults supporting the validity of this biomarker in the diagnosis of antibody-medicated rejection (ABMR) and T-cell-mediated rejection (TCMR), which supports its use in clinical settings [72, 75–77]. In a prospective observation multicenter study, Bloom et al. found that elevated dd-cfDNA levels in the plasma of KT recipients were associated with active rejection status, with an estimated NPV 84% and PPV 61% at a cutoff of 1.0% of dd-cfDNA [72]. This is consistent with prior reports from single-center studies. Donor-derived cfDNA was better in identifying ABMR and high grades of TCMR, but did not perform well with a lower grade of cellular rejection [72, 78]. Again, dd-cfDNA may also be helpful in determining the clinical significance of emergence of dnDSA that warrants further evaluation for ABMR [44].

Serial monitoring of dd-cfDNA may be useful in detecting early rejection or graft injury and guide the decision to obtain kidney biopsies, which continues to be the gold standard to diagnose and grade rejection. Given the high NPV of this test, detecting low levels of dd-cfDNA may allow avoiding unnecessary kidney biopsies, especially in patients who are high risk for complications with the biopsy itself or at risk for sedation and anesthesia. In the right clinical settings, the stability of this biomarker, which can be assessed monthly, may allow safe tapering and modification of immunosuppressive medications to avoid long-term side effects (including CNI toxicity) and ultimately improve long-term patient and graft survival. At this point, pediatric data are limited to small sample sizes and single-center studies in different solid organ transplant populations [73, 79, 80]. Based on adult data, cutoff

(>1% dd-cfDNA) has been found to be associated with allograft injury/rejection, with a sensitivity of 89% and specificity of 73% [81]. This cutoff has not been validated in pediatric populations. Younger children who receive adult-sized kidneys with higher graft-to-body ratios may have a higher baseline dd-cfDNA compared to older children and adults who have a better matched kidney-to-body size.

Puliyanda et al. recently published the first study to evaluate the use of dd-cfDNA in pediatric KT recipients [79]. In their sample of 67 patients who received dd-cfDNA for frequent monitoring or when suspicious for clinical rejection, the authors found that dd-cfDNA >1% was diagnostic of rejection, with a sensitivity of 86% and specificity of 100%. Donor-derived cfDNA in their study was highly predictive of histological rejection on biopsies and superior to other indicators like graft dysfunction or antibody positivity alone. This is especially important in children in whom creatinine may lag behind allograft injury due to having an adult-sized graft in a smaller body [82, 83]. With more data emerging, dd-cfDNA has the potential to be integrated in clinical and immune monitoring post-transplant, along with other biomarkers, to improve early detection of subclinical rejection and improve outcomes.

Urinary Biomarkers

Urinary chemokines are associated with activation of cytotoxic T cells, mediate inflammatory response, and were found to correlate with acute kidney injury, inflammation, and rejection in both adult and pediatric kidney transplant recipients [4, 64]. The most promising chemokines in predicting evolution, severity, and resolution of rejection with treatment are chemokine (C-X-C motif) ligand (CXCL)9 and CXCL10 [64, 65, 84]. Multiple studies in adults showed that serial monitoring of urinary biomarkers was superior to serum creatine in monitoring for allograft inflammation over time and more predictive of long-term adverse outcome [66, 85, 86]. Similarly in pediatric patients, Mincham et al. recently found that change in urinary CXCL10-to-creatinine ratio (CXCL10/Cr) and not change in estimated (e) GFR in pediatric KT recipients correlated with the change in acuity of inflammation and degree of rejection found on the allograft biopsies [87]. Furthermore, Mockler et al. found that elevated CXCL10 at 6 months post-transplant in pediatric KT recipients was associated with worse graft function and higher risk for graft loss at 36 months [88]. Finally, Blydt-Hansen et al. recently published the results of a multicenter observational study evaluating the effects of urinary biomarkers in 97 pediatric KT recipients. CXCL10/Cr predicted acute clinical and subclinical rejection and elevated mean CXCL10/Cr correlated with first-year eGFR decline, highlighting the effect of persistent subclinical inflammation on allograft function. Like other studies, they also found CXCL10/Cr was elevated in patients with BK nephritis [89]. Urinary CXCL10/Cr may improve probability estimates for the risk of rejection when integrated into clinical decision-making [90].

Molecular Diagnostics

Microarray analyses of biopsy tissue have revealed discrepancies between molecular signatures of rejection and/or renal injury and conventional histologic grading [91]. Further, molecular signatures of ongoing renal injury in excess of what is appreciated via histopathologic gradings are associated with progressive decline in graft function and eventual graft failure [92]. Molecular analysis also helps to provide more granular phenotyping of rejection and risk prediction of graft failure, especially in the case of antibody-mediated rejection [91]. The most recent consensus guidelines from the 2017 Banff Conference now incorporate the use of molecular assays in the diagnosis of antibody-mediated rejection, especially in the absence of C4d staining or detectable anti-HLA antibodies [42]. As such, molecular phenotyping of biopsy tissue will likely become more important in clinical decision-making over the coming years.

In addition to molecular diagnostic assays of graft tissue, additional studies focused on narrowing down large genomic datasets to identify specific gene expression panels to be used as non-invasive biomarkers for risk prediction and to inform clinical management [93, 94]. Additional effort is being applied to identify gene sets in peripheral blood [95, 96] or urine [97] to detect subclinical rejection that could inform the timing of diagnostic biopsy for the clinician. It is unclear whether non-invasive gene transcripts from peripheral blood or urine could one day replace invasive biopsy procedures for diagnosis of rejection [98]. In the near future, they are likely best suited to identify patients that would benefit from diagnostic biopsy, which will include broader tissue molecular phenotyping to guide therapy [98].

The Future of Post-transplant Immune Monitoring

Post-transplant monitoring for rejection is likely to change radically in the coming decade as non-invasive biomarkers to detect subclinical graft injury/inflammation and molecular diagnostic testing mature and become more available to clinicians. As individual biomarkers and gene sets are validated, there will also be a need for predictive algorithms to integrate clinical and diagnostic variables into a tailored approach to monitoring and treatment to achieve personalized therapy and optimize long-term outcomes for individual patients.

One could imagine that post-transplant monitoring for an individual patient will be tailored based on pre-transplant risk prediction and then altered based on post-transplant events. Pre-transplant risk stratification could determine the initial immunosuppressive regimen and monitoring approach, including the mode (i.e., non-invasive biomarkers vs surveillance biopsy) and frequency of monitoring for rejection. When rejection is suspected, molecular phenotyping of graft tissue holds the exciting possibility to provide insight into rejection phenotypes that can guide targeted treatment and improve long-term outcomes [38]. Bioinformatics approaches can also be leveraged to identify new approaches or repurpose existing therapies

[99, 100] for the prevention and treatment of rejection. In addition, biomarkers to assess pharmacodynamics and predict therapeutic response to treatment for rejection are also attractive. Large collaborative studies and pragmatic clinical trials are needed to determine how best to utilize the myriad of tools that will soon be available for predicting and detecting rejection to ultimately achieve personalized therapy for all children with kidney transplant.

Q&A

1. A 17-year-old young male presents to transplant clinic for routine outpatient visit. He has a history of end-stage kidney disease (ESRD) secondary to renal dysplasia and received a deceased donor kidney transplant 4 years ago. The patient has missed his regular scheduled labs for the last 2 months. On review of prior tacrolimus levels, you noticed large variations in trough levels over the prior 6 months. Labs today showed mildly elevated creatinine and a high tacrolimus trough level. This patient is at high risk for.
   (a) Drug toxicity
   (b) Subclinical and/or acute rejection
   (c) Development of dnDSA
   (d) Worse graft survival
   (e) All the above

   The correct answer is: e

   High intra-patient variability (IPV) in tacrolimus (TAC) trough levels measured by standard deviation or coefficient variation of TAC has been found to be associated with increased risk of development of donor-specific antibodies (DSA), allograft dysfunction, and higher risk of rejection and graft loss in both pediatric and adult KT recipients. Non-adherence to immunosuppressive medications has been identified as an important factor contributing to intra-patient variability, especially in adolescents and older children >6 months post-transplant.

   In this scenario, the patient is 17-year-old and missed labs with high variability in TAC levels over the last 6 months period which raise the concern for non-adherence to medications. Elevated creatinine level in this setting is concerning for rejection and/or drug toxicity secondary to elevated TAC level.

   Adolescents are at higher risk of non-adherence to medications and worse graft outcome compared to young children and adults. This patient population warrants closer clinical and immunologic monitoring with close attention to variations in therapeutic drug levels. They also benefit from non-invasive biomarkers to help detect early signs of rejection and allow early intervention.
2. Which of the following statement is INCORRECT regarding surevillance biopsies?
   (a) Surveillance biopsies are useful in detecting early signs of drug toxicity, chronic damage, and subclinical rejection especially in smaller children with adult-sized kidney.

(b) Although associated with minimal complications when performed by experienced personals, it is still not without risk.
(c) Majority of pediatric transplant programs perform surveillance biopsies.
(d) The effectiveness of treatment of subclinical rejection diagnosed on surveillance biopsies on outcome is still unclear.

The correct answer is: c

The utility of performing surveillance biopsies as part of routine post-transplant care in both adult and pediatric centers is debated, with significant variation in adaptation, timing, and management approaches to subclinical rejection. According to a 2017 UNOS survey, 17% of responding centers performed surveillance biopsies on all patients, with 3- and 12-month post-transplant biopsies being the most common. An international pediatric survey reported that 34% of the responding pediatric transplant centers performed surveillance biopsies.

3. Which of the following statements is CORRECT?
(a) DnDSA is uncommon in children.
(b) There is variability in the frequency of monitoring and management of DSA post-pediatric kidney transplant.
(c) Detection of c1q fixation and MFI thresholds are diagnostic of acute clinical ABMR.
(d) The development of dnDSA is always associated with acute clinical ABMR.
(e) Guidelines recommend obtaining dnDSA only with clinical suspicion of clinical rejection.

The correct answer is: b

The presence of anti-human leukocyte antigen (HLA) DSA is not uncommon in children following kidney transplant, with reported frequencies of 15–45% by 1–2 years post-transplant. Consensus guidelines published in 2013 recommended screening for de novo DSA (dnDSA) in non-sensitized patients at least every 3 to 12 months post-transplant and performing a kidney biopsy to evaluate for ABMR when DSA is detected. Despite the presence of such guidelines, there is variability among centers in the frequency of monitoring and management of DSA post-pediatric kidney transplant.

The significance and pathogenicity of DSA antibodies for an individual patient is not always straightforward, especially in the absence of graft dysfunction or histological evidence of rejection on biopsy. Not every patient with dnDSA develops acute ABMR or graft loss. To improve decisions for intervention, in the past decade, there have been several studies aimed at identifying the characteristics of humoral alloimmune responses that are most predictive of pathogenicity. These include evaluation of epitope specificity of the antibody (e.g., HLA class I vs II antigens, native versus denatured antigens), antibody abundance (e.g., median fluorescent intensity (MFI), dilution titrations), and ability to interact with complement as determined by antibody isotype (immunoglobulin (Ig)G subclasses, IgG vs IgM) or via direct testing of ability to fix complement component 1q (C1q) or C3d complement [35]. Of these factors, the ability to interact with complement components appears to be the best predictor of overall graft survival and/or acute antibody-mediated rejection. At this time, however, there has not been widespread adoption of these assays because of concerns about variability between centers and about reliability in results due to interfering substances.

Disclosure Statement The authors have no financial interests or conflicts of interest to disclose.

Bibliography

1. Gulati A, Sarwal MM. Pediatric renal transplantation: an overview and update. Curr Opin Pediatr. 2010;22:189–96.
2. Hart A, Smith JM, Skeans MA, et al. OPTN/SRTR 2016 annual data report: kidney. Am J Transplant. 2018;18(Suppl 1):18–113.
3. Dharnidharka VR, Lamb KE, Zheng J, Schechtman KB, Meier-Kriesche HU. Lack of significant improvements in long-term allograft survival in pediatric solid organ transplantation: a US national registry analysis. Pediatric Transplant. 2015;19:477–83.
4. Dharnidharka VR, Malone A. Biomarkers to detect rejection after kidney transplantation. Pediatric Nephrol (Berlin, Germany). 2018;33:1113–22.
5. de Souza V, Cochat P, Rabilloud M, et al. Accuracy of different equations in estimating GFR in pediatric kidney transplant recipients. Clin J Am Soc Nephrol. 2015;10:463–70.
6. Campagne O, Mager DE, Tornatore KM. Population pharmacokinetics of tacrolimus in transplant recipients: what did we learn about sources of Interindividual variabilities? J Clin Pharmacol. 2019;59:309–25.
7. Prytula AA, Bouts AH, Mathot RA, et al. Intra-patient variability in tacrolimus trough concentrations and renal function decline in pediatric renal transplant recipients. Pediatric Transplant. 2012;16:613–8.
8. Defrancq C, De Wilde N, Raes A, et al. Intra-patient variability in tacrolimus exposure in pediatric liver transplant recipients: evolution, risk factors, and impact on patient outcomes. Pediatric Transplant. 2019;23:e13388.
9. Leino AD, King EC, Jiang W, et al. Assessment of tacrolimus intrapatient variability in stable adherent transplant recipients: establishing baseline values. Am J Transplant. 2019;19:1410–20.
10. Pollock-Barziv SM, Finkelstein Y, Manlhiot C, et al. Variability in tacrolimus blood levels increases the risk of late rejection and graft loss after solid organ transplantation in older children. Pediatric Transplant. 2010;14:968–75.
11. Hsiau M, Fernandez HE, Gjertson D, Ettenger RB, Tsai EW. Monitoring nonadherence and acute rejection with variation in blood immunosuppressant levels in pediatric renal transplantation. Transplantation. 2011;92:918–22.
12. Pizzo HP, Ettenger RB, Gjertson DW, et al. Sirolimus and tacrolimus coefficient of variation is associated with rejection, donor-specific antibodies, and nonadherence. Pediatric Nephrol (Berlin, Germany). 2016;31:2345–52.
13. Solomon S, Colovai A, Del Rio M, Hayde N. Tacrolimus variability is associated with de novo donor-specific antibody development in pediatric renal transplant recipients. Pediatric Nephrol (Berlin, Germany). 2020;35:261–70.
14. Gold A, Tonshoff B, Dohler B, Susal C. Association of graft survival with tacrolimus exposure and late intra-patient tacrolimus variability in pediatric and young adult renal transplant recipients-an international CTS registry analysis. Transpl Int. 2020;33(12):1681–92.
15. Gueta I, Markovits N, Yarden-Bilavsky H, et al. Intrapatient variability in tacrolimus trough levels after solid organ transplantation varies at different postoperative time periods. Am J Transplant. 2019;19:611.

16. Rodrigo E, Segundo DS, Fernandez-Fresnedo G, et al. Within-patient variability in tacrolimus blood levels predicts kidney graft loss and donor-specific antibody development. Transplantation. 2016;100:2479–85.
17. Whalen HR, Glen JA, Harkins V, et al. High intrapatient tacrolimus variability is associated with worse outcomes in renal transplantation using a low-dose tacrolimus immunosuppressive regime. Transplantation. 2017;101:430–6.
18. Knight SR. Intrapatient variability in tacrolimus exposure - a useful tool for clinical practice? Transpl Int. 2016;29:1155–7.
19. Rusai K, Dworak J, Potemkina A, et al. Donor-specific HLA antibodies and graft function in kidney-transplanted children - the Vienna cohort. Pediatric Transplant. 2016;20:507–14.
20. Ginevri F, Nocera A, Comoli P, et al. Posttransplant de novo donor-specific hla antibodies identify pediatric kidney recipients at risk for late antibody-mediated rejection. Am J Transplant. 2012;12:3355–62.
21. Filler G, Todorova EK, Bax K, Alvarez-Elias AC, Huang SH, Kobrzynski MC. Minimum mycophenolic acid levels are associated with donor-specific antibody formation. Pediatric Transplant. 2016;20:34–8.
22. Kim JJ, Balasubramanian R, Michaelides G, et al. The clinical spectrum of de novo donor-specific antibodies in pediatric renal transplant recipients. Am J Transplant. 2014;14:2350–8.
23. Loupy A, Hill GS, Jordan SC. The impact of donor-specific anti-HLA antibodies on late kidney allograft failure. Nat Rev Nephrol. 2012;8:348–57.
24. Cioni M, Nocera A, Innocente A, et al. De novo donor-specific HLA antibodies developing early or late after transplant are associated with the same risk of graft damage and loss in nonsensitized kidney recipients. J Immunol Res. 2017;2017:1747030.
25. Aubert O, Loupy A, Hidalgo L, et al. Antibody-mediated rejection due to preexisting versus De novo donor-specific antibodies in kidney allograft recipients. J Am Soc Nephrol. 2017;28:1912–23.
26. Viglietti D, Loupy A, Vernerey D, et al. Value of donor-specific anti-HLA antibody monitoring and characterization for risk stratification of kidney allograft loss. J Am Soc Nephrol. 2017;28:702–15.
27. Tait BD, Susal C, Gebel HM, et al. Consensus guidelines on the testing and clinical management issues associated with HLA and non-HLA antibodies in transplantation. Transplantation. 2013;95:19–47.
28. Parajuli S, Reville PK, Ellis TM, Djamali A, Mandelbrot DA. Utility of protocol kidney biopsies for de novo donor-specific antibodies. Am J Transplant. 2017;17:3210–8.
29. Athavale D, Worthington J, Webb NJ, Roberts D, Martin S, Shenoy M. Pediatric kidney recipients may benefit from monitoring for donor-specific antibodies. Pediatric Transplant. 2014;18:258–65.
30. Reed EF, Rao P, Zhang Z, et al. Comprehensive assessment and standardization of solid phase multiplex-bead arrays for the detection of antibodies to HLA. Am J Transplant. 2013;13:1859–70.
31. Greenshields A, Bray RA, Gebel HM, Liwski RS. Getting on target: development of the novel, prozone-resistant, dual antibody rapid test (DART) for the LABScreen single antigen bead (SAB) assay. Human Immunol. 2019;80:468–77.
32. Maillard N, Mariat C. Solid-phase bead-based assays limitations are not restricted to inter-laboratory variability. Am J Transplant. 2013;13:3049.
33. Tambur AR, Herrera ND, Haarberg KM, et al. Assessing antibody strength: comparison of MFI, C1q, and titer information. Am J Transplant. 2015;15:2421–30.
34. Ma J, Patel A, Tinckam K. Donor-specific antibody monitoring: where is the beef? Adv Chronic Kidney Dis. 2016;23:317–25.
35. Filippone EJ, Farber JL. The humoral theory of transplantation: epitope analysis and the pathogenicity of HLA antibodies. J Immunol Res. 2016;2016:5197396.
36. Hayde N, Solomon S, Caglar E, Ge J, Qama E, Colovai A. C1q-binding DSA and allograft outcomes in pediatric kidney transplant recipients. Pediatric Transplant. 2020;25(2):e13885.

37. Freitas MC, Rebellato LM, Ozawa M, et al. The role of immunoglobulin-G subclasses and C1q in de novo HLA-DQ donor-specific antibody kidney transplantation outcomes. Transplantation. 2013;95:1113–9.
38. Lefaucheur C, Viglietti D, Hidalgo LG, et al. Complement-activating anti-HLA antibodies in kidney transplantation: allograft gene expression profiling and response to treatment. J Am Soc Nephrol. 2018;29:620–35.
39. Cai J, Terasaki PI, Zhu D, et al. Complement-fixing antibodies against denatured HLA and MICA antigens are associated with antibody mediated rejection. Exp Mol Pathol. 2016;100:45–50.
40. Taylor CJ, Kosmoliaptsis V, Martin J, et al. Technical limitations of the C1q single-antigen bead assay to detect complement binding HLA-specific antibodies. Transplantation. 2017;101:1206–14.
41. Loupy A, Haas M, Solez K, et al. The Banff 2015 kidney meeting report: current challenges in rejection classification and prospects for adopting molecular pathology. Am J Transplant. 2017;17:28–41.
42. Haas M, Loupy A, Lefaucheur C, et al. The Banff 2017 kidney meeting report: revised diagnostic criteria for chronic active T cell-mediated rejection, antibody-mediated rejection, and prospects for integrative endpoints for next-generation clinical trials. Am J Transplant. 2018;18:293–307.
43. Louis K, Hertig A, Taupin JL, et al. Markers of graft microvascular endothelial injury may identify harmful donor-specific anti-HLA antibodies and predict kidney allograft loss. Am J Transplant. 2019;19:2434–45.
44. Jordan SC, Bunnapradist S, Bromberg JS, et al. Donor-derived cell-free DNA identifies antibody-mediated rejection in donor specific antibody positive kidney transplant recipients. Transplant Direct. 2018;4:e379.
45. Strommen AM, Moss MC, Goebel J, Bock M. Donor-specific antibodies in a pediatric kidney transplant population-prevalence and association with antiproliferative drug dosing. Pediatric Transplant. 2019;23:e13511.
46. Pearl MH, Chen L, ElChaki R, et al. Endothelin type a receptor antibodies are associated with angiotensin II type 1 receptor antibodies, vascular inflammation, and decline in renal function in pediatric kidney transplantation. Kidney Int Rep. 2020;5:1925–36.
47. Pearl MH, Zhang Q, Palma Diaz MF, et al. Angiotensin II type 1 receptor antibodies are associated with inflammatory cytokines and poor clinical outcomes in pediatric kidney transplantation. Kidney Int. 2018;93:260–9.
48. Zou Y, Stastny P, Susal C, Dohler B, Opelz G. Antibodies against MICA antigens and kidney-transplant rejection. N Eng J Med. 2007;357:1293–300.
49. Pineda S, Sigdel TK, Chen J, Jackson AM, Sirota M, Sarwal MM. Novel non-histocompatibility antigen mismatched variants improve the ability to predict antibody-mediated rejection risk in kidney transplant. Front Immunol. 2017;8:1687.
50. Fichtner A, Susal C, Schroder C, et al. Association of angiotensin II type 1 receptor antibodies with graft histology, function and survival in paediatric renal transplant recipients. Nephrol Dial Transplant. 2018;33:1065–72.
51. Freischlag K, Pearl MH, Chambers ET. The clinical impact of non-HLA antibodies in solid organ transplantation. Clin Transpl. 2016;32:31–43.
52. Bjerre A, Tangeraas T, Heidecke H, Dragun D, Dechend R, Staff AC. Angiotensin II type 1 receptor antibodies in childhood kidney transplantation. Pediatric Transplant. 2016;20:627–32.
53. Pinelli DF, Friedewald JJ, Haarberg KMK, et al. Assessing the potential of angiotensin II type 1 receptor and donor specific anti-endothelial cell antibodies to predict long-term kidney graft outcome. Human Immunol. 2017;78:421–7.
54. Rush D, Nickerson P, Gough J, et al. Beneficial effects of treatment of early subclinical rejection: a randomized study. J Am Soc Nephrol. 1998;9:2129–34.
55. Racusen LC. Protocol transplant biopsies in kidney allografts: why and when are they indicated? Clin J Am Soc Nephrol. 2006;1:144–7.

56. Mehta R, Cherikh W, Sood P, Hariharan S. Kidney allograft surveillance biopsy practices across US transplant centers: a UNOS survey. Clin Transpl. 2017;35(4):e14225.
57. Nazario M, Nicoara O, Becton L, et al. Safety and utility of surveillance biopsies in pediatric kidney transplant patients. Pediatric Transplant. 2018;22:e13178.
58. Dharnidharka VR, Vyas N, Gaut JP, Walther L, Hmiel SP. The utility of surveillance biopsies in pediatric kidney transplantation. Pediatric Nephrol (Berlin, Germany). 2018;33:889–95.
59. Odum JD, Kats A, VanSickle JS, et al. Characterizing the frequency of modifiable histological changes observed on surveillance biopsies in pediatric kidney allograft recipients. Pediatric Nephrol (Berlin, Germany). 2020;35:2173–82.
60. Landsberg A, Riazy M, Blydt-Hansen TD. Yield and utility of surveillance kidney biopsies in pediatric kidney transplant recipients at various time points post-transplant. Pediatric Transplant. 2020;25(2):e13869.
61. Hymes LC, Greenbaum L, Amaral SG, Warshaw BL. Surveillance renal transplant biopsies and subclinical rejection at three months post-transplant in pediatric recipients. Pediatric Transplant. 2007;11:536–9.
62. Zotta F, Guzzo I, Morolli F, Diomedi-Camassei F, Dello SL. Protocol biopsies in pediatric renal transplantation: a precious tool for clinical management. Pediatric Nephrol (Berlin, Germany). 2018;33:2167–75.
63. Seifert ME, Yanik MV, Feig DI, et al. Subclinical inflammation phenotypes and long-term outcomes after pediatric kidney transplantation. Am J Transplant. 2018;18:2189–99.
64. Jackson JA, Kim EJ, Begley B, et al. Urinary chemokines CXCL9 and CXCL10 are non-invasive markers of renal allograft rejection and BK viral infection. Am J Transplant. 2011;11:2228–34.
65. Schaub S, Nickerson P, Rush D, et al. Urinary CXCL9 and CXCL10 levels correlate with the extent of subclinical tubulitis. Am J Transplant. 2009;9:1347–53.
66. Sureshkumar KK, Marcus RJ. Urinary biomarkers as predictors of long-term allograft function after renal transplantation. Transplantation. 2010;90:688–9.
67. Suthanthiran M, Schwartz JE, Ding R, et al. Urinary-cell mRNA profile and acute cellular rejection in kidney allografts. N Eng J Med. 2013;369:20–31.
68. Lui YY, Chik KW, Chiu RW, Ho CY, Lam CW, Lo YM. Predominant hematopoietic origin of cell-free DNA in plasma and serum after sex-mismatched bone marrow transplantation. Clin Chem. 2002;48:421–7.
69. Rhodes A, Wort SJ, Thomas H, Collinson P, Bennett ED. Plasma DNA concentration as a predictor of mortality and sepsis in critically ill patients. Crit Care. 2006;10:R60.
70. Tug S, Helmig S, Deichmann ER, et al. Exercise-induced increases in cell free DNA in human plasma originate predominantly from cells of the haematopoietic lineage. Exerc Immunol Rev. 2015;21:164–73.
71. Beck J, Bierau S, Balzer S, et al. Digital droplet PCR for rapid quantification of donor DNA in the circulation of transplant recipients as a potential universal biomarker of graft injury. Clin Chem. 2013;59:1732–41.
72. Bloom RD, Bromberg JS, Poggio ED, et al. Cell-free DNA and active rejection in kidney allografts. J Am Soc Nephrol. 2017;28:2221–32.
73. Preka E, Ellershaw D, Chandler N, et al. Cell-free DNA in pediatric solid organ transplantation using a new detection method of separating donor-derived from recipient cell-free DNA. Clin Chem. 2020;66:1300–9.
74. Sharon E, Shi H, Kharbanda S, et al. Quantification of transplant-derived circulating cell-free DNA in absence of a donor genotype. PLoS Comput Biol. 2017;13:e1005629.
75. Beck J, Oellerich M, Schulz U, et al. Donor-derived cell-free DNA is a novel universal biomarker for allograft rejection in solid organ transplantation. Transplant Proc. 2015;47:2400–3.
76. Gielis EM, Ledeganck KJ, De Winter BY, et al. Cell-free DNA: an upcoming biomarker in transplantation. Am J Transplant. 2015;15:2541–51.
77. Knight SR, Thorne A, Lo Faro ML. Donor-specific cell-free DNA as a biomarker in solid organ transplantation. A systematic review. Transplantation. 2019;103:273–83.
78. Whitlam JB, Ling L, Skene A, et al. Diagnostic application of kidney allograft-derived absolute cell-free DNA levels during transplant dysfunction. Am J Transplant. 2019;19:1037–49.

79. Puliyanda DP, Swinford R, Pizzo H, Garrison J, De Golovine AM, Jordan SC. Donor-derived cell-free DNA (dd-cfDNA) for detection of allograft rejection in pediatric kidney transplants. Pediatric Transplant. 2020;25(2):e13850.
80. Ragalie WS, Stamm K, Mahnke D, et al. Noninvasive assay for donor fraction of cell-free DNA in pediatric heart transplant recipients. J Am Coll Cardiol. 2018;71:2982–3.
81. Sigdel TK, Archila FA, Constantin T, et al. Optimizing detection of kidney transplant injury by assessment of donor-derived cell-free DNA via massively multiplex PCR. J Clin Med 2018;8(1):19.
82. Birk PE, Stannard KM, Konrad HB, et al. Surveillance biopsies are superior to functional studies for the diagnosis of acute and chronic renal allograft pathology in children. Pediatric Transplant. 2004;8:29–38.
83. Birk PE. Surveillance biopsies in children post-kidney transplant. Pediatric Nephrol (Berlin, Germany). 2012;27:753–60.
84. Blydt-Hansen TD, Gibson IW, Gao A, Dufault B, Ho J. Elevated urinary CXCL10-to-creatinine ratio is associated with subclinical and clinical rejection in pediatric renal transplantation. Transplantation. 2015;99:797–804.
85. Ho J, Wiebe C, Rush DN, et al. Increased urinary CCL2: Cr ratio at 6 months is associated with late renal allograft loss. Transplantation. 2013;95:595–602.
86. Hricik DE, Nickerson P, Formica RN, et al. Multicenter validation of urinary CXCL9 as a risk-stratifying biomarker for kidney transplant injury. Am J Transplant. 2013;13:2634–44.
87. Mincham CM, Gibson IW, Sharma A, et al. Evolution of renal function and urinary biomarker indicators of inflammation on serial kidney biopsies in pediatric kidney transplant recipients with and without rejection. Pediatric Transplant. 2018;22:e13202.
88. Mockler C, Sharma A, Gibson IW, et al. The prognostic value of urinary chemokines at 6 months after pediatric kidney transplantation. Pediatr Transplant. 2018;22:e13205.
89. Blydt-Hansen TD, Sharma A, Gibson IW, et al. Validity and utility of urinary CXCL10/Cr immune monitoring in pediatric kidney transplant recipients. Am J Transplant. 2020;21(4):1545–55.
90. Lamarche C, Sharma AK, Goldberg A, Wang L, Blydt-Hansen TD. Biomarker implementation: evaluation of the decision-making impact of CXCL10 testing in a pediatric cohort. Pediatric Transplant. 2020;25(3):e13908.
91. Loupy A, Lefaucheur C, Vernerey D, et al. Molecular microscope strategy to improve risk stratification in early antibody-mediated kidney allograft rejection. J Am Soc Nephrol. 2014;25:2267–77.
92. Halloran PF, Famulski KS, Reeve J. Molecular assessment of disease states in kidney transplant biopsy samples. Nat Rev Nephrol. 2016;12:534–48.
93. Sigdel TK, Bestard O, Tran TQ, et al. A computational gene expression score for predicting immune injury in renal allografts. PLoS One. 2015;10:e0138133.
94. Khatri P, Roedder S, Kimura N, et al. A common rejection module (CRM) for acute rejection across multiple organs identifies novel therapeutics for organ transplantation. J Exp Med. 2013;210:2205–21.
95. Shaw BI, Cheng DK, Acharya CR, et al. An age-independent gene signature for monitoring acute rejection in kidney transplantation. Theranostics. 2020;10:6977–86.
96. Zhang W, Yi Z, Keung KL, et al. A peripheral blood gene expression signature to diagnose subclinical acute rejection. J Am Soc Nephrol. 2019;30:1481–94.
97. Suthanthiran M, Schwartz JE, Ding R, et al. Urinary-cell mRNA profile and acute cellular rejection in kidney allografts. N Engl J Med. 2013;369:20–31.
98. Verma A, Muthukumar T, Yang H, et al. Urinary cell transcriptomics and acute rejection in human kidney allografts. JCI Insight. 2020;6(8):e588.
99. Roedder S, Kimura N, Okamura H, Hsieh SC, Gong Y, Sarwal MM. Significance and suppression of redundant IL17 responses in acute allograft rejection by bioinformatics based drug repositioning of fenofibrate. PLoS One. 2013;8:e56657.
100. Yi Z, Keung KL, Li L, et al. Key driver genes as potential therapeutic targets in renal allograft rejection. JCI Insight. 2020;5(15):e136220.

Rejection Challenges: Diagnosis and Management

3

Samantha Lang, Maziar Riazy, and Tom D. Blydt-Hansen

A Brief History of Rejection

The Second World War heralded the first breakthrough that rejection is caused by immune mechanisms when Peter Medawar and Thomas Gibson attempted, without success, to treat burns victims using skin allografts. Subsequent research demonstrated that where autografts rapidly stabilized, skin allografts were infiltrated with native monocytes and lymphocytes, leading to vascular and lymphatic proliferation and progressive destruction. These findings and other contemporary research cemented our understanding that the basis of rejection is immunological [1].

Research in the decade after the war led further to an understanding of the importance of cellular immune processes in rejection pathophysiology [2]. Prior to this, rejection was thought to be entirely humoral, with Medawar searching but failing to find a single causative antibody [3]. Despite progressive improvements in understanding the mechanisms for rejection, effective treatment remained elusive. In the face of almost guaranteed failure, nine experimental kidney transplantations were nonetheless performed in France in 1951, justified on the grounds that no treatments for kidney failure existed and life-expectancy was short for these patients [4]. All of these people died within weeks secondary to rejection. Without effective anti-rejection treatment, successful transplantation could only be achieved by avoiding

S. Lang
Department of Experimental Medicine, University of British Columbia, Vancouver, BC, Canada
e-mail: Samantha.lang@bcchr.ca

M. Riazy
Department of Pathology and Laboratory Medicine, University of British Columbia, Vancouver, BC, Canada
e-mail: MRiazy1@providencehealth.bc.ca

T. D. Blydt-Hansen (✉)
Department of Pediatrics, University of British Columbia, Vancouver, BC, Canada
e-mail: Tom.BlydtHansen@cw.bc.ca

K. E. Twombley (ed.), *Challenges in Pediatric Kidney Transplantation*,
https://doi.org/10.1007/978-3-030-74783-1_3

alloreactivity entirely. It was on this basis that the first successful kidney transplant was performed in 1954 between identical twins [5].

Continued efforts to treat or prevent rejection were directed at suppressing the immune response, and led to the use of total body irradiation, 6-mercaptapurine, or azathioprine [6]. Although an improvement, these therapies yielded maximum survival of only 6 months, and many considered abandoning human transplantation.

In a medical breakthrough, Thomas Starzl, at a conference in 1963, reported that the addition of high dose prednisone to azathioprine reversed rejection, extending one-year survival rates above 70% [7]. Starzl's contribution salvaged transplantation as a viable treatment for kidney failure, and corticosteroids still form the basis of rejection treatment today. This was followed by a further breakthrough in the late 1960s, with the discovery of antilymphocyte serum that depletes effector T cells through opsonization-induced apoptosis. Anti-lymphocyte therapies also remain an effective tool in the management of severe or steroid-resistant cellular rejection [8].

Since the advent of pediatric transplantation in the mid-1960s [9, 10], pediatric recipients have faced unique challenges related to growth [11, 12], neurocognitive issues [13], and size mismatch [14]. Specific to rejection, advances in treatment for children tend to lag behind adult protocols due to biases that interventions must be demonstrated to be both safe and efficacious in adults before pediatric trials are commenced [9].

Over the last 70 years, our understanding of rejection has greatly improved and become more nuanced. With advances in induction and maintenance immunosuppression protocols, the incidence of clinical acute rejection has improved from an almost universal certainty to less than 15% in the first post-transplant year [15–17]. However, beyond improvements in first year survival, the rate of subsequent progressive allograft failure has improved little in the last two decades. Chronic forms of rejection (chronic, active antibody/T cell-mediated rejection) remain the leading cause of graft loss, responsible for 38.5% of graft failures [15, 18, 19]. Indeed, the incidence of late acute rejection in children appears now to be increasing [15, 17], which is concerning as late rejection episodes portend a poorer prognosis [20–25]. Some of this increase may be improved ascertainment; ongoing research has led to better characterization of acute and progressive forms of allograft injury.

As we continue to improve our understanding of the mechanisms that underlie inflammation and alloimmune regulation, more targeted treatments may be possible that disrupt chronic inflammatory signaling. Such treatments should not only suppress inflammation but also promote ongoing tolerance, and would represent another significant milestone in the goal of controlling rejection at all phases of the alloimmune pathway.

An Evolving Paradigm of Rejection: From Discreet Episodic Events to a Fluctuating Continuum of Immune Alloreactivity

Rejection is broadly defined as the cognate immunological response by the transplant recipient to the donor kidney and may include cellular (T cell-mediated) or humoral (antibody-mediated) responses. A biopsy is needed to confirm the diagnosis, classify type and severity, and direct treatment.

Kidney function is routinely relied upon as a marker of graft stability: deterioration guides biopsy indication and a return to baseline function is used to signal resolution. This reliance on creatinine misses early subclinical rejection *and* rejection that persists at a lower intensity following treatment. The perception of short-lived functional disturbances belies the possibility of persistent underlying inflammation, lending the impression that rejection is episodic. Later onset of functional decline is attributed to the acquisition of donor-specific antibody, antibody-mediated rejection, and chronic, active T cell-mediated rejection, often without accounting for the indolent nature of inflammation that may have persisted. Advances in the detection of subclinical inflammation have challenged the notion that stable creatinine equates to low allograft risk.

It is now better understood that early rejection episodes and later, more chronic forms of rejection are interrelated and may evolve – one into the other – on a continuum of alloimmune response. Early acute rejection is directly associated with later development of donor-specific antibodies and chronic inflammation in areas of interstitial fibrosis and tubular atrophy (i-IFTA). In the time interval after initial rejection "episodes" are detected and treated, there may be further maturation of residual alloimmune reactivity until it manifests again clinically as chronic forms of antibody-mediated or T cell-mediated rejection, which remain the leading causes of allograft failure.

The adoption of surveillance biopsies in some pediatric transplant centers has led to greater ascertainment of rejection, albeit still episodic, with early rejection rates as high as 40% [26, 27]. By definition, subclinical rejection is detected at a lower level of severity that is not yet causing allograft acute kidney injury. Untreated subclinical rejection is clearly associated with subsequent risk of graft function deterioration (clinical rejection) and adversely impacts graft survival. However, even with treatment, subclinical rejection has a worse allograft outcome compared to children with no rejection. As with clinical rejection, this may be due in part to failure to confirm that alloreactive inflammation has been fully suppressed with treatment. Studies that evaluate follow-up biopsies after treatment identify over 50% with persisting rejection after initial treatment [26, 28–31].

Recent data evaluating chemokine profiles post-transplant identify elevated risk for rejection and graft failure starting in the first weeks after transplant, and that those with persistently greater inflammatory signaling over time do more poorly [32]. This fluctuating inflammatory burden is currently difficult to identify and track, but may become more easily detected as better non-invasive monitoring tools become routinely available in the clinic. The paradigm may therefore need to shift, to consider rejection as a manifestation of a constantly evolving alloimmune response. Immunosuppression and adaptive regulatory responses that suppress inflammation compete with persistent allograft antigen stimulation that sustains the cytotoxic effector responses. The consequence is inflammation that waxes and wanes, and periodically is sufficiently severe as to cause overt dysfunction. The following sections apply this conceptualization to the monitoring and management of different forms of rejection in children.

Pathophysiology of Alloimmune Activation and Downstream Processes

Allorecognition refers to the immunological response to tissues or cells from a member of the same species, which are not recognized as self. Alloimmune-mediated injury begins with T cell recognition of donor HLA alloantigens, which initiates cognate T cell activation and mediates an acute anti-donor tissue inflammatory response. Once activated, resolution depends on intensification of immunosuppression and sustainment of adaptive regulatory responses that are concurrently initiated to ultimately resolve inflammation. However, insufficient suppression of inflammation and continued presentation of alloantigen may favor persistence of the cognate effector response. This complex series of immune responses may evolve over time from acute to more chronic forms of rejection; and with better understanding there may be opportunities for more targeted therapies, depending on the phase of alloimmune maturation. What follows is a simplified model of rejection pathogenesis and its potential for resolution or propagation.

T Cell Development and Activation

CD4+ T cells are activated in a three-stage process. **Signal 1** is T cell receptor (TCR) binding: Dendritic cells and other antigen presenting cells (APC) present class II HLA with donor antigens to naïve T cells in secondary lymphoid organs (SLO) (Fig. 3.1) [33]. In the early post-transplant period, donor-derived APCs play a large role in presenting intact class II HLA molecules to naïve T cells after migrating to SLO from the allograft, in a process known as direct allorecognition [34]. Donor APCs present an array of intact donor alloantigens capable of sensitizing a broad range of T cells, and induce an early polyclonal T cell response that is strongly associated with acute rejection [35]. In animal models with acute rejection, up to 90% of T cells are responsive to intact donor antigen [36]. Recipient APCs can acquire intact class II HLA from donor APCs or graft cells expressing class II HLA [37], which can then present intact alloantigen in a process known as semi-direct allorecognition. In indirect allorecognition, donor alloantigens (both class I and

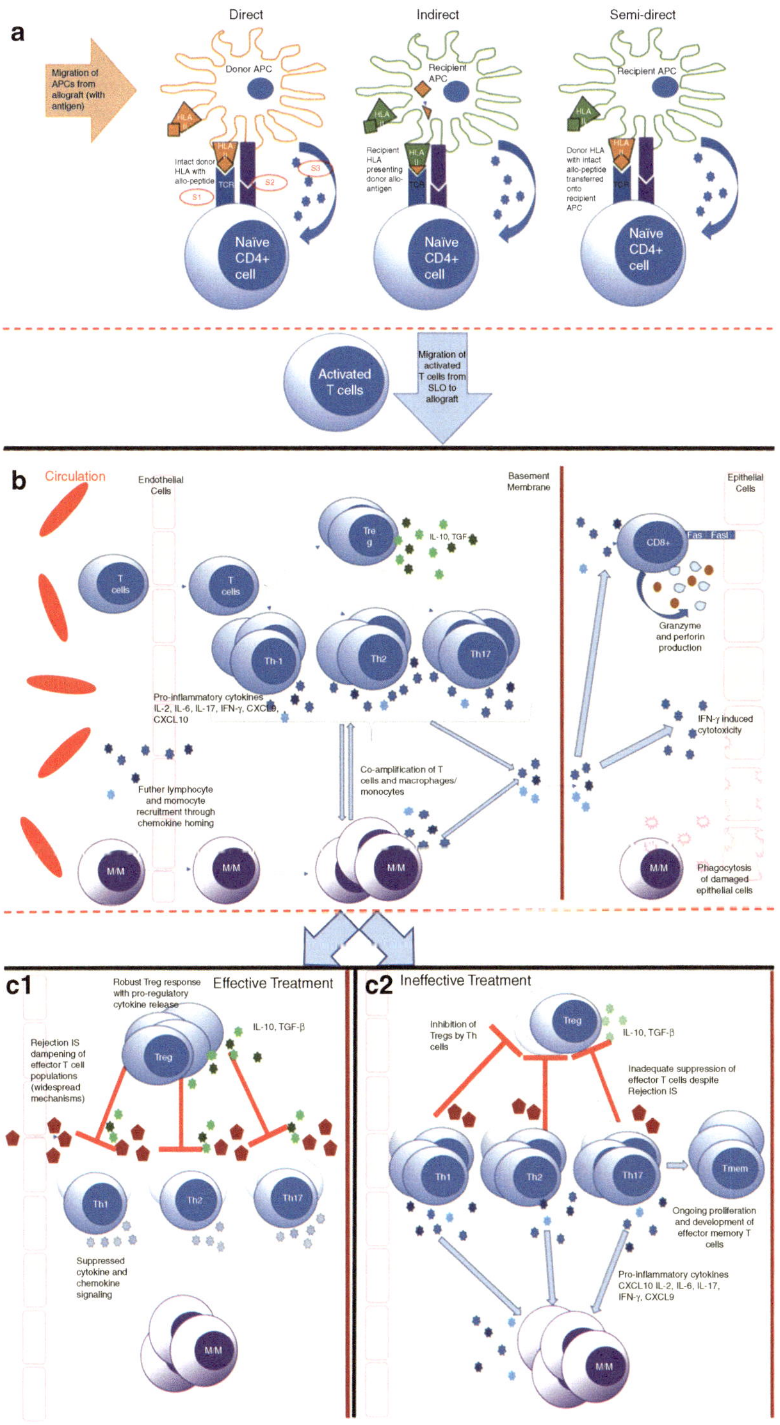
a
Direct
Indirect
Semi-direct
Migration of APCs from allograft (with antigen)
Donor APC
Recipient APC
Recipient APC
Intact donor HLA with allo-peptide
Recipient HLA presenting donor allo-antigen
Donor HLA with intact allo-peptide transferred onto recipient APC
S1
S2
S3
TCR
Naïve CD4+ cell
Activated T cells
Migration of activated T cells from SLO to allograft
b
Circulation
Endothelial Cells
Basement Membrane
Epithelial Cells
T cells
Treg
IL-10, TGF-β
CD8+
Fas
FasL
Granzyme and perforin production
Th-1
Th2
Th17
Pro-inflammatory cytokines IL-2, IL-6, IL-17, IFN-γ, CXCL9, CXCL10
IFN-γ induced cytotoxicity
Co-amplification of T cells and macrophages/ monocytes
Futher lymphocyte and momocyte recruitment through chemokine homing
M/M
Phagocytosis of damaged epithelial cells
c1
Effective Treatment
Robust Treg response with pro-regulatory cytokine release
IL-10, TGF-β
Rejection IS dampening of effector T cell populations (widespread mechanisms)
Th1
Th2
Th17
Suppressed cytokine and chemokine signaling
M/M
c2
Ineffective Treatment
Inhibition of Tregs by Th cells
Treg
IL-10, TGF-β
Inadequate suppression of effector T cells despite Rejection IS
Th1
Th2
Th17
Tmem
Ongoing proliferation and development of effector memory T cells
Pro-inflammatory cytokines CXCL10 IL-2, IL-6, IL-17, IFN-γ, CXCL9
M/M

(continued)

Fig. 3.1 (**a**) Naïve T cells circulate in lymph and secondary lymphoid organs (SLO). Donor (orange) and recipient (green) antigen-presenting cells (APC) deliver antigen from the tissues to the SLOs for T cell surveillance. Naïve T cell activation occurs in response to three signals—S1: interaction between donor HLA antigen on APC and T cell receptor; S2: co-stimulation; S3: cytokines produced by immune cells within the lymph. Direct allorecognition: donor APCs (orange) present intact HLA (orange) to recipient TCR. Indirect allorecognition: recipient APCs (green) present internalized, processed donor HLA allopeptide segments (orange) to TCR. Semi-direct allorecognition: recipient APC (green) acquires intact donor HLA (orange) from donor APC, which is then presented to the TCR. Once activated, T cells exit the lymph and migrate to the allograft. (**b**) Activated T cells (cytotoxic CD8+ and CD4+ helper T cells) home to the allograft. T cells proliferate and mature in response to exposure to their cognate antigen. Inflammatory cytokines produced by CD4+ effector cells upregulate macrophage and monocyte activation and recruit further innate and adaptive cells. Monocytes and macrophages produce cytokines that further drive T cell proliferation. Epithelial cell injury in T-cell mediated rejection occurs via several mechanisms: CD8+ cells bind via the Fas-Fas Ligand, inducing apoptosis, and release perforins and toxic granzymes that cause cell lysis; IFN-γ released by Th cells damages cell integrity; macrophages and monocytes phagocytose cellular debris. IL-2 and IFN-γ induce proliferation of regulatory T cells (Tregs) aimed at commencing self-resolution. (**c1**) Effective rejection immunosuppression (IS) that is delivered early in the rejection trajectory alongside a robust regulatory T cell (Treg) response drives adequate suppression of effector T cells. Effector suppression downregulates inflammatory cytokine signaling, minimizing further innate and adaptive cell recruitment. Tregs induce Th apoptosis through cell-cell contact and the release of pro-regulatory cytokines (IL-10 and TGF-β). Corticosteroids and other anti-lymphocyte therapies induce a range of anti-T cell and anti-inflammatory responses. (**c2**) When rejection treatment is ineffective due to an inability to fully suppress effector T cells and the development of T cell memory (which is less responsive to treatment), there is ongoing recruitment, proliferation, and maturation of effector populations. Production of IL-6 in response to persistent antigenic stimulation inhibits Tregs in favor of Thl7 development and induces conversion of mature Tregs to Th17 cells, further propagating an inflammatory response

class II HLA) are internalized and processed by recipient APCs and then presented to T cells as peptide fragments within the recipient class II HLA molecules. Direct allorecognition is eliminated over the first few months' post-transplant as donor APCs are depleted, and thereafter semi-direct and indirect allorecognition predominate.

Following ligation of the TCR to its antigen, **signal 2** involves secondary ligand-receptor binding between the APC and T cell, known as co-stimulation, which is critical to complete T cell activation. Inadequate provision of this second signal results in T cell anergy. Thus, co-stimulatory pathways represent important potential targets to induce more regulatory alloimmune responses. Key co-stimulatory ligands include CD28:CD80/CD86 and CD40:CD154. The second signal also prompts the production of cytokines that further propagate the cognate alloimmune response – including interleukin-2 (IL-2), which is a key promoter of T cell survival and proliferation.

The cytokine microenvironment provides **signal 3,** which directs differentiation of the activated T cells into various T helper cell subsets (Th cells). An environment rich in IL-12 and IFN-γ drives Th1 production, IL-4 is critical to the development of Th2 cells, and IL-21, IL-6, and transforming growth factor beta (TGF-β) promote

Th17 cells [38–43]. An environment rich in IL-2 and TGF-β (conditional on the absence of IL-6) directs regulatory T cell (Treg) development, with evidence of contributions by other pro-tolerant cytokines such as IL-10 [44]. Nuances in the strength and duration of TCR stimulation are also key to Th cell differentiation [45, 46].

Similar to CD4+ cells, naïve CD8+ cells are activated in SLO through contact with APCs. APCs present intact donor class I HLA antigens to CD8+ cells through direct allorecognition or processed class I HLA peptide segments through indirect or semi-direct allorecognition, and CD8+ activation is further stimulated by IL-12 [47].

The concept of rejection prophylaxis with induction and maintenance immunosuppression is directed toward primary prevention of cognate T cell activation. Once acute rejection is manifest, cognate T cell activation, differentiation, and propagation of the anti-donor antigen response are by definition already well-established, necessitating a different treatment approach that seeks to quell the inflammatory response and restore alloimmune quiescence within the allograft.

T Cell Migration and Mechanisms of Injury in T Cell-Mediated Rejection with the Allograft

Once activated in SLO, T cells gain expression of adhesion factors that enable tissue migration. They return to circulation via the thoracic duct, adhere to endothelium, and migrate within tissues in search of their cognate antigen. Allograft localization is facilitated by expression of homing programs that reflect the site of priming (regional lymph nodes) and allograft inflammation from ischemia reperfusion injury (or other forms of subsequent allograft injury), which upregulates adhesion molecules on renal vascular endothelium [48]. The intensity of T cell proliferation in the SLO in response to the amount of antigen is also a factor. Upon TCR ligation of its cognate antigen, activated T helper (CD4+) and cytotoxic (CD8+) T cells are induced to proliferate in situ, and collectively produce an array of pro-inflammatory cytokines/chemokines (IL-2, IL-6, IL-17, IFN-γ, CXCL9, CXCL10) that recruit innate immune cells (natural killer cells and phagocytic monocytes) (Fig. 3.1). The innate arm of this response is also activated by damage-associated molecular patterns (DAMPs) induced by ischemia or other events and are recognized by pattern recognition receptors (PRR) on phagocytic cells causing up-regulation of costimulatory molecules and secretion of pro-inflammatory cytokines [49]. In concert, both an innate and adaptive component further promotes the influx of activated B and T cells to sustain the effector response [50, 51].

Cellular injury occurs through CD4+ production of cytotoxic cytokines capable of inducing apoptosis such as IFN-γ and by direct interaction between primed CD8+ T cells and donor tissues, including tubular epithelial cells (Fig. 3.1) [33,

52, 53]. Cytotoxic T cells induce apoptosis through Fas-Fas ligand binding and release granzymes and perforins that damage cell integrity and cause lysis [52]. Monocytes and macrophages (type 1) trafficked to the graft perpetuate adaptive effector responses in their role as APCs and produce a further abundance of proinflammatory mediators including cytokines such as IL-1 and TNF-α that reinforce ongoing macrophage responses; IL-6 and IL-23 that promote development and survival of Th17 cells; and IL-12 and IFN-γ that perpetuate ongoing Th1 responses [54, 55].

The cognate immune response evolved as an effective, intense, but targeted anti-pathogen response that is programmed for self-resolution. Some of the same signals that instigate the primary effector response, such as IL-2, also initiate a recovery response dominated by co-localized proliferation of Treg cells [56, 57]. Normally, as the source of novel antigen is destroyed and antigen-mediated effector cell signalling abates, Tregs restrain the effector response by inducing Th cell apoptosis via direct contact and via the release of pro-regulatory cytokines such as TGF-β and IL-10 (Fig. 3.1) [58]. Despite the depletion of the majority of effector T cells through this process, a small proportion survive as long-lived memory T cells [59]. Phagocytic monocytes and macrophages (type 2) play a major role in the late inflammatory stages of injury repair through production of IL-10 and TGF-β, clearance of cellular debris and fibrogenesis, followed by an anti-fibrotic response that restores tissue in scarless healing [55, 60, 61].

In the setting of transplantation, persistence of the novel (donor) antigen presents a unique challenge for immune resolution, since it may perpetuate reactive cognate effector cell signalling. The combination of intensified immunosuppression and intra-graft Treg proliferation may not be sufficient to regain complete control over expanded effector T cell populations (Fig. 3.1). Macrophages and monocytes accumulate in the interstitium and tubules and are unable to progress beyond fibrosis and angiogenesis, contributing over time to scarring and chronic inflammatory injury [54]. Ultimately, prolonged and sustained exposure to donor HLA antigen [62, 63] and inflammatory cytokines like IFN-γ [64, 65] promotes the development of memory $CD4^+$ T cells generated from effector cells, and evolution of chronic inflammation.

B Cell Development and Activation

Naïve B cells develop in the bone marrow and migrate to SLO. The B cell receptor (BCR) is a membrane-bound immunoglobulin that recognizes free soluble antigen in its native form within the lymph or antigen presented by APCs, which is captured from the APC by the B cell and internalized [66]. Initial activation follows similar stages as their T cell counterparts: BCR/antibody affinity, costimulatory or co-inhibitory signals (including ICOS, CD40 ligand, and CD80 and CD86) [67, 68], and then cytokine microenvironment-mediated differentiation. Early B cell activation is promoted by primed T cells via production of B cell activation factor (BAFF) [69].

Following initial activation, immature B cells either develop into marginal B cells or follicular B cells. Follicular B cells, having internalized either soluble antigen or antigen presented on dendritic cells, migrate to the T-B zone of germinal centers within SLO [70]. B cells are one of the few cell types capable of antigen presentation via class II HLA molecules to CD4+ cells [70, 71]. Cognate B cells present their internalized antigen peptides for follicular T cell recognition [66]. Here, the relative preponderance of follicular T helper cells (TfH) and follicular regulatory cells (TfR) determines B cell fate. TfH cells bind follicular B cells, produce IL-4 and IL-21, and provide co-stimulation via the CD154, all of which promote B cell activation (Fig. 3.2) [72]. TfR cells suppress IL-21 and IL-4, express co-inhibitors CTLA-4 and PD-1, and inhibit B cell metabolism [73, 74]. Dominant regulatory influence dramatically suppresses antibody production [73, 75]. Sufficient B-TfH cell affinity results in somatic hypermutation with positive selection for B cells with the highest antibody-antigen affinity, which become antibody producing plasma cells or memory B cells capable of exerting a potent and persisting anti-graft response [71, 76, 77].

Although B cells can be activated directly in the absence of TfH cell interaction, this process results in short-lived (maximum 14 days) extra-follicular plasmablasts, only capable of producing antibody from their original repertoire (Fig. 3.2) [78]. Robust B cell responses develop secondary to TfH cell-mediation and reciprocally promote ongoing T cell activation through their antigen presenting role. Organized intra-graft B cell clusters such as in B cell-rich rejection function as antigen presenting centers and provide co-stimulation to co-aggregated CD4+ T cells [79–82].

Regulatory B cells also exist and may dampen B and T cell responses. Regulatory B cells both produce IL-10 and stimulate IL-10 production by CD4+ cells [83]. Higher levels of regulatory or transitional B cells have also been shown to protect against AMR [84]. As at every stage of the alloimmune continuum, it is the balance of effector and regulatory responses that determines the clinical outcome.

Alloantibodies and Antibody-Mediated Rejection

Antibodies are soluble mediators of the humoral immune system generated either by immature plasmablasts or by mature, more durable plasma cells. Donor-specific antibodies may develop against class I or class II HLA. Class I antigens are expressed by virtually all nucleated cells, whereas class II are constitutively expressed on APCs and can be induced on other cell types during times of inflammation, particularly vascular endothelium. Antibodies against non-HLA alloantigens, such as major-histocompatibility-complex class I–related chain A (MICA) or

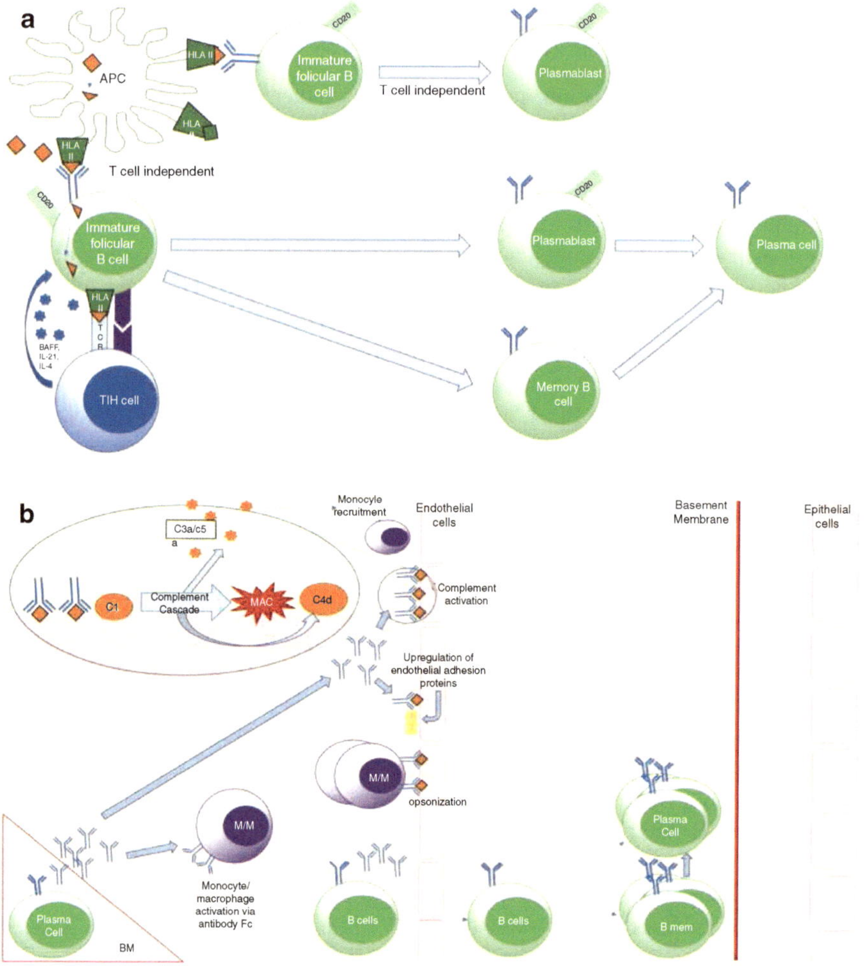

Fig. 3.2 (**a**) Immature follicular B cells within germinal centers of the SLOs bind soluble donor antigen (orange) or extract antigen from APCs (recipient APC shown in figure (green)) using surface antibody. In T cell-independent processes, B cells develop into short-lived plasmablasts. T follicular helper cells produce IL-4, IL-21, and BAFF required for B cell activation and provide B cell co-stimulation. TfH support induces B cell somatic hypermutation important for development into plasma and memory cells, which lose expression of CD20. B cells reciprocally promote ongoing T cell activation through presentation of internalized antigen via class II HLA. (**b**) Long-lived plasma cells migrate to their niche, often bone marrow (BM), where they produce high affinity anti-allograft antibody. B cells including plasma cells also migrate into the allograft. Antibody-mediated injury occurs through complement dependent and independent pathways. Antibody activation of complement induces the complement cascade, culminating in the membrane attack complex (MAC). MAC lyses endothelial cells. Byproducts of complement activation include C3a/C5a (home innate cells and upregulate adhesion markers on endothelial tissue) and C4d (useful diagnostic marker due to covalent binding of endothelium). Antibody signaling independent of complement induces injury through crosstalk with innate cells. The constant portion of the antibody (Fc) activates monocytes and macrophages, inducing innate cell-mediated inflammation, known as antibody-cell-dependent cytotoxicity. Monocytes and macrophages also recognize and induce apoptosis in cells opsonized with antibody

autoantibodies, such as anti-endothelial cell antibodies and angiotensin type 1 receptor antibodies, can play an important role in mediating the intensity or severity of antibody-mediated rejection and in some cases are directly implicated in AMR, in the absence of alloantibody detection [85].

Allograft directed antibodies bind the capillary endothelium and inflict damage via complement dependent and independent pathways (Fig. 3.2) [71, 86]. With a high-enough density of antibody-binding, complement fixation leads to formation of the membrane attack complex (C5b-C9) resulting in cell lysis [87]. Complement activation by-products include C4d, C3a, and C5a. C3a and C5a are chemokines for macrophage and neutrophils and induce endothelial cells to release adhesion molecules and pro-inflammatory cytokines. C4d is particularly useful as a diagnostic marker, since it binds covalently to the endothelium and can be detected for days following antibody binding [88, 89]. Complement driven endothelial damage also triggers the release of Von Willebrand factor leading to platelet activation and the formation of microthrombi [86, 90].

Antibodies are also involved in an array of complement-independent signaling. Following antibody binding, endothelial cells undergo cytoskeletal reorganization that stabilizes the endothelium for leukocyte tethering and triggers endothelial proliferation [91, 92]. Antibodies bind and activate NK cells and macrophages using the antibody Fc portion, leading to antibody-cell-dependent cytotoxicity [91, 93–95]. Activation of the coagulation cascade can lead to the deposition of platelets and microthrombi, amplifying vascular injury and leading to arteriolar necrosis [96].

Alloimmune Chronicity

The transition from acute to chronic allograft inflammation is complex and incompletely understood. Persistence of alloantigen and insufficient suppression of inflammation may permit continued signalling from cytokines such as IL-6, which tip the balance from regulatory to effector cell differentiation. IL-6 simultaneously inhibits Treg development [97] and stimulates transformation of Tregs into Th17 cells [50, 98]. High levels of Th17 and inadequate Treg responses have been associated with chronic rejection [99–104]. Effector B cell production of immunoglobulins as well as B cell maturation are also stimulated by IL-6 [105, 106]. As with Tregs, regulatory B cells are also reduced in chronic AMR (0.98%) compared to stable allografts (2.81%) [107]. This disequilibrium between effector and regulatory response is mirrored in the innate immune response, where expanded populations of intragraft monocytes and macrophages are associated with chronic rejection and express higher levels of PAI-1 mRNA, which is a critical mediator for fibrogenesis [55].

The activation and proliferation of effector responses are inherently associated with the development of immune memory, which likely has a principal role in maintaining chronic forms of rejection. Both memory B and T cells deliver swifter and more effective anti-graft responses, require lower doses of antigen for activation, and are more refractory to standard treatments [108]. Chronic, active TCMR is associated with an upregulation of RNA that characterizes CD8+ cytotoxic memory T cells [109] and a greater proportion of IL-17 producing memory T cells [103]. Memory B cells make up a higher proportion of B cells in chronic rejection [110] and are seen in 80% of biopsies with chronic rejection [111]. These memory cell populations may be not be accessible to lymphocyte depleting therapies, which have renewed efforts to identify alternative treatment strategies that target the signalling pathways that sustain chronic inflammation for tertiary prevention.

Detecting Rejection and Monitoring Its Course

Histological confirmation on kidney biopsy remains the gold standard for rejection diagnosis. The phase at which the rejection process is detected may be relevant to its potential reversibility. Within the allograft, the first signals may be gene expression, followed by cytokine and chemokine production, and alterations in tissue metabolism that result from alloreactive T cell infiltration. With time, inflammatory cells continue to infiltrate and accrue, such that they are detectable histologically, along with their interactions with the tubular epithelium, arterial vasculature, or capillary endothelium. As tissue injury ensues, damage ultimately progresses to clinically detectable acute kidney injury (AKI). The introduction of novel, clinically accessible monitoring tools has the potential to shift the diagnostic paradigm upstream, which may improve early ascertainment and treatment outcomes.

Clinical Monitoring and Biopsy Indication

A mainstay of clinical monitoring for allograft injury includes surveillance of serum creatinine, proteinuria, and donor-specific antibodies (DSA) [112, 113]. Serum creatinine should be monitored daily to weekly for the first few months after transplant, with tapering of frequency to every 1–3 months after the first year, depending on clinical stability [113]. Detection of AKI with serum creatinine elevation is the most common indication for kidney biopsy, after other causes of AKI have been excluded such as functional, infectious, obstructive, or drug-related causes. Persistent rise in serum creatinine of 10–25% above baseline is usually sufficient to indicate a biopsy, a lower threshold than the 33–50% rise recommended for pediatric non-transplant AKI diagnosis [114, 115]. This lower threshold implicitly acknowledges a fundamental limitation of functional monitoring, which is that significant injury must accrue *before* kidney dysfunction becomes manifest [116–119]. This problem is most pronounced in younger children, where functional impairment can be masked by compensation from large adult donor kidney mass relative to pediatric body size [14].

Although published guidelines set the minimum standard at every 3–12 months, monitoring for proteinuria is commonly obtained in children at every clinic visit for surveillance. This may also include monitoring of urine albumin to creatinine ratio, which may be more sensitive for detection of hyperfiltration injury associated with progression of allograft chronic kidney disease. Worsening proteinuria should indicate a kidney biopsy to evaluate for recurrence of primary kidney disease, de novo glomerular disease, or antibody-mediated rejection (AMR). In the setting of AMR, proteinuria usually manifests later with progression to chronic AMR and transplant glomerulopathy, and so is not sensitive for early AMR detection.

Many pediatric transplant programs now include regular monitoring for de novo donor-specific antibody (*dn*DSA) as part of standard care. The most recent consensus guideline was published by The Transplantation Society in 2013 [112], and recommended active testing only at times when risk for AMR is increased, in addition to annual sampling. The argument against more frequent testing relates to cost-benefit in the face of ineffective treatment. With the advent of improving treatments for AMR, more frequent surveillance is better justified, and many pediatric programs routinely test for DSA every 3–6 months. Onset of *dn*DSA should be verified by repeat testing in the absence of other clinical findings and, when persistent, identifies AMR in over 40% of cases [120]. The onset of *dn*DSA is associated with development of AMR within 12 months, eGFR decline, and future graft loss [121, 122]. AMR detected by DSA-indicated biopsies was associated with a greater than 5-fold reduction in graft failure, compared to otherwise clinically indicated biopsy AMR cases [123]. Detection of *dn*DSA early in the evolution of antibody-mediated injury affords opportunity to modify immunosuppression and mitigate progression, and is an important recent addition to routine surveillance for rejection.

Surveillance Biopsies

Despite greatly improved ascertainment rates for rejection with surveillance biopsies, less than half of centers include them as standard practice [26, 124]. The procedure-related risk is very low, and more often the arguments against adoption relate to cost and burden on patients and families [125, 126].

There is no universally accepted protocol for rejection surveillance using biopsies, and yield may depend upon timing. Ascertainment of subclinical rejection fluctuates between 14% and 43% in the first year [26, 27, 124, 127–130]. In children receiving IL-2 receptor antibody induction, the biopsy time point with the greatest yield for TCMR diagnosis was at 6 months (43%), whereas biopsies at 3 or 12 months identified rejection in 15% and 21% of biopsies, respectively [27]. In the setting of depletional antibody induction with anti-thymocyte globulin, similar rates of subclinical TCMR are noted; however the onset is shifted later and peaks instead at the 12-month biopsy (31%), relative to the 6-month time point (14%) [131].

The clinical utility of surveillance biopsies was first established in a landmark clinical trial by Rush et al. [117] demonstrating improved allograft outcome in the surveillance group where rates of subclinical rejection approached 30%. With decline of subclinical rejection rates in low-risk adults to less than 5% [132, 133], continued use protocol surveillance may no longer be justified. However, even with modern immunosuppression, subclinical TCMR rates in children persist at >30% in the first post-transplant year and are associated with progression to late acute TCMR, AMR, chronic forms of rejection, and allograft failure [128, 134, 135]. The benefits of treating subclinical TCMR parallel those related to treating TCMR on clinically indicated biopsies: reduction of subsequent clinical rejection, chronic tubulointerstitial damage, functional decline, and allograft failure [128, 129, 136–138].

Follow-Up Biopsies

The prevailing wisdom that return to baseline creatinine is highly correlated with histological resolution has never been corroborated. To the contrary, several studies evaluating serum creatinine monitoring for TCMR treatment show that it correlates poorly with histological severity at diagnosis and does not reliably predict resolution on subsequent biopsy [28, 116, 139, 140]. Almost by definition, a creatinine-based approach to monitoring subclinical rejection treatment response is nonsensical.

This has led to the adoption of follow-up biopsies in some centers, to more effectively monitor treatment response. The timing varies from 1 to 3 months after treatment and identifies high rates (46–65%) of persistent subclinical TCMR [26, 28–31, 140]. The risk that persisting TCMR may evolve to more chronic rejection is highlighted by rapid development of chronic inflammation (i-IFTA) in 61% of follow-up biopsies at a median of 3 months later [141]. One-year biopsies in patients with prior TCMR identified >50% with i-IFTA-like changes and 8% with transplant glomerulopathy [29]. In the same study, resolution of rejection at 1 year was associated with similarly favorable outcome as patients who had not experienced rejection, whereas i-IFTA-like changes at 1 year were associated four-fold hazard of graft failure.

While follow-up biopsies provide critical information regarding treatment efficacy and ongoing risk for chronic inflammation, there are practical limits to the number of biopsies that will be tolerable in a single patient. This provides the strongest rationale for the need of better surrogate biomarkers that are non-invasive, and which may be used both for diagnosis and treatment monitoring.

Biomarkers for Rejection

Although biomarkers may not supplant biopsy to confirm diagnosis, a blended approach is likely to follow soon where biomarkers indicate high risk for rejection and need for confirmatory biopsy, and additionally indicate low risk such that surveillance biopsy may be safely deferred. The ideal biomarkers will be non-invasive and identify rejection early in its evolution, prior to functional deterioration. This permits prompt treatment that limits allograft injury and mitigates entrenchment of chronic inflammation. Rather than any one biomarker, a combination of biomarkers that evaluate different aspects of the alloimmune response will be optimal to most completely evaluate and monitor alloimmune reactivity.

Gene Expression Signatures

These panels are designed to identify patterns of gene expression using multi-gene panels that associate with rejection. TruGraf™ is a 200-gene peripheral blood-based test that differentiates acute rejection, non-rejection-related graft damage, and stable grafts [142, 143]. It has been proposed as a "rule-out" test for rejection with a negative predictive value of >90%, facilitating decisions to avoid intervention or surveillance biopsy [144]. A different 17-gene signature blood panel (kSORT) has been evaluated, but failed to demonstrate robust clinical utility post-implementation [145]. Finally, a 3-gene urinary panel (CD3ε mRNA, CXCL10 mRNA, and 18S ribosomal RNA) was able to differentiate clinical TCMR samples from those without (AUC 0.74) and from AMR in adults (AUC 0.78) [146]. Notwithstanding their potential, neither the TruGraf™ nor the urinary panel has yet been validated in children or for diagnosis of subclinical rejection.

Chemokines

Chemokines (**chemo**tactic cyto**kines**) are a family of signaling molecules that induce chemotaxis. Urinary C-X-C motif chemokines 9 and 10 (CXCL9, CXCL10) are produced during acute inflammation, stimulated by IFN-γ, and mediate T cell homing to the allograft via the CXCR3 receptor expressed on leukocytes [147–151]. Elevated levels of urinary CXCL9 and CXCL10 are associated with acute rejection [152–161], subclinical rejection [157, 162], and decline in kidney function [153, 159, 163]. There is mixed evidence as to which is superior in predicting AMR [156, 164], and both had augmented success when combined with *dn*DSA monitoring [156, 164]. BKV viremia and nephropathy can also cause elevated CXCL10 levels and is an important differential diagnosis to consider when interpreting CXCL10 results [152, 165–167].

The clinical utility of urinary CXCL10 has been validated in children [168] but is not yet implemented for clinical use. It is sensitive to detection of subclinical and borderline TCMR [169–171], and responsive to changes in histological inflammation intensity after treatment of rejection on follow-up biopsy [28, 168]. Persistent elevation of CXCL10 in the first post-transplant year is associated with eGFR decline in the same time period and may be a potent indicator for immunosuppression titration, to target unresolved inflammation [168, 172].

Metabolomics

Tissue metabolism is strongly influenced by changes in homeostasis, and stereotypic changes in relative metabolite concentrations in biofluids such as urine can be used to detect different types of tissue injury such as TCMR. Machine learning approaches have enabled the development of urine metabolite risk scores in children capable of detecting subclinical TCMR, borderline TCMR, and AMR [116, 173], in addition to allograft AKI and chronic changes of IFTA, glomerulosclerosis, and declining GFR [174–176]. The specificity of a metabolomics approach may be superior to chemokine biomarkers, with the ability to distinguish acute rejection from BKVN [177]. Ho et al. reported that the combination of urinary CXCL10 and a metabolite rejection risk score was more accurate than either individually [178]. By combining a metabolomics approach with other biomarkers such as CXCL10, different aspects of the inflammatory response may be tested to enhance biomarker accuracy and precision.

Cell-Free DNA

Blood-based donor-derived cell-free DNA (dd-cfDNA) identifies donor DNA that is released with transplant tissue damage and is therefore more downstream from immune signaling, inflammatory cell infiltration, and related changes in tissue metabolism. Although two assays are currently approved for clinical use, their utility may be limited to detection of AMR and severe grades of TCMR (Banff ≥1B) [179–181], and do not have sufficient negative predictive value to reliably exclude the possibility rejection [182]. These assays have not been evaluated against surveillance biopsies to detect subclinical rejection, and there is very limited data on their utility in transplanted children [183, 184]. More data will be needed before dd-cfDNA can be recommended for rejection surveillance in children, perhaps in combination with another of the promising biomarkers.

Predisposing Risk Factors for Rejection

Evaluating risk for rejection should incorporate elements that are particular to the recipient, the donor, the extent of alloimmune incompatibility, and then subsequent immunosuppressive management. In reality, we are not yet at a point where we can use this information to proactively personalize immunosuppressive management; however, their consideration influences our index of suspicion as it regards to the intensity of monitoring and indication for kidney biopsy to identify rejection.

Recipient-Related Risks

Patient characteristics including adolescent age, female sex, and black race are associated with increased risk for rejection. Although non-adherence may be confounding, it is important to consider first the biological origins of risk associated with these recipient characteristics.

Females experience higher rates graft loss in both pediatric and adolescent cohorts despite equivalent or better (ages 17 and over) adherence compared with males [185–188]. In contrast to adults, this cannot be attributed to prior sensitization during pregnancy, which is rare in pediatric transplant recipients. In cases with a male donor, H-Y antigens act as an additional alloreactive target [189, 190]. Furthermore, increased T cell alloreactivity has been observed in females, independent of prior pregnancy or male donor [191]. The basis for this sex difference is incompletely understood, but may include estrogen-driven maturation of lymphocytes, increased antibody and cytokine responses, as well as localization of some immune-related genes on the X chromosome [192].

Adolescence is also associated with higher rates of graft loss and rejection [187, 193–195]. Immune-related differences in this age group may drive alloreactivity, and so rejection during adolescence should not be automatically attributed to non-adherence. As opposed to relative immune immaturity that may favor tolerance in transplanted infants [196–198], increase in effector cells and immune activity through adolescence may contribute to greater alloimmune reactivity [199–202]. With further aging in adulthood, gradual immune senescence is associated with decreased absolute numbers of total T cells (CD3+), CD4+, CD8+, naive T cells, and bone marrow progenitor B cells [203, 204], along with declining rejection risk [205]. These changes are independent of sex differences, but may also be influenced by sex hormone production in puberty.

The impact of race and social determinants of health is more complex, since the two factors may be confounding. Black kidney transplant recipients have a higher relative hazard of first rejection, particularly in the USA [17]. This disparity can be explained by more polymorphic HLA in black recipients; ethnicity-based HLA differences that disproportionately advantage white recipients within predominantly white transplant registries; and a potentially higher alloreactivity in black recipients [206–208]. These genetic factors intersect with reduced access to medical insurance, medical care, and affordable medication secondary to higher rates of low socio-economic status in ethnic minority groups [206, 207].

Other recipient factors are emerging as important, although the mechanism by which they prime immunological risk is not clear. Obesity, for example, is associated with acute rejection risk [209] and subsequent allograft failure [209–211]. Vitamin D deficiency has long been linked to inflammation and auto-immune conditions. In kidney transplant recipients, low vitamin D levels are associated with higher rates of rejection, and vitamin D supplementation reduces rejection risk [212, 213]. The immunomodulatory effects of vitamin D are not completely understood but appear to shift T cell populations from a strongly effector profile (Th1/17) to a pro-regulatory response (Treg/Th2) [214]. Recipient inflammatory cell profiles peri-transplant have also been linked to early rejection risk and include low levels of Tregs, poor suppressive Treg function, and high levels of effector cytokines [215–219]. The possibility to use such information to predict rejection risk pre-transplant would substantially advance efforts to tailor immunosuppression to individual risk.

Donor-Recipient Interface

Donor-Related Risks

Increased donor age is a recognized independent risk factor for rejection in recipients of all ages [220–223]. Older donor tissue may be more vulnerable to inflammatory stressors and less able to recover from acute injury [221].

Silent Sensitization

Sensitization refers to elaboration of alloimmune memory responsiveness that develops prior to transplantation and may lead to an accelerated amnestic response to donor HLA antigen after transplantation. Sensitization may result from transfusion of blood products, previous organ transplantation, or pregnancy. In some cases where preformed HLA antibodies are detected, the sensitizing event is obscure and presumed to be heterologous sensitization from infection or vaccination. Silent sensitization refers to an amnestic response that is not detected at the time of transplantation. Red blood cell transfusions increase allosensitization rates by approximately 30% [224], but if screening is not performed within weeks of the exposure, HLA antibody titres may fall to undetectable levels and yet immune memory may persist.

A high level of HLA antibody sensitization is not a significant risk in of itself for adverse outcome, unless the antibody is donor-specific [225, 226]. Although flow-cytometry methods for detecting HLA antibody will sensitively exclude DSA at transplant, historical DSA should also be considered in allocation decisions. Historical DSA is associated with higher rates of both accelerated TCMR and AMR [225, 227], related to activation of memory B or T cell responses that are residual to the initial sensitizing event. In cases of TCMR occurring within 24 hours of transplantation, pre-sensitization is presumed to be a factor but may be difficult to establish with certainty [228].

Clinical testing for donor-specific sensitization only screens for HLA antibody and does not detect cognate B or T cell memory. For example, there is a higher rate of accelerated TCMR with re-transplantation than in a first transplant [229]. Assays that detect B and T cell memory are not available yet in the clinic, but include the IFN-γ Enzyme-Linked Immunospot (ELISPOT) assay, which detects T cell memory by measuring the number or proportion of T cells that rapidly produce IFN-γ in response to donor cell contact [230]. Pre-transplant and early post-transplant ELISPOT reactivity predicts subclinical and clinical TCMR [231–236], and associated kidney function declines following transplantation [231, 234, 235, 237, 238]. Similarly, the B cell IgG ELISPOT could identify cognate memory B cells responsiveness, even after the associated antibody response has become undetectable [239]. B cell priming is associated with AMR development and is predictive of more severe rejection [111, 240]. The availability of additional screening for donor-specific cellular memory responses would provide important complimentary information to HLA antibody screening, to inform allocation decisions and better tailor treatment in the setting of elevated risk.

HLA Mismatch

The benefit of better HLA matching between donor and recipient for rejection risk and graft outcome has been appreciated for decades [241]. Considering the A, B, DR loci in children, the extent of mismatch is not only associated with allograft survival but also with lifetime survival with graft function due to the deleterious impact of mismatching on sensitization and access to re-transplantation [242, 243].

More recently, the focus has shifted to class II mismatch at the DQ and DR loci. Although more precise quantification of mismatch may be ascertained at the epitope level, matching for transplant allocation is still reliant on antigen-level typing. Mismatch at either DQ or DR locus is associated with increased risk for acute rejection [244, 245]. DQ or DR mismatch also accounts for the majority of *dn*DSA risk and antibody-mediated rejection [226, 246], whereas neither HLA-A nor HLA-B mismatch was found to be a significant predictor of *dn*DSA or graft loss [226, 247]. HLA-DQ mismatch is more likely to translate into HLA-DQ *dn*DSA than non-DQ *dn*DSA [248, 249], and is independently associated with increased risk of acute and late rejection and a higher risk of graft loss [249–251].

Pediatric prioritization for allocation is recommended by existing guidelines [113] and may permit selectivity to await minimum levels of matching for pediatric recipients. Several jurisdictions are exploring whether class II matching may be incorporated into standard allocation processes [246, 252, 253], with the promise of mitigating rejection risk and improving allograft survival.

Post-transplant Factors

Delayed graft function (DGF) is defined by the requirement for dialysis within 1 week of transplant. In children, DGF incidence is 4% following living donor, and 5–8% following deceased donor transplantation [254, 255]. DGF is associated with future rejection [256–259] and long-term graft survival. [260] The underlying mechanism of delayed graft function is ischemia reperfusion injury (IRI), leading to innate immune activation and homing of dendritic cells to the allograft, which can precipitate rejection through their role as APCs, activating adaptive immunity [255]. Modifiable risk factors that increase DGF include a long dialysis vintage, longer cold ischemia time, and grafts from older donors [255, 259, 261].

Inadequate immunosuppression for whatever reason increases risk for acute rejection, recognizing that such decisions are a trade-off to deal with adverse symptoms from immunosuppressant toxicity or infectious complications. Increased risk has been demonstrated from insufficient tacrolimus exposure in early [262] or later time periods after transplant [263], and similarly with inadequate early drug exposure to mycophenolate [264] or late drug exposure with dose reductions [265].

Opportunistic viral infections with donor-derived viral pathogens such as cytomegalovirus virus (CMV), Epstein-Barr virus (EBV), and BK virus (BKV) are associated with increased rates of subsequent rejection [256, 266, 267]. This may be due in part to reduction of immunosuppression [268–270], but also to stimulation of the innate immune system, upregulation of pro-inflammatory cytokines, and HLA class II expression, which creates a microenvironment that promotes activation of cognate T cell responses [271, 272]. Cross-reactive memory T cells with specificity to both graft and virus have also been discovered for EBV, CMV, and BKV suggesting a sensitizing role for these viruses through heterologous immunity [273–276].

Non-adherence to treatment is more commonly observed in adolescents compared to in younger children and adults [277–279]. This reality must be placed in the context of need for continued and effective parental supervision into late adolescence, which may be challenged due to adverse home environments [280, 281], parental burnout or competing priorities, and stressors for the adolescent [282, 283]. Non-adherence is an important risk factor associated with late acute and chronic rejection [284–289] and *dn*DSA [226] and is directly implicated in more than a third of pediatric renal allograft losses [18, 277, 278, 290]. The most important aspects of forgetfulness and scheduling [291, 292] can be partially mitigated against by reducing medication complexity [293–295] and employing memory and structured supports such as a pillbox [292] and coaching [296]. But there is no substitute for a redundant system that includes parental or surrogate verification of each intended dose.

Hyperacute Rejection

Hyperacute rejection is the most rapid and severe manifestation of alloimmune response to the kidney transplant. High levels of preformed alloantibody immediately bind vascular endothelium and smooth muscle, triggering diffuse complement-mediated injury. There is subsequent intense neutrophilic infiltration of peritubular and glomerular capillaries, and micro-thrombosis, leading to cortical necrosis [297, 298]. Typically, this becomes immediately evident while the patient is still on the operating table, as the donor graft becoming visibly mottled and dusky with necrosis [297]. The surgeon is left with no option except to remove it.

With improvements in HLA antibody screening and crossmatch, hyperacute rejection is an increasingly rare phenomenon. According to the North American Pediatric Renal Trials and Collaborative Studies (NAPRTCS) 2014 report, of 1018 graft failures since 2000, two were attributed to hyperacute rejection (0.2%) [15]. A

20-year pediatric renal transplant follow-up study in India reported a similarly low rate (0.8%) [299]. In an era where antigen-specific antibody testing is pervasive, the need for donor crossmatch testing has been debated, but is likely to persist in an effort to exclude hyperacute rejection risk in the setting of desensitization protocols or in the setting where a rare donor HLA antigen has not been included on the recipient antibody testing panel.

Acute T Cell-Mediated Rejection (TCMR)

Clinical and Histological Features

Acute T cell-mediated rejection (TCMR) is the most common form of rejection in the early post-transplant period. The clinical suspicion of TCMR is most commonly piqued by a rise in serum creatinine. In an era of modern immunosuppression, more classic features of kidney tenderness, swelling, and fever are rarely seen. In the case of late rejection, where onset may be more indolent, subtle clinical findings associated with progressive tubulointerstitial injury may also raise suspicion, including worsening of anemia, onset of hyperkalemia, or acidosis. None of these clinical signs are specific for rejection.

The diagnosis of TCMR is confirmed histologically. The Banff classification has evolved since the initial working group meeting in 1997 to provide criteria for diagnosis of different subtypes of allograft injury and grading of severity [300]. Each pathological feature is scored from 0 to 3, with 0 indicating minimal or no histologic change and progressively higher scores denoting a greater intensity. These features are then used to classify types of rejection and grade their severity. A detailed review of each criterion is beyond the scope of this chapter. Instead, the principal features will be highlighted in the context of relevant clinical features for each type of rejection. The reader is referred to the 2018 reference guide and the most recent Banff reports, which are regularly updated and provide details of the current classification scheme [301, 302].

The primary pathological features of TCMR are interstitial inflammation outside the fibrotic areas (i-score) and infiltration of mononuclear cells beneath the tubule basement membrane (the basolateral aspect of tubular epithelium), referred to as tubulitis (*t*-score) – Fig. 3.3a. The extent of interstitial inflammation and the intensity of tubulitis within areas of unscarred cortex are used to assign progressively higher Banff *i*- and *t*-scores, which indicate respectively higher grades of severity. A Banff score of *i1t1* or more is generally sufficient to identify suspicion for TCMR diagnosis and is used to dictate need for treatment [303]. A higher grade of TCMR severity is also dictated by the presence of inflammation in the arterial compartment referred to as intimal arteritis (*v*-score), which is characterized by the finding of at least one inflammatory cell undermining the endothelium within arteries that have at least two layers of smooth muscles (*v1*). The intensity of arteritis is denoted by

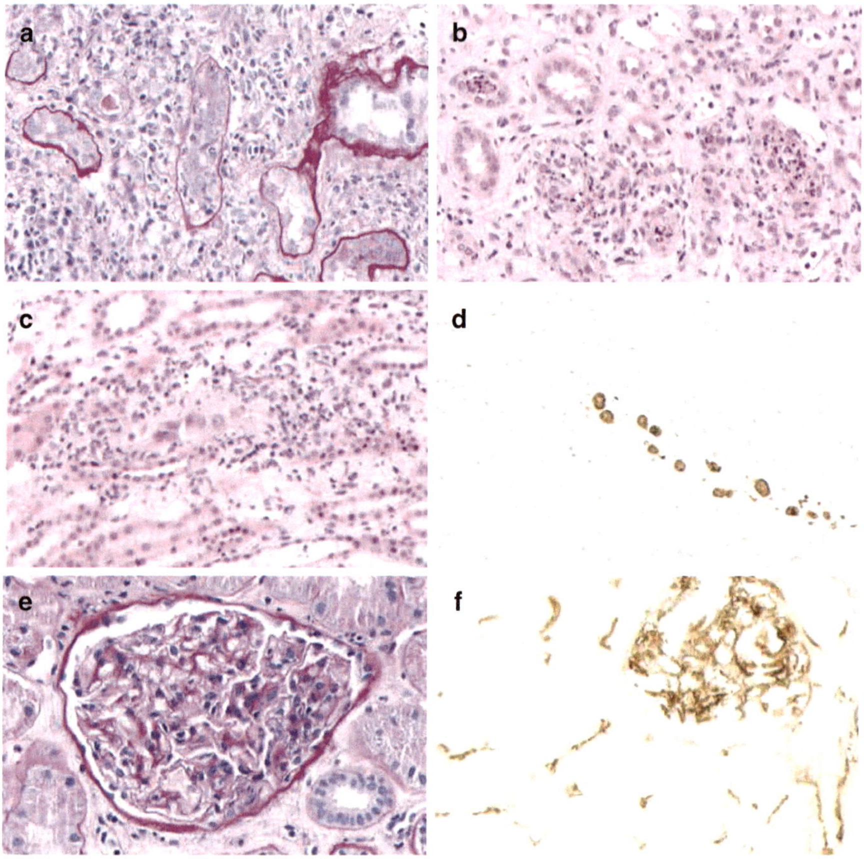

Fig. 3.3 Histologic features of common etiologies with acute inflammation in renal allograft. (**a**) PAS-staining of renal cortex showing acute T cell-mediated rejection. There is moderate to severe lymphocytic tubulitis with severe interstitial inflammation. The inflammation comprises predominantly lymphocytes. (**b**) H&E-stained section of an allograft with pyelonephritis. There is tubulointerstitial inflammation with prominent neutrophilic tubulitis and neutrophilic casts. (C&D) Renal allograft with polyomavirus nephropathy: (**c**) Mild tubulointerstitial inflammation with viral cytopathic changes of enlarged nuclei and vesicular chromatin pattern. (**d**) Immunoperoxidase staining for SV40 T large T antigen (a surrogate marker for BK polyomavirus) is positive in atypical nuclei. (**e** and **f**) Acute antibody-mediated rejection: (**e**) Glomerulitis with segmental near-occlusion of capillary lumen due to endothelial cell swelling and inflammatory influx. (**f**) Indirect evidence of DSA interaction with endothelial cell surface is demonstrated by immunoperoxidase staining for c4d. Frozen sections from the same biopsy as in (**f**) showing diffuse staining of the glomerular capillary walls as well as peritubular capillary basement membranes

higher *v*-scores based on the relative loss of luminal area, the finding of transmural arteritis, or destructive changes (fibrinoid necrosis) extending to arterial smooth muscle layers.

A "borderline" grade for TCMR is assigned in the absence of intimal arteritis, when both inflammation and tubulitis are present but not meeting a minimum Banff score of *i2t2*. This grade is referred to by Banff as "suspicious for acute TCMR." The term "borderline" dates back to the original Banff 1997 criteria, and the ambiguity reflected in the terminology is indicative of the relative lack of data on treatment efficacy and outcome at the time. It is now clear that borderline TCMR is associated with contemporaneous allograft dysfunction and increased risk of subsequent higher grade rejection, progressive tubular atrophy and interstitial fibrosis, de novo donor-specific antibodies, and graft loss [134, 304–306]. Treatment of subclinical TCMR, the majority of which are also borderline grade, reduces inflammation, the risk for persistent rejection, and improves outcome [128, 129, 136, 137]. Given the clinical implications, a "borderline" grade may be better regarded as equivalent to "mild" TCMR. It is on a spectrum of TCMR severity that may warrant a different treatment approach but which, nonetheless, should be regarded as unambiguously pathological.

Isolated tubulitis is a term used to describe the finding of tubulitis in the absence of significant interstitial inflammation ($t > 0$,i0). While the identification of tubulitis seems to indicate that a cognate alloimmune response has been engaged, the absence of associated inflammation suggests that the interaction may not be pathogenic. This is supported by recent reports that isolated tubulitis is not associated with adverse outcomes and that treatment does not positively impact graft function or survival [307, 308]. The existing evidence does not support initiating treatment for isolated tubulitis.

Treatment of TCMR

Corticosteroids

Corticosteroid medications are among the earliest effective treatments for acute rejection. The full breadth of corticosteroid actions is not known but include down-regulation of lymphocyte adhesion, and genomic and non-genomic alteration of cytokines and inflammatory mediators [309]. In autoimmune disorders such as systemic lupus erythematosus, corticosteroids have also been shown to induce Treg expansion [310]. Despite the utility for treating active inflammation, their use is limited by many off-target effects and the serious adverse effects associated with long-term use.

A typical treatment protocol for TCMR would include intravenous (IV) methylprednisolone at a dosage of 10 mg/kg each on three consecutive days, often with an increase in the level of baseline immunosuppression [26]. However, high-quality clinical trials on optimal dose or treatment duration are relatively lacking. Limitations of existing trials include lack of histological confirmation of primary efficacy and absence of long-term outcome data. Early studies that evaluated corticosteroid dosage were completed in the 1970s, in an era with different induction and maintenance immunosuppression, and tested non-inferiority for functional outcomes [311–316]. It is therefore difficult to extrapolate to the modern era. These trials affirmed, however, that risk for corticosteroid toxicity is proportional to the dose, and that gastrointestinal bleeding is reduced by delivering treatment intravenously [317–319].

There is also not a clear consensus on whether or how to provide a taper with oral prednisone following IV methylprednisolone treatment, and little evidence to favor one protocol over another.

Today, IV corticosteroids remain the recommended first-line treatment for acute TCMR, given their efficacy in reversing allograft dysfunction in 60–85% of cases [25, 311, 320]. These results are less promising when kidney biopsy is used to follow-up histology, with identified rates of steroid refractory rejection that range from 13% to over 50% [25, 28, 139].

The effectiveness of corticosteroids as primary treatment is diminished with higher TCMR grade. An adult systematic review reported the rates of refractory rejection measured by clinical resolution: 4% in borderline, 0–25% in Banff grade 1B, 11–20% in Banff 2A, and 38% in Banff 2B [321]. A similar report identified 31% with Banff Grade 1 TCMR who failed to respond, whereas the failure rate was 100% with grade 3 [322]. Histological resolution is also higher in treated borderline cases (56%) compared to Banff grade 1 and above (<30%); and treated borderline rejection was associated with lower rates of subsequent rejection episodes (7%) compared to Banff grade 2 (29%) [29]. Greater TCMR severity also correlated with worse death censored graft survival at 8 years, 71–79% for Banff grade 2 compared to 93% for borderline rejection [321].

Different transplant programs may tailor corticosteroid dosage or use of additional medications based on the histological or clinical severity of rejection, but without strong evidence in support of any one particular protocol. Ideally, future trials will evaluate treatment response stratified for the initial severity of rejection, and target objective measures of primary treatment efficacy and long-term outcomes such as chronic forms of rejection and allograft survival.

Lymphocyte-Depleting Therapies

Lymphocyte-depleting therapies include monoclonal antibodies to discreet T cell antigens or polyclonal antibodies that are elaborated against multiple T cell surface antigen targets. Lymphocyte-depleting therapy is generally reserved for more severe cases or those with corticosteroid refractory rejection. One pediatric study reported a preference for primary treatment with anti-thymocyte globulin (ATG) in those with TCMR with intimal arteritis at diagnosis [323]. After primary treatment with corticosteroids, subsequent deterioration of renal function or worsening renal histology was associated with initiation of anti-lymphocyte treatment rates in 40% and 86% of cases, respectively [324].

The most commonly used polyclonal antibody product is rabbit ATG (thymoglobulin; rATG). Compared to a similar equine polyclonal antibody (ATGAM), rATG has demonstrated superior efficacy in achieving functional and histological recovery and reducing TCMR recurrence, particularly at higher Banff grades [325, 326]. rATG is superior to corticosteroids alone [325, 327–330] for clinical resolution, but is associated with more profound and persisting immunosuppression with increased risk of infectious complications and malignancy. For this reason, IV corticosteroids remain the first-line therapy of choice [331], and rATG is reserved for more severe or refractory cases [332, 333]. The recommended dose for rATG in acute rejection is 1.5 mg/kg for between 5 and 7 doses [334].

The monoclonal antibody muromonab CD3 (Orthoclone OKT3) was previously used to treat rejection, but has been discontinued in the USA due to inferior rejection treatment outcomes [325, 335, 336] and high risk of cytokine release syndrome compared to ATG [337, 338].

Alemtuzumab is a monoclonal anti-CD52 antibody, capable of profound long-term T cell depletion [339]. It has been used for steroid-resistant rejection and severe rejection, stabilizing allograft function in 62.5% of cases [340]. Compared with rATG, alemtuzumab may have a superior adverse effect profile for treatment of steroid resistant rejection in adults, with greater infection-free survival and fewer infusion-related adverse effects [341, 342]. In a small adult case series, alemtuzumab stabilized renal function in 4/5 patients with rATG-refractory rejection [343]. Alemtuzumab also has the potential advantage over rATG of single dose therapy [340, 344]. Similar to rATG, infection-related morbidity may be increased in comparison to treatment with IV methylprednisolone alone [345]. Notwithstanding positive reports, the quality of data on use of alemtuzumab for rejection is limited, and whether it should be preferred over treatment with rATG has not been established.

Late Acute TCMR

Late acute T cell-mediated rejection (LAR) typically presents with declining allograft function, since surveillance biopsies are rare after the first year post-transplant. Earlier detection and treatment of TCMR is known to result in better allograft outcomes [20–25]. LAR may represent a more entrenched immune response that has either failed to completely respond to previous early rejection treatment or has evolved indolently, evading prior detection and treatment. LAR is therefore especially damaging to the allograft, associated more frequently with chronic injury [20, 346], decline in kidney function [20], and inferior graft outcomes [21–24, 127, 347–349]. Compared to children with early TCMR, LAR was associated with double the adjusted hazard of graft failure [350].

TCMR that occurs after the first year may show evidence of B cell reinforcement, in the form of B cell or plasma cell infiltrates, or the presence of *dn*DSA. Compared to early rejection, LAR episodes are more likely to display mixed TCMR/AMR phenotypes and are more commonly associated with concurrent *dn*DSA [351–354]. The true prevalence of mixed rejection is unknown, with rates reported as low as 6% and as high as 96% [18, 353–355], which may represent heterogeneity in methods, cohort, and biopsy sampling/interpretation. Although prior TCMR is a risk factor for *dn*DSA, onset of *dn*DSA may also be detected concurrently [356, 357]. The combination of TCMR and *dn*DSA even without evidence of AMR is associated with a threefold increase in graft failure compared to either DSA or TCMR alone [357]. It is not clear whether anti-lymphocyte therapy with rATG may be effective in such cases, since it is ineffective in depleting B cells or treating antibody-mediated injury. In the setting of mixed rejection, strategies that target both the B cell and T cell-mediated responses may be required.

B Cell-Rich and Plasma Cell-Rich Acute Rejection

B cell- and plasma cell-rich acute rejection (PCAR) have similar morphology to TCMR with the additional finding of B cell and/or mature plasma cell clusters within the allograft. Such infiltrates are evidence of an increasingly robust mixed B and T cell response, even in the absence of DSA or signs of AMR. B cell-rich rejection and PCAR occur later than TCMR commonly occurs [358], are treatment refractory [359, 360], and are associated with a poor prognosis [358–360]. B cell-rich rejection is associated with a 4.5-fold increase in graft loss risk at 2 years post biopsy [361], and as many as half of those with PCAR lose their grafts within 6 months of diagnosis [362]. A study in children showed that those with plasma cell infiltrates had a 71% chance of allograft loss within 2 years compared to 7% for those without [363].

B Cell-Rich Rejection

On light microscopy, B cell-rich rejection is indistinguishable from TCMR without additional immunohistochemical staining for CD20. Finding some scattered intra-graft B cells is common, present in 22–53% of biopsy-proven TCMR [364]. Identification of B cell clusters, however, has been found to strongly associate with steroid resistance, but may be missed at the outset since immunohistochemical staining for CD20 is not routinely performed [360]. Addition of immunohistochemical staining for B cells in cases of steroid-refractory TCMR (Fig. 3.4) may be an important adjuvant to more completely characterize the pathology and likelihood of treatment response.

Rituximab is a CD20 monoclonal antibody that has been evaluated for treatment of B cell-rich rejection [365–367], and treatment leads to depletion of CD20 cells [368]. Zarkhin et al. carried out a randomized trial in 20 children, examining the

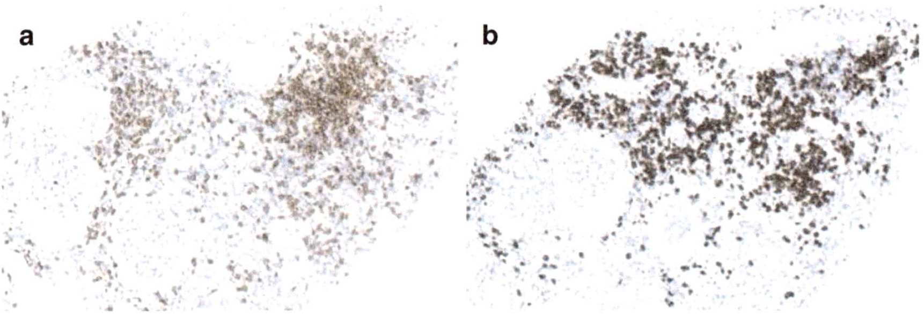

Fig. 3.4 By light microscopy, B cell-rich rejection is indistinguishable from T cell-mediated rejection. However, immunohistochemical staining in this case shows CD3+ staining T cells (**a**) as well as numerous CD20+ staining B cells (**b**)

impact of rituximab compared to pulse IV corticosteroids and/or ATG in acute rejection with B cell infiltrates [369]. Rituximab treatment was associated with improved histology at 6 months follow-up biopsy and superior functional outcome after 12 months. Subsequent B cell repopulation in the rituximab group was predominantly naïve B cells, whereas those treated with IV corticosteroids maintained a high memory-naïve B cell ratio [370]. Further trials are required, but limited evidence would suggest that rituximab may be useful in B cell-rich rejection and has been used safely in a pediatric cohort.

Plasma Cell-Rich Acute Rejection

Plasma cells are long-lived terminally differentiated B cells, which are morphologically distinct and easier to identify on light microscopy. PCAR is diagnosed when plasma cells comprise more than 10% of infiltrating cells in the graft [371] and is detected in 3–5% of biopsies performed for allograft dysfunction [371, 372]. The infiltration of T cells and otherwise classic features of TCMR defines it as a subtype of cellular rejection.

PCAR occurs on average 3 years after transplantation and is associated with DSA in roughly two-thirds of cases [371, 372]. The presence of DSA in PCAR is an important prognostic feature since cases without DSA had substantially better graft survival (82%) than those with DSA (42%) [371]. Yet, in PCAR, the presence of DSA does not necessarily correlate with classical features of AMR. Despite the plasma cell's primary function of antibody production, plasma cell infiltration represents a separate disease entity that can exist independently of both AMR and DSA.

PCAR is associated with a worse prognosis compared to B cell-rich rejection [373]. Plasma cells do not express significant levels of CD20, and so rituximab is not effective for depletion. Adding intravenous immunoglobulin (IVIG) to treatment with IV methylprednisolone has some appeal based on the potential to disrupt B cell maturation to plasma cells, but scant reports on its use are inconclusive [372, 374, 375]. Targeting depletion of plasma cells with proteasome inhibitor medications such as bortezomib may have theoretical rationale, but evidence as to its utility in the setting of PCAR is limited. Alhamoud et al. compared graft outcomes in children with PCAR (treated with IV methylprednisolone 30 mg/kg/dose x5, IVIG, rituximab, and bortezomib) to those with TCMR (treated with IV methylprednisolone) [372]. Graft loss in the PCAR group was 43% at 3 months compared to no graft losses in the TCMR group. However, in those with PCAR who were treatment responsive, eGFR doubled following treatment and matched TCMR controls during subsequent follow-up. However, this study does not parse out the efficacy of bortezomib compared to other therapies, and the use of quadruple immunosuppression was associated with adverse events including infection. Overall, PCAR is a relatively newly recognized rejection type with a poor prognosis. Further study into viable and effective treatment options is needed.

Active Antibody-Mediated Rejection (AMR)

Clinical and Histological Features

Active (or acute) antibody-mediated rejection (AMR) follows the development of donor-specific antibodies, which initiate glomerular injury directly via complement-mediated injury or indirectly via microvascular inflammation. Microvascular inflammation is histologically characterized by endothelial cell swelling and leukocyte congestion of glomerular capillary loops (glomerulitis, *g* score by Banff classification [Fig. 3.3e]) and peritubular capillaries (peritubular capillaritis, *ptc* score by Banff classification). Persistent AMR leads to chronic allograft injury, manifest as transplant glomerulopathy (glomerular basement membrane double-contours, cg by Banff classification [Fig. 3.5d, e]), arterial intimal fibrosis, progressive interstitial fibrosis, and tubular atrophy [226, 376, 377], and is a leading cause of kidney allograft failure [19, 378].

The clinical presentation of AMR depends on the nature of DSA formation. Patients with pre-formed DSA due to prior sensitization may have persistent or rebound of DSA at the time of transplantation. Without prior sensitization, AMR is associated with the development of *dn*DSA. The majority of *dn*DSA form against class II HLA antigens [379]. Class II HLA mismatch therefore serves as a significant risk factor in *dn*DSA development [246, 380]. Additional risk factors for *dn*DSA formation and AMR include non-adherence and prior TCMR [226, 244, 381]. Haas et al. (2017) reported that previous TCMR including borderline changes preceded *dn*DSA driven AMR in 72% of cases [381].

In the setting of desensitization protocols to overcome DSA incompatibility, approximately 30–50% of patients will experience early AMR [382]. This risk is less well-defined when low-level DSA are present and a transplant can proceed without desensitization and with a negative flow crossmatch. Risk for early AMR or TCMR appears to be greater when the DSA is specific for HLA class II [383], in particular when the DSA MFI exceeds 5000 [383–385]. With treatment, however, intermediate term allograft survival in adult recipients appears to be similar [383, 384], but there are no equivalent reports in children. In patients with high levels of HLA sensitization, willingness to cross low-level DSA may be an appealing option to permit more timely access to transplantation, but will require additional vigilance to identify and treat early AMR.

Rates of AMR in children from *dn*DSA are poorly defined and have been estimated as 5–8% [386, 387], but such prevalence estimates will vary dependent on duration of follow-up. Risk of DSA accrues with time at an average rate of approximately 2% per year and is significantly higher in the setting of non-adherence [122]. Subclinical AMR is detected at 1 year on surveillance biopsy in approximately 4% of adult cases with no DSA at transplant, but as high as 48% of cases when DSA is present [135].

In the absence of DSA at transplant, AMR is suspected clinically when there is onset of allograft dysfunction or *dn*DSA identified on surveillance. Proteinuria may also indicate need for investigation but is not usually present at the onset until there

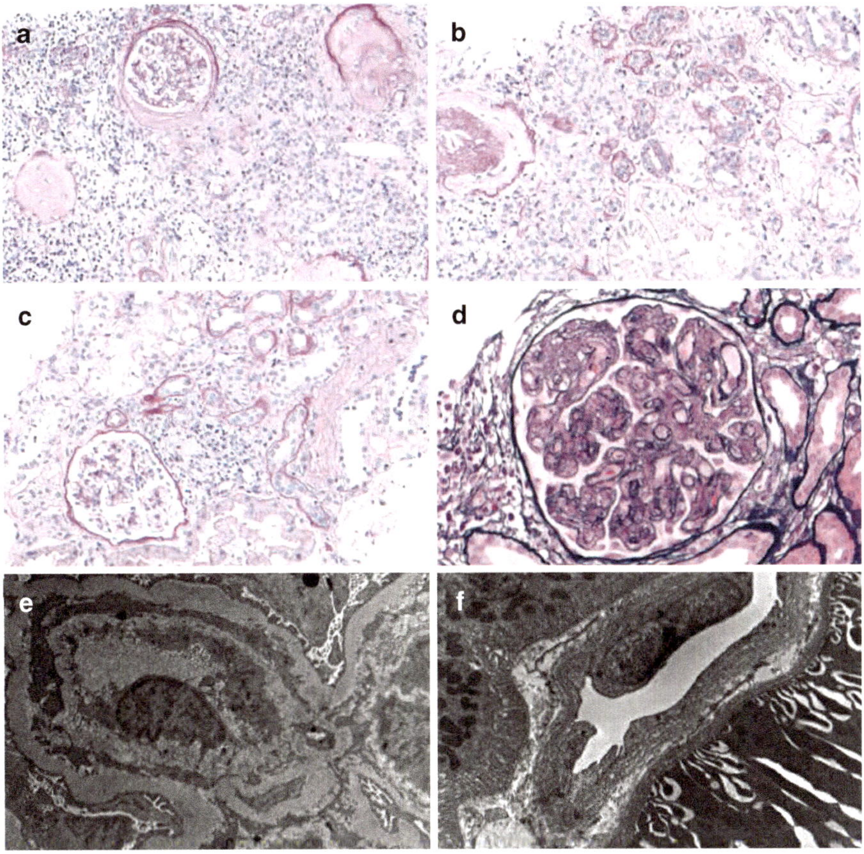

Fig. 3.5 Chronic active rejection. Representative panels (**a**–**c**) are from a biopsy with chronic active T cell-mediated rejection (caTCMR). (**a**) PAS-stained section of cortex with two globally sclerotic glomeruli and an ischemic glomerulus embedded in a portion of cortex with severe chronic tubulointerstitial injury and dense inflammation (i-IFTA). Many tubules show endocrine-type atrophy (lower right) while few partially atrophic tubules are showing moderate to severe tubulitis (top left). (**b**) From the same specimen as in (**a**), this section demonstrates non-atrophic tubules (lower right) adjacent to partially atrophic tubules with corrugated basement membranes, one of which also shows tubulitis (top). The glomerulus to the left is globally sclerotic and is surrounded by background inflammation and endocrine-type atrophic tubules. (**c**) A relatively intact glomerulus and adjacent non-atrophic tubulointerstitium can be seen next to few partially atrophic tubules with thickened and corrugated basement membranes. There is a minute focus of interstitial inflammation and mild tubulitis in a partially atrophic tubules. Panels (**d**–**f**) capture salient features of chronic active antibody-mediated rejection. (**d**) Jones (silver)-staining of this glomerulus highlights capillary loops with global (i.e., more than 50% of capillary loops) double-contours diagnostic of severe transplant glomerulopathy (TG, cg3 by Banff criteria). (**e**) Electron micrograph of a capillary loop double-contour with replication of basement membrane, interpositioning of cellular elements, and swelling of the endothelium with loss of fenestrae. Identification of this change in at least three capillary loops by electron microscopy (in the absence of TG by light microscopy) is sufficient for designation of cg1a by Banff criteria. (**f**) Electron micrograph with severe multilayering of the peritubular capillary basement membranes in chronic active AMR

has already been progression to transplant glomerulopathy. Banff criteria are used for AMR diagnosis [301], which is suspected morphologically by the presence of microvascular inflammation involving the glomerulus (*g*-score) and peritubular capillaries (*ptc*-score). The diagnosis is confirmed by the presence of C4d staining (Fig. 3.3f), or in the presence of DSA, a finding of at least moderate microvascular inflammation or increased expression of gene transcripts in biopsy tissue using classifiers validated for association with AMR. In the absence of microvascular inflammation, intimal arteritis ($v > 0$) or thrombotic microangiopathy or acute tubule injury may also lead to a diagnosis of AMR, provided there is also evidence of DSA and antibody interaction with vascular endothelium and other causes of intimal arteritis, thrombotic microangiopathy, and/or acute tubular injury are excluded.

AMR presenting in the first year after transplant is more likely to be "pure," without associated TCMR [378, 381]. This is more typical of AMR that is associated with preexisting DSA [381], whereas *dn*DSA onset is rare before 6 months post-transplant [354]. Chronic changes such as transplant glomerulopathy are typically absent [377, 388], and the associated DSA may be either class I, class II, or both [378, 388].

AMR presenting after the first year is more likely to present with a mixed picture, with the majority including at least "borderline" TCMR and with predominantly class II DSA [226, 354, 378, 381]. These cases are more likely to also have chronic features including transplant glomerulopathy (Fig. 3.5d, e), IFTA, and multilayering of peritubular capillary basement membrane (Fig. 3.5f) at the time of diagnosis [381].

Treatment of AMR

Data on AMR treatment, on the whole, stems from relatively low-quality evidence, and no medications are FDA approved specifically for use in AMR [389]. There are few RCTs, scarce pediatric data, and no agreed upon standard of care [390]. To further confound interpretation, studies are heterogeneous in regard to early and late AMR, with varying levels of associated TCMR and chronicity at the time of treatment. Treatment strategies are targeted at removing the DSA, removing antibody-producing plasma cells and B cells, and interfering with complement activation in the setting of C4d positive rejection. A combination of plasmapheresis (PP) and intravenous immunoglobulin G (IVIG) has emerged as a standard approach, with or without concomitant treatment with rituximab [391]. A typical treatment regimen may include 1.5x plasma volume removal with PP on a daily or alternate-day basis for 6–8 treatments, with each treatment followed by IVIG at 100–200 mg/kg, and rituximab at 325 mg/m^2 for 1–2 doses. Additional PP/IVIG sessions may be provided depending on the treatment response, based on reduction of the DSA MFI.

Plasmapheresis and IVIG

Whereas plasmapheresis and immunoadsorption are methods of antibody removal, IVIG depletes immature B cells in addition to reducing antibody levels, potentially explaining the complementary effect of using PP and IVIG together [392]. A systematic review pooled the effects of five randomized trials in adults evaluating antibody removal alone and found that when limited to those trials with longer follow-up, antibody removal reduced graft failure rates at 3 years post-diagnosis by half (HR 0.46) [391]. However, treatment with PP alone had inferior graft outcome at 1 year compared to combined treatment with PP and IVIG (46% vs. 90% survival) [393]. Small case series and retrospective reviews also support the use of IVIG and PP to clinically reverse AMR in the majority of patients [394–398].

Rituximab

Rituximab is a humanized monoclonal antibody against CD20. The utility of rituximab in AMR is controversial with disagreement between the two most recent systematic reviews. Macklin et al. reported that four of seven studies demonstrated an improvement in graft survival associated with rituximab use and postulated that rituximab may play a role in the treatment of acute AMR [399]. In contrast Wan et al. reported no additional benefits of rituximab beyond plasmapheresis and IVIG, or in addition to thymoglobulin for mixed TCMR/AMR [391]. The RITUX-ERA multicenter, double blinded, placebo-controlled RCT reported no difference in 1 year graft outcome based on treatment with rituximab [400]. Both groups received corticosteroids, plasma exchange, and IVIG. Long-term outcomes of this trial were recently published: graft survival and kidney function at 7 years were also similar between the intervention and placebo arm [401]. Ahmadi et al. compared IVIG and PP to IVIG, PP, and either high or low dose rituximab. Although not statistically significant, rituximab groups had graft survival over 60% in comparison to 37.5% in the non-rituximab group [402]. Timing may influence rituximab's efficacy, since non-responders were more likely to have proteinuria and a higher grade of inflammation than responders, suggesting rituximab use in the early stages of AMR may be associated with the greater success [403].

Specific to pediatric data, a prospective trial compared rituximab against IV methylprednisolone and/or thymoglobulin rather than IVIG and plasmapheresis. Rituximab improved graft histology and function up to 6 months in cases of acute rejection (including mixed TCMR/AMR) with B cell infiltrates [369]. In a small case series, rituximab was prescribed to three patients with AMR refractory to IV methylprednisolone, IVIG, and plasmapheresis, but disappointingly, two of three continued to have refractory AMR and lost their grafts [387]. In the decision to prescribe rituximab, potential benefit should be weighed against infection risk, which is particularly important when rituximab is combined with other therapies such as bortezomib or lymphocyte depleting agents [404–407].

Bortezomib

Bortezomib induces plasma cell apoptosis, disrupting antibody production. Evidence for its utility in treating AMR is weak. When treatment has been targeted at reducing DSA burden, small case series report limited success [408, 409]. However, in another report it had no benefit in addition to plasmapheresis on *dn*DSA [410].

Small case series using bortezomib in adults that suggest benefit for stabilizing renal function have lacked suitable randomized controls [411–415]. In two small case series, plasma cell-rich AMR was treated with IV methylprednisolone, plasmapheresis, ATG, and rituximab [416, 417]. In the first series, early incorporation of bortezomib was more successful than rescue therapy after initial treatment to achieve plasma cell depletion and stabilizing graft function [417]. In the other series, simultaneous bortezomib administration was successful in stabilizing graft function over the following 2 years [416]. Similarly, small series using bortezomib in children as rescue therapy for refractory AMR have reported improved histology and stabilization of graft function [409, 418, 419]. It may also be that bortezomib is more appropriate in early AMR that is associated with rebound DSA, which may be associated with plasma cell activation and therefore greater susceptibility to bortezomib [410, 420–422].

The BOREJECT trial reports the only randomized evaluation of bortezomib for treatment of late AMR ($n = 44$) compared with placebo, without additional AMR-directed therapies [423]. There was no significant difference from placebo for functional decline or eGFR at 24 months follow-up.

Emerging Treatments

Complement fixation and activation are important mediators of DSA-mediated injury in AMR. Innovative approaches to treatment resistant or severe AMR have targeted inhibition of C1 and C5 complement proteins. Eculizumab is a C5 monoclonal antibody, interrupting complement mediated damage via disruption of the membrane attack complex formation. It has shown promise in treating early AMR and reducing subsequent transplant glomerulopathy but may be most effective in those with prior sensitization and early DSA rebound [424–426]. In one case series, splenectomy was required in combination for greatest short-term efficacy, but was associated with high rates of infection [427]. In a similar approach, two small studies using C1 esterase inhibitors have suggested attenuation of AMR at 6 months [428, 429], but studies that evaluate longer-term efficacy are lacking.

Inhibition of IL-6 activity is emerging as another potential target for treatment. Tocilizumab blocks the IL-6 receptor and has been used more extensively for treatment of chronic AMR, but has been evaluated in one case series with AMR ($n = 7$) and they observed >50% reduction in DSA levels and stabilization of kidney function [430]. As with the inhibitors of complement pathways, more evidence from randomized trials is needed before these treatment approaches can be recommended.

Response to Treatment

Both clinical and subclinical AMR are associated with risk for progression to transplant glomerulopathy and 3.5-fold increased risk of graft loss [135]. Previous transplant and more than one DSA are risk factors for treatment resistant pre-formed DSA [431]. C4d negative AMR is now well recognized as a pathological variant and accounts for 20–60% of all adult AMR cases [432]. There has been some evidence to suggest that C4d positive AMR is a negative prognostic indicator [433], but this has been disputed in several other reports [378, 381, 432, 434, 435]. However, the presence of concurrent TCMR in C4d positive AMR is associated with reduced allograft survival [381, 436]. Patients with IFTA already present at the time of AMR diagnosis also have a worse graft outcome, which is paralleled by a less favorable response to treatment in late compared with early AMR [381, 410, 436–440].

Improvement in DSA MFI with treatment indicates superior treatment efficacy and is an independent predictor of graft survival [381]. Indeed, successful *dn*DSA clearance is associated with 100% graft survival at 2 years [227, 379, 381]. Risk factors for treatment-resistant DSA include class II antibodies, late AMR onset, and higher antibody levels [227, 379, 420, 431, 441]. Late presenting *dn*DSA, which are more likely to be class II antibodies, are particularly problematic for future allograft survival [227, 379, 442]. In a cohort of pediatric renal transplant recipients, older age also predicted *dn*DSA persistence [379].

Active surveillance for DSA may improve outcome. Early AMR detection was associated with better DSA response to bortezomib than late AMR. Those patients who experience a > 50% fall in DSA within 2 weeks of treatment had improved allograft survival over those whose DSA did not substantially reduce [438]. Persistent DSA predisposed to further AMR episodes and more rapid kidney function decline [227, 379, 381, 439]. Once persistent DSA are established, management becomes particularly challenging as the intensive treatments required to clear them place patients at significant risk for complications from over-immunosuppression [443].

Chronic Active TCMR

Chronic active TCMR (caTCMR) is diagnosed histologically [Fig. 3.5a–c] and is defined by chronic inflammatory changes in areas of IFTA, involving the interstitium (*i*-IFTA) and tubules (*t*-IFTA). IFTA represents scaring, as a consequence of earlier injury, whereas *i*-IFTA represents active inflammation in areas of already injured renal cortex. The presence of *i*-IFTA is generally associated with larger areas of damaged cortex compared to cases with IFTA with no additional inflammation. Finding caTCMR is associated with a worse allograft outcome. Three-year survival in transplant recipients with *i*-IFTA falls to 62% versus 82% for those without, with similar findings for individuals with *t*-IFTA [141, 433].

Clinical and Histological Features

The term "creatinine creep" has been used to indicate risk for chronic rejection beyond the first post-transplant year. When in doubt, the decision is usually made to biopsy in order to identify treatable pathology in the allograft. In a phenomenon that is unique to pediatric transplantation, the cause for this gradual rise in serum creatinine must be distinguished from the expected creatinine rise that occurs with growth and accrual of muscle mass over time. We accommodate for this clinically by reporting renal function as a function of body surface area (BSA) with glomerular filtration rate adjusted for BSA (GFR; ml/min/1.73 m^2), which can be measured or estimated using standardized equations (eGFR) [444]. However, there is also a relative, non-pathological gradual decline in eGFR that becomes apparent with growth and increasing BSA. Since the transplanted kidney is usually from an adult donor, it is mature and already hypertrophied to meet adult-sized GFR needs, and thus has a very limited capacity for additional adaptive hyperfiltration as the small child recipient grows to adulthood. The result is that the underlying unadjusted GFR (ml/min) may remain stable as the eGFR (size-adjusted to BSA) appears to be in gradual decline – especially during the adolescent growth spurt. With this in mind, evaluating for stability or decline of the unadjusted GFR over time may provide additional context in the decision whether or not to biopsy.

Chronic active TCMR may also be found in the context of acute TCMR, where a more sudden rise in serum creatinine acts as an indication to biopsy, uncovering both pathological processes. Attention to the deleterious impact of inflammation in areas of IFTA is a more recent phenomenon [445]. Whereas pathological evaluation of acute rejection changes is restricted to the unscarred cortex, caTCMR is characterized by the amount of total inflammation (*ti* score), and within areas of IFTA, the amount of inflammation (*i*-IFTA score) and tubulitis (*t*-IFTA score) [302]. Although closely associated with TCMR, *i*-IFTA is also seen with BK virus nephropathy and AMR, [446] and thus the requirement for both *i*-IFTA and *t*-IFTA for diagnosis. Tubulitis within IFTA is indeed strongly associated with *i*-IFTA, and the majority of those with *i*-IFTA have concurrent *t*-IFTA [141, 433, 445]. The current minimum criteria for caTCMR diagnosis are a matter of ongoing debate and currently require at least moderate level of tubulitis in non-atrophic or partially atrophic tubules ($t \geq 2$) as well as interstitial inflammation in at least 25% of scarred cortical parenchyma (*i*-IFTA≥2). However, even mild inflammation (*i*-IFTA1) is associated with adverse outcome and should likely be considered as potentially pathogenic [433, 447]. Moreover, in the right clinical setting and exclusion of other causes, diagnosis of caTCMR may be invoked even in the absence of *i*-IFTA/*t* requirements. The latter requires the histologic vascular changes of intimal fibrosis associated with mononuclear cell infiltration and neointima formation (grade II by Banff criteria) [302].

The link between fibrosis and inflammation with outcome was first reported in 2005 by Cosio et al. [448], but criteria for caTCMR diagnosis were only first introduced in the Banff 2015 Kidney Meeting report. [449] Indicators of chronic inflammation such as *i*-IFTA have now been independently associated with increased risk of allograft failure [134, 141, 445, 450, 451]. Early *i*-IFTA (at 1 year) is associated with accelerated IFTA, arterial fibrointimal hyperplasia, and chronic glomerulopathy with functional decline [134]. In patients with early TCMR, the finding of *i*-IFTA on posttreatment biopsy was common (61%) and was associated with accelerated progression of IFTA and decreased allograft survival compared to those without [141]. In the setting of late acute TCMR, the presence of *i*-IFTA is an independent determinant of subsequent graft loss, although it is not directly associated with acute TCMR treatment response [25]. In addition, treatment of late acute rejection does not seem to modify the attributable risk for graft failure when *i*-IFTA is present [445].

The major risk for early caTCMR relates to acute allograft inflammation. One-year surveillance biopsies in adults identified *i*-IFTA rates of 26–32%, which were strongly associated with the presence, number, and severity of early TCMR episodes [134, 141]. Additional determinants of early i-IFTA risk include BK virus nephropathy, HLA-B, and HLA-DR mismatch, whereas protective factors were ongoing treatment with oral corticosteroids or inosine-5′monophosphate dehydrogenase (IMPDH) inhibitor therapy [141].

In the setting of late *i*-IFTA detection with *i*-IFTA≥1, rates of concurrent acute rejection are high with 46% exhibiting TMCR (including 15% with borderline) and 32% with AMR; so accounting for a small number with both AMR and TCMR (16%), only 38% had no acute features of rejection [447]. The hazard for graft failure is approximately fourfold increased when *i*-IFTA presents with either C4d+ (36%) or DSA+ (43%), and is worst when both are present [433].

Management

There is no agreed upon treatments for caTCMR, in part because it is a relatively new diagnostic entity. There have been no clinical trials and scant reports that evaluate the outcome in respect to treatment that has been received. Since caTCMR often presents in the context of acute AMR or TCMR, it is tempting to propose that treatment of the acute component may affect outcome. There is little data in support of this, however, and one study that evaluated treatment of acute rejection did not modify outcome [445].

In an absence of evidence, clinicians may consider optimization of immunosuppression. This must be individualized to the patient and weighed against potential increased risk for adverse effects. For calcineurin inhibitors, tacrolimus has been associated with lower rates of *i*-IFTA than the cyclosporine, and tacrolimus may protect against ongoing *i*-IFTA progression [134, 141]. IMPDH inhibitors and corticosteroids are considered anti-proliferative or anti-inflammatory, and their active use has also been associated with reduced risk for *i*-IFTA [141]. Whether conversion to or intensification of these medication classes is warranted to suppress chronic inflammation needs to be urgently evaluated.

Conversion from tacrolimus to an mTOR inhibitor has been tested in small studies as an intervention to either prevent or mitigate IFTA [452–457]. None of these studies have evaluated the potential effect on *i*-IFTA and progression. Caution is advised in particular for early conversion, given a relative lack of benefit and potential increased risk for IFTA progression and incident *dn*DSA [454, 455]. Similarly, mTOR inhibitors have been associated with proteinuria, which may already be manifest in patients with caTCMR if there is associated transplant glomerulopathy [454, 458, 459]. The potential appeal may be in the purported immunoregulatory benefits of mTOR inhibitors [460]. Small studies have evaluated rescue therapy to "treat" IFTA with some success in improving graft function [452, 453, 458], although these studies were predicated on the notion of resolving CNI toxicity. It is not known whether patients in these trials had *i*-IFTA, and whether mTOR inhibitor may be useful in selected populations without concurrent DSA or proteinuria.

With a better understanding of the risk factors and pathogenesis, it is likely that treatment options will become better defined with time. Rather than immunosuppression, it is possible that immunomodulatory therapies may be more effective, such as are now being employed for treatment of chronic autoimmune disorders. Until then, aggressive treatment should be weighed in light of prevailing risk factors such as C4d or DSA positivity, against the likelihood of treatment success and the risks associated with drug toxicity and adverse effects from excess immunosuppression.

Chronic Active AMR

Chronic active AMR (caAMR) is the final phase of continued, progressive alloimmune injury that starts either with pre-sensitization against donor HLA or post-transplant alloimmune activation in the form of acute TCMR. Each may lead to either rebound or de novo DSA production, respectively, that may then progress to active AMR (often with concurrent chronic T cell-mediated inflammation) and further with progressive damage over time to caAMR. The hallmark feature of caAMR is transplant glomerulopathy (TG) (Fig. 3.5d, e], which is a consequence of chronic damage to the glomerular basement membrane from unremitting active AMR [461]. The term "active" requires that there is also an ongoing, acute injury process, as indicated by evidence of both DSA and antibody-mediated injury [301]. The development of caAMR signals a poor prognosis. Redfield et al. [462] reported that of 1722 transplants, 7% were diagnosed with caAMR at a mean of 5.6 years after transplant and had a median allograft survival of just 1.9 years after diagnosis. In a smaller cohort, caAMR ($n = 41$) was identified at median of 6.3 years post-transplant, with 63% progressing to allograft failure at median 3.3 years after diagnosis [463]. Chronic, active AMR is the commonest finding on indication biopsies performed prior to graft failure and is the leading cause of graft loss in the modern transplant era [18].

In the prevailing literature, risk and outcome of caAMR are more often discussed with reference to the characteristic feature of TG. Transplant glomerulopathy is a late-presenting lesion, with median time from transplant to diagnosis of 2.8–7.1 years, which varies in part due to timing of ascertainment [462, 464, 465]. The prevalence of TG on indication biopsy also varies, increasing with time post-transplant. The DeKAF study reported a prospective cohort, using the first clinical indication biopsy after transplant, and a cross-sectional cohort reporting on late indication biopsies in patients with good allograft function (serum creatinine <2.0 mg/dl) [466]. In the prospective cohort, the mean time to biopsy was 1 year and the prevalence of TG was 27%. In the cross-sectional cohort, the median time to biopsy was 7.5 years and prevalence of TG was 67% [447]. In a surveillance biopsy series, Stegall et al. [467] reported TG prevalence of 12% at 10 years (in surviving transplants). This section will review the clinical features and management of caAMR and the impact of concurrent clinical and histological features on outcome.

Clinical and Histological Features

An insidious rise in creatinine, years after transplant, may be the only presenting feature of caAMR, highlighting the importance of *dn*DSA screening to identify AMR early and before there has been progression of TG. Patients with TG may also present with proteinuria or worsening hypertension [377]. Proteinuria is relatively non-specific, but is usually associated with allograft pathology and should indicate need for additional testing to determine the etiology, including biopsy [468]. The prevalence ranges from 7% to 45%, depending on the definition and timing post-transplant [469]. In patients with at least moderate proteinuria (>1500 mg/day), 80% were found to have glomerular disease on biopsy [470]. In this cohort, 11% were reported with TG, and an additional 50% had either acute rejection or chronic allograft nephropathy.

The diagnosis of caAMR is confirmed histologically using Banff criteria [301]. Chronic tissue injury must be accompanied by evidence of active antibody-mediated injury processes such as with AMR, including (1) evidence of antibody interaction with vascular endothelium and (2) evidence of circulating DSA or equivalent. Chronicity is usually denoted by proliferation of capillary basement membranes, which in the glomerulus is identified by TG (cg score [Fig. 3.5d]) and in the peritubular capillaries by evidence for basement membrane multilayering by electron microscopy (*ptcml* score [Fig. 3.5f]). Arterial intimal fibrosis of new onset, excluding other causes, may also be used to indicate chronicity. Early ultrastructural changes associated with TG are readily detected by electron microscopy and accrue with time, and so assessment of multilayering of glomerular basement membrane permits earlier detection of TG and diagnosis of caAMR than reliance on light microscopy alone (Fig. 3.5e) [471].

It is also important to consider in the differential diagnosis that there are other causes of TG, which will affect treatment choices and prognostication. In a series of 417 biopsies with TG, although 76% were consistent with caAMR, 16% showed thrombotic microangiopathy (TMA) lesions, 12% showed a membranoproliferative glomerulonephritis (MPGN) pattern, and (16%) remained equivocal with no specific causes identified [464]. An earlier series also showed association with pre-transplant hepatitis C infection [377]. In the absence of an alloimmune etiology, outcome of transplant glomerulopathy is dictated by the underlying cause. In a small series by Torres et al. [472], patients with TG were both C4d and DSA negative, were of older age, had lower interstitial and microvascular inflammation scores, and had longer allograft survival.

Risk for development of caAMR is not surprisingly strongly associated with prior identification of AMR [473], although a substantial proportion present without a prior clinical diagnosis. In keeping with risk from AMR, development of de novo HLA class II DSA is also a major risk factor for TG [377, 473]. The risk is accentuated in patients with prior sensitization; and in those with AMR at 3 months post-transplant, 43% had developed transplant glomerulopathy at 1 year [474]. In later presenting caAMR, prior acute rejection is an additional risk factor [377]. In a series of 797 patients without pre-sensitization, patients with early TCMR had significantly higher rates of HLA class II DSA (21%) and TG (8%) was seen more often at 1 and 2 year biopsies, compared to those without early TCMR (11% and 1%, respectively) [29].

In a recent series, it is relatively uncommon that TG presents as an isolated finding, accounting for as few as 16% of indication biopsies [464]. In a series of biopsies with confirmed caAMR, concurrent histologic abnormalities included concurrent intimal arteritis (v-lesion; 27%), tubulitis (9%), and IFTA of at least mild (57%) or moderate-severe (23%) severity [463]. This series did not report *i*-IFTA rates; however in the DeKAF prospective cohort, 48% of biopsies with Banff cg >0 (mean 1-year post-transplant) had at least Banff *i*-IFTA1; and in the cross-sectional cohort, the rate was 75% [447]. Neither of these series reported TCMR grade in relation to TG.

The prognosis for patients with caAMR is related in part to the presence of potentially reversible inflammation and the extent of chronic damage that may be considered irreversible. More advanced TG is associated with poorer allograft function and proteinuria at the time of diagnosis, and with subsequent allograft failure [377, 475, 476]. Clinical features of advanced chronicity such as proteinuria [476, 477] and worse kidney function at the time of diagnosis [477, 478] are independent risk factors for allograft failure. Prognostic histological indicators include arteriolar hyalinosis [476] and IFTA severity [381, 463, 476]. Indeed, when the extent of IFTA is considered in patients with active AMR, TG drops off as an independent predictor of allograft failure [381]. These histological indicators can be used in combination with the above clinical indicators along with total inflammation (*ti*) and arteritis (*v*) Banff scores to predict risk for allograft failure [464, 477].

From the perspective of acute inflammation, the presence of C4d staining in the peritubular capillaries (Fig. 3.3f) has been associated with particularly poor outcomes [478, 479], and is also associated with higher levels of HLA class II DSA [473]. In an archetypal analysis of outcome using 552 biopsies with TG, Aubert et al. [464] identified five archetypes, of which the worst prognosis was in patients typified by advanced clinical and histological chronicity (15% of patients). In contrast, the second worst was typified by less chronicity but the highest acute inflammatory scores (*i*, *t*, *v*, *ptc* and *g*-scores) and with c4d deposition (12% of patients). Relatively less inflammation and chronicity defined the remaining archetypes, which were associated with better prognosis. These data suggest that a subgroup of patients with advanced chronicity at diagnosis may not benefit from treatment, but that among the rest, the severity of tubulointerstitial and microvascular acute inflammation is most directly associated with progression and may be amenable to intervention.

Management

As with treatment of AMR, the available evidence to guide treatment of caAMR is weak and inconclusive. With progression of glomerular pathology to include TG, the extent of chronic injury is by definition more advanced. Because there may also be serious infection and malignancy risks associated with most of these treatment approaches, it is important to identify those patients who are unlikely to benefit. For this reason, aggressive treatment in patients who already manifest signs of advanced chronic injury on clinical assessment and histology (as described above) may be associated with more harm than benefit [480, 481]. This approach is endorsed by The Transplantation Society's (TTS) international consensus guideline regarding the treatment of caAMR [390]. It recommends that those with extensive chronicity but minimal inflammation may be a subset of patients in whom treatment confers a high risk of toxicity with little chance of improving allograft longevity [390].

There was also agreement that the current goals of management must focus on stabilizing further deterioration of histology, DSA, and kidney function [390]. However, the consensus concluded a lack of evidence prevents recommendation of any specific therapy or combination of therapies based on these criteria. As such, the expert consensus recommends optimizing maintenance immunosuppression with close monitoring of tacrolimus levels and to re-commence steroids (if on a steroid-free regimen) [390].

The TTS guideline also acknowledges that patients most likely to benefit from treatment include those with high levels of active inflammation and relative preservation of allograft function, in order to slow graft decline [390]. This is highlighted by Haas et al. [381], where the response of AMR to treatment with PP, IVIG, and rituximab was predicted by efficacy of removing DSA (median Banff scores $g = 1$ and $ptc = 2$), with poor response predicted by the severity of IFTA, and not the presence or absence of TG. For the most part, treatments directed to the inflammatory process in caAMR are the same as those for AMR and extends to include treatment of concurrent TCMR when it is present. For AMR, this includes various combinations of IVIG, PP, and/or rituximab [480–485].

In a study exclusively of patients with caAMR by Kahwaji et al. [486], stabilization of kidney function with IVIG and rituximab treatment was restricted to those with more severe microvascular injury (*ptc* score ≥ 2 or $g + ptc$ score ≥ 4). This subset had relatively preserved kidney function at treatment onset (mean serum creatinine 2.1 and 2.3 mg/dL, respectively), and reduction of *g* and *ptc* score was restricted to patients treated with rituximab. By contrast, IVIG and rituximab demonstrated no efficacy in another study where the mean $g + ptc$ score for the cohort was <1 [484]. Moreso et al. [485] conducted a small (n = 25) trial of rituximab and IVIG vs. placebo and did not demonstrate a difference; however this result is confounded by more advanced chronicity in the patients assigned to intervention (eGFR 35 vs. 45 ml/min/1.73 m^2 and $ci + ct$ score 3.0 vs. 2.4 for intervention vs. control). These studies exemplify the importance of identifying and stratifying for caAMR subgroups based on inflammation and chronicity when evaluating therapeutic efficacy.

In adults, triple therapy for caAMR using plasmapheresis/plasma exchange, IVIG, and rituximab positively impacted graft survival compared to placebo in two reports [381, 487]. In a larger cohort comparing non-randomized controls (n = 62), there was no difference with this combination therapy; however the treatment group may have had more severe disease prior to treatment (C4d + 83% vs. 44% in controls) [488]. In all of these studies, a higher rate of infections requiring hospitalization was observed in the treatment arms, highlighting the need to carefully select which patients would be suitable for such intensive management.

Emerging Therapies

Interleukin-6 (IL-6) activity inhibition is a novel immune modulator therapy for treating caAMR [489, 490]. Tocilizumab is an IL-6 receptor blocker and is well-studied for treatment of autoimmune diseases such as arthritis [491]. Receptor blockade leads to high levels of IL-6 circulation, which in the event of missing or stopping medication could lead to rebound phenomena [490]. Clazakizumab is a monoclonal antibody against IL-6 that is currently undergoing clinical trials and may be preferred over tocilizumab due to its ability to directly block IL-6, and avoid excess IL-6 production that occurs when the IL-6 receptor is blocked.

Tocilizumab was offered as a rescue therapy to 32 adult and 4 pediatric patients with caAMR (DSA positive and TG present) that did not respond to IV corticosteroids, IVIG, and rituximab with or without plasmapheresis or eculizumab [492]. There was no control group, but the study saw significant fall in C4d deposition and *g*/*ptc* scores on post-treatment biopsy, a reduction in DSA at 2 years, and 90% graft survival as far out as 6 years post treatment. Estimated GFR was maintained in both adults and children following treatment for 18 months. Lavacca et al. in 2020 replicated these findings, also demonstrating improvements in histology and C4d deposition, reduction in DSA, and stabilized renal function [493]. Randomized trials for IL-6 blockade in caAMR are still required. Three randomized trials are either recruiting or underway to establish the efficacy of tocilizumab or clazakizumab in chronic and late AMR, respectively [494, 495].

Post Rejection Infection Prophylaxis

Opportunistic infections that are amenable to anti-infective prophylaxis with treatment of rejection include cytomegalovirus (CMV), herpes simplex virus (HSV), and *Pneumocystis jiroveci* pneumonia (PJP). In addition, viral disease activity from donor-derived infections such as with BK virus (BKV) and Epstein-Barr virus (EBV) may flare in response to intensified immunosuppression. In general, rates of opportunistic viral infections have risen over time with the introduction of tacrolimus and mycophenolic acid formulations and the increased use of multi-modal maintenance immunosuppressive regimens [496–500]. Further intensification of immunosuppression to treat rejection is therefore an independent risk factor for infection.

Viral opportunistic infections are both more common and more serious when donor-derived infections are transmitted with transplantation to virus naïve recipients [501–504]. In recipients with prior acquired immunity, there still remains some risk due to reinfection or viral re-activation. The impact of opportunistic infection on transplant outcomes is significant: mortality rates for PJP in transplant recipients are as high as 44% [505–508], EBV is a prominent risk factor for post-transplant lymphoproliferative disorder (PTLD) [509], and BKV nephropathy is an important cause of graft loss [510]. Factors that predict increased risk and severity of opportunistic infections with rejection treatment include the use of intravenous corticosteroids, lymphocyte depletion therapy, and lymphopenia [503, 511–514].

After treatment of rejection, additional screening for EBV, CMV, and BKV is recommended in addition to baseline monitoring, in order to pre-emptively identify incipient viremia [515, 516]. In the event of rising viral titers, the approach is tailored to the specific infection. In the cases of EBV and BKV there is a lack of evidence to support the use of anti-viral prophylaxis post-rejection treatment. Management of viremia is therefore targeted to adjustment of maintenance immunosuppression in order to permit an effective cognate anti-virus response [113, 268–270, 517].

In the case of CMV, valganciclovir is effective at preventing CMV disease, and can be used as prophylaxis when rejection treatment is initiated in high-risk recipients (donor positive, recipient naïve). Donor-derived CMV infection can still occur on valganciclovir prophylaxis, but symptomatic infection and CMV disease are rare [268, 518]. The incidence of CMV infection overall in the first year with prophylaxis is 21% but CMV disease is only 10% [504]. According to the International Consensus Guidelines on the Management of Cytomegalovirus in Solid-organ Transplantation, valganciclovir prophylaxis should be re-implemented in children following rejection requiring treatment with IV steroids or a T cell depleting antibody [519]. There is inadequate data to recommend a specific duration in children, and this is likely to vary on a center by center basis, but periods of long prophylaxis up to 200 days have been shown to be well tolerated and safe [519, 520]. In adults, the KDOQI guidelines recommend valganciclovir for 6 weeks following the use of anti-lymphocyte therapy [517]. In cases where valganciclovir is not tolerated (e.g., neutropenia), letermovir has been used successfully for CMV prophylaxis in hematopoietic stem cell transplants [521–523].

In most cases, prophylaxis for herpes simplex virus (HSV) overlaps with CMV, and HSV is successfully suppressed from 9.8% without prophylaxis to 3% with valganciclovir [524]. However, in instances where donor and recipient are seronegative for CMV, CMV prophylaxis is not required [519]. In the case of HSV, reactivation is the main concern in patients who have been previously exposed, and so if valganciclovir is not indicated for CMV prophylaxis, then acyclovir prophylaxis should be given after treatment for rejection in order to mitigate the risk of HSV reactivation [525–527].

Rates of *Pneumocystis jiroveci* pneumonia (PJP) in transplant recipients prior to widespread prophylaxis were between 5 and 15% [514]. *Pneumocystis jiroveci* pneumonia prophylaxis with trimethoprim-sulfamethoxazole has been consistently shown to be highly effective, reducing PJP occurrence by 85% [528]. The KDIGO guidelines recommend that trimethoprim-sulfamethoxazole prophylaxis for PJP should be restarted following treatment for rejection and continued for 3–4 months [529]. Despite this, almost one third of pediatric solid organ transplant providers do not re-start PJP prophylaxis for any reason (including rejection) following completion of initial post-transplant prophylaxis [530].

Special Circumstances: Infection and Rejection

AGPN and Rejection

Acute graft pyelonephritis (AGPN) is usually easy to differentiate from acute rejection clinically, based on urinary symptoms of lower urinary tract infection such as dysuria, frequency, urgency, and cloudy urine, and the addition of symptoms of allograft inflammation that may include allograft tenderness, fever, and malaise. Diagnosis is usually confirmed with mid-stream or catheterized urine culture and finding of abundant leukocytes on urine analysis. The risk for AGPN may be increased in kidney transplant recipients due to vesicoureteral reflux in the transplanted ureter, which is common.

Diagnosis is sometimes confounded in children who depend on intermittent bladder catheterization to evacuate the bladder, where there may be chronic low-grade pyuria or asymptomatic bacteriuria. This is particularly the case when the bladder has been surgically augmented with bowel. Classical symptoms and signs of AGPN may also be attenuated in the transplant recipient. Immunosuppression with corticosteroids in the first post-transplant months and after treatment for rejection may obscure the typical signs of inflammation. The use of prophylactic antibiotics such as PJP prophylaxis may partially treat urinary tract infection and inhibit growth of susceptible bacteria in urine culture.

In a small number of cases, the only clinical sign of AGPN is allograft dysfunction, and the diagnosis is only made on kidney biopsy. Over 70% of AGPN episodes identified on kidney biopsy are associated with a negative urine culture [531]. Subclinical pyelonephritis has also been rarely detected on surveillance kidney biopsy [131].

APGN can occur simultaneously alongside rejection. In a study of biopsy proven AGPN, 37% of cases also had histological evidence of acute rejection [532]. The distinctive histological features of pyelonephritis include neutrophilic interstitial inflammation, neutrophilic tubulitis with or without neutrophil casts, and microabscesses (Fig. 3.3b) [531]. Lymphocytic infiltration may accompany neutrophilic infiltration in pyelonephritis and doesn't necessarily indicate rejection, although areas of pure mononuclear cell infiltration and associated tubulitis apart from areas with neutrophil involvement may imply an additional alloimmune process [533].

Follow-up biopsies comparing patients with AGPN to a control group showed that the AGPN group had higher rates of tubulitis, especially in patients whose creatinine did not resolve post-infection [534]. Another study showed a rejection rate of 22% in biopsies performed soon after AGPN [535].

AGPN may also precipitate a rejection episode, although the temporal association is difficult to confirm definitively [535–538]. Activation of the cell-mediated immune reactivity is initiated in association with the immune response to the bacterial pathogen. This includes upregulation of macrophages and dendritic cells, upregulation of adhesion molecules, and production of pro-inflammatory cytokines within the allograft, which may also activate endothelial cell expression of class II HLA [535, 539].

When both AGPN and acute rejection are diagnosed concurrently, treatment should be first for AGPN. This should include hospitalization for IV antibiotics, either guided by urine/blood culture results or for cases with a negative culture, prescribed empirically [529]. Successful treatment of AGPN and rejection with simultaneous administration of steroids and antibiotics have been reported [532]; however the preference may be to delay rejection treatment if kidney function is sufficiently stable, in order to suppress the active infection before initiating intensified immunosuppression. In cases where a diagnosis of rejection is unclear, a follow-up biopsy may be preferred after 6–8 weeks if the kidney function has stabilized, in order to evaluate for APGN-instigated or ongoing rejection.

BK Virus and Rejection

BK virus (BKV) is a member of the polyoma virus family and is sometimes referred to simply as polyoma virus. BKV infects the majority of individuals asymptomatically during childhood [540, 541] and then establishes latent infection in the urinary tract [542, 543]. BKV infection can therefore be transmitted to the recipient with kidney transplantation. Active infection that is donor derived is usually manifested in the first several months post-transplant. It is heralded by onset of viruria followed by viremia, which may progress to renal parenchymal infection known as BKV nephropathy (BKVN) [544]. BKVN is associated with poor graft outcomes [545–549]. Lack of prior or waning immunity may be identified by serological testing for BKV IgG and is most common in transplant recipients less than 5 years of age [550]. Seronegativity of the recipient has been associated with increased likelihood of developing BKV nephropathy [501, 550]. The incidence of BKVN has risen since the introduction of more potent immunosuppressants [496–499, 551] and currently affects between 3% and 8% in the pediatric renal transplant population [501, 552, 553].

The time period of greatest early rejection risk and manifestation of BKVN post-transplant are relatively superimposed. As a form of viral interstitial nephritis, BKVN is associated with interstitial inflammation and tubulitis that may be indistinguishable for TCMR [548, 554, 555]. The hallmark of BKVN on kidney biopsy is the presence of abnormally large nuclei with or without viral intranuclear inclusions that resemble tumor cells (Fig. 3.3c) and is confirmed by positive SV40 large T antigen (a surrogate marker for BKV infection) immunoperoxidase staining of infected tubule cells (Fig. 3.3d) [548, 555]. The features of AMR are histologically distinct, and should not be confused with BKVN.

Control of BKVN ultimately requires the recipient to mount a cognate response to the viral infection and suppress viral replication [165, 548, 554, 556, 557]. Direct antiviral therapy with medications like cidofovir is usually avoided due to their nephrotoxicity. Treatment is therefore directed at reducing immunosuppression. This creates a paradox in some cases, if there is concern that rejection is present concurrently. There are no trials or even large observational studies that guide treatment in this instance. There are several reports of success in managing simultaneous BKV and rejection with early pulse steroids followed by down-titration immunosuppression [544, 558, 559]. However, others have reported adverse outcomes when any attempt was made to treat the rejection before the BKVN was under control [496, 513, 555, 560–562]. This may be due to steroid-response elements in the BKV virome that may induce viral proliferation or reactivation [563] and exacerbate nephropathy. Howell et al. showed improvement in 4/6 patients that were managed with reduced maintenance MMF, regardless of whether steroids were given or not; the 2/6 who had significant graft decline both had in common no reduction in their baseline immunosuppression and the use of IV methylprednisolone [556].

In cases where mycophenolic acid medications are withdrawn, leflunomide may be considered as an alternative antimetabolite that maintains a lower level of immunosuppression and also has purported anti-viral activity. Leflunomide is an inhibitor of human dihydroorotate dehydrogenase leading to selective inhibition of the mTOR signalling pathway. Although there are multiple case series reporting efficacy, the quality of evidence is low [564]. Its use may also be associated with anemia and liver toxicity, and so although it is used in such scenarios, caution and monitoring for signs of toxicity are required.

Treatment with IVIG has also been used in refractory BKVN and in cases where there is suspected concurrent TCMR. The level of evidence is similarly low, comprised mostly of small case series and without controlled trials [565–569]. The rationale is to provide passive immunization with BKV-specific neutralizing antibodies in pooled IVIG. Indeed, significant increases in titers are observed in kidney transplant recipients post-IVIG administration [570]. In a recent randomized pilot clinical trial in patients with low levels of BKV neutralizing antibodies at transplant, IVIG prophylaxis was associated with a fivefold reduction in BKV viremia after 12 months compared to a similarly high-risk control group [571]. Adverse effects of IVIG are mostly infusion related and in general treatment is well tolerated.

Overall, the ability to make definitive treatment recommendations is limited by low level of available evidence. Resolution of BKV viremia in higher-risk individuals can take months. Safe reintroduction of immunosuppression is usually guided by attainment of persistently low-level if not absent viremia, with frequent monitoring for rebound viremia. Similar to AGPN, concern about BKV infection instigating alloimmune reactivity may be an abiding concern even after BKV viremia is cleared. Evidence of rejection following reduction in immunosuppression can be as high as

25% [548]. In such cases, a follow-up biopsy may be considered once BKV viremia is resolved, and full maintenance immunosuppression has been restored, to identify subclinical rejection. In addition, regular HLA antibody monitoring should be initiated with reduction of immunosuppression, to identify early onset of DSA that may result [334].

Case Studies

1. A 13-year-old girl with end-stage kidney disease with a hypoplastic solitary kidney is 2 years post-transplant and presents with a 40% rise in serum creatinine over a 1-month period and was subsequently diagnosed with grade 1B TCMR on biopsy. Following treatment with IV methylprednisolone, her creatinine initially fell but did not return to baseline and has begun climbing again after 2 months. What is the most appropriate next step in her management?
   (a) Ongoing close monitoring of creatinine.
   (b) Treat with a second course of IV methylprednisolone empirically.
   (c) Treat with ATG empirically.
   (d) Follow-up biopsy.
2. A 4-year-old boy with end-stage kidney failure from ANCA vasculitis presents with BKV viremia first detected at 5 months post-kidney transplant and progressively increasing viral load (2 log-fold) over the ensuing 4 weeks. There has been a ~10% increase from his baseline serum creatinine at the time of his 6-month surveillance biopsy. At the time of the biopsy, his MMF dose has already been reduced by half. The histology shows foci of moderate interstitial inflammation and tubulitis (i2t2), which extends into the medulla. There is associated viral cytopathic change in tubule epithelial cells in areas of inflammation, and SV40 stain is positive, confirming BKV nephropathy. The pathologist is equivocal about whether there is TCMR that is distinct from the BKV nephropathy. Acknowledging that good-quality evidence in this circumstance is limited, what is the safest way to proceed in the first instance?
   (a) Further reduce baseline immunosuppression in order to control BKVN. Discontinue MMF and consider substituting leflunomide. Consider adding regular IVIG treatment until viremia is cleared. Closely monitor creatinine and serial BKV viral loads every 2 weeks. Consider a follow-up biopsy once BKV viremia has resolved, if creatinine has not definitively returned to baseline to identify ongoing TCMR.
   (b) Manage BKVN with anti-viral medication and augment baseline immunosuppression to target TCMR. Closely monitor creatinine and serial BKV viral loads every 2 weeks, and arrange follow-up biopsy to ensure resolution of viremia.
   (c) Treat acute TCMR in the first instance with IV methylprednisolone and augmentation of baseline immunosuppression. Closely monitor creatinine and serial BKV viral loads every 2 weeks, and reduce immunosuppression if viremia intensifies.

(d) Maintain the current immunosuppression to balance risk of BVK and rejection, and follow serum creatinine. If creatinine further increases, then treat for rejection with IV methylprednisolone.

3. A 15-year-old boy, with posterior urethral valves, is 6 years post-kidney transplant. He had grade 1A TCMR at 8 months post-transplant that was treated with IV corticosteroids, with return to baseline creatinine. In the last 2 years, his tacrolimus levels have been in the 4–5 μg/L range. His creatinine has been slowly creeping higher for the past 12 months, and initially evaluated for worsening obstructive uropathy as the cause. But in the last 3 months the rate of increase is greater, and he has developed hypertension; and he is now nearly double the baseline from 2 years earlier. Because of onset of low-grade proteinuria, DSA screening was obtained and identified a single class II DSA at high MFI (>10,000). You arrange a biopsy, which shows evidence of caAMR, i2, t1, *g*2, *ptc*3, C4d+, *cg*1, and mild IFTA (ci1ct1), i-IFTA0. How do you proceed?
   (a) caAMR has no effective treatments, so continue on current immunosuppression to avoid effects from drug toxicity. Counsel the family regarding the inevitable caAMR progression and implications of sensitization on re-transplantation.
   (b) Optimize baseline immunosuppression and trial treatment for the active AMR component with plasmapheresis and IVIG. Follow DSA for treatment response.
   (c) Optimize baseline immunosuppression and trial treatment for the active TCMR, since this is likely the primary cause of acute allograft dysfunction.
   (d) Optimize baseline immunosuppression. Initiate treatment to address inflammation from both active AMR and TCMR, with IV methylprednisolone, plasmapheresis, and IVIG. Follow DSA and consider additional treatment based on treatment response.

Answers:

1. (d)

Monitoring of kidney function is valuable, but obtaining a kidney biopsy to confirm diagnosis and severity of rejection is an important consideration before initiating treatment. ATG may be required in cases of steroid refractory rejection, depending on the ongoing severity of inflammation. If there has been significant improvement in histology but persisting rejection changes, a second course of treatment with corticosteroids may be preferred. Late acute rejection has a higher rate of chronic inflammation, and changes related to i-IFTA should be reviewed. In the setting of persisting inflammation, identification of plasma cell infiltrates and additional staining to identify B cell clusters may provide additional information on prognosis and consideration of additional targeted treatment approaches. In the setting of chronic inflammation, intensification of baseline immunosuppression should also be considered. Late acute rejection is also associated with a higher risk of developing donor-specific HLA antibodies, and the patient should be screened and monitored after rejection.

2. (a)

The optimal treatment for concurrent BKVN and TCMR is unknown. It is difficult to assign etiology of the interstitial nephritis to an alloimmune vs. viral process with certainty. However, it should be clear that some component of the inflammatory response is related to viral nephropathy. Options to further reduce immunosuppression include discontinuation of MMF, dose reduction of tacrolimus, or both. Leflunomide may be used as an alternative anti-metabolite with potential direct anti-viral activity, but careful monitoring for lymphopenia, anemia, and hepatotoxicity is warranted. Due to the long half-life, toxicity may take several weeks to recover once it is manifest. IVIG may be used safely to passively provide anti-BKV antibody and is relatively low-risk, other than the requirement for infusion and risk for infusion-related side effects. It is unclear if there is additional IVIG activity for treating TCMR. Treatment with high-dose corticosteroids may be considered as a last resort, but in most cases the BKV nephropathy will resolve over several months without it; and there is concern that steroids may directly exacerbate the viral nephropathy. Regular monitoring for onset of donor-specific HLA antibodies should be performed while immunosuppression is reduced. Once BKV viremia has resolved, gradual re-titration to full immunosuppression while monitoring for rebound viremia is advised. Clinicians may also consider at that time to perform a surveillance biopsy to ensure that post-resolution of BKV, there is not subclinical rejection.

3. (d)

This person has a new diagnosis of caAMR with relatively low chronicity and high microvascular inflammation. He also has concurrent TCMR that is borderline grade. He is at risk due to previous early rejection and relative underimmunosuppression. Although not conclusively demonstrated in the literature, this subgroup may be most amenable to treatment of active inflammation – targeting both the AMR and TCMR aspects. Adding rituximab to initial therapy with plasmapheresis and IVIG may also be considered. Sustained decrease in DSA is an indicator of primary treatment efficacy. A follow-up biopsy may also be considered to evaluate treatment response. In the setting of refractory DSA and continued AMR, there is increasing evidence that novel treatments that inhibit IL-6 may be effective but at this point should still be considered investigational.

References

1. Medawar PB. The behaviour and fate of skin autografts and skin homografts in rabbits: a report to the War Wounds Committee of the Medical Research Council. J Anat. 1944;78(Pt 5):176.
2. Mitchison NA. Passive transfer of transplantation immunity. Proc. R. Soc. London, Ser. B. 1954;142(906):72–87.
3. Barker CF, Markmann JF. Historical overview of transplantation. Cold Spring Harb Perspect Med. 2013;3(4):a014977.
4. Kuss R. Human renal transplantation memories, 1951 to 1981. In: Terasaki P, editor. History of transplantation: thirty-five recollections. Los Angeles: UCLA Tissue Typing Laboratory; 1991. p. 37–59.

5. Murray JE, Merrill J, Harrison J, Carpenter C. Renal homotransplantation in identical twins. J Am Soc Nephrol. 2001;12(1):201–4.
6. Murray JE, Merrill JP, Harrison JH, Wilson RE, Dammin GJ. Prolonged survival of human-kidney homografts by immunosuppressive drug therapy. N Engl J Med. 1963;268(24):1315–23.
7. Starzl TE, Marchioro TL, Waddell WR. The reversal of rejection in human renal homografts with subsequent development of homograft tolerance. Surg Gynecol Obstetr. 1963;117:385.
8. Martin WJ. Experimental studies relating to the production and clinical testing of anti-human lymphocyte serum. Med J Aust. 1969;2(9):450–5.
9. Verghese PS. Pediatric kidney transplantation: a historical review. Pediatr Res. 2017;81(1–2):259–64.
10. Starzl TE, Marchioro TL, Porter KA, Faris TD, Carey TA. The role of organ transplantation in pediatrics. Pediatr Clin N Am. 1966;13:381.
11. Lilly JR, Giles G, Hurwitz R, Schroter G, Takagi H, Gray S, et al. Renal homotransplantation in pediatric patients. Pediatrics. 1971;47(3):548.
12. Cho MH. Pediatric kidney transplantation is different from adult kidney transplantation. Korean J Pediatr. 2018;61(7):205–9.
13. Holmberg C, Jalanko H. Long-term effects of paediatric kidney transplantation. Nat Rev Nephrol. 2016;12(5):301–11.
14. Bunchman TE, Fryd DS, Sibley RK, Mauer SM. Manifestations of renal allograft rejection in small children receiving adult kidneys. Pediatr Nephrol. 1990;4(3):255–8.
15. NAPRTCS NCS. Annual transplant report.2014.
16. Matas AJ, Smith J, Skeans M, Thompson B, Gustafson S, Stewart D, et al. OPTN/SRTR 2013 annual data report: kidney. Am J Transplant. 2015;15(S2):1–34.
17. Chua A, Cramer C, Moudgil A, Martz K, Smith J, Blydt-Hansen T, et al. Kidney transplant practice patterns and outcome benchmarks over 30 years: the 2018 report of the NAPRTCS. Pediatr Transplant. 2019;23(8):e13597.
18. Sellares J, De Freitas D, Mengel M, Reeve J, Einecke G, Sis B, et al. Understanding the causes of kidney transplant failure: the dominant role of antibody-mediated rejection and nonadherence. Am J Transplant. 2012;12(2):388–99.
19. Gaston RS, Cecka JM, Kasiske BL, Fieberg AM, Leduc R, Cosio FC, et al. Evidence for antibody-mediated injury as a major determinant of late kidney allograft failure. Transplantation. 2010;90(1):68–74.
20. Rodrigues CA, Franco MF, Cristelli MP, Pestana JOM, Tedesco-Silva H. Clinicopathological characteristics and effect of late acute rejection on renal transplant outcomes. Transplantation. 2014;98(8):885–92.
21. Eid L, Tuchman S, Moudgil A. Late acute rejection: incidence, risk factors, and effect on graft survival and function. Pediatr Transplant. 2014;18(2):155–62.
22. El-Zoghby ZM, Stegall MD, Lager DJ, Kremers WK, Amer H, Gloor JM, et al. Identifying specific causes of kidney allograft loss. Am J Transplant. 2009;9(3):527–35.
23. Naesens M, Kuypers DRJ, De Vusser K, Evenepoel P, Claes K, Bammens B, et al. The histology of kidney transplant failure: a long-term follow-up study. Transplantation. 2014;98(4):427–35.
24. Gaston RS, Fieberg A, Hunsicker L, Kasiske BL, Leduc R, Cosio FG, et al. Late graft failure after kidney transplantation as the consequence of late versus early events. Am J Transplant. 2018;18(5):1158–67.
25. Bouatou Y, Viglietti D, Pievani D, Louis K. Duong Van Huyen JP, Rabant M, et al. response to treatment and long-term outcomes in kidney transplant recipients with acute T cell–mediated rejection. Am J Transplant. 2019;19(7):1972–88.
26. Hoffmann AJ, Gibson IW, Ho J, Nickerson P, Rush D, Sharma A, et al. Early surveillance biopsy utilization and management of pediatric renal allograft acute T cell–mediated rejection in Canadian centers: Observations from the PROBE multicenter cohort study. Pediatr Transplant. 2021;25:e13870.

27. Landsberg A, Riazy M, Blydt-Hansen TD. Yield and utility of surveillance kidney biopsies in pediatric kidney transplant recipients at various time points post-transplant. Pediatr Transplantat. 2021;25:e13869.
28. Mincham CM, Gibson IW, Sharma A, Wiebe C, Mandal R, Rush D, et al. Evolution of renal function and urinary biomarker indicators of inflammation on serial kidney biopsies in pediatric kidney transplant recipients with and without rejection. Pediatr Transplant. 2018;22(5):e13202.
29. El Ters M, Grande JP, Keddis MT, Rodrigo E, Chopra B, Dean PG, et al. Kidney allograft survival after acute rejection, the value of follow-up biopsies. Am J Transplant. 2013;13(9):2334–41.
30. Kee TY-S, Chapman JR, O'Connell PJ, Fung CL-S, Allen RD, Kable K, et al. Treatment of subclinical rejection diagnosed by protocol biopsy of kidney transplants. Transplantation. 2006;82(1):36–42.
31. Odum JD, Kats A, VanSickle JS, Chadha V, Brewer B, Staggs VS, et al. Characterizing the frequency of modifiable histological changes observed on surveillance biopsies in pediatric kidney allograft recipients. Pediatr Nephrol. 2020;35(11):2173–82.
32. Blydt-Hansen T, Sharma A, Gibson IW, Wiebe C, Sharma AP, Langlois V, et al. Validity and utility of urinary CXCL10/Cr immune monitoring in pediatric kidney transplant recipients. Am J Transplant. 2021;21(4):1545–55.
33. Nankivell BJ, Alexander SI. Rejection of the kidney allograft. N Engl J Med. 2010;363(15):1451–62.
34. Marino J, Paster J, Benichou G. Allorecognition by T Lymphocytes and allograft rejection. Front Immunol. 2016;7:582.
35. Benichou G. Direct and indirect antigen recognition: the pathways to allograft immune rejection. Front Biosci. 1999;4:D476–80.
36. Benichou G, Valujskikh A, Heeger PS. Contributions of direct and indirect T cell alloreactivity during allograft rejection in mice. J Immunol. 1999;162(1):352–8.
37. Afzali B, Lechler RI, Hernandez-Fuentes MP. Allorecognition and the alloresponse: clinical implications. Tissue Antigens. 2007;69(6):545–56.
38. Yamane H, Paul WE. Cytokines of the γ c family control CD4+ T cell differentiation and function. Nat Immunol. 2012;13(11):1037–44.
39. O'Garra A, Murphy K. Role of cytokines in determining T-lymphocyte function. Curr Opin Immunol. 1994;6(3):458–66.
40. O'Garra A. Cytokines induce the development of functionally heterogeneous T helper cell subsets. Immunity. 1998;8(3):275–83.
41. Bradley LM, Dalton DK, Croft M. A direct role for IFN-gamma in regulation of Th1 cell development. J Immunol. 1996;157(4):1350–8.
42. Louten J, Boniface K, de Waal Malefyt R. Development and function of TH17 cells in health and disease. J Allergy Clin Immunol. 2009;123(5):1004–11.
43. Afkarian M, Sedy JR, Yang J, Jacobson NG, Cereb N, Yang SY, et al. T-bet is a STAT1-induced regulator of IL-12R expression in naive CD4+ T cells. Nat Immunol. 2002;3(6):549–57.
44. Lee H-M, Bautista JL, Hsieh C-S. Chapter 2 – Thymic and peripheral differentiation of regulatory T cells. In: Alexander R, Shimon S, editors. Advances in immunology, vol. 112. Academic Press; 2011. p. 25–71.
45. Brogdon JL, Leitenberg D, Bottomly K. The potency of TCR signaling differentially regulates NFATc/p activity and early IL-4 transcription in naive CD4+ T cells. J Immunol. 2002;168(8):3825–32.
46. Constant S, Pfeiffer C, Woodard A, Pasqualini T, Bottomly K. Extent of T cell receptor ligation can determine the functional differentiation of naive CD4+ T cells. J Exp Med. 1995;182(5):1591–6.
47. Curtsinger JM, Schmidt CS, Mondino A, Lins DC, Kedl RM, Jenkins MK, et al. Inflammatory cytokines provide a third signal for activation of naive $CD4^+$ and $CD8^+$ T cells. J Immunol. 1999;162(6):3256–62.

48. Masopust D, Schenkel JM. The integration of T cell migration, differentiation and function. Nat Rev Immunol. 2013;13(5):309–20.
49. Moreau A, Varey E, Anegon I, Cuturi M-C. Effector mechanisms of rejection. Cold Spring Harb Perspect Med. 2013;3(11):a015461.
50. Atalar K, Afzali B, Lord G, Lombardi G. Relative roles of Th1 and Th17 effector cells in allograft rejection. Curr Opin Organ Transplant. 2009;14(1):23–9.
51. Liao W, Lin J-X, Leonard WJ. IL-2 family cytokines: new insights into the complex roles of IL-2 as a broad regulator of T helper cell differentiation. Curr Opin Immunol. 2011;23(5):598–604.
52. Barry M, Bleackley RC. Cytotoxic T lymphocytes: all roads lead to death. Nat Rev Immunol. 2002;2(6):401–9.
53. Liu Z, Fan H, Jiang S. CD4+ T-cell subsets in transplantation. Immunol Rev. 2013;252(1):183–91.
54. Li J, Li C, Zhuang Q, Peng B, Zhu Y, Ye Q, et al. The evolving roles of macrophages in organ transplantation. J Immunol Res. 2019;2019:1–11.
55. Salehi S, Reed EF. The divergent roles of macrophages in solid organ transplantation. Curr Opin Organ Transplant. 2015;20(4):446.
56. Dummer CD, Carpio VN, Goncalves LF, Manfro RC, Veronese FV. FOXP3+ regulatory T cells: from suppression of rejection to induction of renal allograft tolerance. Transpl Immunol. 2012;26(1):1–10.
57. Stenard F, Nguyen C, Cox K, Kambham N, Umetsu DT, Krams SM, et al. Decreases in circulating CD4+CD25hiFOXP3+ cells and increases in intragraft FOXP3+ cells accompany allograft rejection in pediatric liver allograft recipients. Pediatr Transplant. 2009;13(1):70–80.
58. Scheffold A, Murphy KM, Höfer T. Competition for cytokines: T reg cells take all. Nat Immunol. 2007;8(12):1285–7.
59. Sprent J, Surh CD. T cell memory. Annu Rev Immunol. 2002;20(1):551–79.
60. Lech M, Anders H-J. Macrophages and fibrosis: How resident and infiltrating mononuclear phagocytes orchestrate all phases of tissue injury and repair. Biochim Biophys Acta. 2013;1832(7):989–97.
61. Oishi Y, Manabe I. Macrophages in inflammation, repair and regeneration. Int Immunol. 2018;30(11):511–28.
62. Kim C, Wilson T, Fischer KF, Williams MA. Sustained interactions between T cell receptors and antigens promote the differentiation of CD4+ memory T cells. Immunity. 2013;39(3):508–20.
63. Obst R, van Santen H-M, Mathis D, Benoist C. Antigen persistence is required throughout the expansion phase of a CD4+ T cell response. J Exp Med. 2005;201(10):1555–65.
64. Whitmire JK, Eam B, Benning N, Whitton JL. Direct interferon-γ signaling dramatically enhances $CD4^+$ and $CD8^+$ T cell memory. J Immunol. 2007;179(2):1190–7.
65. Whitmire JK, Benning N, Eam B, Whitton JL. Increasing the CD4+ T cell precursor frequency leads to competition for IFN-γ thereby degrading memory cell quantity and quality. J Immunol. 2008;180(10):6777–85.
66. Avalos A, Ploegh H. Early BCR events and antigen capture, processing, and loading on MHC class II on B cells. Front Immunol. 2014;5:92.
67. Cornell LD, Smith RN, Colvin RB. Kidney transplantation: mechanisms of rejection and acceptance. Annu Rev Pathol Mech Dis. 2008;3:189–220.
68. McAdam AJ, Greenwald RJ, Levin MA, Chernova T, Malenkovich N, Ling V, et al. ICOS is critical for CD40-mediated antibody class switching. Nature. 2001;409(6816):102–5.
69. Nardelli B, Belvedere O, Roschke V, Moore PA, Olsen HS, Migone TS, et al. Synthesis and release of B-lymphocyte stimulator from myeloid cells. Blood. 2001;97(1):198–204.
70. Chong AS. B cells as antigen-presenting cells in transplantation rejection and tolerance. Cell Immunol. 2020;349:104061.
71. Colvin RB, Smith RN. Antibody-mediated organ-allograft rejection. Nat Rev Immunol. 2005;5(10):807–17.
72. Crotty S. Follicular helper CD4 T cells (Tfh). Annu Rev Immunol. 2011;29:621–63.

73. Sage PT, Ron-Harel N, Juneja VR, Sen DR, Maleri S, Sungnak W, et al. Suppression by T(FR) cells leads to durable and selective inhibition of B cell effector function. Nat Immunol. 2016;17(12):1436–46.
74. Sage PT, Sharpe AH. T follicular regulatory cells. Immunol Rev. 2016;271(1):246–59.
75. Mohammed MT, Sage PT. Follicular T-cell regulation of alloantibody formation. Curr Opin Organ Transplant. 2020;25(1):22–6.
76. Noelle RJ, Snow EC, Uhr JW, Vitetta ES. Activation of antigen-specific B cells: role of T cells, cytokines, and antigen in induction of growth and differentiation. Proc Nat Acad Sci. 1983;80(21):6628–31.
77. Steele DJ, Laufer TM, Smiley ST, Ando Y, Grusby MJ, Glimcher LH, et al. Two levels of help for B cell alloantibody production. J Exp Med. 1996;183(2):699–703.
78. Martin F, Oliver AM, Kearney JF. Marginal zone and B1 B cells unite in the early response against T-independent blood-borne particulate antigens. Immunity. 2001;14(5):617–29.
79. Martins H, Silva C, Martini D, Noronha I, editors. Detection of B lymphocytes (CD20+) in renal allograft biopsy specimens. Transplantation proceedings. Elsevier; 2007.
80. Muorah MR, Brogan PA, Sebire NJ, Trompeter RS, Marks SD. Dense B cell infiltrates in paediatric renal transplant biopsies are predictive of allograft loss. Pediatr Transplant. 2009;13(2):217–22.
81. Segerer S, Schlöndorff D. B cells and tertiary lymphoid organs in renal inflammation. Kidney Int. 2008;73(5):533–7.
82. Tsai EW, Ettenger RB. B cells and rejection: is there a link? Meaning and management of rejection characterized by steroid-resistance and B-cell infiltrates. Pediatr Transplant. 2009;13(2):150–4.
83. Shiu KY, McLaughlin L, Rebollo-Mesa I, Zhao J, Burton H, Douthwaite H, et al. Graft dysfunction in chronic antibody-mediated rejection correlates with B-cell–dependent indirect antidonor alloresponses and autocrine regulation of interferon-γ production by Th1 cells. Kidney Int. 2017;91(2):477–92.
84. Shabir S, Girdlestone J, Briggs D, Kaul B, Smith H, Daga S, et al. Transitional B lymphocytes are associated with protection from kidney allograft rejection: a prospective study. Am J Transplant. 2015;15(5):1384–91.
85. Cox ST, Stephens HA, Fernando R, Karasu A, Harber M, Howie AJ, et al. Major histocompatibility complex class I-related chain A allele mismatching, antibodies, and rejection in renal transplantation. Hum Immunol. 2011;72(10):827–34.
86. McCaughan JA, O'Rourke DM, Courtney AE. The complement cascade in kidney disease: from sideline to center stage. Am J Kidney Dis. 2013;62(3):604–14.
87. Benzaquen LR, Nicholson-Weller A, Halperin JA. Terminal complement proteins C5b-9 release basic fibroblast growth factor and platelet-derived growth factor from endothelial cells. J Exp Med. 1994;179(3):985–92.
88. Collins AB, Schneeberger EE, Pascual MA, Saidman SL, Williams WW, Tolkoff-Rubin N, et al. Complement activation in acute humoral renal allograft rejection: diagnostic significance of C4d deposits in peritubular capillaries. J Am Soc Nephrol. 1999;10(10):2208–14.
89. Böhmig GA, Exner M, Habicht A, Schillinger M, Lang U, Kletzmayr J, et al. Capillary C4d deposition in kidney allografts: a specific marker of alloantibody-dependent graft injury. J Am Soc Nephrol. 2002;13(4):1091–9.
90. Baldwin WM, Ota H, Rodriguez ER. Complement in transplant rejection:diagnostic and mechanistic considerations. Springer Semin Immunopathol. 2003;25(2):181–97.
91. Valenzuela NM, Reed EF. Antibodies in transplantation: the effects of HLA and non-HLA antibody binding and mechanisms of injury. Transplantation immunology. Springer; 2013. p. 41–70.
92. Valenzuela NM, Reed EF. Antibodies to HLA molecules mimic agonistic stimulation to trigger vascular cell changes and induce allograft injury. Curr Transplant Rep. 2015;2(3):222–32.
93. Lee C-Y, Lotfi-Emran S, Erdinc M, Murata K, Velidedeoglu E, Fox-Talbot K, et al. The involvement of FcR mechanisms in antibody-mediated rejection. Transplantation. 2007;84(10):1324–34.

94. Yuan FF, Watson N, Sullivan JS, Biffin S, Moses J, Geczy AF, et al. Association of Fc gamma receptor IIA polymorphisms with acute renal-allograft rejection. Transplantation. 2004;78(5):766–9.
95. Fadel FI, Elshamaa MF, Salah A, Elghoroury EA, El-Rahman SA, Ibrahim MH, et al. FcγRIIa defunctioning polymorphism in paediatric patients with renal allograft. Cent Eur J Immunol. 2017;42(4):363–9.
96. Loupy A, Lefaucheur C. Antibody-mediated rejection of solid-organ allografts. N Engl J Med. 2018;379(12):1150–60.
97. Kimura A, Kishimoto T. IL-6: regulator of Treg/Th17 balance. Eur J Immunol. 2010;40(7):1830–5.
98. Lee YK, Mukasa R, Hatton RD, Weaver CT. Developmental plasticity of Th17 and Treg cells. Curr Opin Immunol. 2009;21(3):274–80.
99. Braudeau C, Racape M, Giral M, Louis S, Moreau A, Berthelot L, et al. Variation in numbers of CD4+CD25highFOXP3+ T cells with normal immuno-regulatory properties in long-term graft outcome. Transpl Int. 2007;20(10):845–55.
100. Carmona-Escamilla MA, Queipo G, Garcia-Mosqueda LA, Garcia-Covarrubias L, Fonseca-Sanchez MA, Villanueva-Ortega E, et al. Peripheral blood regulatory T cells are diminished in kidney transplant patients with chronic allograft nephropathy. Transplant Proc. 2018;50(2):444–8.
101. Xu Y, Jin J, Wang H, Shou Z, Wu J, Han F, et al. The regulatory/cytotoxic infiltrating T cells in early renal surveillance biopsies predicts acute rejection and survival. Nephrol Dial Transplant. 2012;27(7):2958–65.
102. Piloni D, Morosini M, Magni S, Balderacchi A, Scudeller L, Cova E, et al. Analysis of long term CD4+CD25highCD127- T-reg cells kinetics in peripheral blood of lung transplant recipients. BMC Pulm Med. 2017;17(1):102.
103. Chung BH, Kim KW, Kim B-M, Doh KC, Cho M-L, Yang CW. Increase of Th17 cell phenotype in kidney transplant recipients with chronic allograft dysfunction. PLoS One. 2015;10(12):e0145258.
104. Ma L, Zhang H, Hu K, Lv G, Fu Y, Ayana DA, et al. The imbalance between Tregs, Th17 cells and inflammatory cytokines among renal transplant recipients. BMC Immunol. 2015;16(1):56.
105. Kishimoto T, Akira S, Taga T. Interleukin-6 and its receptor: a paradigm for cytokines. Science. 1992;258(5082):593–7.
106. Wang H, Guan Q, Lan Z, Li S, Ge W, Chen H, et al. Prolonged renal allograft survival by donor interleukin-6 deficiency: association with decreased alloantibodies and increased intragraft T regulatory cells. Am J Physiol Renal Physiol. 2012;302(2):F276–F83.
107. Salehi S, Shahi A, Afzali S, Keshtkar AA, Farashi Bonab S, Soleymanian T, et al. Transitional immature regulatory B cells and regulatory cytokines can discriminate chronic antibody-mediated rejection from stable graft function. Int Immunopharmacol. 2020;86:106750.
108. Ingulli E. Mechanism of cellular rejection in transplantation. Pediatr Nephrol. 2010;25(1):61.
109. Curci C, Sallustio F, Serino G, De Palma G, Trpevski M, Fiorentino M, et al. Potential role of effector memory T cells in chronic T cell-mediated kidney graft rejection. Nephrol Dial Transplant. 2016;31(12):2131–42.
110. Nouël A, Ségalen I, Jamin C, Doucet L, Caillard S, Renaudineau Y, et al. B cells display an abnormal distribution and an impaired suppressive function in patients with chronic antibody–mediated rejection. Kidney Int. 2014;85(3):590–9.
111. Luque S, Lúcia M, Melilli E, Lefaucheur C, Crespo M, Loupy A, et al. Value of monitoring circulating donor-reactive memory B cells to characterize antibody-mediated rejection after kidney transplantation. Am J Transplant. 2019;19(2):368–80.
112. Tait BD, Susal C, Gebel HM, Nickerson PW, Zachary AA, Claas FH, et al. Consensus guidelines on the testing and clinical management issues associated with HLA and non-HLA antibodies in transplantation. Transplantation. 2013;95(1):19–47.
113. Kidney Disease: Improving Global Outcomes (KDIGO) Transplant Work Group. KDIGO clinical practice guideline for the care of kidney transplant recipients. Am J Transplant. 2009;9(Suppl 3):S1–155.

114. Akcan-Arikan A, Zappitelli M, Loftis LL, Washburn KK, Jefferson LS, Goldstein SL. Modified RIFLE criteria in critically ill children with acute kidney injury. Kidney Int. 2007;71(10):1028–35.
115. Group AKIW. Kidney disease: improving global outcomes (KDIGO) acute kidney injury work group. KDIGO clinical practice guideline for acute kidney injury. Kidney Int Suppl. 2012;2:1–138.
116. Blydt-Hansen TD, Sharma A, Gibson IW, Mandal R, Wishart DS. Urinary metabolomics for noninvasive detection of borderline and acute T cell-mediated rejection in children after kidney transplantation. Am J Transplant. 2014;14(10):2339–49.
117. Rush D, Nickerson P, Gough J, McKenna R, Grimm P, Cheang M, et al. Beneficial effects of treatment of early subclinical rejection: a randomized study. J Am Soc Nephrol. 1998;9(11):2129–34.
118. Naesens M, Kambham N, Concepcion W, Salvatierra O Jr, Sarwal M. The evolution of non-immune histological injury and its clinical relevance in adult-sized kidney grafts in pediatric recipients. Am J Transplant. 2007;7(11):2504–14.
119. Dart AB, Schall A, Gibson IW, Blydt-Hansen TD, Birk PE. Patterns of chronic injury in pediatric renal allografts. Transplantation. 2010;89(3):334–40.
120. Bertrand D, Gatault P, Jauréguy M, Garrouste C, Sayegh J, Bouvier N, et al. Protocol biopsies in patients with subclinical de novo donor-specific antibodies after kidney transplantation: a multicentric study. Transplantation. 2020;104(8):1726–37.
121. Ginevri F, Nocera A, Comoli P, Innocente A, Cioni M, Parodi A, et al. Posttransplant de novo donor-specific HLA antibodies identify pediatric kidney recipients at risk for late antibody-mediated rejection. Am J Transplant. 2012;12(12):3355–62.
122. Wiebe C, Gibson IW, Blydt-Hansen TD, Pochinco D, Birk PE, Ho J, et al. Rates and determinants of progression to graft failure in kidney allograft recipients with de novo donor-specific antibody. Am J Transplant. 2015;15(11):2921–30.
123. Parajuli S, Joachim E, Alagusundaramoorthy S, Blazel J, Aziz F, Garg N, et al. Subclinical antibody-mediated rejection after kidney transplantation: treatment outcomes. Transplantation. 2019;103(8):1722–9.
124. Nazario M, Nicoara O, Becton L, Self S, Hill J, Mack E, et al. Safety and utility of surveillance biopsies in pediatric kidney transplant patients. Pediatr Transplant. 2018;22(4):e13178.
125. Birk PE, Blydt-Hansen TD, Dart AB, Kaita LM, Proulx C, Taylor G. Low incidence of adverse events in outpatient pediatric renal allograft biopsies. Pediatr Transplant. 2007;11(2):196–200.
126. Rose EM, Kennedy SE, Mackie FE. Surveillance biopsies after paediatric kidney transplantation: a review. Pediatr Transplant. 2016;20(6):748–55.
127. Hymes LC, Warshaw BL, Hennigar RA, Amaral SG, Greenbaum LA. Prevalence of clinical rejection after surveillance biopsies in pediatric renal transplants: does early subclinical rejection predispose to subsequent rejection episodes? Pediatr Transplant. 2009;13(7):823–6.
128. Seifert ME, Yanik MV, Feig DI, Hauptfeld-Dolejsek V, Mroczek-Musulman EC, Kelly DR, et al. Subclinical inflammation phenotypes and long-term outcomes after pediatric kidney transplantation. Am J Transplant. 2018;18(9):2189–99.
129. Kanzelmeyer NK, Ahlenstiel T, Drube J, Froede K, Kreuzer M, Broecker V, et al. Protocol biopsy-driven interventions after pediatric renal transplantation. Pediatr Transplant. 2010;14(8):1012–8.
130. Zotta F, Guzzo I, Morolli F, Diomedi-Camassei F, Dello SL. Protocol biopsies in pediatric renal transplantation: a precious tool for clinical management. Pediatr Nephrol. 2018;33(11):2167–75.
131. Dharnidharka VR, Dharnidharka VR, Vyas N, Vyas N, Gaut JP, Gaut JP, et al. The utility of surveillance biopsies in pediatric kidney transplantation. Pediatr Nephrol. 2018;33(5):889–95.
132. Rush D, Arlen D, Boucher A, Busque S, Cockfield SM, Girardin C, et al. Lack of benefit of early protocol biopsies in renal transplant patients receiving TAC and MMF: a randomized study. Am J Transplant. 2007;7(11):2538–45.
133. Nankivell BJ, Borrows RJ, Fung CLS, O'Connell PJ, Allen RDM, Chapman JR. Natural history, risk factors, and impact of subclinical rejection in kidney transplantation. Transplantation. 2004;78(2):242–9.

134. Nankivell BJ, Shingde M, Keung KL, Fung CL, Borrows RJ, O'Connell PJ, et al. The causes, significance and consequences of inflammatory fibrosis in kidney transplantation: the Banff i-IFTA lesion. Am J Transplant. 2018;18(2):364–76.
135. Loupy A, Vernerey D, Tinel C, Aubert O, van Huyen J-PD, Rabant M, et al. Subclinical rejection phenotypes at 1 year post-transplant and outcome of kidney allografts. J Am Soc Nephrol. 2015;26(7):1721–31.
136. Seikku P, Krogerus L, Jalanko H, Holmberg C. Better renal function with enhanced immunosuppression and protocol biopsies after kidney transplantation in children. Pediatr Transplant. 2005;9(6):754–62.
137. Kurtkoti J, Sakhuja V, Sud K, Minz M, Nada R, Kohli H, et al. The utility of 1-and 3-month protocol biopsies on renal allograft function: a randomized controlled study. Am J Transplant. 2008;8(2):317–23.
138. Hymes LC, Greenbaum L, Amaral SG, Warshaw BL. Surveillance renal transplant biopsies and subclinical rejection at three months post-transplant in pediatric recipients. Pediatr Transplant. 2007;11(5):536–9.
139. Birk PE, Stannard KM, Konrad HB, Blydt-Hansen TD, Ogborn MR, Cheang MS, et al. Surveillance biopsies are superior to functional studies for the diagnosis of acute and chronic renal allograft pathology in children. Pediatr Transplant. 2004;8(1):29–38.
140. Gaber LW, Moore LW, Gaber AO, Tesi RJ, Meyer J, Schroeder TJ. Correlation of histology to clinical rejection reversal: a thymoglobulin multicenter trial report. Kidney Int. 1999;55(6):2415–22.
141. Lefaucheur C, Gosset C, Rabant M, Viglietti D, Verine J, Aubert O, et al. T cell–mediated rejection is a major determinant of inflammation in scarred areas in kidney allografts. Am J Transplant. 2018;18(2):377–90.
142. Kurian S, Williams A, Gelbart T, Campbell D, Mondala T, Head S, et al. Molecular classifiers for acute kidney transplant rejection in peripheral blood by whole genome gene expression profiling. Am J Transplant. 2014;14(5):1164–72.
143. Marsh CL, Kurian SM, Rice JC, Whisenant TC, David J, Rose S, et al. Application of TruGraf v1: a novel molecular biomarker for managing kidney transplant recipients with stable renal function. Transplant Proc. 2019;51(3):722–8.
144. First M, Kleiboeker S, Rose S, Friedewald J, Abecassis M. The real-life experience of developing and commercializing TruGraf, a validated non-invasive transplant biomarker. J Biochem Analyt Stud. 2020;4(2) https://doi.org/10.16966/2576-5833.123.
145. Van Loon E, Giral M, Anglicheau D, Lerut E, Dubois V, Rabeyrin M, et al. Diagnostic performance of kSORT, a blood-based mRNA assay for noninvasive detection of rejection after kidney transplantation: a retrospective multicenter cohort study. Am J Transplant. 2020;21(2):740–50.
146. Suthanthiran M, Schwartz JE, Ding R, Abecassis M, Dadhania D, Samstein B, et al. Urinary-cell mRNA profile and acute cellular rejection in kidney allografts. N Engl J Med. 2013;369(1):20–31.
147. Dufour JH, Dziejman M, Liu MT, Leung JH, Lane TE, Luster AD. IFN-γ-inducible protein 10 (IP-10; CXCL10)-deficient mice reveal a role for IP-10 in effector T cell generation and trafficking. J Immunol (1950). 2002;168(7):3195–204.
148. El-Sawy T, Fahmy NM, Fairchild RL. Chemokines: directing leukocyte infiltration into allografts. Curr Opin Immunol. 2002;14(5):562–8.
149. Miura M, Morita K, Kobayashi H, Hamilton TA, Burdick MD, Strieter RM, et al. Monokine induced by IFN-gamma is a dominant factor directing T cells into murine cardiac allografts during acute rejection. J Immunol (1950). 2001;167(6):3494–504.
150. Panzer U, Reinking RR, Steinmetz OM, Zahner G, Sudbeck U, Fehr S, et al. CXCR3 and CCR5 positive T-cell recruitment in acute human renal allograft rejection. Transplantation. 2004;78(9):1341–50.
151. Qin S, Rottman JB, Myers P, Kassam N, Weinblatt M, Loetscher M, et al. The chemokine receptors CXCR3 and CCR5 mark subsets of T cells associated with certain inflammatory reactions. J Clin Invest. 1998;101(4):746–54.

152. Jackson JA, Kim EJ, Begley B, Cheeseman J, Harden T, Perez SD, et al. Urinary chemokines CXCL9 and CXCL10 are noninvasive markers of renal allograft rejection and BK viral infection. Am J Transplant. 2011;11(10):2228–34.
153. Hricik DE, Nickerson P, Formica RN, Poggio ED, Rush D, Newell KA, et al. Multicenter validation of urinary CXCL9 as a risk-stratifying biomarker for kidney transplant injury. Am J Transplant. 2013;13(10):2634–44.
154. Hu H, Aizenstein BD, Puchalski A, Burmania JA, Hamawy MM, Knechtle SJ. Elevation of CXCR3-binding chemokines in urine indicates acute renal-allograft dysfunction. Am J Transplant. 2004;4(3):432–7.
155. Rush D, Somorjai R, Cecka MJ, Cosio F, Gaston R, Gourishankar S, et al. Urine magnetic resonance spectroscopy (UMRS): results from the deterioration of kidney allograft function (DeKAF) study. Am J Transplant. 2009;9(S2):350.
156. Rabant M, Amrouche L, Lebreton X, Aulagnon F, Benon A, Sauvaget V, et al. Urinary C-X-C motif chemokine 10 independently improves the noninvasive diagnosis of antibody–mediated kidney allograft rejection. J Am Soc Nephrol. 2015;26(11):2840–51.
157. Rabant M, Amrouche L, Morin L, Bonifay R, Lebreton X, Aouni L, et al. Early low urinary CXCL9 and CXCL10 might predict immunological quiescence in clinically and histologically stable kidney recipients. Am J Transplant. 2016;16(6):1868–81.
158. Tatapudi RR, Muthukumar T, Dadhania D, Ding R, Li B, Sharma VK, et al. Noninvasive detection of renal allograft inflammation by measurements of mRNA for IP-10 and CXCR3 in urine. Kidney Int. 2004;65(6):2390–7.
159. Matz M, Beyer J, Wunsch D, Mashreghi M-F, Seiler M, Pratschke J, et al. Early post-transplant urinary IP-10 expression after kidney transplantation is predictive of short-and long-term graft function. Kidney Int. 2006;69(9):1683–90.
160. Millán O, Budde K, Sommerer C, Aliart I, Rissling O, Bardaji B, et al. Urinary miR-155-5p and CXCL10 as prognostic and predictive biomarkers of rejection, graft outcome and treatment response in kidney transplantation. Br J Clin Pharmacol. 2017;83(12):2636–50.
161. Raza A, Firasat S, Khaliq S, Aziz T, Mubarak M, Naqvi SA, et al. The association of urinary interferon-gamma inducible protein-10 (IP10/CXCL10) levels with kidney allograft rejection. Inflamm Res. 2017;66(5):425–32.
162. Hirt-Minkowski P, Amico P, Ho J, Gao A, Bestland J, Hopfer H, et al. Detection of clinical and subclinical tubulo-interstitial inflammation by the urinary CXCL10 chemokine in a real-life setting. Am J Transplant. 2012;12(7):1811–23.
163. Hirt-Minkowski P, Rush DN, Gao A, Hopfer H, Wiebe C, Nickerson PW, et al. Six-month urinary CCL2 and CXCL10 levels predict long-term renal allograft outcome. Transplantation. 2016;100(9):1988–96.
164. Mühlbacher J, Doberer K, Kozakowski N, Regele H, Camovic S, Haindl S, et al. Non-invasive chemokine detection: improved prediction of antibody-mediated rejection in donor-specific antibody-positive renal allograft recipients. Front Med. 2020;7:114.
165. Schaub S, Hirsch HH, Dickenmann M, Steiger J, Mihatsch MJ, Hopfer H, et al. Reducing immunosuppression preserves allograft function in presumptive and definitive polyomavirus-associated nephropathy. Am J Transplant. 2010;10(12):2615–23.
166. Handschin J, Hirt-Minkowski P, Hönger G, Mitrovic S, Savic Prince S, Ho J, et al. Technical considerations and confounders for urine CXCL10 chemokine measurement. Transplant Direct. 2020;6(1):e519.
167. Weseslindtner L, Hedman L, Wang Y, Strassl R, Helanterä I, Aberle SW, et al. Longitudinal assessment of the CXCL10 blood and urine concentration in kidney transplant recipients with BK polyomavirus replication—a retrospective study. Transpl Int. 2020;33(5):555–66.
168. Blydt-Hansen T, Sharma A, Gibson IW, Wiebe C, Sharma AP, Langlois V, et al. Validity and utility of urinary CXCL10/Cr immune monitoring in pediatric kidney transplant recipients. Am J Transplant. 2021;21(4):1545–55.
169. Ho J, Rush DN, Karpinski M, Storsley L, Gibson IW, Bestland J, et al. Validation of urinary CXCL10 as a marker of borderline, subclinical, and clinical tubulitis. Transplantation. 2011;92(8):878–82.

170. Blydt-Hansen TD, Gibson IW, Gao A, Dufault B, Ho J. Elevated urinary CXCL10-to-creatinine ratio is associated with subclinical and clinical rejection in pediatric renal transplantation. Transplantation. 2015;99(4):797–804.
171. Schaub S, Nickerson P, Rush D, Mayr M, Hess C, Golian M, et al. Urinary CXCL9 and CXCL10 levels correlate with the extent of subclinical tubulitis. Am J Transplant. 2009;9(6):1347–53.
172. Mockler C, Sharma A, Gibson IW, Gao A, Wong A, Ho J, et al. The prognostic value of urinary chemokines at 6 months after pediatric kidney transplantation. Pediatr Transplant. 2018;22(5):e13205.
173. Blydt-Hansen TD, Sharma A, Gibson IW, Wishart DS, Mandal R, Ho J, et al. Urinary metabolomics for noninvasive detection of antibody-mediated rejection in children after kidney transplantation. Transplantation. 2017;101(10):2553.
174. Archdekin B, Sharma A, Gibson IW, Rush D, Wishart DS, Blydt-Hansen TD. Non-invasive differentiation of non-rejection kidney injury from acute rejection in pediatric renal transplant recipients. Pediatr Transplant. 2019;23(3):e13364.
175. Landsberg A, Sharma A, Gibson IW, Rush D, Wishart DS, Blydt-Hansen TD. Non-invasive staging of chronic kidney allograft damage using urine metabolomic profiling. Pediatr Transplant. 2018;22(5):e13226.
176. Bassi R, Niewczas MA, Biancone L, Bussolino S, Merugumala S, Tezza S, et al. Metabolomic profiling in individuals with a failing kidney allograft. PLoS One. 2017;12(1):e0169077.
177. Sigdel TK, Schroeder AW, Yang JYC, Sarwal RD, Liberto JM, Sarwal MM. Targeted urine metabolomics for monitoring renal allograft injury and immunosuppression in pediatric patients. J Clin Med. 2020;9(8):2341.
178. Ho J, Sharma A, Mandal R, Wishart DS, Wiebe C, Storsley L, et al. Detecting renal allograft inflammation using quantitative urine metabolomics and CXCL10. Transplant Direct. 2016;2(6):e78.
179. Bloom RD, Bromberg JS, Poggio ED, Bunnapradist S, Langone AJ, Sood P, et al. Cell-free DNA and active rejection in kidney allografts. J Am Soc Nephrol. 2017;28(7):2221–32.
180. Knight SR, Thorne A, Faro MLL. Donor-specific cell-free DNA as a biomarker in solid organ transplantation. A systematic review. Transplantation. 2019;103(2):273–83.
181. Xiao H, Gao F, Pang Q, Xia Q, Zeng X, Peng J, et al. Diagnostic accuracy of donor-derived cell-free DNA in renal-allograft rejection: a meta-analysis. Transplantation. 2020; https://doi.org/10.1097/TP.0000000000003443.
182. Crew RJ, Khairallah P, Husain SA. Cell-free DNA: proceed, but with caution. J Am Soc Nephrol. 2020; https://doi.org/10.1681/ASN.2020060915.
183. Stoltz D, Brubaker A, Grskovic M, Woodward R, Gallo A, editors. Donor-derived cell-free DNA parallels increases in donor specific antibodies in pediatric kidney transplant recipients. Am J Transplant; 2017, Wiley, Hoboken.
184. Stoltz D, Brubaker A, Grskovic M, Woodward R, Gallo A, editors. Donor-derived cell-free DNA predicts biopsy-proven acute cellular rejection in pediatric kidney transplant recipients. Am J Transplant; 2017, Wiley, Hoboken.
185. Bobanga ID, Vogt BA, Woodside KJ, Cote DR, Dell KM, Cunningham RJ 3rd, et al. Outcome differences between young children and adolescents undergoing kidney transplantation. J Pediatr Surg. 2015;50(6):996–9.
186. Lepeytre F, Dahhou M, Zhang X, Boucquemont J, Sapir-Pichhadze R, Cardinal H, et al. Association of sex with risk of kidney graft failure differs by age. J Am Soc Nephrol. 2017;28(10):3014–23.
187. Smith JM, Martz K, Blydt-Hansen TD. Pediatric kidney transplant practice patterns and outcome benchmarks, 1987-2010: a report of the North American Pediatric Renal Trials and Collaborative Studies. Pediatr Transplant. 2013;17(2):149–57.
188. Boucquemont J, Pai ALH, Dharnidharka VR, Hebert D, Furth SL, Foster BJ. Gender differences in medication adherence among adolescent and young adult kidney transplant recipients. Transplantation. 2019;103(4):798–806.

189. Tan JC, Wadia PP, Coram M, Grumet FC, Kambham N, Miller K, et al. HY antibody development associates with acute rejection in female patients with male kidney transplants. Transplantation. 2008;86(1):75.
190. Gratwohl A, Döhler B, Stern M, Opelz G. HY as a minor histocompatibility antigen in kidney transplantation: a retrospective cohort study. Lancet. 2008;372(9632):49–53.
191. Mifsud NA, Purcell AW, Chen W, Holdsworth R, Tait BD, McCluskey J. Immunodominance hierarchies and gender bias in direct TCD8-cell alloreactivity. Am J Transplant. 2008;8(1):121–32.
192. Selmi C. The X in sex: how autoimmune diseases revolve around sex chromosomes. Best Pract Res Clin Rheumatol. 2008;22(5):913–22.
193. Andreoni KA, Forbes R, Andreoni RM, Phillips G, Stewart H, Ferris M. Age-related kidney transplant outcomes: health disparities amplified in adolescence. JAMA Intern Med. 2013;173(16):1524–32.
194. Smith JM, Ho P, McDonald RA. Renal transplant outcomes in adolescents: a report of the North American Pediatric Renal Transplant Cooperative Study. Pediatr Transplant. 2002;6(6):493–9.
195. Chinnakotla S, Verghese P, Chavers B, Rheault MN, Kirchner V, Dunn T, et al. Outcomes and risk factors for graft loss: lessons learned from 1,056 pediatric kidney transplants at the University of Minnesota. J Am Coll Surg. 2017;224(4):473–86.
196. West LJ. B-cell tolerance following ABO-incompatible infant heart transplantation. Transplantation. 2006;81(3):301–7.
197. West LJ, Pollock-Barziv SM, Dipchand AI, Lee KJ, Cardella CJ, Benson LN, et al. ABO-incompatible heart transplantation in infants. N Engl J Med. 2001;344(11):793–800.
198. West LJ, Pollock-Barziv SM, Lee KJ, Dipchand AI, Coles JG, Ruiz P. Graft accommodation in infant recipients of ABO-incompatible heart transplants: donor ABH antigen expression in graft biopsies. J Heart Lung Transplant. 2001;20(2):222.
199. Ettenger RB, Blifeld C, Prince H, Gradus DB-E, Cho S, Sekiya N, et al. The pediatric nephrologist's dilemma: growth after renal transplantation and its interaction with age as a possible immunologic variable. J Pediatr. 1987;111(6):1022–5.
200. Scornik JC, Pfaff WW, Howard RJ, Fennell RS, Ramos E, Peterson JC, et al. Increased antibody responsiveness to blood transfusions in pediatric patients. Transplantation. 1994;58(12):1361–5.
201. Shearer WT, Rosenblatt HM, Gelman RS, Oyomopito R, Plaeger S, Stiehm ER, et al. Lymphocyte subsets in healthy children from birth through 18 years of age: the pediatric AIDS clinical trials group P1009 study. J Allergy Clin Immunol. 2003;112(5):973–80.
202. Bartlett JA, Schleifer SJ, Demetrikopoulos MK, Delaney BR, Shiflett SC, Keller SE. Immune function in healthy adolescents. Clin Diagn Lab Immunol. 1998;5(1):105–13.
203. Wikby A, Mansson IA, Johansson B, Strindhall J, Nilsson SE. The immune risk profile is associated with age and gender: findings from three Swedish population studies of individuals 20-100 years of age. Biogerontology. 2008;9(5):299–308.
204. Weng NP. Aging of the immune system: how much can the adaptive immune system adapt? Immunity. 2006;24(5):495–9.
205. Klein SL, Marriott I, Fish EN. Sex-based differences in immune function and responses to vaccination. Trans R Soc Trop Med Hyg. 2015;109(1):9–15.
206. Malek SK, Keys BJ, Kumar S, Milford E, Tullius SG. Racial and ethnic disparities in kidney transplantation. Transpl Int. 2011;24(5):419–24.
207. Kasiske BL, Neylan JF, Riggio RR, Danovitch GM, Kahana L, Alexander SR, et al. The effect of race on access and outcome in transplantation. N Engl J Med. 1991;324(5):302–7.
208. Roberts JP, Wolfe RA, Bragg-Gresham JL, Rush SH, Wynn JJ, Distant DA, et al. Effect of changing the priority for HLA matching on the rates and outcomes of kidney transplantation in minority groups. N Engl J Med. 2004;350(6):545–51.
209. Kaur K, Jun D, Grodstein E, Singer P, Castellanos L, Teperman L, et al. Outcomes of underweight, overweight, and obese pediatric kidney transplant recipients. Pediatr Nephrol. 2018;33(12):2353–62.

210. Ladhani M, Lade S, Alexander SI, Baur LA, Clayton PA, McDonald S, et al. Obesity in pediatric kidney transplant recipients and the risks of acute rejection, graft loss and death. Pediatr Nephrol. 2017;32(8):1443–50.
211. Winnicki E, Dharmar M, Tancredi DJ, Nguyen S, Butani L. Effect of BMI on allograft function and survival in pediatric renal transplant recipients. Pediatr Nephrol. 2018;33(8):1429–35.
212. Tanaci N, Karakose H, Guvener N, Tutuncu NB, Colak T, Haberal M. Influence of 1,25-dihydroxyvitamin D3 as an immunomodulator in renal transplant recipients: a retrospective cohort study. Transplant Proc. 2003;35(8):2885–7.
213. Cianciolo G, Galassi A, Capelli I, Angelini ML, La Manna G, Cozzolino M. Vitamin D in kidney transplant recipients: mechanisms and therapy. Am J Nephrol. 2016;43(6):397–407.
214. Guillot X, Semerano L, Saidenberg-Kermanac'h N, Falgarone G, Boissier M-C. Vitamin D and inflammation. Joint Bone Spine. 2010;77(6):552–7.
215. Nguyen MT, Fryml E, Sahakian SK, Liu S, Cantarovich M, Lipman M, et al. Pretransplant recipient circulating CD4+CD127lo/− tumor necrosis factor receptor 2+ regulatory T cells: a surrogate of regulatory T cell-suppressive function and predictor of delayed and slow graft function after kidney transplantation. Transplantation. 2016;100(2):314–24.
216. Nguyen M-T, Sahakian S, Liu S, Wang Y, Tchervenkov J, Paraskevas S. Pre-transplant circulating TNFR2+ regulatory T cells predict acute rejection within the first 6 months after kidney transplantation. Am J Transplant. 2017;17(suppl 3)., Wiley, Hoboken.
217. San Segundo D, Millan O, Munoz-Cacho P, Boix F, Paz-Artal E, Talayero P, et al. High proportion of pretransplantation activated regulatory T cells (CD4+CD25highCD62L+CD45RO+) predicts acute rejection in kidney transplantation: results of a multicenter study. Transplantation. 2014;98(11):1213–8.
218. Haouami Y, Dhaouadi T, Sfar I, Bacha M, Gargah T, Bardi R, et al. The role of IL-23/IL-17 axis in human kidney allograft rejection. J Leukoc Biol. 2018;104(6):1229–39.
219. Millan O, Rafael-Valdivia L, San Segundo D, Boix F, Castro-Panete MJ, Lopez-Hoyos M, et al. Should IFN-gamma, IL-17 and IL-2 be considered predictive biomarkers of acute rejection in liver and kidney transplant? Results of a multicentric study. Clin Immunol. 2014;154(2):141–54.
220. Tullius SG, Tran H, Guleria I, Malek SK, Tilney NL, Milford E. The combination of donor and recipient age is critical in determining host Immunoresponsiveness and renal transplant outcome. Ann Surg. 2010;252(4):662–74.
221. de Fijter JW, Mallat MJ, Doxiadis II, Ringers J, Rosendaal FR, Claas FH, et al. Increased immunogenicity and cause of graft loss of old donor kidneys. J Am Soc Nephrol. 2001;12(7):1538–46.
222. Hricik DE, Poggio ED, Woodside KJ, Sarabu N, Sanchez EQ, Schulak JA, et al. Effects of cellular sensitization and donor age on acute rejection and graft function after deceased-donor kidney transplantation. Transplantation. 2013;95(10):1254–8.
223. Lebranchu Y, Baan C, Biancone L, Legendre C, Morales JM, Naesens M, et al. Pretransplant identification of acute rejection risk following kidney transplantation. Transpl Int. 2014;27(2):129–38.
224. Karpinski M, Pochinco D, Dembinski I, Laidlaw W, Zacharias J, Nickerson P. Leukocyte reduction of red blood cell transfusions does not decrease allosensitization rates in potential kidney transplant candidates. J Am Soc Nephrol. 2004;15(3):818–24.
225. Dunn TB, Noreen H, Gillingham K, Maurer D, Ozturk OG, Pruett TL, et al. Revisiting traditional risk factors for rejection and graft loss after kidney transplantation. Am J Transplant. 2011;11(10):2132–43.
226. Wiebe C, Gibson IW, Blydt-Hansen TD, Karpinski M, Ho J, Storsley LJ, et al. Evolution and clinical pathologic correlations of de novo donor-specific HLA antibody post kidney transplant. Am J Transplant. 2012;12(5):1157–67.
227. Redondo-Pachón D, Pérez-Sáez MJ, Mir M, Gimeno J, Llinás L, García C, et al. Impact of persistent and cleared preformed HLA DSA on kidney transplant outcomes. Hum Immunol. 2018;79(6):424–31.

228. Maruyama M, Kenmochi T, Saigo K, Akutsu N, Iwashita C, Ohtsuki K, et al. Acute cellular rejection occurring on the first day after living-related renal transplantation: a case report. Clin Transpl. 2006;20:38–41.
229. Zhu L, Fu C, Lin K, Wang Z, Guo H, Chen S, et al. Patterns of early rejection in renal retransplantation: a single-center experience. J Immunol Res. 2016;2016:2697860.
230. Heeger PS, Greenspan NS, Kuhlenschmidt S, Dejelo C, Hricik DE, Schulak JA, et al. Pretransplant frequency of donor-specific, IFN-gamma-producing lymphocytes is a manifestation of immunologic memory and correlates with the risk of posttransplant rejection episodes. J Immunol (1950). 1999;163(4):2267–75.
231. Nickel P, Presber F, Bold G, Biti D, Schonemann C, Tullius SG, et al. Enzyme-linked immunosorbent spot assay for donor-reactive interferon-gamma-producing cells identifies T-cell presensitization and correlates with graft function at 6 and 12 months in renal-transplant recipients. Transplantation. 2004;78(11):1640–6.
232. Kim S, Oh E, Kim M, Park Y, Han K, Yang H, et al., editors. Pretransplant donor-specific interferon-γ ELISPOT assay predicts acute rejection episodes in renal transplant recipients. Transplant Proc. 2007;39(10):3057–60, Elsevier.
233. Kim Y, Park K-H, Chung BH, Choi B-S, Yang CW, Kim J-I, et al. Pretransplant IFN-γ ELISPOT assay as a potential screening test to select immunosuppression protocols for patients receiving basiliximab induction therapy. Transl Res. 2012;160(3):230–6.
234. Gandolfini I, Crespo E, Baweja M, Jarque M, Donadei C, Luque S, et al. Impact of preformed T-cell alloreactivity by means of donor-specific and panel of reactive T cells (PRT) ELISPOT in kidney transplantation. PLoS One. 2018;13(7):e0200696.
235. Bestard O, Crespo E, Stein M, Lucia M, Roelen D, de Vaal Y, et al. Cross-validation of IFN-γ Elispot assay for measuring alloreactive memory/effector T cell responses in renal transplant recipients. Am J Transplant. 2013;13(7):1880–90.
236. Crespo E, Lucia M, Cruzado JM, Luque S, Melilli E, Manonelles A, et al. Pre-transplant donor-specific T-cell alloreactivity is strongly associated with early acute cellular rejection in kidney transplant recipients not receiving T-cell depleting induction therapy. PLoS One. 2015;10(2):e0117618.
237. Hricik DE, Rodriguez V, Riley J, Bryan K, Tary-Lehmann M, Greenspan N, et al. Enzyme linked immunosorbent spot (ELISPOT) assay for interferon-gamma independently predicts renal function in kidney transplant recipients. Am J Transplant. 2003;3(7):878–84.
238. Augustine JJ, Siu DS, Clemente MJ, Schulak JA, Heeger PS, Hricik DE. Pre-transplant IFN-gamma ELISPOTs are associated with post-transplant renal function in African American renal transplant recipients. Am J Transplant. 2005;5(8):1971–5.
239. Crespo M, Heidt S, Redondo D, Pascual J. Monitoring B cell subsets and alloreactivity in kidney transplantation. Transplant Rev. 2015;29(2):45–52.
240. Lúcia M, Luque S, Crespo E, Melilli E, Cruzado JM, Martorell J, et al. Preformed circulating HLA-specific memory B cells predict high risk of humoral rejection in kidney transplantation. Kidney Int. 2015;88(4):874–87.
241. Sanfilippo F, Vaughn WK, Spees EK, Light JA, LeFor WM. Benefits of HLA-A and HLA-B matching on graft and patient outcome after cadaveric-donor renal transplantation. N Engl J Med. 1984;311(6):358–64.
242. Foster BJ, Dahhou M, Zhang X, Platt RW, Smith JM, Hanley JA. Impact of HLA mismatch at first kidney transplant on lifetime with graft function in young recipients. Am J Transplant. 2014;14(4):876–85.
243. Hardy BE, Shah T, Cicciarelli J, Lemley KV, Hutchinson IV, Cho YW. Kidney transplantation in children and adolescents: an analysis of United Network for Organ Sharing Database. Transplant Proc. 2009;41(5):1533–5.
244. Wiebe C, Nevins TE, Robiner WN, Thomas W, Matas AJ, Nickerson P. The synergistic effect of class II HLA epitope-mismatch and nonadherence on acute rejection and graft survival. Am J Transplant. 2015;15(8):2197–202.

245. Vu LT, Baxter-Lowe LA, Garcia J, McEnhill M, Summers P, Hirose R, et al. HLA-DR matching in organ allocation: balance between waiting time and rejection in pediatric kidney transplantation. Arch Surg (Chicago 1960). 2011;146(7):824–9.
246. Wiebe C, Pochinco D, Blydt-Hansen TD, Ho J, Birk PE, Karpinski M, et al. Class II HLA epitope matching-a strategy to minimize De novo donor-specific antibody development and improve outcomes. Am J Transplant. 2013;13(12):3114–22.
247. Shi X, Lv J, Han W, Zhong X, Xie X, Su B, et al. What is the impact of human leukocyte antigen mismatching on graft survival and mortality in renal transplantation? A meta-analysis of 23 cohort studies involving 486,608 recipients. BMC Nephrol. 2018;19(1):116–0.
248. Tagliamacco A, Cioni M, Comoli P, Ramondetta M, Brambilla C, Trivelli A, et al. DQ molecules are the principal stimulators of de novo donor-specific antibodies in nonsensitized pediatric recipients receiving a first kidney transplant. Transpl Int. 2014;27(7):667–73.
249. DeVos JM, Gaber AO, Knight RJ, Land GA, Suki WN, Gaber LW, et al. Donor-specific HLA-DQ antibodies may contribute to poor graft outcome after renal transplantation. Kidney Int. 2012;82(5):598–604.
250. Leeaphorn N, Pena JRA, Thamcharoen N, Khankin EV, Pavlakis M, Cardarelli F. HLA-DQ mismatching and kidney transplant outcomes. Clin J Am Soc Nephrol. 2018;13(5):763–71.
251. Lim WH, Chapman JR, Coates PT, Lewis JR, Russ GR, Watson N, et al. HLA-DQ mismatches and rejection in kidney transplant recipients. Clin J Am Soc Nephrol. 2016;11(5):875–83.
252. Bryan CF, Chadha V, Warady BA. Donor selection in pediatric kidney transplantation using DR and DQ eplet mismatching: a new histocompatibility paradigm. Pediatr Transplant. 2016;20(7):926–30.
253. Kausman JY, Walker AM, Cantwell LS, Quinlan C, Sypek MP, Ierino FL. Application of an epitope-based allocation system in pediatric kidney transplantation. Pediatr Transplant. 2016;20(7):931–8.
254. Van Arendonk KJ, Boyarsky BJ, Orandi BJ, James NT, Smith JM, Colombani PM, et al. National trends over 25 years in pediatric kidney transplant outcomes. Pediatrics. 2014;133(4):594–601.
255. Grenda R. Delayed graft function and its management in children. Pediatr Nephrol. 2017;32(7):1157–67.
256. do Nascimento Ghizoni Pereira L, Tedesco-Silva H Jr, Koch-Nogueira PC. Acute rejection in pediatric renal transplantation: Retrospective study of epidemiology, risk factors, and impact on renal function. Pediatr Transplant. 2020;25:e13856.
257. Wu WK, Famure O, Li Y, Kim SJ. Delayed graft function and the risk of acute rejection in the modern era of kidney transplantation. Kidney Int. 2015;88(4):851–8.
258. Weber S, Dienemann T, Jacobi J, Eckardt KU, Weidemann A. Delayed graft function is associated with an increased rate of renal allograft rejection: a retrospective single center analysis. PLoS One. 2018;13(6):e0199445.
259. Mogulla MR, Bhattacharjya S, Clayton PA. Risk factors for and outcomes of delayed graft function in live donor kidney transplantation – a retrospective study. Transplant Int. 2019;32(11):1151–60.
260. Yarlagadda SG, Coca SG, Formica RN Jr, Poggio ED, Parikh CR. Association between delayed graft function and allograft and patient survival: a systematic review and meta-analysis. Nephrol Dial Transplant. 2009;24(3):1039–47.
261. Lauronen J, Peräsaari JP, Saarinen T, Jaatinen T, Lempinen M, Helanterä I. Shorter cold ischemia time in deceased donor kidney transplantation reduces the incidence of delayed graft function especially among highly sensitized patients and kidneys from older donors. Transplant Proc. 2020;52(1):42–9.
262. Larkins N, Matsell DG. Tacrolimus therapeutic drug monitoring and pediatric renal transplant graft outcomes. Pediatr Transplant. 2014;18(8):803–9.
263. Wiebe C, Rush DN, Nevins TE, Birk PE, Blydt-Hansen T, Gibson IW, et al. Class II Eplet mismatch modulates tacrolimus trough levels required to prevent donor-specific antibody development. J Am Soc Nephrol. 2017;28(11):3353–62.

264. Kiberd BA, Lawen J, Fraser AD, Keough-Ryan T, Belitsky P. Early adequate mycophenolic acid exposure is associated with less rejection in kidney transplantation. Am J Transplant. 2004;4(7):1079–83.
265. Bunnapradist S, Lentine KL, Burroughs TE, Pinsky BW, Hardinger KL, Brennan DC, et al. Mycophenolate mofetil dose reductions and discontinuations after gastrointestinal complications are associated with renal transplant graft failure. Transplantation. 2006;82(1):102–7.
266. Alexopoulos E, Papadimitriou M, Reinke P, Volk H-D. Late-acute renal allograft rejection and symptomless cytomegalovirus infection. Lancet. 1995;345(8952):794.
267. Babel N, Schwarzmann F, Prang N, Jaeger M, Wolf H, Kern F, et al. Association between Epstein-Barr virus infection and late acute transplant rejection in long-term transplant patients. Transplantation. 2001;72(4):736–9.
268. Paulsen G, Cumagun P, Mixon E, Fowler K, Feig D, Shimamura M. Cytomegalovirus and Epstein-Barr virus infections among pediatric kidney transplant recipients at a center using universal Valganciclovir Prophylaxis. Pediatr Transplant. 2019;23:e13382.
269. Allen UD, Preiksaitis JK, Practice ASTIDCo. Epstein-Barr virus and posttransplant lymphoproliferative disorder in solid organ transplantation. Am J Transplant. 2013;13(Suppl 4):107–20.
270. Hirsch HH, Randhawa PS. BK polyomavirus in solid organ transplantation-guidelines from the American Society of Transplantation Infectious Diseases Community of Practice. Clin Transpl. 2019;33(9):e13528.
271. Borchers AT, Perez R, Kaysen G, Ansari AA, Gershwin ME. Role of cytomegalovirus infection in allograft rejection: a review of possible mechanisms. Transpl Immunol. 1999;7(2):75–82.
272. Martin-Gandul C, Mueller NJ, Pascual M, Manuel O. The impact of infection on chronic allograft dysfunction and allograft survival after solid organ transplantation. Am J Transplant. 2015;15(12):3024–40.
273. Stranavova L, Pelak O, Svaton M, Hruba P, Fronkova E, Slavcev A, et al. Heterologous cytomegalovirus and Allo-reactivity by shared t-cell receptor repertoire in kidney transplantation. Front Immunol. 2019;10:2549.
274. Burrows S, Khanna R, Burrows J, Moss D. An alloresponse in humans is dominated by cytotoxic T lymphocytes (CTL) cross-reactive with a single Epstein-Barr virus CTL epitope: implications for graft-versus-host disease. J Exp Med. 1994;179(4):1155–61.
275. Gaston JS, Rickinson AB, Epstein MA. Cross-reactivity of self-HLA-restricted Epstein-Barr virus-specific cytotoxic T lymphocytes for Allo-HLA determinants. J Exp Med. 1983;158(6):1804–21.
276. Zeng G, Huang Y, Huang Y, Lyu Z, Lesniak D, Randhawa P. Antigen-specificity of T cell infiltrates in biopsies with T cell–mediated rejection and BK polyomavirus viremia: analysis by next generation sequencing. Am J Transplant. 2016;16(11):3131–8.
277. Dobbels F, Ruppar T, De Geest S, Decorte A, Van Damme-Lombaerts R, Fine R. Adherence to the immunosuppressive regimen in pediatric kidney transplant recipients: a systematic review. Pediatr Transplant. 2010;14(5):603–13.
278. Butler JA, Roderick P, Mullee M, Mason JC, Peveler RC. Frequency and impact of nonadherence to immunosuppressants after renal transplantation: a systematic review. Transplantation. 2004;77(5):769–76.
279. Weng FL, Chandwani S, Kurtyka KM, Zacker C, Chisholm-Burns MA, Demissie K. Prevalence and correlates of medication non-adherence among kidney transplant recipients more than 6 months post-transplant: a cross-sectional study. BMC Nephrol. 2013;14(1):261.
280. Bullington P, Pawola L, Walker R, Valenta A, Briars L, John E. Identification of medication non-adherence factors in adolescent transplant patients: the patient's viewpoint. Pediatr Transplant. 2007;11(8):914–21.
281. Foulkes L-M, Boggs SR, Fennell RS, Skibinski K. Social support, family variables, and complicance in renal transplant children. Pediatr Nephrol. 1993;7(2):185–8.
282. Shaw RJ, Palmer L, Blasey C, Sarwal M. A typology of non-adherence in pediatric renal transplant recipients. Pediatr Transplant. 2003;7(6):489–93.

283. Dobbels F, Damme-Lombaert RV, Vanhaecke J, Geest SD. Growing pains: non-adherence with the immunosuppressive regimen in adolescent transplant recipients. Pediatr Transplant. 2005;9(3):381–90.
284. Morrissey P, Reinert S, Yango A, Gautam A, Monaco A, Gohh R, editors. Factors contributing to acute rejection in renal transplantation: the role of noncompliance. Transplant Proc; 2005; 37(5):2044-2047: Elsevier.
285. Lerut E, Kuypers DR, Verbeken E, Cleutjens J, Vlaminck H, Vanrenterghem Y, et al. Acute rejection in non-compliant renal allograft recipients: a distinct morphology. Clin Transpl. 2007;21(3):344–51.
286. Hsiau M, Fernandez HE, Gjertson D, Ettenger RB, Tsai EW. Monitoring nonadherence and acute rejection with variation in blood immunosuppressant levels in pediatric renal transplantation. Transplantation. 2011;92(8):918–22.
287. Gaston R, Hudson S, Ward M, Jones P, Macon R. Late renal allograft loss: noncompliance masquerading as chronic rejection. Transplant Proc. 1999;31(4A):21S–3S.
288. Pollock-BarZiv SM, Finkelstein Y, Manlhiot C, Dipchand AI, Hebert D, Ng VL, et al. Variability in tacrolimus blood levels increases the risk of late rejection and graft loss after solid organ transplantation in older children. Pediatr Transplant. 2010;14(8):968–75.
289. Vanhove T, Vermeulen T, Annaert P, Lerut E, Kuypers DR. High intrapatient variability of tacrolimus concentrations predicts accelerated progression of chronic histologic lesions in renal recipients. Am J Transplant. 2016;16(10):2954–63.
290. Solomon S, Colovai A, Del Rio M, Hayde N. Tacrolimus variability is associated with de novo donor-specific antibody development in pediatric renal transplant recipients. Pediatr Nephrol. 2020;35(2):261–70.
291. Simons LE, McCormick ML, Mee LL, Blount RL. Parent and patient perspectives on barriers to medication adherence in adolescent transplant recipients. Pediatr Transplant. 2009;13(3):338–47.
292. Zelikovsky N, Schast AP, Palmer J, Meyers KE. Perceived barriers to adherence among adolescent renal transplant candidates. Pediatr Transplant. 2008;12(3):300–8.
293. Srivastava K, Arora A, Kataria A, Cappelleri JC, Sadosky A, Peterson AM. Impact of reducing dosing frequency on adherence to oral therapies: a literature review and meta-analysis. Patient Prefer Adherence. 2013;7:419.
294. Min S-I, Ha J, Kang HG, Ahn S, Park T, Park D, et al. Conversion of twice-daily tacrolimus to once-daily tacrolimus formulation in stable pediatric kidney transplant recipients: pharmacokinetics and efficacy. Am J Transplant. 2013;13(8):2191–7.
295. Sabbatini M, Garofalo G, Borrelli S, Vitale S, Torino M, Capone D, et al. Efficacy of a reduced pill burden on therapeutic adherence to calcineurin inhibitors in renal transplant recipients: an observational study. Patient Prefer Adherence. 2014;8:73.
296. Foster BJ, Pai ALH, Zelikovsky N, Amaral S, Bell L, Dharnidharka VR, et al. A randomized trial of a multicomponent intervention to promote medication adherence: the teen adherence in kidney transplant effectiveness of intervention trial (TAKE-IT). Am J Kidney Dis. 2018;72(1):30–41.
297. Kissmeyer-Nielsen F, Olsen S, Petersen VP, Fjeldborg O. Hyperacute rejection of kidney allografts, associated with pre-existing humoral antibodies against donor cells. Lancet. 1966;288(7465):662–5.
298. Williams GM, Hume DM, Hudson RP Jr, Morris PJ, Kano K, Milgrom F. Hyperacute renal-homograft rejection in man. N Engl J Med. 1968;279(12):611–8.
299. Meena J, Sinha A, Hari P, Dinda AK, Khandelwal P, Goswami S, et al. Pediatric kidney transplantation: experience over two decades. Asian J Pediatr Nephrol. 2018;1(1):22.
300. Racusen LC, Solez K, Colvin RB, Bonsib SM, Castro MC, Cavallo T, et al. The Banff 97 working classification of renal allograft pathology. Kidney Int. 1999;55(2):713–23.
301. Loupy A, Haas M, Roufosse C, Naesens M, Adam B, Afrouzian M, et al. The Banff 2019 kidney meeting report (I): updates on and clarification of criteria for T cell- and antibody-mediated rejection. Am J Transplant. 2020;20(9):2318–31.

302. Roufosse C, Simmonds N, Clahsen-van Groningen M, Haas M, Henriksen KJ, Horsfield C, et al. A 2018 reference guide to the Banff classification of renal allograft pathology. Transplantation. 2018;102(11):1795–814.
303. Becker J, Chang A, Nickeleit V, Randhawa P, Roufosse C. Banff borderline changes suspicious for acute T cell–mediated rejection: where do we stand? Am J Transplant. 2016;16(9):2654–60.
304. Nankivell BJ, Agrawal N, Sharma A, Taverniti A, P'Ng CH, Shingde M, et al. The clinical and pathological significance of borderline T cell–mediated rejection. Am J Transplant. 2019;19(5):1452–63.
305. Masin-Spasovska J, Spasovski G, Dzikova S, Petrusevska G, Dimova B, Lekovski L, et al. The evolution of untreated borderline and subclinical rejections at first month kidney allograft biopsy in comparison with histological changes at 6 months protocol biopsies. Prilozi. 2005;26(1):25.
306. Mehta RB, Tandukar S, Jorgensen D, Randhawa P, Sood P, Puttarajappa C, et al. Early subclinical tubulitis and interstitial inflammation in kidney transplantation have adverse clinical implications. Kidney Int. 2020;98(2):436–47.
307. Dale LA, Brennan C, Batal I, Morris H, Jain NG, Valeri A, et al. Treatment of borderline infiltrates with minimal inflammation in kidney transplant recipients has no effect on allograft or patient outcomes. Clin Transpl. 2020;34(9):e14019.
308. Nankivell BJ, P'Ng CH, Chapman JR. Does tubulitis without interstitial inflammation represent borderline acute T cell mediated rejection? Am J Transplant. 2019;19(1):132–44.
309. Rhen T, Cidlowski JA. Antiinflammatory action of glucocorticoids — new mechanisms for old drugs. N Engl J Med. 2005;353(16):1711–23.
310. Mathian A, Jouenne R, Chader D, Cohen-Aubart F, Haroche J, Fadlallah J, et al. Regulatory T cell responses to high-dose methylprednisolone in active systemic lupus erythematosus. PLoS One. 2015;10(12):e0143689.
311. Alarcon-Zurita A, Ladefoged J. Treatment of acute allograft rejection with high doses of corticosteroids. Kidney Int. 1976;9(4):351–4.
312. Orta-Sibu N, Chantler C, Bewick M, Haycock G. Comparison of high-dose intravenous methylprednisolone with low-dose oral prednisolone in acute renal allograft rejection in children. Br Med J (Clin Res Ed). 1982;285(6337):258–60.
313. Kauffman JH, Stromstad S, Sampson D, Stawicki A, editors. Randomized steroid therapy of human kidney transplant rejection. Transplant Proc. 1979;11(1):36–8.
314. Stromstad S, Kauffman H, Sampson D, Stawicki A, editors. Randomized steroid therapy of human kidney transplant rejection. Surg Forum. 1978;29:376–7.
315. De Backer D, Abramowicz D, De Pauw L, Viseur P, Vanherweghem J, Kinnaert P, et al. High or low dose steroid therapy for acute renal transplant rejection after prophylactic OKT3 treatment: a prospective randomized study. Transplant Int. 1992;5:437–9.
316. Lui S, Sweny P, Scoble J, Varghese Z, Moorhead J, Fernando O. Low-dose vs high-dose intravenous methylprednisolone therapy for acute renal allograft rejection in patients receiving cyclosporin therapy. Nephrol Dial Transplant. 1989;4(5):387–9.
317. Feduska NJ, Turcotte JG, Gikas PW, Bacon GE, Penner JA. Reversal of renal allograft rejection with intravenous methylprednisolone "pulse" therapy. J Surg Res. 1972;12(3):208–15.
318. Gray D, Daar A, Shepherd H, Oliver D, Morris P. Oral versus intravenous high-dose steroid treatment of renal allograft rejection: the big shot or not? Lancet. 1978;311(8056):117–8.
319. Mussche M, Ringoir S, Lameire N. High intravenous doses of methylprednisolone for acute cadaveric renal allograft rejection. Nephron. 1976;16(4):287–91.
320. Mittal R, Agarwal S, Dash S, Saxena S, Tiwari S, Mehta S, et al. Clinical profile and course and outcome of late acute rejection episodes in living-related-donor renal allograft recipients. Nephron. 1995;71(1):40–3.
321. Lamarche C, Côté J-M, Sénécal L, Cardinal H. Efficacy of acute cellular rejection treatment according to Banff score in kidney transplant recipients: a systematic review. Transplant Direct. 2016;2(12):e115.

322. Mazzucchi E, Lucon AM, Nahas WC, Neto ED, de Castro MCR, Saldanha LB, et al. Histologic outcome of acute cellular rejection in kidney transplantation after treatment with methylprednisolone. Transplant Proc. 2000;32(4):784–5.
323. Chen J, Liverman R, Garro R, Jernigan S, Travers C, Winterberg PD. Acute cellular rejection treatment outcomes stratified by Banff grade in pediatric kidney transplant. Pediatr Transplant. 2019;23(2):e13334.
324. Leblanc J, Subrt P, Pare M, Hartell D, Senecal L, Blydt-Hansen T, et al. Practice patterns in the treatment and monitoring of acute T cell-mediated kidney graft rejection in Canada. Can J Kidney Health Dis. 2018;5:2054358117753616.
325. Uslu A, Nart A. Treatment of first acute rejection episode: systematic review of level I evidence. Transplant Proc. 2011;43(3):841–6, Elsevier.
326. Gaber AO, First MR, Tesi RJ, Gaston RS, Mendez R, Mulloy LL, et al. Results of the double-blind, randomized, multicenter, phase iii clinical trial of thymoglobulin versus Atgam in the treatment of acute graft rejection episodes after renal transplantation. Transplantation. 1998;66(1):29–37.
327. Hoitsma AJ, Reekers P, Kreeftenberg JG, van Lier HJ, Capel PJ, Koene RA. Treatment of acute rejection of cadaveric renal allografts with rabbit antithymocyte globulin. Transplantation. 1982;33(1):12–6.
328. Hoitsma AJ, van Lier HJ, Reekers P, Koene RA. Improved patient and graft survival after treatment of acute rejections of cadaveric renal allografts with rabbit antithymocyte globulin. Transplantation. 1985;39(3):274–9.
329. Theodorakis J, Schneeberger H, Illner W, Stangl M, Zanker B, Land W. Aggressive treatment of the first acute rejection episode using first-line anti-lymphocytic preparation reduces further acute rejection episodes after human kidney transplantation. Transpl Int. 1998;11(1):S86–S9.
330. Streem SB, Novick AC, Braun WE, Steinmuller D, Greenstreet R. Low-dose maintenance prednisone and antilymphoblast globulin for the treatment of acute rejection. A steroid-sparing approach to immunosuppressive therapy. Transplantation. 1983;35(5):420–4.
331. Webster AC, Wu S, Tallapragada K, Park MY. Polyclonal and monoclonal antibodies for treating acute rejection episodes in kidney transplant recipients. Cochrane Database Syst Rev. 2017;7:CD004756.
332. Shinn C, Malhotra D, Chan L, Cosby RL, Shapiro JI. Time course of response to pulse methylprednisolone therapy in renal transplant recipients with acute allograft rejection. Am J Kidney Dis. 1999;34(2):304–7.
333. Bamoulid J, Staeck O, Crépin T, Halleck F, Saas P, Brakemeier S, et al. Anti-thymocyte globulins in kidney transplantation: focus on current indications and long-term immunological side effects. Nephrol Dial Transplant. 2016;32(10):1601–8.
334. Cooper JE. Evaluation and treatment of acute rejection in kidney allografts. Clin J Am Soc Nephrol. 2020;15(3):430–8.
335. Lye W, Vathsala A, Lee W, Leong S, editors. Low-dose OKT3 is not effective in the treatment of steroid-resistant acute renal allograft rejections. Transplant Proc. 1998;30(7):3106–7.
336. Davies S, Brown E, Woodrow D, Phillips M, Gower P. The high failure rate of OKT3 in the treatment of acute renal allograft rejection resistant to steroids with or without antithymocyte globulin. Transplantation. 1991;52(4):746–9.
337. Kainz A, Korbély R, Soleiman A, Mayer B, Oberbauer R. Antithymocyte globulin use for treatment of biopsy confirmed acute rejection is associated with prolonged renal allograft survival. Transpl Int. 2010;23(1):64–70.
338. Mariat C, Alamartine E, Diab N, de Filippis JP, Laurent B, Berthoux F. A randomized prospective study comparing low-dose OKT3 to low-dose ATG for the treatment of acute steroid-resistant rejection episodes in kidney transplant recipients. Transpl Int. 1998;11(3):231–6.
339. Bloom DD, Hu H, Fechner JH, Knechtle SJ. T-lymphocyte alloresponses of Campath-1H-treated kidney transplant patients. Transplantation. 2006;81(1):81–7.
340. Basu A, Ramkumar M, Tan H, Khan A, McCauley J, Marcos A, et al., editors. Reversal of acute cellular rejection after renal transplantation with Campath-1H. Transplant Proc. 2005;37(2):923–6, Elsevier.

341. Van Der Zwan M, Groningen C-V, Marian C, van den Hoogen MW, Kho MM, Roodnat JI, et al. Comparison of alemtuzumab and anti-thymocyte globulin treatment for acute kidney allograft rejection. Front Immunol. 2020;11:1332.
342. Van den Hoogen M, Hesselink D, Van Son W, Weimar W, Hilbrands L. Treatment of steroid-resistant acute renal allograft rejection with alemtuzumab. Am J Transplant. 2013;13(1):192–6.
343. Csapo Z, Benavides-Viveros C, Podder H, Pollard V, Kahan B, editors. Campath-1H as rescue therapy for the treatment of acute rejection in kidney transplant patients. Transplantat Proc. 2005;37(5):2032–6, Elsevier.
344. Magliocca JF, Knechtle SJ. The evolving role of alemtuzumab (Campath-1H) for immunosuppressive therapy in organ transplantation. Transpl Int. 2006;19(9):705–14.
345. Clatworthy MR, Friend PJ, Calne RY, Rebello PRU, Hale G, Waldmann H, et al. Alemtuzumab (CAMPATH-1H) for the treatment of acute rejection in kidney transplant recipients: Long-term follow-up. Transplantation. 2009;87(7):1092–5.
346. Sijpkens YW, Doxiadis II, Van Kemenade FJ, Zwinderman AH, De Fijter JW, Claas FH, et al. Chronic rejection with or without transplant vasculopathy. Clin Transpl. 2003;17(3):163–70.
347. Kunchala R, Gudipati A, Guditi S, Taduri G, Raju S, Uppin M. Late acute rejection in renal allografts: clinical, pathologic, and follow-up data from a single tertiary care center. Indian J Transplant. 2018;12(1):48–52.
348. Massy ZA, Guijarro C, Kasiske BL. Clinical predictors of chronic renal allograft rejection. Kidney Int Suppl. 1995;52:S85.
349. Wu O, Levy AR, Briggs A, Lewis G, Jardine A. Acute rejection and chronic nephropathy: a systematic review of the literature. Transplantation. 2009;87(9):1330–9.
350. Tejani A, Sullivan EK. The impact of acute rejection on chronic rejection: a report of the North American Pediatric Renal Transplant Cooperative Study. Pediatr Transplant. 2000;4(2):107–11.
351. Randhawa P. T-cell-mediated rejection of the kidney in the era of donor-specific antibodies: diagnostic challenges and clinical significance. Curr Opin Organ Transplant. 2015;20(3):325–32.
352. Okada M, Kamei K, Matsuoka K, Ito S. Development of antibody mediated rejection shortly after acute cellular rejection in a pediatric kidney transplantation recipient. CEN Case Rep. 2018;7(2):288–91.
353. Lefaucheur C, Loupy A, Vernerey D, Duong-Van-Huyen J-P, Suberbielle C, Anglicheau D, et al. Antibody-mediated vascular rejection of kidney allografts: a population-based study. Lancet. 2013;381(9863):313–9.
354. Dörje C, Midtvedt K, Holdaas H, Naper C, Strøm EH, Øyen O, et al. Early versus late acute antibody-mediated rejection in renal transplant recipients. Transplantation. 2013;96(1):79–84.
355. Halloran P, Merino Lopez M, Barreto PA. Identifying subphenotypes of antibody-mediated rejection in kidney transplants. Am J Transplant. 2016;16(3):908–20.
356. Charnaya O, Tuchman S, Moudgil A. Results of early treatment for de novo donor-specific antibodies in pediatric kidney transplant recipients in a cross-sectional and longitudinal cohort. Pediatr Transplant. 2018;22(2):e13108.
357. Cherukuri A, Mehta R, Sharma A, Sood P, Zeevi A, Tevar AD, et al. Post-transplant donor specific antibody is associated with poor kidney transplant outcomes only when combined with both T-cell–mediated rejection and non-adherence. Kidney Int. 2019;96(1):202–13.
358. Jiqiu W, Jinsong C, Dongrui C, MingChao Z, Shuming J, Zhi-Hong L. CD20+ B-cell infiltration is related to the time after transplant and poor prognosis of acute cellular rejection in renal transplant. Exp Clin Transplant. 2013;11:412–7.
359. Zarkhin V, Kambham N, Li L, Kwok S, Hsieh S-C, Salvatierra O, et al. Characterization of intra-graft B cells during renal allograft rejection. Kidney Int. 2008;74(5):664–73.
360. Lu Y, Li B, Shen Q, Wang R, Chen Z, Jiang H, et al. Effects of CD20+ B-cell infiltration into allografts on kidney transplantation outcomes: a systematic review and meta-analysis. Oncotarget. 2017;8(23):37935.

361. Tsai EW, Rianthavorn P, Gjertson DW, Wallace WD, Reed EF, Ettenger RB. CD20+ lymphocytes in renal allografts are associated with poor graft survival in pediatric patients. Transplantation. 2006;82(12):1769–73.
362. Desvaux D, Le Gouvello S, Pastural M, Abtahi M, Suberbielle C, Boeri N, et al. Acute renal allograft rejections with major interstitial oedema and plasma cell-rich infiltrates: high γ-interferon expression and poor clinical outcome. Nephrol Dial Transplant. 2004;19(4):933–9.
363. Dufek S, Khalil A, Mamode N, Sebire NJ, Marks SD. Plasma-cell-rich infiltrates in paediatric renal transplant biopsies are associated with increased risk of renal allograft failure. Pediatr Nephrol. 2017;32(4):679–84.
364. Zarkhin V, Chalasani G, Sarwal MM. The yin and yang of B cells in graft rejection and tolerance. Transplant Rev. 2010;24(2):67–78.
365. Alausa M, Almagro U, Siddiqi N, Zuiderweg R, Medipalli R, Hariharan S. Refractory acute kidney transplant rejection with CD20 graft infiltrates and successful therapy with rituximab. Clin Transpl. 2005;19(1):137–40.
366. Lehnhardt A, Mengel M, Pape L, Ehrich J, Offner G, Strehlau J. Nodular B-cell aggregates associated with treatment refractory renal transplant rejection resolved by rituximab. Am J Transplant. 2006;6(4):847–51.
367. Vega J, Goecke H, Carrasco A, Escobar C, Escobar M, Espinosa R, et al. Rituximab in the treatment of acute cellular rejection of renal allograft with CD20-positive clusters in the infiltrate. Clin Exp Nephrol. 2011;15(2):308–11.
368. Steinmetz OM, Lange-Hüsken F, Turner J-E, Vernauer A, Helmchen U, Stahl RAK, et al. Rituximab removes intrarenal B cell clusters in patients with renal vascular allograft rejection. Transplantation. 2007;84(7):842–50.
369. Zarkhin V, Li L, Kambham N, Sigdel T, Salvatierra O, Sarwal M. A randomized, prospective trial of rituximab for acute rejection in pediatric renal transplantation. Am J Transplant. 2008;8(12):2607–17.
370. Zarkhin V, Lovelace PA, Li L, Hsieh S-C, Sarwal MM. Phenotypic evaluation of B-cell subsets after rituximab for treatment of acute renal allograft rejection in pediatric recipients. Transplantation. 2011;91(9):1010–8.
371. Abbas K, Mubarak M, Zafar MN, Aziz T, Abbas H, Muzaffar R, et al. Plasma cell-rich acute rejections in living-related kidney transplantation: a clinicopathological study of 50 cases. Clin Transpl. 2015;29(9):835–41.
372. Alhamoud I, Huang R, Lacelle C, Burguete D, Hendricks AR, Torrealba JR, et al. Allograft outcomes of treated children with kidney transplant who developed plasma cell-rich acute rejection (PCAR): a single center's experience. Pediatr Transplant. 2019;23(6):e13500.
373. Hasegawa J, Honda K, Omoto K, Wakai S, Shirakawa H, Okumi M, et al. Clinical and pathological features of plasma cell-rich acute rejection after kidney transplantation. Transplantation. 2018;102(5):853–9.
374. Adrogue HE, Soltero L, Land GA, Ramanathan V, Truong LD, Suki WN. Immunoglobulin therapy for plasma cell-rich rejection in the renal allograft. Transplantation. 2006;82(4):567–9.
375. Lara EP, García EH, Fuentes MCR, Molina MC, Guindo MCDG, Ortega AO, editors. Plasma cell-rich acute rejection in renal transplantation: a case report. Transplantation Proceedings. 2020;52(2):512–4, Elsevier.
376. Hill GS, Nochy D, Bruneval P, Duong van Huyen JP, Glotz D, Suberbielle C, et al. Donor-specific antibodies accelerate arteriosclerosis after kidney transplantation. J Am Soc Nephrol. 2011;22(5):975–83.
377. Gloor JM, Sethi S, Stegall MD, Park WD, Moore SB, DeGoey S, et al. Transplant glomerulopathy: subclinical incidence and association with alloantibody. Am J Transplant. 2007;7(9):2124–32.
378. Einecke G, Sis B, Reeve J, Mengel M, Campbell PM, Hidalgo LG, et al. Antibody-mediated microcirculation injury is the major cause of late kidney transplant failure. Am J Transplant. 2009;9(11):2520–31.

379. Kim J, Balasubramanian R, Michaelides G, Wittenhagen P, Sebire N, Mamode N, et al. The clinical spectrum of de novo donor-specific antibodies in pediatric renal transplant recipients. Am J Transplant. 2014;14(10):2350–8.
380. Wiebe C, Kosmoliaptsis V, Pochinco D, Gibson IW, Ho J, Birk PE, et al. HLA-DR/DQ molecular mismatch: a prognostic biomarker for primary alloimmunity. Am J Transplant. 2019;19(6):1708–19.
381. Haas M, Mirocha J, Reinsmoen NL, Vo AA, Choi J, Kahwaji JM, et al. Differences in pathologic features and graft outcomes in antibody-mediated rejection of renal allografts due to persistent/recurrent versus de novo donor-specific antibodies. Kidney Int. 2017;91(3):729–37.
382. Marfo K, Lu A, Ling M, Akalin E. Desensitization protocols and their outcome. Clin J Am Soc Nephrol. 2011;6(4):922–36.
383. Kwon H, Kim YH, Choi JY, Shin S, Jung JH, Park SK, et al. Impact of pretransplant donor-specific antibodies on kidney allograft recipients with negative flow cytometry cross-matches. Clin Transpl. 2018;32(6):e13266.
384. Adebiyi OO, Gralla J, Klem P, Freed B, Davis S, Wiseman AC, et al. Clinical significance of pretransplant donor-specific antibodies in the setting of negative cell-based flow cytometry crossmatching in kidney transplant recipients. Am J Transplant. 2016;16(12):3458–67.
385. Kwon H, Kim YH, Kim JY, Choi JY, Shin S, Jung JH, et al. The results of HLA-incompatible kidney transplantation according to pre-transplant crossmatch tests: donor-specific antibody as a prominent predictor of acute rejection. Clin Transpl. 2019;33(5):e13533.
386. Twombley K, Thach L, Ribeiro A, Joseph C, Seikaly M. Acute antibody-mediated rejection in pediatric kidney transplants: a single center experience. Pediatr Transplant. 2013;17(7):E149–E55.
387. Gulleroglu K, Baskin E, Bayrakci US, Turan M, Ozdemir BH, Moray G, et al. Antibody-mediated rejection and treatment in pediatric patients: one center's experience. Exp Clin Transplant. 2013;11(5):404–7.
388. Bagnasco SM, Zachary AA, Racusen LC, Arend LJ, Carter-Monroe N, Alachkar N, et al. Time course of pathologic changes in kidney allografts of positive crossmatch HLA-incompatible transplant recipients. Transplantation. 2014;97(4):440–5.
389. Velidedeoglu E, Cavaillé-Coll MW, Bala S, Belen OA, Wang Y, Albrecht R. Summary of 2017 FDA public workshop: antibody-mediated rejection in kidney transplantation. Transplantation. 2018;102(6):e257–e64.
390. Schinstock CA, Mannon RB, Budde K, Chong AS, Haas M, Knechtle S, et al. Recommended treatment for antibody-mediated rejection after kidney transplantation: the 2019 expert consensus from the Transplantion Society Working Group. Transplantation. 2020;104(5):911–22.
391. Wan SS, Ying TD, Wyburn K, Roberts DM, Wyld M, Chadban SJ. The treatment of antibody-mediated rejection in kidney transplantation: an updated systematic review and meta-analysis. Transplantation. 2018;102(4):557–68.
392. Simon HU, Späth PJ. IVIG – mechanisms of action. Allergy. 2003;58(7):543–52.
393. Slatinska J, Honsova E, Burgelova M, Slavcev A, Viklicky O. Plasmapheresis and intravenous immunoglobulin in early antibody-mediated rejection of the renal allograft: a single-center experience. Ther Apher Dial. 2009;13(2):108–12.
394. Ibernon M, Gil-Vernet S, Carrera M, Seron D, Moreso F, Bestard O, et al., editors. Therapy with plasmapheresis and intravenous immunoglobulin for acute humoral rejection in kidney transplantation. Transplant Proc. 2005;37(9):3743–5, Elsevier.
395. Suaywan K, Nimkietkajorn V, Luesutthiviboon L. Intensive plasmapheresis and intravenous immunoglobulin for treatment of antibody-mediated rejection after kidney transplant. Exp Clin Transplant. 2014;4:328–33.
396. Montgomery RA, Zachary AA, Racusen LC, Leffell MS, King KE, Burdick J, et al. Plasmapheresis and intravenous immune globulin provides effective rescue therapy for refractory humoral rejection and allows kidneys to be successfully transplanted into cross-match-positive recipients. Transplantation. 2000;70(6):887–95.
397. Gubensek J, Buturovic-Ponikvar J, Kandus A, Arnol M, Kovac J, Marn-Pernat A, et al., editors. Plasma exchange and intravenous immunoglobulin in the treatment of antibody-mediated

rejection after kidney transplantation: a single-center historic cohort study. Transplantation Proceedings. 2013;45(4):1524–7, Elsevier.
398. Brown C, Abraham K, O'Kelly P, Conlon P, Walshe J, editors. Long-term experience of plasmapheresis in antibody-mediated rejection in renal transplantation. Transplant Proc. 2009;41(9):3690–2, Elsevier.
399. Macklin PS, Morris PJ, Knight SR. A systematic review of the use of rituximab for the treatment of antibody-mediated renal transplant rejection. Transplant Rev. 2017;31(2):87–95.
400. Sautenet B, Blancho G, Büchler M, Morelon E, Toupance O, Barrou B, et al. One-year results of the effects of rituximab on acute antibody-mediated rejection in renal transplantation: RITUX ERAH, a multicenter double-blind randomized placebo-controlled trial. Transplantation. 2016;100(2):391–9.
401. Bailly E, Ville S, Blancho G, Morelon E, Bamoulid J, Caillard S, et al. An extension of the RITUX-ERAH study, multicenter randomized clinical trial comparing rituximab to placebo in acute antibody-mediated rejection after renal transplantation. Transpl Int. 2020;33(7):786–95.
402. Ahmadi F, Dashti-Khavidaki S, Khatami M, Gatmiri M, Ahmadi F, Mahdavi-Mazdeh M, et al. Comparing plasmapheresis plus IVIg with plasmapheresis plus IVIg plus rituximab on the management of suspicious antibody-mediated acute rejection in kidney transplant recipients. Int J Organ Transplant Med. 2019;10(3):127.
403. Immenschuh S, Zilian E, Dämmrich ME, Schwarz A, Gwinner W, Becker JU, et al. Indicators of treatment responsiveness to rituximab and plasmapheresis in antibody-mediated rejection after kidney transplantation. Transplantation. 2015;99(1):56–62.
404. Waiser J, Duerr M, Schönemann C, Rudolph B, Wu K, Halleck F, et al. Rituximab in combination with bortezomib, plasmapheresis, and high-dose IVIG to treat antibody-mediated renal allograft rejection. Transplant Direct. 2016;2(8):e91.
405. Gulleroglu K, Baskin E, Moray G, Ozdemir H, Arslan H, Haberal M. Rituximab therapy and infection risk in pediatric renal transplant patients. Exp Clin Transplant. 2016;14(2):172–5.
406. Scemla A, Loupy A, Candon S, Mamzer M-F, Martinez F, Zuber J, et al. Incidence of infectious complications in highly sensitized renal transplant recipients treated by rituximab: a case-controlled study. Transplantation. 2010;90(11):1180–4.
407. Baskin E, Gulleroglu K, Bayrakci U, Aktas S, Moray G, Ozdemir H, et al. Rituximab therapy and infection risk in pediatric renal transplant patients: 1899. Transplantation. 2012;94(10S):73.
408. De Sousa-Amorim E, Revuelta I, Diekmann F, Cofan F, Lozano M, Cid J, et al. Bortezomib for refractory acute antibody-mediated rejection in kidney transplant recipients: a single-Centre case series. Nephrology. 2016;21(8):700–4.
409. Roberti I, Vyas S. Successful treatment of severe acute antibody-mediated rejection of renal allografts with bortezomib–a report of two pediatric cases. Pediatr Transplant. 2015;19(8):E189–E92.
410. Gupta G, Jawdeh BGA, Racusen LC, Bhasin B, Arend LJ, Trollinger B, et al. Late antibody-mediated rejection in renal allografts: outcome after conventional and novel therapies. Transplantation. 2014;97(12):1240–6.
411. Nigos JG, Arora S, Nath P, Hussain SM, Marcus RJ, Ko TY, et al. Treatment of antibody-mediated rejection in kidney transplant recipients: a single-center experience with a bortezomib-based regimen. Exp Clin Transplant. 2012;10(6):609–13.
412. Méndez JB, LLY L, Díaz MS, Curiel IT, Galindo-Lopéz R, Córdova AB, et al., editors. Antibody-mediated rejection treatment with bortezomib in renal transplant recipients: a single-center 24-month follow-up case report. Transplant Proc. 2020;52(4):1123–6, Elsevier.
413. Kolonko A, Słabiak-Błaż N, Karkoszka H, Więcek A, Piecha G. The preliminary results of Bortezomib used as a primary treatment for An early acute antibody-mediated rejection after kidney transplantation-a single-center case series. J Clin Med. 2020;9(2):529.
414. Kizilbash S, Claes D, Ashoor I, Chen A, Jandeska S, Matar RB, et al. Bortezomib in the treatment of antibody-mediated rejection in pediatric kidney transplant recipients: a multicenter Midwest Pediatric Nephrology Consortium study. Pediatr Transplant. 2017;21(3):e12873.

415. Waiser J, Budde K, Schütz M, Liefeldt L, Rudolph B, Schönemann C, et al. Comparison between bortezomib and rituximab in the treatment of antibody-mediated renal allograft rejection. Nephrol Dial Transplant. 2012;27(3):1246–51.
416. Abbas K, Mubarak M, Zafar MN, Musharraf W, Imam M, Aziz T, et al. Management of plasma cell-rich acute rejection in living-related kidney transplant: role of proteasome inhibitor. Exp Clin Transplant. 2019;17(1):42–6.
417. Tasaki M, Saito K, Nakagawa Y, Ikeda M, Imai N, Ito Y, et al., editors. Bortezomib eliminates plasma cells from a renal graft in plasma cell–rich acute rejection. Transplant Proc. 2019;51(6):1732–8, Elsevier.
418. Pearl MH, Nayak AB, Ettenger RB, Puliyanda D, Diaz MFP, Zhang Q, et al. Bortezomib may stabilize pediatric renal transplant recipients with antibody-mediated rejection. Pediatr Nephrol. 2016;31(8):1341–8.
419. Nguyen S, Gallay B, Butani L. Efficacy of bortezomib for reducing donor-specific antibodies in children and adolescents on a steroid minimization regimen. Pediatr Transplant. 2014;18(5):463–8.
420. Walsh RC, Brailey P, Girnita A, Alloway RR, Shields AR, Wall GE, et al. Early and late acute antibody-mediated rejection differ immunologically and in response to proteasome inhibition. Transplantation. 2011;91(11):1218–26.
421. Flechner SM, Fatica R, Askar M, Stephany BR, Poggio E, Koo A, et al. The role of proteasome inhibition with bortezomib in the treatment of antibody-mediated rejection after kidney-only or kidney-combined organ transplantation. Transplantation. 2010;90(12):1486–92.
422. Lee J, Kim BS, Park Y, Lee JG, Lim BJ, Jeong HJ, et al. The effect of Bortezomib on antibody-mediated rejection after kidney transplantation. Yonsei Med J. 2015;56(6):1638–42.
423. Eskandary F, Regele H, Baumann L, Bond G, Kozakowski N, Wahrmann M, et al. A randomized trial of bortezomib in late antibody-mediated kidney transplant rejection. J Am Soc Nephrol. 2018;29(2):591–605.
424. Tan EK, Bentall A, Dean PG, Shaheen MF, Stegall MD, Schinstock CA. Use of eculizumab for active antibody-mediated rejection that occurs early post–kidney transplantation: a consecutive series of 15 cases. Transplantation. 2019;103(11):2397–404.
425. Chehade H, Rotman S, Matter M, Girardin E, Aubert V, Pascual M. Eculizumab to treat antibody-mediated rejection in a 7-year-old kidney transplant recipient. Pediatrics (Evanston). 2015;135(2):e551–e5.
426. Haas M. Eculizumab as primary therapy for active antibody-mediated rejection of renal allografts: a matter of timing, severity, and donor-specific antibodies. Transplantation. 2019;103(11):2219–20.
427. Orandi BJ, Zachary AA, Dagher NN, Bagnasco SM, Garonzik-Wang JM, Van Arendonk KJ, et al. Eculizumab and splenectomy as salvage therapy for severe antibody-mediated rejection after HLA-incompatible kidney transplantation. Transplantation. 2014;98(8):857–63.
428. Montgomery RA, Orandi BJ, Racusen L, Jackson AM, Garonzik-Wang JM, Shah T, et al. Plasma-derived C1 esterase inhibitor for acute antibody-mediated rejection following kidney transplantation: results of a randomized double-blind placebo-controlled pilot study. Am J Transplant. 2016;16(12):3468–78.
429. Viglietti D, Gosset C, Loupy A, Deville L, Verine J, Zeevi A, et al. C1 inhibitor in acute antibody-mediated rejection nonresponsive to conventional therapy in kidney transplant recipients: a pilot study. Am J Transplant. 2016;16(5):1596–603.
430. Pottebaum AA, Venkatachalam K, Liu C, Brennan DC, Murad H, Malone AF, et al. Efficacy and safety of tocilizumab in the treatment of acute active antibody-mediated rejection in kidney transplant recipients. Transplant Direct. 2020;6(4):e543.
431. Caillard S, Becmeur C, Gautier-Vargas G, Olagne J, Muller C, Cognard N, et al. Pre-existing donor-specific antibodies are detrimental to kidney allograft only when persistent after transplantation. Transpl Int. 2017;30(1):29–40.
432. Sai K, Omoto K, Shimizu T, Honda K, Tanabe K. The impact of C4d-negative acute antibody-mediated rejection on short-term prognosis among kidney transplant recipients. Nephrology (Carlton). 2015;20(Suppl 2):16–9.

433. Matas AJ, Fieberg A, Mannon RB, Leduc R, Grande J, Kasiske BL, et al. Long-term follow-up of the DeKAF cross-sectional cohort study. Am J Transplant. 2019;19(5):1432–43.
434. Orandi BJ, Alachkar N, Kraus ES, Naqvi F, Lonze BE, Lees L, et al. Presentation and outcomes of C4d-negative antibody-mediated rejection after kidney transplantation. Am J Transplant. 2016;16(1):213–20.
435. Loupy A, Hill GS, Suberbielle C, Charron D, Anglicheau D, Zuber J, et al. Significance of C4d Banff scores in early protocol biopsies of kidney transplant recipients with preformed donor-specific antibodies (DSA). Am J Transplant. 2011;11(1):56–65.
436. Matignon M, Muthukumar T, Seshan SV, Suthanthiran M, Hartono C. Concurrent acute cellular rejection is an independent risk factor for renal allograft failure in patients with C4d-positive antibody-mediated rejection. Transplantation. 2012;94(6):603–11.
437. Okada M, Tomosugi T, Futamura K, Hiramitsu T, Goto N, Narumi S, et al. Mid-term outcomes after treatment for antibody-mediated rejection by De novo donor-specific HLA antibody in renal transplant recipients: does early treatment lead to better outcomes? Transplant Proc. 2020;52(10):3051–7.
438. Everly MJ, Everly JJ, Arend LJ, Brailey P, Susskind B, Govil A, et al. Reducing de novo donor-specific antibody levels during acute rejection diminishes renal allograft loss. Am J Transplant. 2009;9(5):1063–71.
439. Lefaucheur C, Nochy D, Hill G, Suberbielle-Boissel C, Antoine C, Charron D, et al. Determinants of poor graft outcome in patients with antibody-mediated acute rejection. Am J Transplant. 2007;7(4):832–41.
440. Rafiq MA, De Boccardo G, Schröppel B, Bromberg JS, Sehgal V, Dinavahi R, et al. Differential outcomes in 3 types of acute antibody-mediated rejection. Clin Transpl. 2009;23(6):951–7.
441. Zachary AA, Montgomery RA, Leffell MS. Factors associated with and predictive of persistence of donor-specific antibody after treatment with plasmapheresis and intravenous immunoglobulin. Hum Immunol. 2005;66(4):364–70.
442. Touzot M, Couvrat-Desvergnes G, Castagnet S, Cesbron A, Renaudin K, Cantarovich D, et al. Differential modulation of donor-specific antibodies after B-cell depleting therapies to cure chronic antibody mediated rejection. Transplantation. 2015;99(1):63–8.
443. Zhang R. Donor-specific antibodies in kidney transplant recipients. Clin J Am Soc Nephrol. 2018;13(1):182–92.
444. Schwartz GJ, Munoz A, Schneider MF, Mak RH, Kaskel F, Warady BA, et al. New equations to estimate GFR in children with CKD. J Am Soc Nephrol. 2009;20(3):629–37.
445. Mannon RB, Matas AJ, Grande J, Leduc R, Connett J, Kasiske B, et al. Inflammation in areas of tubular atrophy in kidney allograft biopsies: a potent predictor of allograft failure. Am J Transplant. 2010;10(9):2066–73.
446. Halloran PF, Matas A, Kasiske BL, Madill-Thomsen KS, Mackova M, Famulski KS. Molecular phenotype of kidney transplant indication biopsies with inflammation in scarred areas. Am J Transplant. 2019;19(5):1356–70.
447. Helgeson ES, Mannon R, Grande J, Gaston RS, Cecka MJ, Kasiske BL, et al. I-IFTA and chronic active T cell-mediated rejection: a tale of 2 (DeKAF) cohorts. Am J Transplant. 2020; https://doi.org/10.1111/ajt.16352.
448. Cosio FG, Grande JP, Wadei H, Larson TS, Griffin MD, Stegall MD. Predicting subsequent decline in kidney allograft function from early surveillance biopsies. Am J Transplant. 2005;5(10):2464–72.
449. Loupy A, Haas M, Solez K, Racusen L, Glotz D, Seron D, et al. The Banff 2015 kidney meeting report: current challenges in rejection classification and prospects for adopting molecular pathology. Am J Transplant. 2017;17(1):28–41.
450. Matas AJ, Leduc R, Rush D, Cecka JM, Connett J, Fieberg A, et al. Histopathologic clusters differentiate subgroups within the nonspecific diagnoses of CAN or CR: preliminary data from the DeKAF study. Am J Transplant. 2010;10(2):315–23.
451. Mengel M, Reeve J, Bunnag S, Einecke G, Jhangri GS, Sis B, et al. Scoring total inflammation is superior to the current Banff inflammation score in predicting outcome and the degree of molecular disturbance in renal allografts. Am J Transplant. 2009;9(8):1859–67.

452. Chen J, Li L, Wen J, Tang Z, Ji S, Sha G, et al. Observation of efficacy and safety of converting the calcineurin inhibitor to sirolimus in renal transplant recipients with chronic allograft nephropathy. Transplant Proc. 2008;40(5):1411–5.
453. Das U, Dakshinamurty KV. Safety and efficacy of everolimus in chronic allograft nephropathy. Saudi J Kidney Dis Transplant. 2013;24(5):910–6.
454. de Sandes-Freitas TV, Felipe CR, Campos ÉF, de Lima MG, Soares MF, de Franco MF, et al. Subclinical lesions and donor-specific antibodies in kidney transplant recipients receiving tacrolimus-based immunosuppressive regimen followed by early conversion to sirolimus. Transplantation. 2015;99(11):2372–81.
455. Heilman RL, Cortese C, Geiger XJ, Younan K, Wadei HM, Mai ML, et al. Impact of early conversion from tacrolimus to sirolimus on chronic allograft changes in kidney recipients on rapid steroid withdrawal. Transplantation. 2012;93(1):47–53.
456. Pankewycz O, Leca N, Kohli R, Weber-Shrikant E, Said M, Alnimri M, et al. Conversion to low-dose tacrolimus or rapamycin 3 months after kidney transplantation: a prospective, protocol biopsy-guided study. Transplant Proc. 2011;43(2):519–23.
457. Uslu A, Töz H, Sen S, Alkan FT, Nart A, Aykas A, et al. Late conversion from calcineurin inhibitor-based to sirolimus-based immunosuppression due to chronic toxicity: a prospective study with protocol biopsy amendment. Transplant Proc. 2009;41(2):756–63.
458. Abramowicz D, Hadaya K, Hazzan M, Broeders N, Hoang AD, Ghisdal L, et al. Conversion to sirolimus for chronic renal allograft dysfunction: risk factors for graft loss and severe side effects. Nephrol Dial Transplant. 2008;23(11):3727–9.
459. Liew A, Chiang GS, Vathsala A. Factors associated with proteinuria in renal transplant recipients treated with sirolimus. Transpl Int. 2009;22(3):313–22.
460. Gong N, Chen Z, Wang J, Fang A, Li Y, Xiang Y, et al. Immunoregulatory effects of sirolimus vs. tacrolimus treatment in kidney allograft recipients. Cell Immunol. 2015;297(2):87–93.
461. Sijpkens YW, Joosten SA, Wong MC, Dekker FW, Benediktsson H, Bajema IM, et al. Immunologic risk factors and glomerular C4d deposits in chronic transplant glomerulopathy. Kidney Int. 2004;65(6):2409–18.
462. Redfield RR, Ellis TM, Zhong W, Scalea JR, Zens TJ, Mandelbrot D, et al. Current outcomes of chronic active antibody mediated rejection – a large single center retrospective review using the updated BANFF 2013 criteria. Hum Immunol. 2016;77(4):346–52.
463. Sablik KA, Clahsen-van Groningen MC, Damman J, Roelen DL, Betjes MGH. Banff lesions and renal allograft survival in chronic-active antibody mediated rejection. Transpl Immunol. 2019;56:101213.
464. Aubert O, Higgins S, Bouatou Y, Yoo D, Raynaud M, Viglietti D, et al. Archetype analysis identifies distinct profiles in renal transplant recipients with transplant glomerulopathy associated with allograft survival. J Am Soc Nephrol. 2019;30(4):625–39.
465. Abreu R, Carvalho F, Viana H, Mesquita I, Possante M, Aires I, et al. Morphologic patterns and treatment of transplant glomerulopathy: a retrospective analysis. Clin Transplant. 2017;31(4) https://doi.org/10.1111/ctr.12915.
466. Gourishankar S, Leduc R, Connett J, Cecka JM, Cosio F, Fieberg A, et al. Pathological and clinical characterization of the 'troubled transplant': data from the DeKAF study. Am J Transplant. 2010;10(2):324–30.
467. Stegall MD, Cornell LD, Park WD, Smith BH, Cosio FG. Renal allograft histology at 10 years after transplantation in the tacrolimus era: evidence of pervasive chronic injury. Am J Transplant. 2018;18(1):180–8.
468. Myslak M, Amer H, Morales P, Fidler ME, Gloor JM, Larson TS, et al. Interpreting post-transplant proteinuria in patients with proteinuria pre-transplant. Am J Transplant. 2006;6(7):1660–5.
469. Knoll GA. Proteinuria in kidney transplant recipients: prevalence, prognosis, and evidence-based management. Am J Kidney Dis. 2009;54:1131–44.
470. Amer H, Fidler ME, Myslak M, Morales P, Kremers WK, Larson TS, et al. Proteinuria after kidney transplantation, relationship to allograft histology and survival. Am J Transplant. 2007;7(12):2748–56.

471. Grodsky JD, Craver RD, Ashoor IF. Early identification of transplant glomerulopathy in pediatric kidney transplant biopsies: a single-center experience with electron microscopy analysis. Pediatr Transplant. 2019;23(5):e13459.
472. Torres IB, Salcedo M, Moreso F, Sellarés J, Castellá E, Azancot MA, et al. Comparing transplant glomerulopathy in the absence of C4d deposition and donor-specific antibodies to chronic antibody-mediated rejection. Clin Transpl. 2014;28(10):1148–54.
473. Issa N, Cosio FG, Gloor JM, Sethi S, Dean PG, Moore SB, et al. Transplant glomerulopathy: risk and prognosis related to anti-human leukocyte antigen class II antibody levels. Transplantation. 2008;86(5):681–5.
474. Loupy A, Suberbielle-Boissel C, Hill GS, Lefaucheur C, Anglicheau D, Zuber J, et al. Outcome of subclinical antibody-mediated rejection in kidney transplant recipients with preformed donor-specific antibodies. Am J Transplant. 2009;9(11):2561–70.
475. Cosio FG, Gloor JM, Sethi S, Stegall MD. Transplant glomerulopathy. Am J Transplant. 2008;8(3):492–6.
476. John R, Konvalinka A, Tobar A, Kim SJ, Reich HN, Herzenberg AM. Determinants of long-term graft outcome in transplant glomerulopathy. Transplantation. 2010;90(7):757–64.
477. Patri P, Seshan SV, Matignon M, Desvaux D, Lee JR, Lee J, et al. Development and validation of a prognostic index for allograft outcome in kidney recipients with transplant glomerulopathy. Kidney Int. 2016;89(2):450–8.
478. Kieran N, Wang X, Perkins J, Davis C, Kendrick E, Bakthavatsalam R, et al. Combination of peritubular c4d and transplant glomerulopathy predicts late renal allograft failure. J Am Soc Nephrol. 2009;20(10):2260–8.
479. Sharif A, Kraus ES, Zachary AA, Lonze BE, Nazarian SM, Segev DL, et al. Histologic phenotype on 1-year posttransplantation biopsy and allograft survival in HLA-incompatible kidney transplants. Transplantation. 2014;97(5):541–7.
480. Billing H, Rieger S, Susal C, Waldherr R, Opelz G, Wuhl E, et al. IVIG and rituximab for treatment of chronic antibody-mediated rejection: a prospective study in paediatric renal transplantation with a 2-year follow-up. Transplant Int. 2012;25(11):1165–73.
481. Billing H, Rieger S, Ovens J, Süsal C, Melk A, Waldherr R, et al. Successful treatment of chronic antibody-mediated rejection with IVIG and rituximab in pediatric renal transplant recipients. Transplantation. 2008;86(9):1214–21.
482. Fehr T, Rusi B, Fischer A, Hopfer H, Wuthrich RP, Gaspert A. Rituximab and intravenous immunoglobulin treatment of chronic antibody-mediated kidney allograft rejection. Transplantation. 2009;87(12):1837–41.
483. An GH, Yun J, Hong YA, Khvan M, Chung BH, Choi BS, et al. The effect of combination therapy with rituximab and intravenous immunoglobulin on the progression of chronic antibody mediated rejection in renal transplant recipients. J Immunol Res. 2014;2014:828732.
484. Bachelet T, Nodimar C, Taupin JL, Lepreux S, Moreau K, Morel D, et al. Intravenous immunoglobulins and rituximab therapy for severe transplant glomerulopathy in chronic antibody-mediated rejection: a pilot study. Clin Transpl. 2015;29(5):439–46.
485. Moreso F, Crespo M, Ruiz JC, Torres A, Gutierrez-Dalmau A, Osuna A, et al. Treatment of chronic antibody mediated rejection with intravenous immunoglobulins and rituximab: a multicenter, prospective, randomized, double-blind clinical trial. Am J Transplant. 2018;18(4):927–35.
486. Kahwaji J, Najjar R, Kancherla D, Villicana R, Peng A, Jordan S, et al. Histopathologic features of transplant glomerulopathy associated with response to therapy with intravenous immune globulin and rituximab. Clin Transpl. 2014;28(5):546–53.
487. Nair P, Gheith O, Al-Otaibi T, Mostafa M, Rida S, Sobhy I, et al. Management of chronic active antibody-mediated rejection in renal transplant recipients: single-center experience. Exp Clin Transplant. 2019;17(Suppl 1):113–9.
488. Piñeiro GJ, De Sousa-Amorim E, Solé M, Ríos J, Lozano M, Cofán F, et al. Rituximab, plasma exchange and immunoglobulins: an ineffective treatment for chronic active antibody-mediated rejection. BMC Nephrol. 2018;19(1):261.

489. Jordan SC, Ammerman N, Choi J, Huang E, Peng A, Sethi S, et al. Novel therapeutic approaches to allosensitization and antibody-mediated rejection. Transplantation. 2019;103(2):262–72.
490. Mayer KA, Doberer K, Eskandary F, Halloran PF, Böhmig GA. New concepts in chronic antibody-mediated kidney allograft rejection: prevention and treatment. Curr Opin Organ Transplant. 2021;26(1):97–105.
491. Jordan SC, Choi J, Kim I, Wu G, Toyoda M, Shin B, et al. Interleukin-6, a cytokine critical to mediation of inflammation, autoimmunity and allograft rejection: therapeutic implications of IL-6 receptor blockade. Transplantation. 2017;101(1):32–44.
492. Choi J, Aubert O, Vo A, Loupy A, Haas M, Puliyanda D, et al. Assessment of tocilizumab (anti-interleukin-6 receptor monoclonal) as a potential treatment for chronic antibody-mediated rejection and transplant glomerulopathy in HLA-sensitized renal allograft recipients. Am J Transplant. 2017;17(9):2381–9.
493. Lavacca A, Presta R, Gai C, Mella A, Gallo E, Camussi G, et al. Early effects of first-line treatment with anti-interleukin-6 receptor antibody tocilizumab for chronic active antibody-mediated rejection in kidney transplantation. Clin Transplant. 2020;34:e13908.
494. Eskandary F, Dürr M, Budde K, Doberer K, Reindl-Schwaighofer R, Waiser J, et al. Clazakizumab in late antibody-mediated rejection: study protocol of a randomized controlled pilot trial. Trials. 2019;20(1):1–13.
495. ClinicalTrials.gov. ClinicalTrials.gov is a database of privately and publicly funded clinical studies conducted around the world.
496. Binet I, Nickeleit V, Hirsch HH, Prince O, Dalquen P, Gudat F, et al. Polyomavirus disease under new immunosuppressive drugs: a cause of renal graft dysfunction and graft loss. Transplantation. 1999;67(6):918–22.
497. Hirsch HH, Vincenti F, Friman S, Tuncer M, Citterio F, Wiecek A, et al. Polyomavirus BK replication in de novo kidney transplant patients receiving tacrolimus or cyclosporine: a prospective, randomized, multicenter study. Am J Transplant. 2013;13(1):136–45.
498. Borni-Duval C, Caillard S, Olagne J, Perrin P, Braun-Parvez L, Heibel F, et al. Risk factors for BK virus infection in the era of therapeutic drug monitoring. Transplantation. 2013;95(12):1498–505.
499. Pham P-TT, Reddy UG. Immunosuppression and risk of polyomavirus BK replication. Nat Rev Nephrol. 2013;9(3):135–6.
500. Lufft V, Kliem V, Behrend M, Pichlmayr R, Koch KM, Brunkhorst R. Incidence of Pneumocystis carinii pneumonia after renal transplantation. Impact of immunosuppression. Transplantation. 1996;62(3):421–3.
501. Smith JM, McDonald RA, Finn LS, Healey PJ, Davis CL, Limaye AP. Polyomavirus nephropathy in pediatric kidney transplant recipients. Am J Transplant. 2004;4(12):2109–17.
502. Schnitzler MA, Lowell JA, Hardinger KL, Boxerman SB, Bailey TC, Brennan DC. The association of cytomegalovirus sero-pairing with outcomes and costs following cadaveric renal transplantation prior to the introduction of oral ganciclovir CMV prophylaxis. Am J Transplant. 2003;3(4):445–51.
503. Jordan CL, Taber DJ, Kyle MO, Connelly J, Pilch NW, Fleming J, et al. Incidence, risk factors, and outcomes of opportunistic infections in pediatric renal transplant recipients. Pediatr Transplant. 2016;20(1):44–8.
504. Kranz B, Vester U, Wingen AM, Nadalin S, Paul A, Broelsch CE, et al. Acute rejection episodes in pediatric renal transplant recipients with cytomegalovirus infection. Pediatr Transplant. 2008;12(4):474–8.
505. Mortari N, Freire M, Azevedo LS, De Paula FJ, Caiaffa-filho H, Nahas W, et al. Risk factors for mortality among kidney transplant recipients with Pneumocystis jirovecii infection. Transplantation. 2018;102(Suppl 7S-1):S361.
506. Borstnar S, Lindic J, Tomazic J, Kandus A, Pikelj A, Prah J, et al. Pneumocystis Jirovecii pneumonia in renal transplant recipients: a National Center Experience. Transplant Proc. 2013;45(4):1614–7.

507. Gordon SM, LaRosa SP, Arroliga AC, Avery RK, Longworth DL. Should prophylaxis for Pneumocystis carinii pneumonia in solid organ transplant recipients ever be discontinued? Clin Infect Dis. 1999;28(2):240–6.
508. Saltzman RW, Albin S, Russo P, Sullivan KE. Clinical conditions associated with PCP in children. Pediatr Pulmonol. 2012;47(5):510–6.
509. Le J, Durand C, Agha I, Brennan DC. Epstein-Barr virus and renal transplantation. Transplant Rev. 2016;31(1):55–60.
510. Fogeda M, Muñoz P, Luque A, Morales MD, Bouza E, Group BKVS, et al. Cross-sectional study of BK virus infection in pediatric kidney transplant recipients. Pediatr Transplant. 2007;11(4):394–401.
511. Lee SH, Huh KH, Joo DJ, Kim MS, Kim SI, Lee J, et al. Risk factors for Pneumocystis jirovecii pneumonia (PJP) in kidney transplantation recipients. Sci Rep. 2017;7(1):1–8.
512. Razonable RR, Rivero A, Rodriguez A, Wilson J, Daniels J, Jenkins G, et al. Allograft rejection predicts the occurrence of late-onset cytomegalovirus (CMV) disease among CMV-mismatched solid organ transplant patients receiving prophylaxis with oral ganciclovir. J Infect Dis. 2001;184(11):1461–4.
513. Boonyapredee M, Knight K, Little D. Increased BK viremia and progression to BK-virus nephropathy following high-dose intravenous immunoglobulin for acute cellular rejection. Mil Med. 2014;179(6):e699–702.
514. Fishman JA, Gans H, Practice tAIDCo. Pneumocystis jiroveci in solid organ transplantation: guidelines from the American Society of Transplantation Infectious Diseases Community of Practice. Clin Transplant. 2019;33(9):e13587.
515. Al Khasawneh E, Araya CE, Dharnidharka VR. Missed viral surveillance testing visits associate with full blown viral diseases in children receiving kidney transplants. Pediatr Transplant. 2013;17(2):129–32.
516. Smith JM, Dharnidharka VR. Viral surveillance and subclinical viral infection in pediatric kidney transplantation. Pediatr Nephrol (Berlin, West). 2015;30(5):741–8.
517. Bia M, Adey DB, Bloom RD, Chan L, Kulkarni S, Tomlanovich S. KDOQI US commentary on the 2009 KDIGO clinical practice guideline for the care of kidney transplant recipients. Am J Kidney Dis. 2010;56(2):189–218.
518. Razonable RR. Management strategies for cytomegalovirus infection and disease in solid organ transplant recipients. Infect Dis Clin. 2013;27(2):317–42.
519. Kotton CN, Kumar D, Caliendo AM, Huprikar S, Chou S, Danziger-Isakov L, et al. The third international consensus guidelines on the management of cytomegalovirus in solid-organ transplantation. Transplantation. 2018;102(6):900–31.
520. Varela-Fascinetto G, Benchimol C, Reyes-Acevedo R, Genevray M, Bradley D, Ives J, et al. Tolerability of up to 200 days of prophylaxis with valganciclovir oral solution and/or film-coated tablets in pediatric kidney transplant recipients at risk of cytomegalovirus disease. Pediatr Transplant. 2017;21(1):e12833.
521. Bansal R, Gordillo CA, Abramova R, Assal A, Mapara MY, Pereira MR, et al. Extended letermovir administration, beyond day 100, is effective for CMV prophylaxis in patients with graft versus host disease. Transpl Infect Dis. 2020:e13487. https://doi.org/10.1111/tid.13487.
522. Marty FM, Ljungman PT, Chemaly RF, Wan H, Teal VL, Butterton JR, et al. Outcomes of patients with detectable CMV DNA at randomization in the phase III trial of letermovir for the prevention of CMV infection in allogeneic hematopoietic cell transplantation. Am J Transplant. 2020;20(6):1703–11.
523. Ljungman P, Schmitt M, Marty FM, Maertens J, Chemaly RF, Kartsonis NA, et al. A mortality analysis of letermovir prophylaxis for cytomegalovirus (CMV) in CMV-seropositive recipients of allogeneic hematopoietic cell transplantation. Clin Infect Dis. 2020;70(8):1525–33.
524. Martin-Gandul C, Stampf S, Héquet D, Mueller NJ, Cusini A, van Delden C, et al. Preventive strategies against cytomegalovirus and incidence of α-herpesvirus infections in solid organ transplant recipients: a nationwide cohort study. Am J Transplant. 2017;17(7):1813–22.
525. Wilck MB, Zuckerman RA. Herpes simplex virus in solid organ transplantation. Am J Transplant. 2013;13(s4):121–7.

526. Lee DH, Zuckerman RA. Herpes simplex virus infections in solid organ transplantation: guidelines from the American Society of Transplantation Infectious Diseases Community of Practice. Clin Transpl. 2019;33(9):e13526.
527. Slifkin M, Doron S, Snydman DR. Viral prophylaxis in organ transplant patients. Drugs. 2004;64(24):2763–92.
528. Stern A, Green H, Paul M, Vidal L, Leibovici L. Prophylaxis for pneumocystis pneumonia (PCP) in non-HIV immunocompromised patients. Cochrane Database Syst Rev. 2014;(10):CD005590.
529. Kidney Disease: Improving Global Outcomes Transplant Work Group. KDIGO clinical practice guideline for the care of kidney transplant recipients. Am J Transplant. 2009;9(Suppl 3):S1.
530. Paulsen G, Michaels MG, Danziger-Isakov L, Dipchand AI, Green M, McCulloch M. Variability of Pneumocystis jirovecii prophylaxis use among pediatric solid organ transplant providers. Pediatr Transplant. 2020;24(1):e13609.
531. Idrees M, Sadiq S, Ali T, Rehman I, Akhtar S. Biopsy-proven acute graft pyelonephritis: a retrospective study from Sindh institute of urology and transplantation. Saudi J Kidney Dis Transpl. 2020;31(2):415–22.
532. Powers HR, Hellinger W, Cortese C, Wadei HM. 2659. Retrospective review of biopsy proven acute graft pyelonephritis in renal transplant patients. Open Forum Infect Dis. 2019;6(Suppl 2):S930.
533. Mohamed N, Aggarwal V, Cole E, John R. Histopathologic detection of rejection in acute allograft pyelonephritis. Transplantation. 2012;94(7):e46–7.
534. Cartery C, Guilbeau-Frugier C, Esposito L, Sallusto F, Guitard J, Cardeau-Desangles I, et al. Systematic kidney biopsies after acute allograft pyelonephritis. Exp Clin Transplant. 2013;11(3):239–44.
535. Audard V, Amor M, Desvaux D, Pastural M, Baron C, Philippe R, et al. Acute graft pyelonephritis: a potential cause of acute rejection in renal transplant. Transplantation. 2005;80(8):1128–30.
536. Kamath NS, John GT, Neelakantan N, Kirubakaran MG, Jacob CK. Acute graft pyelonephritis following renal transplantation. Transpl Infect Dis. 2006;8(3):140–7.
537. Singh R, Geerlings SE, Bemelman FJ. Asymptomatic bacteriuria and urinary tract infections among renal allograft recipients. Curr Opin Infect Dis. 2015;28(1):112–6.
538. Singh R, Geerlings SE, Peters-Sengers H, Idu MM, Hodiamont CJ, Ten Berge IJ, et al. Incidence, risk factors, and the impact of allograft pyelonephritis on renal allograft function. Transpl Infect Dis. 2016;18(5):647–60.
539. Ahmed EB, Alegre M-L, Chong AS. Role of bacterial infections in allograft rejection. Expert Rev Clin Immunol. 2008;4(2):281–93.
540. Gardner SD. Prevalence in England of antibody to human polyomavirus (B.K.). Br Med J. 1973;1(5845):77–8.
541. Brown P, Tsai T, Gajdusek DC. Seroepidemiology of human papovaviruses. Discovery of virgin populations and some unusual patterns of antibody prevalence among remote peoples of the world. Am J Epidemiol. 1975;102(4):331.
542. Boldorini R, Veggiani C, Barco D, Monga G. Kidney and urinary tract polyomavirus infection and distribution: molecular biology investigation of 10 consecutive autopsies. Arch Pathol Lab Med. 2005;129(1):69–73.
543. Heritage J, Chesters PM, McCance DJ. The persistence of papovavirus BK DNA sequences in normal human renal tissue. J Med Virol. 1981;8(2):143.
544. Hirsch HH, Knowles W, Dickenmann M, Passweg J, Klimkait T, Mihatsch MJ, et al. Prospective study of polyomavirus type BK replication and nephropathy in renal-transplant recipients. N Engl J Med. 2002;347(7):488–96.
545. Drachenberg CB, Papadimitriou JC, Hirsch HH, Wali R, Crowder C, Nogueira J, et al. Histological patterns of polyomavirus nephropathy: correlation with graft outcome and viral load. Am J Transplant. 2004;4(12):2082–92.
546. Binet I, Nickeleit V, Hirsch HH. Polyomavirus infections in transplant recipients. Curr Opin Organ Transplant. 2000;5(3):210–6.

547. Nickeleit V, Hirsch HH, Zeiler M, Gudat F, Prince O, Thiel G, et al. BK-virus nephropathy in renal transplants-tubular necrosis, MHC-class II expression and rejection in a puzzling game. Nephrol Dial Transplant. 2000;15(3):324–32.
548. Randhawa PS, Finkelstein S, Scantlebury V, Shapiro R, Vivas C, Jordan M, et al. Human polyoma virus-associated interstitial nephritis in the allograft kidney. Transplantation. 1999;67(1):103.
549. Geetha D, Geetha D, Talusan Y, Racusen L, Ratner L. Human polyoma virus causing renal allograft dysfunction. Transplantation. 2000;69(supplement):S387.
550. Ali AM, Gibson IW, Birk P, Blydt-Hansen TD. Pretransplant serologic testing to identify the risk of polyoma BK viremia in pediatric kidney transplant recipients. Pediatr Transplant. 2011;15(8):827–34.
551. Gard L, van Doesum W, Niesters HG, van Son WJ, Diepstra A, Stegeman CA, et al. A delicate balance between rejection and BK polyomavirus associated nephropathy; a retrospective cohort study in renal transplant recipients. PLoS One. 2017;12(6):e0178801.
552. Todd AR, Langlois V, Tellier R, Robinson L, Hébert D. The prevalence of BK viremia and urinary viral shedding in a pediatric renal transplant population: a single-center retrospective analysis. Pediatr Transplant. 2006;10(5):586–92.
553. Herman J, Van Ranst M, Snoeck R, Beuselinck K, Lerut E, Van Damme-Lombaerts R. Polyomavirus infection in pediatric renal transplant recipients: evaluation using a quantitative real-time PCR technique. Pediatr Transplant. 2004;8(5):485–92.
554. McGilvray ID, Lajoie G, Humar A, Cattral MS. Polyomavirus infection and acute vascular rejection in a kidney allograft: coincidence or mimicry? Am J Transplant. 2003;3(4):501–4.
555. Drachenberg CB, Beskow CO, Cangro CB, Bourquin PM, Simsir A, Fink J, et al. Human polyoma virus in renal allograft biopsies: morphological findings and correlation with urine cytology. Hum Pathol. 1999;30(8):970–7.
556. Howell DN, Smith SR, Butterly DW, Klassen PS, Krigman HR, Burchette JJL, et al. Diagnosis and management of BK polyomavirus interstitial nephritis in renal transplant recipients. Transplantation. 1999;68(9):1279–88.
557. Egli A, Köhli S, Dickenmann M, Hirsch HH. Inhibition of polyomavirus BK-specific T-cell responses by immunosuppressive drugs. Transplantation. 2009;88(10):1161–8.
558. Mayr M, Nickeleit V, Hirsch HH, Dickenmann M, Mihatsch MJ, Steiger J. Polyomavirus BK nephropathy in a kidney transplant recipient: critical issues of diagnosis and management. Am J Kidney Dis. 2001;38(3):e13.1–e.5.
559. Kim YJ, Jeong JC, Koo TY, Kwon HY, Han M, Jeon HJ, et al. Impact of combined acute rejection on BK virus-associated nephropathy in kidney transplantation. J Korean Med Sci. 2013;28(12):1711–5.
560. Tanabe T, Shimizu T, Sai K, Miyauchi Y, Shirakawa H, Ishida H, et al. BK polyomavirus nephropathy complicated with acute T-cell-mediated rejection in a kidney transplant recipient: a case report. Clin Transpl. 2011;25:39–43.
561. Celik B, Shapiro R, Vats A, Randhawa PS. Polyomavirus allograft nephropathy: sequential assessment of histologic viral load, tubulitis, and graft function following changes in immunosuppression. Am J Transplant. 2003;3(11):1378–82.
562. Hussain S, Bresnahan BA, Cohen EP, Hariharan S. Rapid kidney allograft failure in patients with polyoma virus nephritis with prior treatment with antilymphocyte agents. Clin Transpl. 2002;16(1):43–7.
563. Moens U, Subramaniam N, Johansen B, Johansen T, Traavik T. A steroid hormone response unit in the late leader of the noncoding control region of the human polyomavirus BK confers enhanced host cell permissivity. J Virol. 1994;68(4):2398–408.
564. Schneidewind L, Neumann T, Dräger DL, Kranz J, Hakenberg OW. Leflunomide in the treatment of BK polyomavirus associated nephropathy in kidney transplanted patients – a systematic review. Transplant Rev. 2020;34(4):100565.
565. Anyaegbu EI, Almond PS, Milligan T, Allen WR, Gharaybeh S, Al-Akash SI. Intravenous immunoglobulin therapy in the treatment of BK viremia and nephropathy in pediatric renal transplant recipients. Pediatr Transplant. 2012;16(1):E19–24.

566. Hwang SD, Lee JH, Lee SW, Kim JK, Kim MJ, Song JH. High-dose intravenous immunoglobulin treatment of polyomavirus nephropathy developing after T cell-mediated rejection treatment: a case report. Transplant Proc. 2018;50(8):2575–8.
567. Matsumura S, Kato T, Taniguchi A, Kawamura M, Nakazawa S, Namba-Hamano T, et al. Clinical efficacy of intravenous immunoglobulin for BK polyomavirus-associated nephropathy after living kidney transplantation. Ther Clin Risk Manag. 2020;16:947–52.
568. Shah T, Vu D, Naraghi R, Campbell A, Min D. Efficacy of intravenous immunoglobulin in the treatment of persistent BK viremia and BK virus nephropathy in renal transplant recipients. Clin Transpl. 2014:109–16.
569. Vu D, Shah T, Ansari J, Naraghi R, Min D. Efficacy of intravenous immunoglobulin in the treatment of persistent BK viremia and BK virus nephropathy in renal transplant recipients. Transplant Proc. 2015;47(2):394–8.
570. Velay A, Solis M, Benotmane I, Gantner P, Soulier E, Moulin B, et al. Intravenous immunoglobulin administration significantly increases BKPyV genotype-specific neutralizing antibody titers in kidney transplant recipients. Antimicrob Agents Chemother. 2019;63(8):e00393-19.
571. Benotmane I, Solis M, Velay A, Cognard N, Olagne J, Gautier Vargas G, et al. Intravenous immunoglobulin as a preventive strategy against BK virus viremia and BKV-associated nephropathy in kidney transplant recipients – results from a proof-of-concept study. Am J Transplant. 2021;21(1):329–37.

Part II

Infectious Challenges

Pretransplant Donor and Recipient Infectious Challenges

4

Sarah Kizilbash and Jodi M. Smith

Pretransplant Infectious Disease Evaluation

Infections are one of the leading causes of death in pediatric kidney transplant recipients [1]. Candidates awaiting kidney transplant are at an increased risk of infections due to immunological abnormalities resulting from the chronic kidney disease [2]. Furthermore, patients on dialysis are at risk of unique infections such as catheter-associated access site infections, bloodstream infections, and peritonitis. Congenital anomalies of the kidney and the urinary tract (CAKUT) are frequently associated with urinary tract infections and colonization with multidrug-resistant organisms. Identification and treatment of active and latent infections prior to transplant are critical for preventing overwhelming posttransplant infections.

The goals of pretransplant infectious disease evaluation are to identify and treat active and latent infections, to identify colonization patterns with multidrug-resistant organisms, and to assess immunity against vaccine-preventable diseases. The evaluation informs perioperative antibiotic management plan to prevent perioperative infections and an antimicrobial prophylaxis plan to prevent posttransplant reactivation of latent infections. Additionally, pretransplant evaluation is aimed at screening potential donors for active or latent infections to prevent posttransplant donor-derived infections.

S. Kizilbash
Department of Pediatrics, University of Minnesota, Minneapolis, MN, USA

J. M. Smith (✉)
Department of Pediatrics, Seattle Children's Hospital/University of Washington, Seattle, WA, USA
e-mail: jodi.smith@seattlechildrens.org

K. E. Twombley (ed.), *Challenges in Pediatric Kidney Transplantation*,
https://doi.org/10.1007/978-3-030-74783-1_4

Evaluation of the Pediatric Kidney Transplant Candidate

Pretransplant evaluation includes a detailed medical history, physical examination, laboratory investigations (serological and molecular diagnostic tests), and radiographic studies. Medical history should focus on current and past infections, animal exposure, travel to or residence in areas with unique endemic infections, exposure to tuberculosis, lifestyle history, risk factors for HIV and other sexually transmitted diseases, risk factors of hepatitis viruses, and history of conditions predisposing to infections (urinary tract anomalies, Mitrofanoff, neurogenic bladder, vesicoureteral reflux, clean intermittent catheterization). All access sites and indwelling catheters should be examined for signs of infection.

Active infections are a contraindication to transplant and must be adequately treated or controlled prior to the transplant [3]. Active infections should be ruled out with tests including blood cultures, urine cultures, stool cultures, and respiratory cultures/PCR tests as clinically indicated. Table 4.1 lists organisms for which routine pretransplant screening is recommended [4]. Screening for additional organisms (Table 4.2) is considered depending on candidate's risk factors such as exposure to areas with unique endemic infections [3, 4].

HIV and Hepatitis Viruses

As indicated in Table 4.1, all transplant candidates need pretransplant screening for HIV, hepatitis B, and hepatitis C viruses. Although active HIV infection is not a contraindication, the patient should be on adequate viral suppression therapy prior to transplant [3]. Hepatitis B-positive patients must undergo evaluation for active liver disease and must also be treated with antiviral therapy prior to transplant. Once started, the therapy for hepatitis B should continue indefinitely pre- and

Table 4.1 Standard pretransplant infectious disease screening for transplant candidates

Infections	Tests
Human immunodeficiency virus	HIV antibody/antigen Nucleic acid amplification testing
Cytomegalovirus	IgG
Epstein-Barr virus	VCA IgG, IgM
Hepatitis B virus	HBsAg, HBcAb IgM and IgG, HBsAb Nucleic acid amplification testing
Hepatitis C virus	HCV antibody Nucleic acid amplification testing
Toxoplasma	IgG
Syphilis	Rapid Plasma Reagin, or Venereal Disease Research Laboratory
Tuberculosis	Purified protein derivative or Interferon gamma release assay Chest radiograph
Urinary infection	Urine culture
Bloodstream infection	Blood culture

Table 4.2 Pretransplant infectious disease screening for candidates from endemic areas

Infection	Tests
Strongyloides	Serology
Trypanosoma cruzi	Serology
Coccidioides	Serology, antigen enzyme immunoassay
Histoplasma	Serology, antigen enzyme immunoassay
Blastomyces	Antigen enzyme immunoassay
Malaria	Blood smear

posttransplant [5]. Patients with no evidence of viremia but positive hepatitis B core antibody may develop hepatitis B reactivation posttransplant. Although routine prophylaxis is not recommended in these patients due to the low incidence of reactivation, it may be considered with agents such as lamivudine [5]. Kidney transplant candidates with hepatitis C viremia should be evaluated for liver disease. [3] These patients should also be considered for direct-acting antiviral therapy prior to transplant [3].

Cytomegalovirus/Epstein-Barr Virus Serostatus of Donor and Recipient

CMV and EBV are common viral complications posttransplant. Knowledge of the donor and recipient serostatus helps to guide both viral surveillance and prophylaxis strategies posttransplant. A primary viral infection is defined as infection in a recipient who is seronegative at the time of transplant. Reactivation infection occurs in the setting of a patient who is seropositive. Pediatric patients are at higher risk for primary infection due to higher rates of recipient seronegativity at the time of transplant. Recent US data demonstrated that 43% of pediatric kidney transplant recipient were EBV seronegative and 62% were CMV seronegative at the time of transplant [6]. The combination of a donor who was positive for cytomegalovirus and a pediatric recipient who was negative occurred in 39% of deceased donor transplants and in 29% of living donor transplants. The combination of a donor who was positive for Epstein-Barr virus and a recipient who was negative occurred in 37% of deceased donor transplants and in 52% of living donor transplants. [6]

Cytomegalovirus

CMV, a DNA virus of the herpes virus family, is perhaps the single most important pathogen in solid organ transplantation [8, 9]. Its importance lies in the fact that CMV not only causes significant morbidity by direct infection but its immunomodulatory effects also predispose to other infectious complications. Consensus guidelines from AST, KDIGO, and the Transplantation Society International CMV Consensus Group recommend universal prophylaxis for high-risk patients (seronegative recipients of seropositive organs or seropositive recipients of seropositive organs in the setting of anti-T-cell antibody immunosuppression), based on the available data suggesting better graft survival and clinical outcomes [8, 9]. Recommendations guide the duration of therapy based on the serostatus of the donor and recipient [8, 9]. For CMV D+/R- patients, 3–6 months of prophylaxis with oral ganciclovir or valganciclovir is recommended. For CMV R+ patients, 3 months is recommended, but 6 months should be considered if anti-lymphocyte induction is used. No prophylaxis is recommended in the CMV D−/R- patient. In addition, treatment of rejection with anti-lymphocyte antibodies in at-risk recipients (D+/R-) should prompt re-initiation of prophylaxis or preemptive therapy for 1–3 months [8, 9].

The timing and frequency of screening for CMV is largely center-specific and influenced by donor and recipient CMV serostatus, as well as whether universal or preemptive therapy is employed. Published guidelines recommend regular monitoring using a quantitative viral load assay for the first year posttransplant; however, the duration and frequency may vary depending on the type of CMV prevention strategy [8, 9].

Epstein-Barr Virus

For EBV, the primary goal of viral surveillance is to prevent the development of posttransplant lymphoproliferative disorder (PTLD). Awareness of risk factors associated with PTLD guides viral surveillance strategies. Numerous risk factors have been identified including young age, Caucasian race, male gender, specific immunosuppressive medications, and type of organ transplanted [7–10]. However, primary EBV infection is considered to be the most important. Due to the seroepidemiology of primary EBV infection, pediatric patients are often EBV seronegative making them an exceptionally vulnerable population. Surveillance strategies differ based on recipient serostatus. KDIGO recommends the following posttransplant EBV schedule for high-risk D+/R- patients: once in the first week after transplant, at least monthly for the first 3–6 months, and then at least every 3 months until the end of the first year with re-initiation of monitoring after treatment for acute rejection. While the D−/R− patient might be at decreased risk of developing EBV disease compared to D+/R−, they are still at increased risk relative to the R+ patient and therefore warrant close monitoring. Some centers may choose to measure EBV loads more frequently. Beyond the first year, selective monitoring, such as in those with persistently high viral loads or in those with higher than normal immunosuppression, may be performed based on center preferences. Some centers recommend continued monitoring for an indefinite period for all patients. For seropositive individuals, selective monitoring may be considered.

Mycobacterium tuberculosis

Tuberculosis (TB) is the second most common infectious cause of death across the world [5, 11]. It is caused by members of the *M. tuberculosis* complex, most commonly *Mycobacterium tuberculosis*. Transplant recipients are at a particularly increased risk with a 4–30 times higher incidence compared with the general population [6, 12]. The prevalence of TB in the developed world among transplant recipients is estimated to be 1.2–6.4% [13].

In most cases, posttransplant TB is caused by reactivation of the latent disease. However, donor transmission and primary exposure posttransplant may also play a role [8, 14]. Risk factors for TB include history of residence outside the United States, homelessness, incarceration, cigarette smoking, chronic kidney disease, and exposure to a known case of TB [12]. Pretransplant screening for TB should include a detailed history of TB risk factors for all candidates and living donors. All candidates and living donors should undergo purified protein-derived test or interferon gamma release assay test (IGRAs). Since end-stage renal disease may be associated with anergy resulting in false negative tests, all candidates should also undergo chest radiographs [3]. Conventional PPD is considered positive if there is >5 mm induration at 48 to 72 hours [11]. Patients with negative results should be considered for a second skin test 2 weeks later, as false negative may become positive due to "immune boosting" for remote exposures [15]. The IGRA test is more sensitive compared with PPD in patients with end-stage renal disease and those who are immunocompromised. IGRA is also the preferred test in the setting of Bacillus Calmette-Guerin (BCG) vaccination [15, 16]. All patients who are immunocompromised at the time of evaluation, such as those with nephrotic syndrome or those on treatment for autoimmune diseases, should be evaluated with a combination of IGRA, chest radiograph, detailed history, and ascertainment of risk factors for TB [17]. Candidates with latent TB should initiate treatment prior to or immediately following the transplant in low-prevalence areas [3]. Commonly used regimen includes isoniazid for 6–9 months. For patients who develop toxicity to isoniazid, alternative regimens, such as rifampin for 4 months, may be considered in consultation with infectious disease experts [12].

Although successful treatment of active TB is possible posttransplant, it is complicated by drug toxicities and drug-drug interactions. KDIGO recommends completion of treatment for active TB prior to transplant [3]. The treatment regimen (isoniazid, rifampin, pyrazinamide, and ethambutol) in transplant recipients is the same as that in the general population. The usual duration is 6 months; however, it may be 20 months long for multidrug-resistant TB [12, 18]. Directly observed therapy (DOT) programs have improved treatment adherence and should be considered for transplant candidates/recipients.[6, 12]

Since TB may be transmitted to recipients via transplantation [14], active donor TB is a contraindication to donation. All living donors should complete therapy for active or latent TB prior to donation. Candidates who receive organs from donors with untreated TB must complete treatment for latent TB posttransplant [4]. All candidates with a pretransplant TB history must be vigilantly followed for disease reactivation during the first year posttransplant.

Fungal Infections and Endemic Mycoses

Transplant recipients are at an increased risk of invasive fungal infections. Risk factors for posttransplant fungal infections include environmental exposures, pretransplant colonization, and the state of net immunosuppression [2, 19]. Fungal infections in transplant recipients may be broadly divided into two categories: reactivation of fungi not causing invasive disease in an immunocompetent host and disseminated infection with fungi that are geographically limited. Candidiasis is the most common fungal infection in pediatric kidney transplant recipients [20]. While pretransplant fungal colonization is not a contraindication to transplant, active fungal infections must be treated prior to the transplant [3]. Posttransplant antifungal prophylaxis should be modified based on pretransplant colonization patterns and susceptibilities.

Endemic mycoses refer to fungi that are restricted to certain geographic regions with a worldwide distribution. The most common endemic mycoses in the United States include histoplasmosis, blastomycosis, and coccidioidomycosis. *Histoplasma* and *Blastomyces* are found in the Mississippi and the Ohio River Valleys, while *Coccidioides* is endemic in the Southwestern United States and areas of California's Central Valley. Endemic mycoses account for 5% of the fungal infections in solid organ recipients in the United States [4, 21]. Although rare, endemic mycoses can cause severe and disseminated disease in transplant recipients [19, 22]. Reactivation of pretransplant latent disease and donor transmission are preventable causes of posttransplant disease. Hence, pretransplant screening of donors and recipients is necessary.

Histoplasmosis is the most common endemic mycosis in transplant recipients in the United States. It is caused by *H. capsulatum* and is acquired via inhalation through the pulmonary route. Environmental exposures include disrupted soil around construction sites, caves inhabited by bats, chicken coops, and other buildings where birds live [26]. Pretransplant screening should begin with a detailed history about former and current areas of residence, a detailed travel history, and history of environmental exposures. Radiographs of candidates from endemic areas may show old and healed lesions of histoplasmosis such as calcified granulomata in the lungs, liver, and spleen. Evidence of old but healed infection is not a contraindication to transplant [21]. Although routine posttransplant prophylaxis for histoplasmosis is not recommended, azole prophylaxis may be considered for seropositive transplant recipients and recipients of organs from seropositive donors to prevent posttransplant reactivation [21]. Recipients at risk of posttransplant histoplasmosis should be vigilantly followed posttransplant.

Coccidioidomycosis is caused by *Coccidioides immitis* and *Coccidioides posadasii*, and it is also acquired via inhalation [23]. The incidence of coccidioidomycosis in transplant recipients in endemic areas is 1.45–6.9% [24]. Coccidioidomycosis may also be acquired through donor transmission or reactivation of a latent infection. It usually manifests within the first year posttransplant as disseminated disease associated with a mortality rate of ~30% [21]. Pretransplant screening of candidates is challenging, as serology may be negative in patients with end-stage renal disease.

Antigen testing, direct visualization, PCR, and culture are other diagnostic strategies that may be used. Candidates with active disease must complete treatment prior to transplant. It is recommended that all candidates from endemic regions receive 6–12 months of azole prophylaxis. Recipients of organs from donors with prior infection should also receive azole prophylaxis [21].

Blastomycosis is caused by *Blastomyces dermatitidis*. Blastomycosis in solid organ recipients is exceedingly rare [24]. Routine prophylaxis to prevent posttransplant infection is not recommended [21].

Parasitic Infections

Parasitic infections are increasingly being recognized as a cause of morbidity and mortality in transplant recipients. Like other infections, parasitic disease may occur by reactivation of a dormant infection or may be acquired from the donor through transplantation.

Toxoplasmosis is the most prevalent parasitic infection worldwide. It is estimated to affect 30–50% of the world's population [25]. Infection rates in the United States are estimated to be 11% [26]. The American Society of Transplantation Infectious Diseases Community of Practice recommends screening of all donors and recipients for *Toxoplasma* using serology [4]. While all solid organ recipients are at an increased risk of developing toxoplasmosis, the risk is the highest in heart transplant recipients [27]. Seronegative recipients who receive organs from seronegative donors (D+/R-) are at the highest risk of disease reactivation. It is recommended that all D+/R- and all seropositive recipients receive prophylaxis with Bactrim to prevent disease reactivation. Those who are allergic to Bactrim may be treated with dapsone for prophylaxis [26]. Bactrim and dapsone also have the advantage of providing protection against *Pneumocystis jirovecii* infection.

Strongyloides stercoralis, an intestinal parasite, is another common parasite that may cause disseminated infection in transplant recipients. It is estimated to infect 30–100 million individuals worldwide [28, 29]. In the United States, the prevalence is <6%, and it is mostly seen in the immigrant population in the Southeastern Unites States [29]. A recent retrospective study of 1689 adult kidney transplant candidates, referred to a transplant center in Texas from July 2012 to June 2017, showed a seropositivity rate of 9.9% [30]. *Strongyloides* may cause a chronic infection in human hosts that may persist for decades with few to no symptoms. However, in the setting of posttransplant immunosuppression, *Strongyloides* may cause a disseminated disease with mortality rates ranging from 50% to 89% [30, 31]. Due to the disease severity in transplant setting, all candidates and prospective donors residing in endemic areas are required to complete pretransplant screening for *Strongyloides* [32]. Serology screening is much more sensitive than stool screening. Patients who test positive must complete treatment with ivermectin or thiabendazole prior to transplant [32].

Based on epidemiological risk factors, other parasites for which pretransplant screening may be considered include malaria, *Trypanosoma*, *Cryptosporidium* sp.,

Giardia lamblia, *Schistosoma*, and *Entamoeba histolytica*. KDIGO recommends malaria screening with a blood smear for candidates with exposure to endemic areas. Patients screening positive should be adequately treated prior to transplant [3].

COVID-19

The coronavirus disease 2019 (COVID-19), characterized by significant respiratory and multiorgan disease, is caused by the novel severe acute respiratory syndrome coronavirus 2 (SARS-COV-2). This virus first emerged in December 2019 in Wuhan, China [33]. As of October 24, 2020, COVID-19 has caused 8.47 million cases in the United States with 223,393 deaths [34].

Droplets expelled during talking, coughing, sneezing, or eating are the most common mode of transmission. Transmission may also occur through aerosol; however, it is unclear if this is a significant mode of transmission outside of laboratory settings. Common symptoms of COVID-19 infection include fever, dry cough, shortness of breath, fatigue, myalgias, nausea and vomiting, diarrhea, headaches, weakness, and rhinorrhea. Common complications include pneumonia, acute respiratory distress syndrome, liver injury characterized by elevation of liver enzymes, cardiac injury marked by troponin elevation, acute heart failure, myocarditis, prothrombotic coagulopathy, acute kidney injury, and acute cerebral vascular disease. Rare complications include cytokine storm and macrophage activating syndrome. Patients become contagious about 2 to 3 days prior to the onset of symptoms until about 8 days after symptom onset [33].

Nearly 80% of patients with COVID-19 have mild manifestations, 15% develop severe illness, and 5% become critical. Data are limited on the impact of COVID-19 on kidney transplant recipients. It is speculated that transplant recipients are at high risk of complications due to their immunocompromised status. However, anecdotal reports describe a mild course in most pediatric kidney transplant recipients.

The American Society of Transplantation has published guidelines to screen donors for COVID-19. According to these guidelines, nucleic acid amplification testing (NAT) for COVID-19 must be performed on at least one sample from the respiratory tract within 3 days of procurement. A second viral test should be considered 24 hours after the first and within 24–48 hours of procurement. For donors with a history of COVID-19, either a negative NAT test should be documented, or the donor should be asymptomatic with the onset of symptoms 21 to 90 days prior to the donation. Living donors should be advised to follow universal masking precautions and strict social distancing for 14 days prior to donation. Donors should also be encouraged to self-quarantine after the pre-operative COVID-19 test [35]. Similarly, all transplant candidates should self-quarantine or follow strict social distancing for a 14-day period prior to the transplant. All candidates should also have a negative NAT test documented prior to surgery.

Urinary Tract Infections

Urinary tract infection (UTI) is the most common bacterial infection in kidney transplant recipients, in both adults and children [36]. UTIs will develop in 20–40% in the first year posttransplant and 40–60% by 3 years posttransplant. UTI is not only a cause of morbidity but is also associated with higher rates of graft loss and patient death [37, 38]. The urogenital tract is the most common entry point for systemic sepsis [39]. Numerous risk factors have been identified for UTIs posttransplant. Urologic anomalies such as neurogenic bladder, urinary tract obstruction, vesicoureteral reflux, bladder augmentation, clean intermittent catheterization, and UTIs prior to transplant have all been associated with an increased risk of UTI posttransplant [10, 40–42]. It is recommended that children with any of these risk factors be referred for urological evaluation prior to transplant to mitigate risk factors for posttransplant recurrent UTIs [3]. KDIGO guidelines do not recommend routine native kidney nephrectomy in children for hydronephrosis/vesicoureteral reflux associated with recurrent UTIs [3]. The European guidelines recommend nephrectomy for children with significant vesicoureteral reflux and recurrent UTIs to decrease the risk of posttransplant urosepsis [43]. Transplant centers vary in their practice regarding nephrectomy for UTIs. A retrospective study by Ghane et al. of 49 pediatric kidney recipients documented nephrectomy for vesicoureteral reflux and recurrent UTIs in 11 recipients [44]. The decision about nephrectomy should be individualized based on risk factors in consultation with transplant surgery and urology.

Not all organisms found in the urine culture are pathogenic. Multiple organisms in a culture likely indicate contamination. Similarly, organisms like *Lactobacillus* and *Gardnerella vaginalis* are unlikely to cause disease [45]. Asymptomatic bacterial and fungal colonization are frequently seen in children with structural abnormalities of the genitourinary system and do not constitute a contraindication to transplant [3].

PHS Increased Risk Donors

The increased risk donor (IRD) classification identifies donors who are most at risk of inadvertently transmitting HIV, hepatitis B, and hepatitis C to recipients via transplantation. This classification does not denote the quality of the donor in relation to graft survival. IRDs may transmit HIV, hepatitis B, and/or hepatitis C infection(s) to recipients through transplantation despite testing negative on enzyme-linked immunosorbent assay (ELISA) and/or viral NAT test due to the inability of these tests to detect window period infections [46]. The window period refers to the interval between virus acquisition and virus detection, and it varies from virus to virus. The Centers for Disease Control and Prevention (CDC) first published criteria to identify IRDs in 1994. The initial intent was to reduce HIV transmission to recipients via transplantation. The criteria were updated in 2013 to also include risk factors for hepatitis B and hepatitis C infections (Table 4.3). [46] As illustrated in

Table 4.3 The Centers for Disease Control and Prevention criteria for increased risk donors

2013 guidelines
Men having sex with men in the preceding 12 months
Non-medical injection drug use in the preceding 12 months
Sex in exchange for money or drugs in the preceding 12 months
Sex with a known or suspected case of HIV, hepatitis B, or hepatitis C in the preceding 12 months
Women who have had sex with a man who had had sex with men in the preceding 12 months
Sex with a person who had sex in exchange for money or drugs in the preceding 12 months
Sex with a person who injected non-medical drugs in the preceding 12 months
A child ≤18 months born to a mother with a known history of or at high risk for HIV, Hepatitis B, or hepatitis C infection
A child breastfed in the preceding 12 months by a mother with a known history of or at high risk for HIV infection
People in a correctional facility for more than 72 consecutive hours in the preceding 12 months
People with a new diagnosis of or who have been treated for syphilis, gonorrhea, chlamydia, or genital ulcers in the preceding 12 months
Hemodiluted deceased donor's blood sample (can result in false negative testing)
People on hemodialysis in the preceding 12 months
When deceased donor's medical or behavior history cannot be ascertained, donor should be considered increased risk

Table 4.3, a donor may be labeled as an IRD for several different exposures, and not all exposures are equal in the term of the risk magnitude. In April 2019, the Advisory Committee for Blood and Tissue Safety and Availability revised the 2013 guidelines and recommended shortening the period for risk ascertainment from 12 months to 3 months prior to donation [47].

Window Period Duration and the Risk of Virus Transmission

The duration of the window period varies based on the test. Since ELISA requires serological conversion prior to detection, the window period is shorter for NAT compared with ELISA. The window period for HIV is 22 days for ELISA but only 5–10 days for NAT. Similarly, the window period for hepatitis B is 38–50 days for ELISA but 20–26 days for NAT. For hepatitis C, NAT reduces the duration of window period by approximately 60 days compared with ELISA [48]. The risk of inadvertent virus transmission is extremely low for exposures that occur more than 3 weeks prior to donation. According to a systemic review and meta-analysis, the risk of an undetected hepatitis C infection ranges from 0.027 to 32.4 per 10,000 IRDs, [49] and the risk of an undetected HIV infection ranges from 0.04 to 4.9 per 10,000 IRDs [50]. The risk of transmitting an undetected hepatitis B infection is also small. In 2007, an IRD, who tested negative on ELISA but retrospectively tested positive on NAT, transmitted HIV and hepatitis C to four solid organ recipients. All four recipients were adult recipients. Pediatric data provides no evidence of HIV, hepatitis B, and/or hepatitis C transmission in children following a kidney transplant. A retrospective study of 11,188 pediatric solid organ transplant recipients, transplanted between 2008 and 2013, found no cases of donor-derived HIV, hepatitis B, or hepatitis C infections in any of the pediatric kidney transplant recipients [51]. Vaccination for hepatitis B and curative direct-acting antiviral therapy for hepatitis C have further mitigated the risks of adverse long-term consequences of an inadvertent transmission.

Outcomes of PHS Increased Risk Donors in Pediatric Kidney Transplantation

According to the 2013 criteria, 20% of all deceased donors in the United States are IRDs [52]. Despite the high proportion of IRDs in the deceased donor pool, only 13% of all pediatric deceased donor kidney transplants in 2015 were IRD transplants [53]. IRDs have a high discard rate despite the growing gap between the organ supply and demand. In 2019, 1010 kidneys form IRDs were discarded [52]. A retrospective study of 45,112 deceased donors showed that IRDs were 8.2% less likely to be used for transplantation compared with non-IRD donors [54]. Concerns about transmitting stigmatized infections and fears of legal repercussions dissuade providers from accepting IRD organs. A recent survey of 22 pediatric nephrologists from 11 UNOS regions showed that only 14% would routinely accept IRD kidneys and 41% would not accept an IRD organ under any circumstances. Only 55% of the respondents were comfortable counseling patients and families about IRDs [55]. Increased education of patients and providers about risks and benefits may improve IRD utilization.

Except for the risk of infection transmission, IRDs are usually high-quality kidneys. IRD donors are more likely to be young, have lower kidney donor profile index scores (KDPI), and have anoxia as their cause of death. [56–58] A pediatric study of 328 IRD recipients found the mean KDPI score of IRD donors to be 19.0 (standard deviation: 15.1) portending excellent graft survival [53].

IRD kidney transplants in children are associated with similar patient and graft survival compared with non-IRD kidney transplants. A retrospective study comparing 328 pediatric IRD recipients with 4850 non-IRD recipients found no difference in patient and graft survival between the groups. This study also found no difference in graft losses and deaths due to infections between IRD and non-IRD recipients. Importantly, the study found a significant survival benefit of IRD transplantation in children compared with remaining on the waiting list for a non-IRD deceased donor transplant [53]. This study illustrates that IRD transplants are beneficial for children. Among pediatric candidates on the deceased donor waiting list, 15–20% wait >3 years, and 20% have PRA of >80% [59]. IRD transplantation should be considered for these children given the survival benefit compared with remaining on the waiting list.

Informed Consent

Public health service (PHS) recommends that informed consent should be obtained from candidates prior to proceeding with an IRD transplant. The risks and benefits of both accepting and rejecting an IRD kidney should be discussed with the candidate. The candidate should be informed that all donors are screened for HIV, hepatitis B, and hepatitis C infections but that no test or screening question can eliminate the risk of infection [60].

Posttransplant Testing

In 2019, the Advisory Committee for Blood and Tissue Safety and Availability recommended that all transplant recipients should undergo testing for HIV, hepatitis B, and hepatitis C 4–6 weeks after the transplant, regardless of the donor's risk profile [47]. Routine posttransplant testing is important for early detection of donor-derived infections to allow timely intervention (viral suppression for HIV and hepatitis B and curative therapy for hepatitis C) to minimize adverse consequences [61]. For all viruses, NAT is the preferred method of testing due to its short window. If a donor-derived HIV, hepatitis B, and/or hepatitis C infection is detected, OPTN, the center that procured organ/tissues, and all centers that transplanted the organ/tissues should be promptly notified [61].

Immunizations

Preparing the Dialysis Patient for Transplantation

Morbidity and mortality from vaccine-preventable illness are significant concerns in the pediatric dialysis population. However, children with ESRD are often under the care of numerous physicians at multiple sites where vaccinations are administered, and the vaccine history in these complex patients may be overlooked. Pediatric dialysis patients should receive routine childhood vaccinations on a timely schedule, and every effort should be made to complete the vaccination program prior to transplantation—using an accelerated schedule if necessary.

Increased adherence to vaccine recommendations has been observed when the nephrologist assumes responsibility for the administration and surveillance of immunizations. In addition, ensuring that family members are up to date with their immunizations will help to maximize the preventive benefits of this intervention. Small studies in pediatric dialysis patients demonstrate vaccine responsiveness, but an important issue still not well studied is the duration of the immunity following vaccination in this patient population. Thus, it is important for practitioners to be diligent, measure titers when possible, and revaccinate to maintain the health of this vulnerable population.

Achieving immunity to vaccine-preventable childhood infections prior to renal transplantation is critical. Ideally, all routine immunizations should be up to date prior to referral for transplant. Particular attention and priority should be given to the live/attenuated vaccines (MMR and varicella) that are generally not recommended following organ transplantation. If no immunization records are available, routine immunizations should be "caught up" according to the recommendations of the AAP and ACIP guidelines [62–64].

Vaccine Schedule: Current American Academy of Pediatrics Recommendations

In general, patients on dialysis should receive the standard immunizations according to the time frames suggested by the Advisory Committee on Immunization Practices (ACIP), the American Academy of Pediatrics (AAP), and the American Academy of Family Physicians [62–64]. Routine childhood immunizations currently include vaccination against diphtheria, *Haemophilus influenzae* type B (HIB), hepatitis A and B, human papillomavirus, influenza, measles, mumps, *Neisseria meningitides*, pertussis, polio, rotavirus, rubella, *Streptococcus pneumoniae*, tetanus, and varicella.

Numerous studies document the safety of vaccination of dialysis patients. Killed or component vaccines have not been associated with any deterioration in dialysis efficacy. Live-virus vaccines have also been shown to be safe in the pediatric dialysis population.

There are several vaccines (e.g., hepatitis B, influenza, and pneumococcus) with specific recommendations in the AAP Red Book for individuals with chronic kidney disease.

Summary of recommendations with end stage kidney disease, including transplant candidates [62–64]

Children and adolescents with chronic or end-stage kidney disease, including kidney transplant candidates, should receive all vaccinations as appropriate for age, exposure history, and immune status. Patients 2 years or older should be given a dose of PPSV23, if not previously given. (Patients with end-stage kidney disease should receive PPSV23 if they have not received a dose within 5 years and have not received two lifetime doses.) PCV13 is administered if not previously received, even for those 6 years or older. When PCV13 and PPSV23 both are indicated, PPSV23 should be given at least 8 weeks after the last PCV13 dose. Kidney transplant candidates who are hepatitis B surface antibody (anti-HBs) negative should receive the hepatitis B vaccine (HepB) series, followed by serologic testing and further doses if serologic test results are negative (as indicated for an immunocompetent vaccinee who remains seronegative). Patients 12 months or older who have not received hepatitis A vaccine (HepA) did not complete the vaccination series or who are seronegative should receive the HepA vaccine series. The MMR vaccine can be given to infants 6 through 11 months of age who are kidney transplant candidates and who are not immunocompromised, repeating the dose at ≥12 months if still awaiting a transplant that will not occur within 4 weeks of vaccination. Living kidney donors should have up-to-date vaccination status. Household members of these patients should be counseled about risks of infection and should have vaccination status made current.

Hepatitis B

Hepatitis B vaccination is recommended for all chronic hemodialysis patients. Vaccination is also recommended for chronic kidney disease patients prior to them reaching end stage [65]. Compared to immunocompetent individuals, hemodialysis patients are less likely to have protective levels of antibody after vaccination with standard vaccine dosages. Protective levels of antibody developed in 67–86% of hemodialysis patients who received 3–4 doses in various dosages and schedules [66]. Higher seroprotection rates have been identified in patients with chronic kidney failure who were vaccinated prior to reaching end stage and starting dialysis. Based on this, higher vaccine dosages or an increased number of doses are recommended for those on hemodialysis. Testing after vaccination is recommended for hemodialysis patients to determine their response to the vaccine. Testing should be performed 1–2 months after administration of the last dose of the vaccine series by using a method that allows determination of a protective level of anti-HBs (e.g., >10 mIU/mL). If the patient has anti-HB levels of <10 mIU/mL after the primary vaccine series, they should be revaccinated with a second hepatitis B vaccination series. Administration of three or four doses on an appropriate schedule followed by anti-HB testing 1–2 months after the third dose is usually more practical than serologic testing after one or more doses of vaccine [66]. For hemodialysis patients, the need for booster doses should be assessed annually by testing for antibody to hepatitis B surface antigen. A booster dose should be administered when anti-HB levels decline to <10 mIU/mL [66].

Influenza Vaccine

Children with kidney failure are identified to be at high risk for severe complications of influenza. [67]

Therefore, annual influenza vaccination is recommended with the inactivated vaccine. Live attenuated influenza vaccine is not generally recommended for children on dialysis. To allow time for production of protective antibody levels, vaccination should ideally occur before onset of influenza activity in the community. Therefore, vaccination should start as soon as vaccine is available.

Pneumococcal Vaccine [68, 69]

For children ages 2–5 yrs. on dialysis or posttransplant:

1. Administer one dose of PCV13 if any incomplete schedule of three doses of PCV (PCV7 and/or PCV13) were received previously.

2. Administer two doses of PCV13 at least 8 weeks apart if unvaccinated or any incomplete schedule of fewer than three doses of PCV (PCV7 and/or PCV13) were received previously.
3. Administer one supplemental dose of PCV13 if four doses of PCV7 or other age-appropriate complete PCV7 series was received previously.
4. The minimum interval between doses of PCV (PCV7 or PCV13) is 8 weeks.
5. For children with no history of PPSV23 vaccination, administer PPSV23 at least 8 weeks after the most recent dose of PCV13.

For children ages 6 to 18 yrs. on dialysis or posttransplant:

1. If neither PCV13 nor PPSV23 has been received previously, administer one dose of PCV13 now and one dose of PPSV23 at least 8 weeks later.
2. If PCV13 has been received previously but PPSV23 has not, administer one dose of PPSV23 at least 8 weeks after the most recent dose of PCV13.
3. If PPSV23 has been received but PCV13 has not, administer one dose of PCV13 at least 8 weeks after the most recent dose of PPSV23.

For children ages 6 to 18 yrs. on dialysis or posttransplant who have not received PPSV23, administer one dose of PPSV23. If PCV13 has been received previously, then PPSV23 should be administered at least 8 weeks after any prior PCV13 dose.

A single revaccination with PPSV23 should be administered 5 years after the first dose.

Special Situations [70, 71]

In heavily immunosuppressed patients, live vaccines are usually not recommended. This is primarily a safety concern, because persons who have altered immunocompetence and receive live vaccines might be at increased risk for an adverse reaction because of uninhibited growth of the attenuated live virus or bacteria. Vaccines might also be less effective in this population. Inactivated vaccines might best be deferred during a period of altered immunocompetence due to concern about their effectiveness. Additionally, if an inactivated vaccine is administered during the period of altered immunocompetence, it might need to be repeated after immune function has improved. For the purpose of the AAP Redbook, high-level immunosuppression is defined as receiving daily corticosteroid therapy at a dose ≥20 mg (or > 2 mg/kg/day for patients weighing <10 kg) of prednisone or equivalent for ≥14 days or receiving certain biologic immune modulators, for example, tumor necrosis factor-alpha (TNF-α) antagonists (e.g., adalimumab, certolizumab, infliximab, etanercept, and golimumab) or anti-B-lymphocyte monoclonal antibodies (e.g., rituximab), and low-level immunosuppression is defined as receiving a lower daily dose of systemic corticosteroid than for high-level immunosuppression for ≥14 days or receiving alternate-day corticosteroid therapy and receiving methotrexate at a dosage of ≤0.4 mg/kg/week, azathioprine at a dosage of ≤3 mg/kg/day, or 6-mercaptopurine at a dosage of ≤1.5 mg/kg/day [71]. Live-virus vaccination should be deferred for at least 1 month after discontinuation of high-dose systemically absorbed corticosteroid therapy administered for ≥14 days. In general, live vaccines should be withheld 3 months following biologic immune modulators, and both inactivated and live vaccines should be withheld at least 6 months following therapy with anti-B-cell antibodies.

Household/Live Donor Vaccination

In an effort to protect the dialysis patients from infection, especially if live vaccines are contraindicated for the patient, every effort should be made to ensure that all household contacts are fully vaccinated per standard vaccine schedules. If time permits, potential live organ donors (who may not be household members) should also be fully vaccinated per standard vaccine schedules.

Live Vaccines

Varicella Vaccine

Administer a two-dose series of varicella vaccine at ages 12 through 15 months and 4 through 6 years. The second dose may be administered before age 4 years, provided at least 3 months have elapsed since the first dose. If the second dose was administered at least 4 weeks after the first dose, it can be accepted as valid. Immunity to varicella zoster virus (VZV) should be assessed in dialysis patients, and seronegative patients should be re-immunized prior to transplantation. VZV vaccine may be given as early as 9 months of age if early transplant is anticipated. It can be given simultaneously with MMR or at least 4 weeks later. It is generally recommended that transplant not occur for a minimum of 4–6 weeks after varicella immunization due to the live virus it contains.

Measles-Mumps-Rubella Vaccine

Administer a two-dose series of MMR vaccine at ages 12 through 15 months and 4 through 6 years. The second dose may be administered before age 4 years, provided at least 4 weeks have elapsed since the first dose. Immunity to measles and rubella should be assessed prior to transplant in dialysis patients. Immunity to mumps remains more challenging and potentially concerning in view of recent epidemics of mumps in both Europe and the United States, but in general can be assumed to be present in the face of adequate responses to measles and rubella. Seronegative patients should be re-/immunized prior to transplant. MMR is approved for use down to 6 months of age and could be given if early transplant is anticipated, but such patients should still receive the two-dose series once they are greater than 1 year old. Two catch-up doses may be given at least 1 month apart. In general, patients should not undergo transplantation for a minimum of 4–6 weeks after immunization with MMR due to the live viruses it contains.

Recombinant and Inactivated ("Killed") Vaccines

DTaP/Tdap/dT Vaccine

Children aged 2 months to 7 years should be vaccinated according to the routine immunization schedule: Administer a five-dose series of DTaP vaccine at ages 2, 4, 6, 15 through 18 months, and 4 through 6 years. The fourth dose may be administered as early as age 12 months, provided at least 6 months have elapsed since the third dose. However, the fourth dose of DTaP need not be repeated if it was administered at least 4 months after the third dose of DTaP. The fifth dose of DTaP vaccine is not necessary if the fourth dose was administered at age 4 years or older. Patients should receive the Tdap booster by age 11 to 12 years and then every 10 years thereafter. For the catch-up vaccination schedule and for information about the appropriate use of Tdap and Td in older patients, please see CDC/ACIP recommendations [70].

Poliovirus Vaccine

A total of four doses of inactivated trivalent polio vaccine are recommended for all children: Administer a four-dose series of IPV at ages 2, 4, 6 through 18 months, and 4 through 6 years. The final dose in the series should be administered on or after the fourth birthday and at least 6 months after the previous dose. The first three doses can be given a month apart in children over 6 years of age who have not received any vaccines. Oral polio vaccine is no longer recommended in the United States and should not be administered to children awaiting transplantation.

Haemophilus Influenzae Type B Vaccine

Administer a two- or three-dose Hib vaccine primary series and a booster dose (dose 3 or 4 depending on vaccine used in primary series) at age 12 through 15 months to complete a full Hib vaccine series. One booster dose (dose 3 or 4 depending on vaccine used in primary series) of any Hib vaccine should be administered at age 12 through 15 months. The number of vaccinations required and the catch-up immunization schedule with HIB vaccine are influenced by the specific vaccine product used; please see CDC/ACIP guidelines for more detail [62].

Hepatitis A Vaccine

Initiate the two-dose Hep A vaccine series at 12 through 23 months; separate the two doses by 6 to 18 months. In those greater than 2 years old not previously vaccinated, a total of two doses given 6 months apart is recommended.

Hepatitis B Vaccine

A three-dose series should be administered to all children beginning at birth and concluding by 6 months of age. Catch-up immunization should be initiated for all children as soon as possible due to the high risks associated with hepatitis B infection in patients receiving hemodialysis or posttransplant. Response to vaccination can be assessed by determining the antibody level at 1 to 2 months after the third dose, and if <10 mIU/mL, the patient can receive up to three more doses. Please see earlier section which describes repeating the hepatitis B vaccine series.

Meningococcal Vaccine

One dose of meningococcal vaccine is recommended for all adolescents. With high-risk condition (e.g., functional or anatomic asplenia, complement deficiency, HIV infection, eculizumab exposure), vaccination in infancy followed by boosters every 5 years is recommended. Many new meningococcal vaccine formulations and subtypes have been approved recently, and the recommended age ranges have been revised. The CDC/ACIP recommendations should be reviewed for the most up-to-date guidelines [70].

Human Papillomavirus

Administer a three-dose series of HPV vaccine to all adolescents aged 11 through 12 years. Either HPV4 or HPV2 may be used for females, and only HPV4 may be used for males. The vaccine is approved for use starting at age 9 years old. In order to maximize the efficacy of vaccination, consider vaccinating dialysis patients at age 9 in order to increase the chance of completing the series before they are immunosuppressed for organ transplantation [72].

Updating Immunizations for the Dialysis Patient Awaiting Transplant

The immunization status of patients on the transplant waiting list should be monitored and updated as appropriate. Hepatitis B antibody status should be assessed with annual antibody testing and vaccine re-administered using either brand of commercially available vaccine (Recombivax HB or Energix) when antibody levels decline below 10 mIU/mL. Recommendations using Recombivax vaccine include a repeat dose 1 to 2 months after the third dose if the antibody levels decline below 10 mIU/mL. Patients should receive the Tdap booster by age 11 to 16 years and then every 10 years. The influenza vaccine should be given annually once a year to both the patient and his/her family.

Questions

1. Which of the following is a contraindication to transplant?
   (a) Active tuberculosis infection
   (b) HIV infection on antiviral therapy
   (c) CMV seropositivity
   (d) Hepatitis B infection on antiviral therapy

   (a). KDIGO recommends completion of treatment for active TB prior to transplant.

2. Pretransplant testing for the following are recommended for ALL patients except:
   (a) COVID-19
   (b) CMV
   (c) Histoplasmosis
   (d) Hepatitis B
   (c). Histoplasmosis testing is only recommended in endemic areas.
3. All of the following are criteria for increased risk donors except:
   (a) Hemodiluted deceased donor's blood sample.
   (b) When deceased donor's medical or behavior history cannot be ascertained, donor should be considered increased risk.
   (c) Donor on ECMO in the week prior to donation.
   (d) Sex in exchange for money or drugs in the preceding 12 months.
   (c). Donor on ECMO does not place the donor in the increased risk category.
4. All of the following statements about pretransplant vaccination are true except:
   (a) Vaccination of household contacts of dialysis patients is not recommended.
   (b) Hepatitis B antibody status should be assessed with annual antibody testing and vaccine re-administered when antibody levels decline.
   (c) For transplant candidates, priority should be given to the live vaccines since they are generally not recommended following organ transplantation.
   (d) Hepatitis B vaccination is recommended for all chronic hemodialysis patients.
   (a). Household contacts of dialysis patients should be vaccinated to help protect the patient.

References

1. Foster BJ, Dahhou M, Zhang X, Platt RW, Hanley JA. Change in mortality risk over time in young kidney transplant recipients. Am J Transplant. 2011;11:2432–42.
2. Kato S, Chmielewski M, Honda H, et al. Aspects of immune dysfunction in end-stage renal disease. Clin J Am Soc Nephrol. 2008;3:1526–33.
3. Chadban SJ, Ahn C, Axelrod DA, et al. KDIGO clinical practice guideline on the evaluation and management of candidates for kidney transplantation. Transplantation. 2020;104:S11–s103.
4. Malinis M, Boucher HW. Screening of donor and candidate prior to solid organ transplantation-guidelines from the american society of transplantation infectious diseases community of practice. Clin Transpl. 2019;33:e13548.
5. Te H, Doucette K. Viral hepatitis: guidelines by the american society of transplantation infectious disease community of practice. Clin Transpl. 2019;33:e13514.
6. Pereyra F, Rubin RH. Prevention and treatment of cytomegalovirus infection in solid organ transplant recipients. Curr Opin Infect Dis. 2004;17:357–61.
7. Cockfield SM, Preiksaitis JK, Jewell LD, Parfrey NA. Post-transplant lymphoproliferative disorder in renal allograft recipients. Clinical experience and risk factor analysis in a single center. Transplantation. 1993;56:88–96.
8. Walker RC, Paya CV, Marshall WF, et al. Pretransplantation seronegative Epstein-Barr virus status is the primary risk factor for posttransplantation lymphoproliferative disorder in adult heart, lung, and other solid organ transplantations. J Heart Lung Transplant. 1995;14:214–21.
9. Dharnidharka VR, Tejani AH, Ho PL, Harmon WE. Post-transplant lymphoproliferative disorder in the United States: young Caucasian males are at highest risk. Am J Transplant. 2002;2:993–8.

10. Silva A, Rodig N, Passerotti CP, et al. Risk factors for urinary tract infection after renal transplantation and its impact on graft function in children and young adults. J Urol. 2010;184:1462–7.
11. Lewinsohn DM, Leonard MK, LoBue PA, et al. Official american thoracic society/infectious diseases society of america/centers for disease control and prevention clinical practice guidelines: diagnosis of tuberculosis in adults and children. Clin Infect Dis. 2017;64:111–5.
12. Subramanian AK, Theodoropoulos NM. Mycobacterium tuberculosis infections in solid organ transplantation: guidelines from the infectious diseases community of practice of the american society of transplantation. Clin Transpl. 2019;33:e13513.
13. Muñoz P, Rodríguez C, Bouza E. Mycobacterium tuberculosis infection in recipients of solid organ transplants. Clin Infect Dis. 2005;40:581–7.
14. Wolfe CR, Ison MG, Practice tAIDCo. Donor-derived infections: guidelines from the American Society of Transplantation Infectious Diseases Community of Practice. Clin Transplant. 2019;33:e13547.
15. Casas S, Muñoz L, Moure R, et al. Comparison of the 2-step tuberculin skin test and the quantiFERON-TB Gold In-Tube Test for the screening of tuberculosis infection before liver transplantation. Liver Transplant. 2011;17:1205–11.
16. Kim SH, Lee SO, Park JB, et al. A prospective longitudinal study evaluating the usefulness of a T-cell-based assay for latent tuberculosis infection in kidney transplant recipients. Am J Transplant Off J Am Soc Transplant Am Soc Transplant Surg. 2011;11:1927–35.
17. Hasan T, Au E, Chen S, Tong A, Wong G. Screening and prevention for latent tuberculosis in immunosuppressed patients at risk for tuberculosis: a systematic review of clinical practice guidelines. BMJ Open. 2018;8:e022445.
18. Weiss P, Chen W, Cook VJ, Johnston JC. Treatment outcomes from community-based drug resistant tuberculosis treatment programs: a systematic review and meta-analysis. BMC Infect Dis. 2014;14:333.
19. Shoham S, Marr KA. Invasive fungal infections in solid organ transplant recipients. Future Microbiol. 2012;7:639–55.
20. Khan A, El-Charabaty E, El-Sayegh S. Fungal infections in renal transplant patients. J Clin Med Res. 2015;7:371–8.
21. Miller R, Assi M. Endemic fungal infections in solid organ transplant recipients-guidelines from the american society of transplantation infectious diseases community of practice. Clin Transpl. 2019;33:e13553.
22. Rappo U, Beitler JR, Faulhaber JR, et al. Expanding the horizons of histoplasmosis: disseminated histoplasmosis in a renal transplant patient after a trip to Bangladesh. Transplant Infectious Dis. 2010;12:155–60.
23. Nguyen C, Barker BM, Hoover S, et al. Recent advances in our understanding of the environmental, epidemiological, immunological, and clinical dimensions of coccidioidomycosis. Clin Microbiol Rev. 2013;26:505–25.
24. Kauffman CA, Freifeld AG, Andes DR, et al. Endemic fungal infections in solid organ and hematopoietic cell transplant recipients enrolled in the Transplant-Associated Infection Surveillance Network (TRANSNET). Transplant Infectious Dis. 2014;16:213–24.
25. Flegr J, Prandota J, Sovičková M, Israili ZH. Toxoplasmosis—a global threat. Correlation of latent toxoplasmosis with specific disease burden in a set of 88 countries. PLoS One. 2014;9:e90203.
26. La Hoz RM, Morris MI. Tissue and blood protozoa including toxoplasmosis, Chagas disease, leishmaniasis, Babesia, Acanthamoeba, Balamuthia, and Naegleria in solid organ transplant recipients-Guidelines from the American Society of Transplantation Infectious Diseases Community of Practice. Clin Transpl. 2019;33:e13546.
27. Wreghitt TG, Hakim M, Gray JJ, et al. Toxoplasmosis in heart and heart and lung transplant recipients. J Clin Pathol. 1989;42:194–9.
28. Bisoffi Z, Buonfrate D, Montresor A, et al. Strongyloides stercoralis: a plea for action. PLoS Negl Trop Dis. 2013;7:e2214.

29. Center for Disease Control and Prevention. Epidemiology and risk factor – strongyloides. 2020. Accessed 10/24/20, 2020, at https://www.cdc.gov/parasites/strongyloides/epi.html#:~:text=The%20global%20prevalence%20of%20Strongyloidesof%20persons%20sampled%20were%20infected.
30. Al-Obaidi M, Hasbun R, Vigil KJ, et al. Seroprevalence of strongyloides stercoralis and evaluation of universal screening in kidney transplant candidates: a single-center experience in Houston (2012-2017). Open Forum Infect Dis. 2019;6
31. Roxby AC, Gottlieb GS, Limaye AP. Strongyloidiasis in transplant patients. Clin Infect Dis. 2009;49:1411–23.
32. La Hoz RM, Morris MI. Intestinal parasites including Cryptosporidium, Cyclospora, Giardia, and Microsporidia, Entamoeba histolytica, Strongyloides, Schistosomiasis, and Echinococcus: guidelines from the American Society of Transplantation Infectious Diseases Community of Practice. Clin Transpl. 2019;33:e13618.
33. Wiersinga WJ, Rhodes A, Cheng AC, Peacock SJ, Prescott HC. Pathophysiology, transmission, diagnosis, and treatment of coronavirus disease 2019 (COVID-19): a review. JAMA. 2020;324:782–93.
34. Comeau S, Jensen L, Cockfield SM, Sapijaszko M, Gourishankar S. Non-melanoma skin cancer incidence and risk factors after kidney transplantation: a Canadian experience. Transplantation. 2008;86:535–41.
35. SARS-CoV-2 (Coronavirus, 2019-nCoV): Recommendations and Guidance for Organ Donor Testing. 2020. Accessed 10/20/2020, 2020, at https://www.myast.org/sites/default/files/Donor%20Testing_100520_revised_ReadyToPostUpdated10-12.pdf.
36. Chavers BM, Gillingham KJ, Matas AJ. Complications by age in primary pediatric renal transplant recipients. Pediatr Nephrol. 1997;11:399–403.
37. Abbott KC, Swanson SJ, Richter ER, et al. Late urinary tract infection after renal transplantation in the United States. Am J Kidney Dis. 2004;44:353–62.
38. Muller V, Becker G, Delfs M, Albrecht KH, Philipp T, Heemann U. Do urinary tract infections trigger chronic kidney transplant rejection in man? J Urol. 1998;159:1826–9.
39. Wagener MM, Yu VL. Bacteremia in transplant recipients: a prospective study of demographics, etiologic agents, risk factors, and outcomes. Am J Infect Control. 1992;20:239–47.
40. Chuang P, Parikh CR, Langone A. Urinary tract infections after renal transplantation: a retrospective review at two US transplant centers. Clin Transpl. 2005;19:230–5.
41. Takai K, Tollemar J, Wilczek HE, Groth CG. Urinary tract infections following renal transplantation. Clin Transpl. 1998;12:19–23.
42. Kamath NS, John GT, Neelakantan N, Kirubakaran MG, Jacob CK. Acute graft pyelonephritis following renal transplantation. Transpl Infect Dis. 2006;8:140–7.
43. European Best Practice Guidelines for Renal Transplantation. Section IV: Long-term management of the transplant recipient. IV.11 Paediatrics (specific problems). Nephrol Dial Transplant. 2002;17(Suppl 4):55–8.
44. Ghane Sharbaf F, Bitzan M, Szymanski KM, et al. Native nephrectomy prior to pediatric kidney transplantation: biological and clinical aspects. Pediatric Nephrol (Berlin, Germany). 2012;27:1179–88.
45. Goldman JD, Julian K. Urinary tract infections in solid organ transplant recipients: guidelines from the American Society of Transplantation infectious diseases Community of Practice. Clin Transpl. 2019;33:e13507.
46. Understanding the Risk of Transmission of HIV, Hepatitis B, and Hepatitis C from U.S. PHS Increased Risk Donors. at https://optn.transplant.hrsa.gov/media/2270/dtac_guidance_risks_201706.pdf.
47. Jones JM, Kracalik I, Levi ME, et al. Assessing solid organ donors and monitoring transplant recipients for human immunodeficiency virus, hepatitis B virus, and hepatitis C virus infection – U.S. public health service guideline, 2020. MMWR Recomm Rep. 2020;69:1–16.
48. Singer AL, Kucirka LM, Namuyinga R, Hanrahan C, Subramanian AK, Segev DL. The high-risk donor: viral infections in solid organ transplantation. Curr Opin Organ Transplant. 2008;13:400–4.

49. Kucirka LM, Sarathy H, Govindan P, et al. Risk of window period hepatitis-C infection in high infectious risk donors: systematic review and meta-analysis. Am J Transplant Off J Am Soc Transplant Am Soc Transplant Surg. 2011;11:1188–200.
50. Kucirka LM, Sarathy H, Govindan P, et al. Risk of window period HIV infection in high infectious risk donors: systematic review and meta-analysis. Am J Transplant Off J Am Soc Transplant Am Soc Transplant Surg. 2011;11:1176–87.
51. Green M, Covington S, Taranto S, Michaels MG, Wolfe C, Kaul DR. Pediatrics and donor-derived disease transmission: the US OPTN experience. Pediatr Transplant. 2018;22:e13115.
52. Kizilbash SJ, Chavers BM. Strategies to expand the deceased donor pool for pediatric kidney transplant recipients. Kidney 360 2020;1:691–3.
53. Kizilbash SJ, Rheault MN, Wang Q, et al. Kidney transplant outcomes associated with the use of increased risk donors in children. Am J Transplant Off J Am Soc Transplant Am Soc Transplant Surg. 2019;19:1684–92.
54. Duan KI, Englesbe MJ, Volk ML. Centers for disease control 'high-risk' donors and kidney utilization. Am J Transplant Off J Am Soc Transplant Am Soc Transplant Surg. 2010;10:416–20.
55. Anderson B, Jezewski E, Sela N, Westphal S, Hoffman A. Public health service increased risk donor kidney grafts for transplant into children, a survey of pediatric nephrologists. Pediatric Transplantation. n/a:e13863.
56. Kucirka LM, Bowring MG, Massie AB, Luo X, Nicholas LH, Segev DL. Landscape of deceased donors labeled increased risk for disease transmission under new guidelines. Am J Transplant Off J Am Soc Transplant Am Soc Transplant Surg. 2015;15:3215–23.
57. Lonze BE, Dagher NN, Liu M, et al. Outcomes of renal transplants from Centers for Disease Control and Prevention high-risk donors with prospective recipient viral testing: a single-center experience. Arch Surg(Chicago, Ill : 1960). 2011;146:1261–6.
58. Pruett TL, Clark MA, Taranto SE. Deceased organ donors and PHS risk identification: impact on organ usage and outcomes. Transplantation. 2017;101:1670–8.
59. OPTN/SRTR 2018 Annual Data Report: Preface. Am J Transplant. 2020;20(Suppl s1):1–10.
60. Farrugia D, Cheshire J, Mahboob S, et al. Mortality after pediatric kidney transplantation in England—a population-based cohort study. Pediatr Transplant. 2014;18:16–22.
61. Seem DL, Lee I, Umscheid CA, Kuehnert MJ. PHS guideline for reducing human immunodeficiency virus, hepatitis B virus, and hepatitis C virus transmission through organ transplantation. Public Health Rep. (Washington, DC : 1974). 2013;128:247–343.
62. Strikas RA, ACIP, ACIP Child/Adolescent Immunization Work Group. Advisory committee on immunization practices recommended immunization schedules for persons aged 0 through 18 years — United States, 2015. MMWR. 2015;64(04):93–4.
63. Rangel MC, Coronado VG, Euler GL, Strikas RA. Vaccine recommendations for patients on chronic dialysis. The Advisory Committee on Immunization Practices and the American Academy of Pediatrics. Semin Dial. 2000;13:101.
64. Chi C, Patel P, Pilishvili T, et al. ACIP. Guidelines for vaccinating kidney dialysis patients and patients with chronic kidney disease. http://www.cdc.gov/dialysis/PDFs/Vaccinating_Dialysis_Patients_and_Patients_dec2012.pdf.
65. Misurac JM, VanDeVoorde RG, Kallash M, et al. Immunogenicity of Augmented Compared With Standard Dose Hepatitis B Vaccine in Pediatric Patients on Dialysis: a Midwest Pediatric Nephrology Consortium Study. Clin J Am Soc Nephrol. 2017;12(5):772–8. https://doi.org/10.2215/CJN.04750416. Epub 2017 Mar 7.PMID: 28270432.
66. Mast EE, Weinbaum CM, Fiore AE, et al. A comprehensive immunization strategy to eliminate transmission of hepatitis B virus infection in the United States: recommendations of the Advisory Committee on Immunization Practices (ACIP) Part II: immunization of adults. MMWR Recomm Rep. 2006;55(RR-16):1–33.
67. Fiore AE, Uyeki TM, Broder K, et al. Prevention and control of influenza with vaccines: recommendations of the Advisory Committee on Immunization Practices (ACIP), 2010. MMWR Recomm Rep. 2010;59(RR-8):1–62.
68. Centers for Disease Control and Prevention. Use of 13-Valent Pneumococcal Conjugate Vaccine and 23-Valent Pneumococcal Polysaccharide Vaccine for Adults with Immunocompromising

Conditions: Recommendations of the Advisory Committee on Immunization Practices (ACIP). MMWR Morb Mortal Wkly Rep. 2012;61:816–9.
69. Nuorti JP, Whitney CG. Prevention of Pneumococcal Disease Among Infants and Children -Use of 13-Valent Pneumococcal Conjugate Vaccine and 23-Valent Pneumococcal Polysaccharide Vaccine -Recommendations of the Advisory Committee on Immunization Practices (ACIP). MMWR Recomm Rep. 2010;59(RR-11):1–18.
70. https://www.cdc.gov/vaccines/hcp/acip-recs/general-recs/immunocompetence.html.
71. American Academy of Pediatrics. Immunization in special clinical circumstances. In: Pickering L, Baker C, Kimberlin D, Long S, editors. Red book: 2009 Report of the committee on infectious diseases. 28th ed. Elk Grove Village, IL: American Academy of Pediatrics. p. 2009.
72. Nailescu C, Nelson RD, et al. Human papillomavirus vaccination in male and female adolescents before and after kidney transplantation: a pediatric nephrology research consortium study. Front Pediatr. 8:46. https://doi.org/10.3389/fped.2020.00046.

Post-transplant Recipient Infectious Challenges

5

Isa F. Ashoor and Sonia Solomon

Introduction

Significant progress has been made in the field of pediatric transplantation over the past couple of decades as evidenced by an overall decline in early acute rejection rates and improvement in both patient and graft survival [1–3]. This is largely attributed to improvement in surgical techniques, donor and recipient selection, and immunosuppression protocols. Despite that, achievement of tolerance – the holy grail of transplantation medicine – remains elusive, and personalized medicine is still far from routine application. As such, the majority of pediatric kidney transplant recipients continue to receive non-selective immunosuppressive protocols that contribute to an increased risk of opportunistic infections and cancer following transplantation. In fact, infections have surpassed kidney transplant rejection as the most common cause of hospitalization [4]. This chapter will focus on challenges related to the prevention, diagnosis, and treatment of opportunistic post-kidney transplant infections (infections caused by CMV, EBV, and BK virus and PJP), resurgent outbreaks of measles and mumps, cancer risk, specifically post-transplant lymphoproliferative disorder (PTLD), and urinary tract infections (UTIs).

I. F. Ashoor (✉)
Department of Pediatrics, LSU Health and Children's Hospital New Orleans, New Orleans, LA, USA
e-mail: iashoo@lsuhsc.edu

S. Solomon
Department of Pediatric Nephrology, Maria Fareri Children's Hospital/New York Medical College/Westchester Medical Center/Boston Children's Health Physicians, Valhalla, NY, USA
e-mail: ssolomon20@nymc.edu

K. E. Twombley (ed.), *Challenges in Pediatric Kidney Transplantation*,
https://doi.org/10.1007/978-3-030-74783-1_5

Opportunistic Post-Kidney Transplant Infections (CMV, EBV, and BK Virus and PJP)

Cytomegalovirus (CMV)

Cytomegalovirus (CMV) is common in the general population, but it poses a problem in the immunocompromised transplant patients [5, 6]. CMV remains a great contributor to morbidity and mortality. CMV infection is common up to 6 months after transplant without the use of prophylaxis [7]. The majority of pediatric CMV guidelines have been extrapolated from adult research as there is limited data on pediatrics [5].

Risk Factors

Those at highest risk for primary or secondary CMV infection include seronegative recipients of seropositive donors [7, 8]. In pediatrics, about 62% of deceased donor renal transplant recipients and about 32% of living donor renal transplant recipients were seronegative for CMV [9]. Recent studies have demonstrated that risk stratification of seropositive donor to seropositive recipients and seronegative donors to seronegative recipients did not increase transplant wait times and there was no difference in graft outcomes [10]. CMV infections are most often seen after the completion of prophylaxis [7]. Other risk factors include administration of T-cell depleting agents, steroid pulses, graft rejection, coinfection with other herpes viruses, and neutropenia [5, 7]. Zhang et al. demonstrated in murine models that ischemia/reperfusion injury itself is also a risk factor for CMV reactivation [11].

Clinical Presentation

Patients can present with asymptomatic CMV infection which is defined by CMV replication in the absence of clinical symptoms. They may also present with primary infection which can occur with seronegative recipients of seropositive donor organs [6]. Although unusual, primary infection can be secondary to person-to-person contact or blood transfusions [6]. Reactivation of latent infection can also occur depending on the degree of immunosuppression. Superinfection may occur in seropositive donor and seropositive recipient pairs [6]. They may also present with CMV disease which is defined as evidence of CMV infection with symptoms including fever, fatigue, leukopenia, thrombocytopenia, hepatitis, pneumonitis, colitis, retinitis, or encephalitis [5, 7]. It is prudent to be mindful that CMV levels may be low or undetectable in those with GI or CNS disease [7]. In addition, CMV has been known to contribute to acute or chronic nephropathy in kidney transplant recipients [5].

Screening

At this time, the most commonly used assays to monitor CMV infection are the quantitative molecular assays [5, 7]. Quantitative nucleic acid testing (QNAT) CMV DNA assays are frequently used [12]. This testing employs polymerase chain reaction (PCR) to detect CMV DNA in plasma, with higher levels being associated with more severe disease [6]. CMV can be detected in the whole blood or plasma, being cognizant that whole blood assays have higher viral loads than plasma assays [5]. Other assays that have been used to detect CMV include pp65 antigenemia assays and cell culture [5, 13]. pp65 antigenemia assay is based on the presence of infected cells in peripheral blood which is detected by a fluorescence assay [5]. This methodology has higher sensitivity and specificity than cell cultures but is akin to CMV PCR monitoring [5]. Cell culture technique is another traditional method of CMV detection [14]. In this method, clinical specimens are inoculated into human fibroblast cells which then are allowed to incubate for up to 3 weeks [14]. The degree of cytopathic effect CMV demonstrates is associated with CMV titers [14]. Given the length of time needed for definitive results using the traditional tissue culture results, the shell vial assay was developed which uses a centrifuge amplification technique for faster results [14]. The infectivity of CMV within the fibroblasts increases during the centrifugation process [14]. After 16 hours of incubation, CMV viral antigens may be detected by monoclonal antibodies via immunofluorescence [14]. However, tissue diagnosis is important in invasive disease [6, 7]. QNAT is not only used to diagnose CMV disease but it is also used to help guide management [7]. Low-level viremia is defined as a quantitative viral load <2500 IU, but no specific cutoff for initiation of treatment is known and varies by center [7]. Tissue diagnosis is based on the detection of viral inclusion bodies or CMV antigens using DNA hybridization or immunohistochemistry [15]. Frozen biopsy tissue is transferred to slides, in which fluorescently labeled secondary antibodies are used to visualize antibodies against CMV antigens [14]. Light or fluorescent microscopy is used to analyze the slides [14].

Prophylaxis and Preemptive Therapy

Prevention of CMV is attempted with prophylaxis or preemptive therapy [5]. Prophylaxis uses either ganciclovir or valganciclovir. However, the ideal length of prophylaxis remains unknown [16]. Prophylaxis varies by center but is guided by risk stratification, with concern that shorter prophylaxis can increase the risk of CMV detection and disease [17]. A suggested risk-based CMV prophylaxis strategy is summarized in Table 5.1. Donor seropositive/recipient seronegative pairs are the patients at the highest risk. These patients would require CMV prophylaxis for at

Table 5.1 Risk-based prophylaxis strategy for CMV monitoring [7, 12, 18]

Induction with lymphocyte depleting agents	
High risk: D+/R-	Prophylaxis for 6 months
Intermediate risk: D+/R+, D-/R+	Prophylaxis for 6 months
Low risk: D-/R-	Pre-emptive therapy[a]
Induction with IL-2 receptor antibody	
High risk: D+/R-	Prophylaxis for 3–6 months
Intermediate risk: D+/R+, D-/R+	Pre-emptive therapy[a]
Low risk: D-/R-	Pre-emptive therapy[a]

[a]Pre-emptive therapy: CMV monitoring weekly or biweekly from month 1 to 3, followed by monthly monitoring from month 3 to 6

least 3–6 months [7, 12, 19]. More recently, cytomegalovirus cell-mediated immunity (CMI) has been proposed as a factor in determining the duration of prophylaxis [6, 20]. CMV levels should be monitored biweekly or monthly [7]. In intermediate-risk patients (donor seronegative/recipient seropositive or donor seropositive/recipient seropositive), either preemptive therapy or 3 months of prophylaxis can be utilized [5, 7, 12]. Seropositive recipients who received T-cell-depleting agents typically receive at least 6 months of prophylaxis [7, 19]. Moderate- and low-risk patients may require CMV monitoring with levels checked weekly or biweekly [7]. Prophylaxis can be completed with valganciclovir, acyclovir, or ganciclovir [7], but if using valganciclovir, the doses must be adjusted for renal clearance [12].

Preemptive therapy is a cost-effective practice employed by some centers, which is defined by routine strategic monitoring for positive CMV assays. If replication is noted, patients are treated to prevent significant disease [5].

Treatment

It has been noted that CMV disease is not common with prophylaxis. However, after the completion of prophylaxis, the risk of disease increases up to 37% in high-risk patients [7]. If patients have CMV disease, the Kidney Disease Improving Global Outcomes (KDIGO) guidelines recommend weekly monitoring of CMV levels [19]. Adult treatment guidelines include oral valganciclovir or intravenous ganciclovir for a minimum of 2–3 weeks and until there are at least two negative CMV tests a week apart [5–7]. This should be followed by 3 months of prophylaxis [7]. KIDGO recommends that pediatric patients with CMV disease be treated with intravenous (IV) ganciclovir [19]. However, oral valganciclovir is equally effective as IV ganciclovir [7]. If patients have hypogammaglobulinemia, the addition of CMV hyperimmunoglobulin may be of benefit [7]. Providers should be aware of and monitor for CMV ganciclovir antiviral resistance [6, 7]. Common genetic resistance testing can determine common mutations such as the UL97 and UL54 which may guide treatment options in patients that do not respond to first-line treatment [7]. For example, IV ganciclovir cannot be used in UL97 mutations [7]. UL97 mutations lead to impaired phosphorylation of ganciclovir in virus-infected cells, with resultant lack of synthesis to the active form of the drug, ganciclovir triphosphate [21].

Other intravenous treatment options include cidofovir and foscarnet [6, 7]. Of note, multiple studies have demonstrated that mTOR inhibitors can be associated with a lower incidence of CMV infection, which may lead clinicians to use low-dose calcineurin inhibitors and mTOR inhibitors for maintenance immunosuppression in patients at high risk for CMV or post-CMV infection. mTOR inhibitors have been demonstrated to improve CMV-specific effector memory T-cells, increased cytokine release, and improved function of CMV-specific cytotoxic CD 8+ T-cells [22–25].

BK Virus

BK is an abbreviation of the name of the first patient whom the virus was isolated from in 1971 with renal failure and obstruction. BK is a polyomavirus that can infect many species, including humans [7]. Primary infection is typically asymptomatic and is found in up to 80% of healthy adults as they have antibodies against the BK virus [26]. BK virus can cause infection in up to 10% of renal transplant recipients and most occur within the first 2 years after transplant [7, 18]. In pediatrics, BK viremia can occur as early as the first 4 months of post-transplant [26]. In adult patients, 30–60% of transplant recipients will develop viremia which could cause nephropathy [7, 27]. In pediatric patients, 3.8% of patients developed nephropathy and 10–24% developed graft loss [26, 28, 29]. In adults, graft loss ranges from 10% to 60% which can occur secondary to late diagnosis or treatment failure [30, 31]. Fifty percent of renal transplant recipients will have asymptomatic urinary shedding as the virus will become latent in rental tubular cells and ureteral cell layers [7, 30]. Viruria and tubular cell lysis is followed by replication in the interstitium crossing into the peritubular capillaries leading to nephropathy [26]. BK reactivation typically occurs within the tubular cells from the donor kidney [32]. Acute rejection and graft failure have been associated with BK nephropathy 2 years after diagnosis [27, 29].

Risk Factors

Risk factors include deceased donor renal transplants, human leukocyte antigen (HLA) mismatch, donor antibodies positive to BK, younger recipients, T-cell depleting agents, tacrolimus, mycophenolic acid, steroids, obstructive processes as primary disease, ureteric stenting, history of acute rejection, and retransplantation secondary to BK viremia [7, 8, 26, 27]. In a retrospective study in pediatric renal transplant recipients, 78% of patient with viremia and nephropathy had used tacrolimus, whereas 81% of patients with self-limited viremia were treated with mTOR inhibitors and cyclosporine A [33]. Hisadome et al. demonstrates that BK-antibody negative recipients who received a kidney from BK-antibody positive donors were at higher risk for developing decoy cells [34]. However, recipients with pre-transplant BK viruria were not found to have an increased risk of BK viremia or nephropathy post-transplant in a prospective study of pediatric and adult kidney transplant recipients [35]. Adult and pediatric studies have demonstrated that an increase in BK-virus-specific T cells correlates with BK virus clearance. Those with loss of BK-virus-specific T cells were noted to be at increased risk for BK viremia [36–38].

Clinical Presentation

Primary symptoms of BK viremia include viruria and viremia [7, 39]. Without screening of BK viruria or viremia, patients can present with allograft dysfunction or occasionally with ureteric smooth muscle proliferation manifesting as stenosis [7, 40]. Other non-renal symptoms include encephalitis, pneumonitis, polyomavirus-associated multifocal leukoencephalopathy (PML), or hemophagocytic syndrome

[7, 41]. Gold standard of diagnosis requires an allograft biopsy [7]. Renal biopsy may demonstrate intranuclear polyomavirus inclusion bodies in tubular epithelial cells (Fig. 5.1), epithelial cell necrosis, tubulointerstitial nephritis with cytopathic changes, and positive immunohistochemistry staining with antibodies for SV40 large T antigen, BK virus antigen, or in situ hybridization for BK virus nucleic acids [7, 30, 32].

Screening

Standard of care in renal transplant recipients requires frequent monitoring of BK viruria and/or BK viremia and renal dysfunction [7, 18]. Screening varies by center but KIDGO recommendation includes screening monthly for the first 3–6 months, then every 3 months until 12 months, followed by yearly evaluation for the 5 years post-transplant [7, 18, 19, 32]. Screening should also be completed in recipients with worsening allograft function or after treatment of acute rejection [18, 19]. This allows for early detection of virus replication which can lead to reduction in immunosuppression to assist with viral clearance [7]. Screening can include urine cytology for decoy cells and urine, plasma, or whole blood PCR for BK virus [18]. Whether to screen via urine or blood remains controversial. Negative urine studies have nearly 100% negative predictive value [18, 32]. Urine studies look specifically for decoy cells or BK deoxyribonucleic acid (DNA); however, these are less specific [7]. Positive urine tests include the presence of decoy cells or urine BK loads over 7 log gEq/mL or urine DNA load $>10^7$ copies/mL [7, 41]. KDIGO, and other studies, generally suggest plasma levels greater than 10,000 copies/mL and whole blood PCR >1500 copies/mL are considered positive [7, 18, 19, 27]. Studies have demonstrated that BK viruria precedes BK viremia by 4 weeks and that BK viremia precedes BK nephropathy on average by 8 weeks [30].

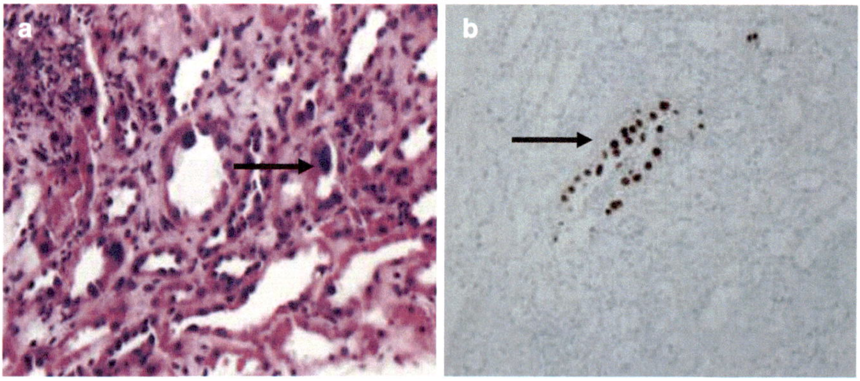

Fig. 5.1 BK virus nephropathy. (**a**) Tubular cell with intranuclear viral inclusion bodies (arrow). (**b**) Positive SV40 immunostaining (arrow) in a patient with BK virus nephropathy

Treatment

Monitoring for plasma BK DNA and appropriate immunosuppressive reduction has been proven to treat BK viremia [27, 30]. Preemptive therapy should be based off of plasma levels as opposed to viruria [30]. Plasma levels should be monitored every 2 weeks to help guide treatment management, and the level to start treatment is center dependent [30]. If there is a rise in serum creatinine, a biopsy should be considered [30]. Once rejection is ruled out and the biopsy is concerning for BK nephropathy, treatment can be initiated; however, if concomitant rejection is present, treatment for rejection should occur first [30]. Treatment for BK nephropathy requires minimizing immunosuppression [7]. The method for minimizing immunosuppression can vary. Options include (1) reduction of calcineurin inhibitors, followed by reduction or discontinuation of anti-metabolite [18, 30], (2) discontinuation of anti-metabolite followed by reduction of calcineurin inhibitors, or (3) reduction of both calcineurin inhibitor (CNI) and anti-metabolite [18, 30]. Reduction of CNI includes decreasing the dose by 15–20%, with goal troughs of less than 6 ng/mL [18, 30, 32, 42]. Other centers may switch from tacrolimus to cyclosporine (goal trough levels of 50–75 ng/mL) or to an mTOR inhibitor (goal trough levels less than 6 ng/mL) [6, 18, 30, 32].

Regardless of the choice of treatment, viral loads, renal function, and drug levels should be monitored frequently [7]. The main risk of minimizing immunosuppression includes rejection [7]. However, the treatment of rejection can subsequently incite flares of BK viremia [7]. If viremia persists in spite of immunosuppression reduction, other adjunctive therapies should be considered. There have been no studies, only case reports, that demonstrate the efficacy of these other therapies in children, which include cidofovir, brincidofovir, leflunomide, fluoroquinolones, or intravenous immunoglobulin G (IVIG) [7, 27, 39]. Much of the data involved in BK viremia are from the adult literature. Cidofovir has been used but needs to be monitored for nephrotoxicity [7, 27]. Brincidofovir is currently undergoing testing in clinical trials as an alternative therapy to cidofovir [27]. Leflunomide has antiviral along with some immunosuppressive properties with few case reports of clearance of viremia in pediatric patients, but adult studies have demonstrated significant side effects with its use [7, 27]. Side effects of leflunomide include diarrhea, nausea, transaminitis, neuropathy, hair loss, visual disturbances, and arthralgia [43]. In a small pediatric case series, 67% of the pediatric transplant patients (six kidney transplant recipients and one lung transplant recipient) responded to leflunomide with concomitant discontinuation of mycophenolate; they suggested a leflunomide target level of 30–40 mg/L [44]. Fluoroquinolones are not routinely recommended with minimal evidence showing little efficacy [27]. Intravenous immunoglobulins in the setting of standard treatment can assist in prolonged clearance in adults, but no difference was seen in graft survival [27]. However, Bentomane et al. demonstrated that treating patients with low titers of BK virus neutralizing antibodies with adjunctive IVIG had similar outcomes compared to those with high neutralizing antibodies, demonstrating that IVIG might be excellent in preventing BK viremia [45]. Another therapy that is currently undergoing investigation is T-cell adoptive immunotherapy [46].

If patients require retransplantation, the ideal time is after immunosuppressive agents have been discontinued for 6 months with low levels of BK viremia and BK viruria [7]. Transplant nephrectomy does not preclude BK viremia in the subsequent transplants, but may be needed if minimizing immunosuppression is not possible or viremia persists [7]. There has been evidence of excellent graft survival following retransplantation after BK nephropathy [47].

Epstein-Barr Virus

Epstein-Barr virus (EBV) is a herpesvirus that is found in the majority of people by the age of 5 years [27]. EBV infection post-transplant can be either primary through oral transmission or secondary as a result of either reactivation of latent virus in seropositive recipients or reactivation of latent disease from a seropositive donor in a seronegative recipient [30]. In pediatric patients, about 40% of deceased donor renal transplant recipients and about 58% of living donor renal transplant recipients were EBV serology negative at the time of transplant [9].

Risk Factors

Risk factors for EBV viremia include deceased donor renal transplant, recipients younger than 5 years old, greater than 5 HLA mismatches, and EBV seronegative recipients [48]. Symptomatic EBV viremia is more frequent in pediatric renal transplant recipients compared to adult renal transplant recipients as it is more likely to be a primary infection in younger patients with developing naive immune systems producing a more robust response [30, 49]. Due to frequent surveillance for EBV viremia, patients may develop subclinical viremia. Li et al. demonstrated the risk factors for subclinical viremia which included EBV seronegative status, recipients less than 5 years old, steroid use, and lack of prophylaxis. They also demonstrated that these patients were at risk of developing hypertension, lower 3-year graft function, high incidence of acute rejection, and high incidence of graft loss [50].

Clinical Presentation

The diagnosis of EBV can be made through symptoms, laboratory values, and imaging [30]. Patients can present with a wide array of symptoms including meningitis, encephalitis, tonsillitis, mononucleosis, diarrhea, pancreatitis, hepatosplenomegaly, atypical lymphocytosis, thrombocytopenia, anemia, adenopathy, allograft dysfunction, disseminated disease, or post-transplant lymphoproliferative disease (PTLD) [27, 30, 51]. In pediatric renal transplant recipients, 35–40% of patients have subclinical viral infection [8]. Renal transplant recipients have a lower incidence of PTLD than other solid organ transplants, given the use of less aggressive immunosuppressive regimens [27, 52]. Further discussion of PTLD can be seen later in this chapter.

Screening

Serologies may not be as useful in immunocompromised patients due to delayed or impaired humoral response after the initiation of immunosuppressive agents [8, 27, 53]; therefore, viral load of EBV DNA is used for serial monitoring [27]. Recipients who were EBV negative at the time of transplant were generally at high risk of having higher viral loads [30].

The goal of frequent monitoring of EBV viremia is to prevent the development of PTLD [18, 54]. KIDGO recommends screening patients at high risk for EBV primary infection/reactivation once in the first week after transplantation, then monthly for the first 3–6 months, then every 3 months until the end of the first year of transplant, and with any episodes of rejection [19].

Whether to use whole blood or plasma remains up for debate, but what is known is that levels should be monitored using the same type assay completed within the same lab to keep consistency [18]. The level to initiate intervention is also not defined and is center specific [18].

Antiviral prophylaxis is controversial without sufficient data to support its use [7, 27]. Often prophylaxis such as ganciclovir or valganciclovir is used in CMV prophylaxis and treatment which may also prevent EBV viremia [27]. However, there are recent studies that do not demonstrate any effect on the prevention of EBV-related PTLD [27]. A systemic review demonstrated that EBV prophylaxis had no effect on the development of PTLD in high-risk EBV patients [55].

Treatment

Treatment for EBV viremia includes reduction of immunosuppression in the setting of viremia, along with antivirals, IVIG, and monoclonal antibodies in severe disease [18]. Patients with primary or secondary EBV viremia can initially be treated with reducing immunosuppression; however, it may not be successful in patients with persistent high viral loads [7, 19, 30]. However, PTLD should be considered in those who remain viremic [7]. Infiltrating PTLD and acute rejection should be considered in patients with rising serum creatinine and viremia [7]. Response of EBV treatment is generally diagnosed by clearance of viremia [30]. Some groups opt to use anti-CD20 monoclonal antibody treatment to deplete B cells that act as the EBV host cell, including as a pre-emptive measure before development of actual viremia [30, 56, 57]. However, data are lacking to determine if this approach leads to sustained viral clearance or simply masks persistent disease [30]. Patients with persistent viremia may require changes in their immunosuppression [30]. If there is coinfection with CMV, this must be treated as well [7]. Further discussion of PTLD can be seen later in this chapter.

Pneumocystis jirovecii pneumonia (PJP)

Pneumocystis jirovecii formerly known as *Pneumocystis carinii* is an opportunistic fungus that invades the alveoli causing an uncommon cause of pneumonia in renal transplant recipients [6]. In adult renal transplant recipients, mortality is high at around 50%. Fortunately, due to prophylaxis, the incidence is low in both pediatric and adult patients [39]. Without PJP prophylaxis, the risk is greatest in the 6 months immediately post-transplant and during other periods of increased immunosuppression [40]. However, since the advent of generalized prophylaxis, the risk of PJP is now highest during the second-year post-transplant as PJP prophylaxis has generally been discontinued by this time and PJP prophylaxis has not been proven to be effective during this year of transplant [58]. Risk factors for PJP include higher donor age, higher recipient age, increased immunosuppression, high-dose steroids, CMV coinfection, lymphopenia, acute rejection, treatment with anti-thymocyte globulin for rejection, and exposure to PJP [6, 59]. Symptoms of PJP include fever, dyspnea, and non-productive cough with hypoxia [39]. CXR and CT scans may demonstrate "ground glass" interstitial infiltrates (Fig. 5.2) [39]. Diagnosis requires a bronchoscopy for sputum, bronchoalveolar lavage, or tissue samples which would then be sent for cytology, PCR, and the Silver or Giemsa stains [6, 39]. Serum-based 1,3, beta-D-glucan, a component of fungal cell wall component, has been utilized in the diagnosis of invasive fungal infections [40, 60]. There have been case reports of using direct metagenomic next-generation sequencing to diagnose PJP in difficult cases [61]. Interestingly, hypercalcemia has been seen in both adult and pediatric PJP patients, which is thought to be secondary to a granulomatous mechanism of PJP [62, 63]. Treatment includes reduction of immunosuppression and high-dose trimethoprim sulfamethoxazole (TMP) along with high-dose steroids in those who are critically ill [6, 39]. Trimethoprim sulfamethoxazole should be given for 14–21 days and the dose should be adjusted for renal function [39]. The low incidence of PJP is noted to be secondary to prophylaxis, which emphasizes the importance of prophylaxis [6]. Prophylaxis should be given for 6–12 months after

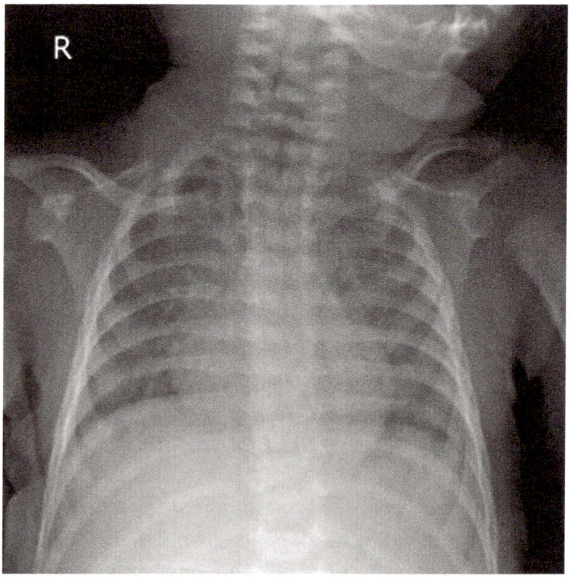

Fig. 5.2 "Ground-glass" appearance on chest X-ray in a child with *Pneumocystis jirovecii pneumonia* (PJP) infection

transplant, especially in patients with robust immunosuppression or after treatment of rejection [6]. Alternatives to trimethoprim sulfamethoxazole, which can be less than ideal, include atovaquone, dapsone, clindamycin, pentamidine (inhaled or IV), or TMP plus dapsone (G6PD should be checked prior to administration) [6, 39, 40, 64].

Resurgent Viral Infection Outbreaks: Measles and Mumps

The past decade has seen a resurgence of some vaccine-preventable infections, such as measles and mumps due to a combination of imported infections from unvaccinated travelers, and waning herd immunity levels in populations with an increasing prevalence of non-vaccinated individuals [65, 66]. Pediatric kidney transplant recipients are particularly vulnerable to measles and mumps infections in communities that experience an outbreak. This is due to a potential lack of vaccination against measles and mumps in recipients who were transplanted at a very young age before completing their primary vaccination series [67]. In those who were previously vaccinated, an impaired antibody response due to chronic kidney disease and/or declining antibody levels due to post-transplant immunosuppression may be other contributing factors [67, 68].

Both measles and mumps are highly contagious and spread via airborne and droplet routes, respectively [69, 70]. Measles can present with a generalized maculopapular rash, fever, cough, coryza, or conjunctivitis in immunocompetent hosts [69]. A more serious presentation of pneumonia and/or meningoencephalitis can be seen in some patients, particularly immunocompromised hosts [71, 72]. Symptoms may take weeks to months to develop in immunosuppressed patients following initial exposure, and progression can be rapid with a high rate of mortality [71]. Treatment is supportive and involves reduction of net immunosuppression. In addition, provision of vitamin A is recommended by the World Health Organization for all affected children older than 1 year of age [69]. Intravenous immunoglobulin and the antiviral ribavirin have been used in the treatment of measles in immunosuppressed patients, though no definitive data exist regarding their efficacy in this setting [71]. A stronger case can be made for the use of immunoglobulin to infer passive immunity to measles in patients who have not received the measles vaccines or have no documented protective antibody titers. Administration of intramuscular or intravenous immunoglobulin within 6–7 days of exposure to a confirmed case of measles provides significant protection against measles and is recommended for most patients [73, 74]. Mumps infection manifests as an acute viral syndrome with fever, fatigue, myalgia, and a viral exanthem and generally follows a benign course in immunocompetent individuals [70]. Swelling of the parotid glans due to parotitis is characteristic, while less frequent but well-described complications include aseptic meningitis, encephalitis, orchitis, and oophoritis [70]. In addition, kidney transplant recipients can experience interstitial nephritis in the allograft that may lead to transplant failure [75]. Treatment is largely supportive in conjunction with reduction of immunosuppression [76].

Due to the lack of effective antiviral therapies for measles and mumps, primary prevention via vaccination is paramount. There is growing evidence that administration of the measles-mumps-rubella (MMR) vaccine can be safe in a subset of kidney transplant recipients who meet specific criteria for low-level immunosuppression [77]. This may be a particularly useful strategy in the context of a community outbreak to protect recipients with missing pre-transplant MMR vaccination or documented suboptimal post-transplant antibody titers [78].

Cancer Risks

The rarity of individual post-kidney transplantation cancer events makes this complication one of the most challenging to address for pediatric nephrologists. A high index of suspicion informed by the recipient risk factor profile for developing a post-transplant malignancy is critical for prevention, early diagnosis, and effective treatment. The following discussion will briefly review the current literature regarding post-kidney transplantation cancer incidence, then focus on recipients' risk assessment for cancer (specifically PTLD), and end with a brief discussion of challenges related to current cancer prevention and treatment strategies.

Cancer Incidence

Cancer events following pediatric kidney transplantation can be divided into two main categories: lymphoproliferative disease (most commonly EBV-driven PTLD) and non-lymphoproliferative solid tumors. PTLD is the most common cancer following pediatric kidney transplantation with an incidence ranging from 1% to 2% in the first 5 years of post-kidney transplantation [79] and a 25-year cumulative incidence of 3.3% as reported by the Australian and New Zealand Dialysis and Transplant Registry [80]. The North American Pediatric Renal Trials and Collaborative Studies (NAPRTCS) registry reported 316 malignancy events over 30 years since its inception in 1987 till the end of 2017, of which 85% were PTLD diagnoses [2]. As for non-lymphoproliferative solid tumors, an analysis of the NAPRTCS registry identified 35 patients with a solid tumor diagnosis in 10,474 registry participants for an observed incidence rate of 72.1 per 100,000-person years. Those events were diagnosed at a median of 726 days post-transplant and represented a 6.7-fold increased risk compared to the general pediatric population [81]. The most common types of solid tumors in this cohort were renal cell carcinoma, followed by thyroid carcinoma and melanoma. Differences in cancer epidemiology could be regional. In an analysis of 1734 pediatric kidney transplant recipients in the Australian and New Zealand Dialysis and Transplant Registry over a median follow-up period of 13.4 years, the most common type of cancer was non-melanoma skin cancer in 196 recipients [82]. This is similar to data reported from adult solid organ recipients where non-melanoma skin cancers (squamous cell and basal cell carcinomas) are the most common types of cancer occurring in up to 15%

of recipients at 15 years of post-transplantation [79]. Of concern is an increase in cancer rates reported in the NAPRTCS registry most recent cohort from 2012 to 2017 after a period of steady decline since 2001. Overall, cancer rates in the most recent NAPRTCS cohort are at 1.03% and 2.31% at 1- and 3-year post-transplantation up from 0.83% and 1.51% in the 2007–2011 cohort [2]. Better understanding of cancer risk factors is needed to reverse this trend.

Cancer Risk Factors

Several large-scale registry analyses and smaller scale observational cohorts have identified a variety of factors that contribute to increased risk of cancer post-kidney transplantation, particularly PTLD.

Immunosuppression Burden

The cumulative burden of immunosuppression refers to both the intensity and duration of immunosuppressive regimen. The effect of immunosuppression duration is reflected in higher risk for post-transplant malignancy with greater time elapsed since the index transplant event as discussed later. Data on the intensity of immunosuppression and its relationship with post-transplant malignancy can be indirectly deduced from worse odds in recipients with fewer HLA matches [83] or recipients of deceased donor grafts relative to living donor grafts [84, 85]. Interestingly, in a study of 195 kidney transplant recipients who consented to electronic monitoring of their medication adherence, and followed up for a median of 10.1 years, those most adherent to their medication regimen had the highest cancer risk at 59.4%. This was significantly higher than the risk in the less adherent groups which ranged from 36.1% to 38.1% [86]. The occurrence of PTLD events was noted to be more common with belatacept treatment, a newer intravenous long-term maintenance immunosuppressive regimen, relative to cyclosporine, particularly in EBV seronegative recipients [87]. A recent Cochrane Database Systematic Review examining the use of belatacept in adult kidney transplantation did not reveal any significant difference in PTLD occurrence relative to those treated with calcineurin inhibitor-based regimens, which may reflect better patient selection for long-term belatacept therapy based on PTLD baseline risk [88].

Various induction therapy regimens have been linked to different cancer risks likely reflecting their contribution to the overall immunosuppression burden, though this relationship may be compounded by the potential higher risk of acute rejection with less potent induction therapies or no induction leading to subsequent escalation of immunosuppressive therapy. No association was found between the use of interleukin-2 receptor antibody (IL2R-Ab) induction and subsequent cancer risk in 461 pediatric kidney transplant recipients in the Australia and New Zealand Dialysis and Transplant registry in comparison to 197 recipients without induction [89].

Polyclonal antibody induction with antithymocyte globulin (ATG) has been linked to increased risk of PTLD relative to IL2R-Ab induction or no induction in an older registry analysis of 59,560 kidney transplant recipients in the Organ

Procurement and Transplantation Network/United Network for Organ Sharing (OPTN/UNOS) databases [90]. The Australian and New Zealand Dialysis and Transplant Registry reported a higher risk for PTLD with any induction agent other than IL2R-Ab induction [80]. However, a recent Cochrane Database Systematic Review that included both adult and pediatric studies revealed uncertain effects of anti-thymocyte globulin (ATG) induction on either early (1–2 years) or late (5 years) malignancy rates [91]. An analysis of the NAPRTCS registry did not reveal a difference in time to development of PTLD between recipients of a low versus high cumulative dose of rabbit ATG induction at a threshold of 7.5 mg per kg of body weight [92]. With an overall trend toward lower cumulative ATG dose exposure and more frequent use of antiviral prophylaxis, PTLD rates with ATG induction have generally remained at less than 1% in kidney transplant recipients [93, 94]. Alemtuzumab is emerging as an induction therapy choice for pediatric recipients on steroid avoidance protocols [95]. Data on PTLD risk with alemtuzumab induction are limited and, so far, uncertain [91]. This will be important to analyze as pediatric experience with this agent grows.

EBV Recipient-Donor Sero-Mismatch

EBV-positive tumors constitute ~50–80% of all PTLD cases [96]. Primary EBV infection in seronegative pediatric and adult recipients of seropositive donor kidneys has been identified as a major risk factor for PTLD [80, 97, 98]. EBV viremia, and specifically a higher EBV viral load peak, has been associated with PTLD development [99], though a clear cut link between the duration of viremia and the EBV viral load threshold at which the PTLD risk starts or increases is a subject of controversy and ongoing research [100]. There have also been cases of PTLD with low viral loads, making diagnosis even more challenging. Another challenging entity is the patient who develops a chronically high viral load (i.e., carrier state) following a primary EBV infection. This chronic high viral load state has been reported in as high as 24% of pediatric recipients in one cohort and may persist for months to years following the primary infection [101]. The risk of subsequent development of PTLD in pediatric recipients with chronic high EBV viral loads remains unclear with two small studies, including a combined total of 30 patients, demonstrating no PTLD development over a median follow-up period of 6.9 and 7.8 years, respectively [101, 102], and spontaneous resolution of the chronic high viral load state in 15 of 16 patients in one study [102].

Time Since Transplant

The risk of cancer increases over time as demonstrated in a retrospective analysis of 884 pediatric kidney transplant recipients at the University of Minnesota between 1963 and 2015, where the overall risk increased from 13% at 20 years of post-transplant to 26% at 30 years [103]. This is supportive of the hypothesis that both aging and cumulative chronic exposure to immunosuppression contribute to loss of anti-tumor surveillance mechanisms.

HLA Haplotypes

An analysis of 9202 pediatric kidney transplant recipients from the Collaborative Transplant Study in Germany identified a higher risk (hazard ratio 2.04) for post-transplant non-Hodgkin's lymphoma in recipients with 2 HLA-DR mismatches relative to those with 0–1 DR mismatches. This finding was consistent across two decades from 1997 to 2007 [104]. Fewer HLA matches were also significantly associated with PTLD development in an analysis of the US Renal Data Systems (USRDS) database involving 25,127 kidney transplant recipients [83]. Those findings may be an indirect reflection of the higher risk for rejection (with subsequent escalation of immunosuppression) in those with 2 HLA-DR mismatches or fewer HLA matches, respectively. In another study looking at novel association of certain HLA antigen types and PTLD, both HLA-B40 and HLA-B8 antigens were associated with increased risk for PTLD in EBV seronegative and EBV seropositive recipients, respectively [85]. Another study suggested a higher risk for PTLD in solid organ transplant recipients with HLA-A1 carrier status presumably due to reduced ability to mount an effective cytotoxic T-cell response in those individuals to control latent EBV infection [105]. In another multi-center case-control study comparing 155 PTLD cases in solid organ transplant recipients with 1996 controls who did not develop PTLD, expression of HLA-A03 or HLA-DR7 was each independently associated with a reduced risk of PTLD, whereas expression of HLA-B18 or HLA B-21 was associated with a higher risk [106].

Pre-transplant Malignancy

The occurrence of pre-transplant malignancy that leads to ESRD requiring kidney transplantation is infrequent. Typical scenarios involve children with a history of bilateral Wilms' tumor or a prior PTLD with subsequent graft failure. Pre transplant kidney candidate evaluation guidelines recommend a minimum waiting period for individual malignancies prior to proceeding with kidney transplantation that is determined based on receipt of curative treatment and in consultation with oncology [107]. This stems from concerns regarding higher risk for cancer recurrence post-transplantation with shorter remission times. The risk of cancer recurrence following kidney transplantation was found to be 2.4% per 100 person-years in a meta-analysis of 39 studies, with a greater risk in those transplanted within 5 years of cancer diagnosis [108]. While data are limited, pediatric recipients with pre-transplant malignancy have comparable patient and graft survival to recipients without that history [109], and no cases of PTLD recurrence have been reported in the NAPRTCS registry [110].

Age

In an analysis of data from the Scientific Registry of Transplant recipients (SRTR), Dharnidharka et al. demonstrated young recipient age (<18 years) as an independent risk factor for PTLD with a 2.81 higher odds relative to other age groups [111]. Further risk stratification within this age group reveals a pattern suggestive of higher risk in adolescents based on a few studies. In a study of 46 EBV seronegative pediatric kidney transplant recipients who developed primary EBV infection, adolescents were significantly more likely to develop PTLD compared to younger transplant recipients [112]. Similarly, in the University of Minnesota cohort of 884 pediatric kidney transplant recipients from 1963 to 2015, older recipient age at transplantation was associated with a higher risk of post-transplant malignancy (34.6% of which was PTLD) with an adjusted hazard ratio of 3.14 for adolescents of ages 14–17 relative to children younger than 3 years [103]. A 2001 analysis of NAPRTCS data did not reveal younger children (0–5 years old) to be at higher risk for PTLD [84]. Taken together, the propensity of adolescents to bear the highest risk may reflect higher incidence of acute rejection in this age group with subsequent escalation of immunosuppression.

Gender

Male gender was found to have 1.4 higher odds relative to female gender for development of PTLD in an analysis of SRTR data from 1988 to 1999 [111]. This was not seen in an analysis of NAPRTCS data from 2001 [84].

Race

African-American race was found to be associated with decreased risk for PTLD [85, 113], whereas Caucasian race was found to have a 2.22 higher odds relative to other race groups for the development of PTLD in an analysis of SRTR data from 1988 to 1999 [111]. The higher risk in Caucasian children was also seen in the NAPRTCS registry [84].

Donor Source

Receipt of a deceased donor kidney transplant has been identified as a risk factor for subsequent development of PTLD compared to receipt of a living donor kidney transplant [84, 85]. However, due to study design limitations, it is unclear if this is independent of immunosuppression burden which is likely higher in deceased donor recipients relative to living donor recipients.

Recombinant Growth Hormone (rGH) Use

Early data from NAPRTCS suggested a possible association of pre-transplant use of rGH and later development of PTLD in patients with chronic kidney disease (CKD) who subsequently go on to receive a kidney transplant [114]. In a more recent study of 650 pediatric kidney transplant recipients in the Australian and New Zealand Dialysis and Transplant registry, this association was not seen with rGH use at any time point in 8 of 20 patients who developed PTLD [115].

Cancer Prevention Strategies

Primary prevention of post-transplant malignancy involves strategies aimed at eliminating or reducing cancer risk factors. This encompasses vaccination against viral-induced tumors. So far, the only effective vaccine for cancer prevention in clinical practice is the human papilloma virus (HPV) vaccine which has shown efficacy in preventing HPV-related disease such as warts and cervical cancer [116]. However, given the immunosuppressed nature of kidney transplant recipients, response to vaccination may be blunted if delivered post-transplantation [117]. Similarly, regular application of sunscreen may be an effective primary prevention strategy for non-melanoma skin cancer in this population [118]. De novo use or conversion to sirolimus as a backbone for the post-transplant immunosuppressive regimen was associated with a 40% reduced risk of post-transplant malignancy in a systematic review of 21 randomized trials involving 5876 kidney transplant recipients [119]. Similarly, early (within 90 days) use of sirolimus-based regimen was associated with a 29% risk reduction of skin cancer in a large registry analysis of 45,164 kidney transplant recipients relative to a tacrolimus-, mycophenolate-, and prednisone-based regimen [120]. However, in both studies, sirolimus was associated with a higher risk of overall mortality from cardiovascular, cerebrovascular, and infectious causes, thus discouraging its use for cancer prevention in this population.

Secondary prevention focuses on early detection of disease or disease-specific surrogate markers with subsequent attempts to reduce progression. Serial monitoring of EBV viral load has been used as a surrogate measure of immunosuppression burden and, by extension, for PTLD risk [121]. This remains the current standard for PTLD prevention due to lack of other specific effective measures, though the exact viremia thresholds at which PTLD risk increases and at which intervention should occur are yet to be determined. Given the variations in EBV viral load monitoring assay techniques between different labs and variable viremia levels in the same patient based on the assay sample source (whole blood, plasma, or peripheral blood mononuclear cells) [100], protocols to guide immunosuppression modulation in response to viral load monitoring are institution specific. Pre-emptive use of rituximab for treatment of EBV viremia to prevent PTLD has been reported in very small-scale pediatric and adult cohorts and requires further study before routine use [57, 122].

Cancer Treatment

Due to the rare nature of post-transplant malignancy in pediatric kidney transplant recipients, a multidisciplinary treatment approach in consultation with an oncologist is desirable for optimal outcomes. With regard to PTLD, the first line of treatment involves reduction of the overall burden of immunosuppression [123]. While there are no standardized protocols, typical approaches include elimination of antimetabolites and reduction of CNI dose or target trough level. EBV-positive tumors and those with CD20-positive expression predict a better survival likely due to rituximab treatment being effective in this subset of patients [124, 125]. Poor prognostic risk factors include central nervous system (CNS) and bone marrow involvement [126, 127]. Infusion of EBV-specific cytotoxic T cells (for EBV-positive tumors) and systemic chemotherapy are additional treatment options for more advanced disease that fails initial reduction of immunosuppression [128, 129].

Cancer Outcomes

In a recent analysis of 1810 children included in the Australian and New Zealand Dialysis and Transplant Registry, who were followed up for a median of 13.4 years, cancer-related deaths accounted for 12% of all mortality events (50 of 431 total deaths) [1]. This was similar to the data from the latest NAPRTCS registry report, where 608 deaths were recorded over a 30-year period of which 68 (11.3%) were attributed to cancer [2]. Of note, the relative risk of dying from the same cancers is higher in pediatric kidney transplant recipients relative to the general pediatric population [130]. This is despite improvements in early detection, prevention, and treatment that have led to an overall improved survival following PTLD diagnosis. In a review of 92 PTLD cases from the NAPRTCS registry, there were 12 deaths, only 10 of which were directly attributable to cancer. Patient survival rates post-PTLD diagnosis in the NAPRTCS registry were 90.6% at 1 year and 87.4% at 5 years, with most recent year of PTLD diagnosis significantly being associated with better patient survival [110].

Urinary Tract Infections (UTI)

UTIs in kidney transplant recipients encompass a spectrum of presentations ranging from lower tract involvement (cystitis), graft infection (pyelonephritis), and urosepsis. By definition, given the immunocompromised nature of kidney transplant recipients, all UTIs in this population are considered complicated UTIs [131].

Prevalence

UTIs are the most common infectious complication following kidney transplantation [8]. A Dutch pediatric cohort study of 234 patients demonstrated an increase in UTI rates over the past 30 years from 3.3 infections per 100 patient years (1980–1989) to 4.4 infections per 100 patient years (2000–2010) [132]. In an analysis of 60,702 recipients in the USRDS database, 32% experienced a UTI in the first-year post-kidney transplantation [133]. Pediatric specific rates vary by cohort examined but are largely similar. In a German cohort of 110 pediatric kidney transplant recipients, febrile UTIs occurred in 36% of children at a median of 0.98 years post-transplantation [134]. In a Canadian cohort of 76 pediatric kidney transplant recipients, UTIs occurred in 28% over a mean follow-up duration of 3.3 years with the majority of episodes occurring in the first year [135]. In another Spanish pediatric prospective cohort of 36 consecutive kidney transplant recipients, 28 UTI episodes were noted during the 2 year follow-up period with seven episodes classified as pyelonephritis [136]. In a Nigerian cohort of 62 children post-kidney transplant, 40.3% developed a UTI over a mean follow-up period of 36.9 months with multiple episodes reported per patient (89 UTI episodes in 25 patients) [137].

Risk Factors

1. *Kidney disease etiology:* Children with underlying urological abnormalities such as obstructive uropathy, neurogenic bladder, and vesicoureteral reflux (VUR) as their etiology for end-stage kidney disease (ESKD) are at higher risk for UTIs [138, 139]. In a study of 155 pediatric kidney transplant recipients, of whom 32 had severe bladder pathology, UTI incidence was significantly higher than those with a normal bladder (68.8% vs 23%) [138]. Similarly, in another study of 117 kidney transplant recipients younger than 20 years old who developed ESKD due to obstructive and reflux uropathy, UTIs were noted in 45% compared to 2% in 117 matched controls whose ESKD was due to other reasons [139].
2. *Ureteral stents:* Placement of a ureteral stent at the time of kidney transplantation to maintain the patency of the donor ureter to recipient bladder anastomosis is a common though not universal practice in kidney transplantation and varies by center. The ureteral stent is generally left in place for up to 6 weeks post-transplantation before removal. The presence of the stent prevents complete closure of the ureteral orifice during bladder contraction, which can lead to vesicoureteral reflux into the graft raising concerns for increased UTI risk. In a single-center study of 129 pediatric kidney transplant recipients over a 10 year period, stent placement was found to be a significant risk factor for early UTI [140]. Early stent removal (defined as less than 15 days post-op) was found to prevent UTIs relative to later removal in a Cochrane Database Systematic Review that included 1127 patients (across five studies, one with pediatric enrollment) with a relative risk of 0.49 for the early removal group [141].
3. *Vesicoureteral reflux and voiding dysfunction:* The UTI frequency was not significantly different in pediatric kidney transplant recipients with VUR (46%) compared to those without VUR (33%) in a study of 67 pediatric patients; however, pyelonephritis accounted for 82% of all UTIs in the VUR group compared to 14% of all UTIs in those without VUR ($p < 0.01$) [142]. Native nephrectomy of refluxing systems prior to kidney transplantation is occasionally recommended to reduce the risk of post-transplant febrile UTI in the native kidney, though the practice is not universal. Small studies have demonstrated some benefit to pre-transplant native nephrectomy or surgical reimplantation of refluxing native ureters, though the contribution of voiding dysfunction management on post-transplant outcomes in those studies makes it difficult to ascertain the specific benefit of surgical intervention [143, 144]. Voiding dysfunction is common after kidney transplantation irrespective of underlying etiology of ESKD. In a study of 68 kidney transplant recipients between 5 and 20 years of age, voiding dysfunction manifested as abnormal bladder capacity, abnormal urine flow, and post-void residual urine in 72% of patients. Notably, voiding dysfunction was as prevalent in those with congenital disorders with urinary tract malformations to those with congenital disorders without urinary tract malformations or those with acquired kidney disorders [145].
4. *Host-pathogen interaction:* The state of overall immunosuppression contributes to the increased UTI risk in kidney transplant recipients due to impaired

systemic and localized host defense mechanisms against bacterial pathogens [131]. Specific pathogen virulence factors may also be at play. In adult kidney transplant patients, use of whole genome sequencing to examine virulence factors in *Escherichia coli* (*E. coli*) isolates from patients with either asymptomatic bacteriuria or pyelonephritis identified a significantly higher prevalence of a gene cluster encoding P fimbriae which allows the *E. coli* to colonize the kidney [146]. There is emerging evidence that alterations in gut microbiota following kidney transplantation, specifically a relative gut abundance of uropathogens such as *E. coli* and Enterococcus species, are associated with an increased risk of UTIs [147].

Prevention

Given the significantly higher risk of UTIs following kidney transplantation in children with underlying urologic abnormalities, a comprehensive pre-transplant urologic evaluation and treatment plan focusing on maximizing bladder capacity and relieving obstructed urinary tracts is desirable [148]. In the post-transplantation period, prevention strategies center around the use of prophylactic antibiotics, management of voiding dysfunction, and surgical techniques to correct VUR into the transplant kidney. The benefit of routine long-term low-dose antibiotic prophylaxis for UTI prevention in otherwise healthy children with primary VUR compared to no treatment remains an area of controversy with a recent Cochrane Database Systematic Review demonstrating minimal or no difference with regard to repeat symptomatic and febrile UTIs in this population [149]. Limited data exist to inform decision-making in the pediatric kidney transplant population. In a small cohort of 18 pediatric kidney transplant recipients with VUR (12 girls and 6 boys), almost all of those who presented with recurrent febrile UTI (8 of 9) required surgical interventions for their VUR, whereas those without recurrent febrile UTIs were successfully managed with bladder training and prophylactic antibiotics [150]. The use of daily trimethoprim-sulfamethoxazole as PJP prophylaxis for the first 6 months post-kidney transplant was not associated with reduction of asymptomatic bacteriuria or UTI risk in one adult study, and instead it was associated with increased bacterial resistance rates [151]. One small retrospective adult study suggested a possible benefit to the use of ciprofloxacin for 30 days in addition to routine PJP prophylaxis for 6 months in reducing UTI risk [152]. Post-transplant VUR surgical correction can be accomplished via minimally invasive techniques such as endoscopic subureteral transurethral injection of dextranomer/hyaluronic acid; however, this carries a potential risk of ureteral obstruction that may require open reimplantation [153]. An open ureteral reimplantation using an extra-vesical approach has been shown to be safe and effective in pediatric patients, though VUR may persist in some cases with lower urinary tract dysfunction [154].

Treatment

There is consensus that all symptomatic urinary tract infections in kidney transplant recipients should be managed with appropriate antibiotic therapy based on culture and sensitivity results [155]. Empiric coverage should be tailored based on local epidemiologic sensitivity patterns and a patient's prior history of UTIs if any. Treatment duration recommendations are not standardized, though it is common to target a longer 14-day treatment course in febrile kidney transplant patients with evidence of graft dysfunction suggestive of graft pyelonephritis. Reduction of immunosuppression is not commonly done. Treatment of asymptomatic bacteriuria is an area of controversy and is discussed below.

Asymptomatic Bacteriuria

The Infectious Diseases Society of America (IDSA) defines asymptomatic bacteriuria (ASB) as the presence of one or more species of bacteria growing in the urine at a significant colony count ($\geq 10^5$ colony-forming units [CFU]/mL), irrespective of the presence of pyuria, in the absence of signs or symptoms attributable to UTI [156]. Data on the risk of progression of ASB into a clinically significant symptomatic UTI are conflicting. In a retrospective cohort of 189 adult kidney transplant recipients of whom 96 developed at least one episode of ASB and received antibiotic treatment, there was a sevenfold higher risk of pyelonephritis compared to recipients without ASB [157]. In another retrospective study of 77 adult kidney transplant recipients who experienced a total of 334 ASB episodes, 30% of ASB episodes were treated with antibiotics. Prior treatment of ASB with antibiotics was not associated with significant difference in subsequent development of symptomatic UTI in that study. Despite the high number of ASB episodes, only four symptomatic UTIs developed in the entire cohort [158]. A Cochrane Database Systematic Review noted an incidence of symptomatic UTIs ranging from 19% to 31% in those with untreated ASB in the qualified studies. Treatment of ASB with antibiotics was not associated with prevention of symptomatic UTI in that review [159]. A randomized controlled trial comparing universal treatment of all ASB episodes occurring between 2 and 24 months post-kidney transplantation in 53 adult recipients to no treatment in 59 controls found no difference in the occurrence of acute pyelonephritis or lower urinary tract infection [160]. Pediatric data are limited. In a single-center retrospective study of 37 pediatric kidney transplant recipients with a total of 171 ASB episodes among them between 2- and 24-months post-kidney transplantation, the majority (95.9%) were left untreated. Of those, 91.5% did not progress to a clinical UTI [161]. The updated 2019 IDSA guidelines recommend against screening and treatment of ASB in kidney transplant recipients beyond 1 month from their kidney transplant surgery and make no recommendations for or against that practice in the first post-transplant month due to insufficient evidence [156].

Outcomes

In an analysis of 870 pediatric kidney transplant recipients in the USRDS database, those with an early UTI (defined as occurring before 6 months of post-kidney transplantation) were found to be at higher risk for graft loss (adjusted hazard ratio of 5.47 [95% CI 1.93–15.4]). However, graft loss risk was not increased in those with a late UTI. Similarly, early but not late hospitalized UTI was associated with a higher risk of post-transplant death. When all UTIs were taken into account regardless of need for hospitalization, neither early nor late UTI had an impact on patient survival [162].

MOC Questions

1. *In which scenario may a patient present with CMV disease but have low viral loads?*
   A. Pneumonitis
   B. Encephalitis
   C. Retinitis
   D. Leukopenia
   Answer: B
   CMV disease is defined as evidence of CMV infection with a multitude of symptoms including fever, fatigue, leukopenia, thrombocytopenia, hepatitis, pneumonitis, colitis, retinitis, or encephalitis. However, CMV viral load levels may be low or undetectable in those with gastrointestinal (GI) or CNS disease
2. *Which of the following represents the cornerstone for treatment of BK viremia post-kidney transplantation?*
   A. Reduction of immunosuppression
   B. Conversion from steroid-free to steroid-based immunosuppression
   C. Leflunomide
   D. Cidofovir
   Answer: A
   Treatment for BK nephropathy requires minimizing immunosuppression. The method for minimizing immunosuppression varies. Options include reducing calcineurin inhibitors, followed by reduction or discontinuation of the anti-metabolite. Other strategies include discontinuation of anti-metabolite followed by reduction of calcineurin inhibitors, while others may reduce both calcineurin inhibitors along with the anti-metabolite. Cidofovir and leflunomide are adjunct treatment options that have been used with variable success. The addition of steroids without discontinuation or lowering of another immunosuppressive drug would be counterproductive as it increases the overall burden of immunosuppression.
3. *Which of the following is the most significant risk factor for development of PTLD following primary EBV infection in a kidney transplant recipient?*
   A. EBV seronegative status at transplantation

B. Non-adherence to immunosuppression
C. mTOR-based maintenance immunosuppression
D. IL-2 receptor antibody induction therapy

Answer: A

Primary EBV infection in seronegative pediatric and adult recipients of seropositive donor kidneys has been identified as a major risk factor for PTLD. Interestingly, in a study of 195 kidney transplant recipients who consented to electronic monitoring of their medication adherence, and followed up for a median of 10.1 years, those most adherent to their medication regimen had the highest cancer risk at 59.4%. This was significantly higher than the risk in the less adherent groups which ranged from 36.1% to 38.1%. De novo use or conversion to sirolimus as a backbone for the post-transplant immunosuppressive regimen was associated with a 40% reduced risk of post-transplant malignancy in a systematic review of 21 randomized trials involving 5876 kidney transplant recipients. Various induction therapy regimens have been linked to different cancer risks likely reflecting their contribution to the overall immunosuppression burden, though this relationship may be compounded by the potential higher risk of acute rejection with less potent induction therapies or no induction leading to subsequent escalation of immunosuppressive therapy. No association was found between the use of interleukin-2 receptor antibody induction and subsequent cancer risk in 461 pediatric kidney transplant recipients in the Australia and New Zealand Dialysis and Transplant registry in comparison to 197 recipients without induction.

4. *Which of the following is associated with a higher UTI risk following pediatric kidney transplantation?*
   A. Asymptomatic bacteriuria
   B. Early ureteral stent removal
   C. Presence of native kidneys
   D. ESKD secondary to congenital anomalies of kidney and urinary tract (CAKUT)

   Answer: D

   Children with underlying urological abnormalities such as obstructive uropathy, neurogenic bladder, and vesicoureteral reflux as their etiology for end-stage kidney disease (ESKD) are at higher risk for UTIs. Data on the risk of progression of asymptomatic bacteriuria (ASB) into a clinically significant symptomatic UTI are conflicting. Pediatric data are limited. In a single-center retrospective study of 37 pediatric kidney transplant recipients with a total of 171 ASB episodes among them between 2- and 24-months post-kidney transplantation, the majority (95.9%) were left untreated. Of those, 91.5% did not progress to a clinical UTI. The presence of a ureteral stent prevents complete closure of the ureteral orifice during bladder contraction which can lead to vesicoureteral reflux into the graft raising concerns for increased UTI risk. In a single-center study of 129 pediatric kidney transplant recipients over a 10-year period, stent placement was found to be a significant risk factor for early UTIs. Early stent removal (defined as less than 15 days post-op) was found to prevent

UTIs relative to later removal in a Cochrane Database Systematic Review that included 1127 patients with a relative risk of 0.49 for the early removal group. Native nephrectomy of refluxing systems prior to kidney transplantation is occasionally recommended to reduce the risk of post-transplant febrile UTI in the native kidney, though the practice is not universal. In the absence of VUR into the native kidneys, the contribution of native nephrectomy to post-transplant UTI prevention is uncertain.

References

1. Francis A, Johnson DW, Melk A, Foster BJ, Blazek K, Craig JC, et al. Survival after kidney transplantation during childhood and adolescence. Clin J Am Soc Nephrol. 2020;15(3):392–400.
2. Chua A, Cramer C, Moudgil A, Martz K, Smith J, Blydt-Hansen T, et al. Kidney transplant practice patterns and outcome benchmarks over 30 years: the 2018 report of the NAPRTCS. Pediatr Transplant. 2019;23(8):e13597.
3. Mumford L, Maxwell H, Ahmad N, Marks SD, Tizard J. The impact of changing practice on improved outcomes of paediatric renal transplantation in the United Kingdom: a 25 years review. Transpl Int. 2019;32(7):751–61.
4. Dharnidharka VR, Stablein DM, Harmon WE. Post-transplant infections now exceed acute rejection as cause for hospitalization: a report of the NAPRTCS. Am J Transplant. 2004;4(3):384–9.
5. Humar A, Snydman D, Practice ASTIDCo. Cytomegalovirus in solid organ transplant recipients. Am J Transplant. 2009;9 Suppl 4:S78–86.
6. Sawinski D, Blumberg EA. Infection in renal transplant recipients. In: Chronic kidney disease, dialysis, and transplantation; 2019. p. 621–38.e6. https://www.elsevier.com/books/chronic-kidney-disease-dialysis-and-transplantation/abrams/978-0-323-52978-5.
7. Fishman JA. Infection in organ transplantation. Am J Transplant. 2017;17(4):856–79.
8. Dandamudi R, Smith J, Dharnidharka VR. Renal transplantation and predisposition to opportunistic infections. Curr Opin Pediatr. 2019;31(2):226–31.
9. Hart A, Smith JM, Skeans MA, Gustafson SK, Wilk AR, Castro S, et al. OPTN/SRTR 2018 annual data report: kidney. Am J Transplant. 2020;20 Suppl s1:20–130.
10. Lockridge J, Roberts D, Olyaei A, Noble BN, Langewisch E, Rehman S, et al. Cytomegalovirus serologic matching in deceased donor kidney allocation optimizes high- and low-risk (D+R- and D-R-) profiles and does not adversely affect transplant rates. Am J Transplant. 2020;20(12):3502–8.
11. Zhang Z, Qiu L, Yan S, Wang JJ, Thomas PM, Kandpal M, et al. A clinically relevant murine model unmasks a "two-hit" mechanism for reactivation and dissemination of cytomegalovirus after kidney transplant. Am J Transplant. 2019;19(9):2421–33.
12. Ganapathi L, Blumenthal J, Alawdah L, Lewis L, Gilarde J, Jones S, et al. Impact of standardized protocols for cytomegalovirus disease prevention in pediatric solid organ transplant recipients. Pediatr Transplant. 2019;23(7):e13568.
13. Rha B, Redden D, Benfield M, Lakeman F, Whitley RJ, Shimamura M. Correlation and clinical utility of pp65 antigenemia and quantitative polymerase chain reaction assays for detection of cytomegalovirus in pediatric renal transplant patients. Pediatr Transplant. 2012;16(6):627–37.
14. Ross SA, Novak Z, Pati S, Boppana SB. Overview of the diagnosis of cytomegalovirus infection. Infect Disord Drug Targets. 2011;11(5):466–74.
15. Azevedo LS, Pierrotti LC, Abdala E, Costa SF, Strabelli TMV, Campos SV, et al. Cytomegalovirus infection in transplant recipients. Clinics (Sao Paulo). 2015;70(7):515–23.

16. Chatani B, Glaberson W, Nemeth Z, Tamariz L, Gonzalez IA. GCV/VCVG prophylaxis against CMV DNAemia in pediatric renal transplant patients: a systematic review and meta-analysis. Pediatr Transplant. 2019;23(6):e13514.
17. Cameron BM, Kennedy SE, Rawlinson WD, Mackie FE. The efficacy of valganciclovir for prevention of infections with cytomegalovirus and Epstein-Barr virus after kidney transplant in children. Pediatr Transplant. 2017;21(1).
18. Smith JM, Dharnidharka VR. Viral surveillance and subclinical viral infection in pediatric kidney transplantation. Pediatr Nephrol. 2015;30(5):741–8.
19. Kasiske BL, Zeier MG, Chapman JR, Craig JC, Ekberg H, Garvey CA, et al. KDIGO clinical practice guideline for the care of kidney transplant recipients: a summary. Kidney Int. 2010;77(4):299–311.
20. Fernández-Ruiz M, Rodríguez-Goncer I, Parra P, Ruiz-Merlo T, Corbella L, López-Medrano F, et al. Monitoring of CMV-specific cell-mediated immunity with a commercial ELISA-based interferon-γ release assay in kidney transplant recipients treated with antithymocyte globulin. Am J Transplant. 2020;20(8):2070–80.
21. Stanat SC, Reardon JE, Erice A, Jordan MC, Drew WL, Biron KK. Ganciclovir-resistant cytomegalovirus clinical isolates: mode of resistance to ganciclovir. Antimicrob Agents Chemother. 1991;35(11):2191–7.
22. Pape L, Ahlenstiel T. mTOR inhibitors in pediatric kidney transplantation. Pediatr Nephrol. 2014;29(7):1119–29.
23. Tedesco-Silva H, Felipe C, Ferreira A, Cristelli M, Oliveira N, Sandes-Freitas T, et al. Reduced incidence of cytomegalovirus infection in kidney transplant recipients receiving everolimus and reduced tacrolimus doses. Am J Transplant. 2015;15(10):2655–64.
24. Hocker B, Zencke S, Pape L, Krupka K, Koster L, Fichtner A, et al. Impact of everolimus and low-dose cyclosporin on cytomegalovirus replication and disease in pediatric renal transplantation. Am J Transplant. 2016;16(3):921–9.
25. Bak S, Tischer S, Dragon A, Ravens S, Pape L, Koenecke C, et al. Selective effects of mTOR inhibitor sirolimus on naïve and CMV-specific T cells extending its applicable range beyond immunosuppression. Front Immunol. 2018;9(2953).
26. Hamasaki Y, Dolan NM, Cubitt D, Breuer J, Sebire NJ, Marks SD. BK viremia and nephropathy in pediatric renal transplant recipients. Pediatr Transplant. 2019;23(5):e13460.
27. Scaggs Huang FA, Danziger-Isakov L. Infectious disease risks in pediatric renal transplantation. Pediatr Nephrol. 2019;34(7):1155–66.
28. Fogeda M, Munoz P, Luque A, Morales MD, Bouza E, Group BKVS. Cross-sectional study of BK virus infection in pediatric kidney transplant recipients. Pediatr Transplant. 2007;11(4):394–401.
29. Smith JM, Dharnidharka VR, Talley L, Martz K, McDonald RA. BK virus nephropathy in pediatric renal transplant recipients: an analysis of the North American Pediatric Renal Trials and Collaborative Studies (NAPRTCS) registry. Clin J Am Soc Nephrol. 2007;2(5):1037–42.
30. Comoli P, Ginevri F. Monitoring and managing viral infections in pediatric renal transplant recipients. Pediatr Nephrol. 2012;27(5):705–17.
31. Ginevri F, De Santis R, Comoli P, Pastorino N, Rossi C, Botti G, et al. Polyomavirus BK infection in pediatric kidney-allograft recipients: a single-center analysis of incidence, risk factors, and novel therapeutic approaches. Transplantation. 2003;75(8):1266–70.
32. Hirsch HH, Brennan DC, Drachenberg CB, Ginevri F, Gordon J, Limaye AP, et al. Polyomavirus-associated nephropathy in renal transplantation: interdisciplinary analyses and recommendations. Transplantation. 2005;79(10):1277–86.
33. Ahlenstiel-Grunow T, Pape L. Immunosuppression, BK polyomavirus infections, and BK polyomavirus-specific T cells after pediatric kidney transplantation. Pediatr Nephrol. 2020;35(4):625–31.
34. Hisadome Y, Noguchi H, Nakafusa Y, Sakihama K, Mei T, Kaku K, et al. Association of pretransplant BK polyomavirus antibody status with BK polyomavirus infection after kidney transplantation: a prospective cohort pilot study of 47 transplant recipients. Transplant Proc. 2020;52(6):1762–8.

35. Verghese PS, Schmeling DO, Filtz EA, Matas AJ, Balfour HH, Jr. The impact of recipient BKV shedding before transplant on BKV viruria, DNAemia, and nephropathy post-transplant: a prospective study. Pediatr Transplant. 2017;21(5).
36. Ahlenstiel-Grunow T, Pape L. Virus-specific T cells in pediatric renal transplantation. Pediatr Nephrol. 2021;36(4):789–96.
37. Ginevri F, Azzi A, Hirsch HH, Basso S, Fontana I, Cioni M, et al. Prospective monitoring of polyomavirus BK replication and impact of pre-emptive intervention in pediatric kidney recipients. Am J Transplant. 2007;7(12):2727–35.
38. Schachtner T, Stein M, Babel N, Reinke P. The loss of BKV-specific immunity from pretransplantation to posttransplantation identifies kidney transplant recipients at increased risk of BKV replication. Am J Transplant. 2015;15(8):2159–69.
39. Cawcutt KA, Zimmer A. Management of infection in patients with kidney transplant. Critical Care Nephrology. 2019:552–60.e1.
40. Fishman JA, Costa SF, Alexander BD. Infection in kidney transplant recipients. In: Kidney transplantation - principles and practice; 2019. p. 517–38. https://www.elsevier.com/books/kidney-transplantation-principles-and-practice/knechtle/978-0-323-53186-3.
41. Hirsch HH, Randhawa P, Practice ASTIDCo. BK virus in solid organ transplant recipients. Am J Transplant. 2009;9 Suppl 4:S136–46.
42. Kumar D, Mian M, Singer L, Humar A. An interventional study using cell-mediated immunity to personalize therapy for Cytomegalovirus infection after transplantation. Am J Transplant. 2017;17(9):2468–73.
43. Sahoo DH, Bandyopadhyay D, Xu M, Pearson K, Parambil JG, Lazar CA, et al. Effectiveness and safety of leflunomide for pulmonary and extrapulmonary sarcoidosis. Eur Respir J. 2011;38(5):1145–50.
44. Launay M, Baudouin V, Guillemain R, Maisin A, Flodrops H, Douez E, et al. Leflunomide for BKvirus: report of seven kidney-transplanted children. Int J Organ Transplant Med. 2018;9(4):178–83.
45. Benotmane I, Solis M, Velay A, Cognard N, Olagne J, Gautier Vargas G, et al. Intravenous immunoglobulins as a preventive strategy against BK virus viremia and BKV-associated nephropathy in kidney transplant recipients-Results from a proof-of-concept study. Am J Transplant. 2021;21(1):329–37.
46. Jahan S, Scuderi C, Francis L, Neller MA, Rehan S, Crooks P, et al. T-cell adoptive immunotherapy for BK nephropathy in renal transplantation. Transpl Infect Dis. 2020;22:e13399.
47. Dharnidharka VR, Cherikh WS, Neff R, Cheng Y, Abbott KC. Retransplantation after BK virus nephropathy in prior kidney transplant: an OPTN database analysis. Am J Transplant. 2010;10(5):1312–5.
48. Laurent A, Klich A, Roy P, Lina B, Kassai B, Bacchetta J, et al. Pediatric renal transplantation: a retrospective single-center study on epidemiology and morbidity due to EBV. Pediatr Transplant. 2018;22(3):e13151.
49. Toyoda M, Moudgil A, Warady BA, Puliyanda DP, Jordan SC. Clinical significance of peripheral blood Epstein-Barr viral load monitoring using polymerase chain reaction in renal transplant recipients. Pediatr Transplant. 2008;12(7):778–84.
50. Li L, Chaudhuri A, Weintraub LA, Hsieh F, Shah S, Alexander S, et al. Subclinical cytomegalovirus and Epstein-Barr virus viremia are associated with adverse outcomes in pediatric renal transplantation. Pediatr Transplant. 2007;11(2):187–95.
51. Lau JSY, Low ZM, Abbott I, Shochet L, Kanellis J, Kitching AR, et al. Epstein-Barr virus encephalitis in solid organ transplantation. New Microbiol. 2017;40(3):212–7.
52. Opelz G, Döhler B. Lymphomas after solid organ transplantation: a collaborative transplant study report. Am J Transplant. 2004;4(2):222–30.
53. Nijland ML, Kersten MJ, Pals ST, Bemelman FJ, Ten Berge IJM. Epstein-Barr virus-positive posttransplant lymphoproliferative disease after solid organ transplantation: pathogenesis, clinical manifestations, diagnosis, and management. Transplant Direct. 2015;2(1):e48-e.
54. Comak E, Akman S, Ongut G, Colak D, Koyun M, Dogan CS, et al. Epstein-Barr virus infection in children with renal transplantation: 17 years experience at a single center. Ren Fail. 2014;36(5):760–6.

55. AlDabbagh MA, Gitman MR, Kumar D, Humar A, Rotstein C, Husain S. The role of antiviral prophylaxis for the prevention of Epstein-Barr virus-associated posttransplant lymphoproliferative disease in solid organ transplant recipients: a systematic review. Am J Transplant. 2017;17(3):770–81.
56. Schachtner T, Reinke P. Pretransplant prophylactic rituximab to prevent Epstein-Barr virus (EBV) viremia in EBV-seronegative kidney transplant recipients from EBV-seropositive donors: results of a pilot study. Transpl Infect Dis. 2016;18(6):881–8.
57. Hyun H, Park E, Cho M, Min SI, Ha J, Kang HJ, et al. Post-transplant lymphoproliferative diseases in pediatric kidney allograft recipients with Epstein-Barr virus viremia. J Korean Med Sci. 2019;34(30):e203.
58. Iriart X, Bouar ML, Kamar N, Berry A. Pneumocystis pneumonia in solid-organ transplant recipients. J Fungi (Basel). 2015;1(3):293–331.
59. Lee SH, Huh KH, Joo DJ, Kim MS, Kim SI, Lee J, et al. Risk factors for Pneumocystis jirovecii pneumonia (PJP) in kidney transplantation recipients. Sci Rep. 2017;7(1):1571.
60. De Vlieger G, Lagrou K, Maertens J, Verbeken E, Meersseman W, Van Wijngaerden E. Beta-D-Glucan detection as a diagnostic test for invasive aspergillosis in immunocompromised critically ill patients with symptoms of respiratory infection: an autopsy-based study. J Clin Microbiol. 2011;49(11):3783.
61. Chen J, He T, Li X, Wang X, Peng L, Ma L. Metagenomic next-generation sequencing in diagnosis of a case of Pneumocystis jirovecii pneumonia in a kidney transplant recipient and literature review. Infect Drug Resist. 2020;13:2829–36.
62. Hamroun A, Lenain R, Bui Nguyen L, Chamley P, Loridant S, Neugebauer Y, et al. Hypercalcemia is common during Pneumocystis pneumonia in kidney transplant recipients. Sci Rep. 2019;9(1):12508.
63. Hocker B, Wendt C, Nahimana A, Tonshoff B, Hauser PM. Molecular evidence of pneumocystis transmission in pediatric transplant unit. Emerg Infect Dis. 2005;11(2):330–2.
64. Quinn M, Fannin JT, Sciasci J, Bragg A, Campbell PK, Carias D, et al. Pentamidine for prophylaxis against Pneumocystis jirovecii pneumonia in pediatric oncology patients receiving immunosuppressive chemotherapy. Antimicrob Agents Chemother. 2018;62(8):e00173–18.
65. Whitaker JA, Poland GA. Measles and mumps outbreaks in the United States: think globally, vaccinate locally. Vaccine. 2014;32(37):4703–4.
66. Gahr P, DeVries AS, Wallace G, Miller C, Kenyon C, Sweet K, et al. An outbreak of measles in an undervaccinated community. Pediatrics. 2014;134(1):e220–8.
67. Höcker B, Aguilar M, Schnitzler P, Pape L, Bald M, König J, et al. Vaccination titres pre- and post-transplant in paediatric renal transplant recipients and the impact of immunosuppressive therapy. Pediatr Nephrol. 2018;33(5):897–910.
68. Prelog M, Pohl M, Ermisch B, Fuchshuber A, Huzly D, Jungraithmayr T, et al. Demand for evaluation of vaccination antibody titers in children considered for renal transplantation. Pediatr Transplant. 2007;11(1):73–6.
69. Moss WJ. Measles. Lancet. 2017;390(10111):2490–502.
70. Hviid A, Rubin S, Mühlemann K. Mumps. Lancet. 2008;371(9616):932–44.
71. Turner A, Jeyaratnam D, Haworth F, Sinha MD, Hughes E, Cohen B, et al. Measles-associated encephalopathy in children with renal transplants. Am J Transplant. 2006;6(6):1459–65.
72. Kidd IM, Booth CJ, Rigden SP, Tong CY, MacMahon EM. Measles-associated encephalitis in children with renal transplants: a predictable effect of waning herd immunity? Lancet England. 2003;362:832.
73. Matysiak-Klose D, Santibanez S, Schwerdtfeger C, Koch J, von Bernuth H, Hengel H, et al. Post-exposure prophylaxis for measles with immunoglobulins revised recommendations of the standing committee on vaccination in Germany. Vaccine. 2018;36(52):7916–22.
74. Young MK, Nimmo GR, Cripps AW, Jones MA. Post-exposure passive immunisation for preventing measles. Cochrane Database Syst Rev. 2014;(4):Cd010056.
75. Baas MC, van Donselaar KA, Florquin S, van Binnendijk RS, ten Berge IJ, Bemelman FJ. Mumps: not an innocent bystander in solid organ transplantation. Am J Transplant. 2009;9(9):2186–9.

76. Park SB, Jin KB, Hwang EA, Han SY, Kim HC, Kim HT, et al. Case of adult mumps infection after renal transplantation. Transplant Proc. 2008;40(7):2442–3.
77. Suresh S, Upton J, Green M, Pham-Huy A, Posfay-Barbe KM, Michaels MG, et al. Live vaccines after pediatric solid organ transplant: proceedings of a consensus meeting, 2018. Pediatr Transplant. 2019;23(7):e13571.
78. Cardemil CV, Dahl RM, James L, Wannemuehler K, Gary HE, Shah M, et al. Effectiveness of a third dose of MMR vaccine for mumps outbreak control. N Engl J Med. 2017;377(10):947–56.
79. Mynarek M, Hussein K, Kreipe HH, Maecker-Kolhoff B. Malignancies after pediatric kidney transplantation: more than PTLD? Pediatr Nephrol. 2014;29(9):1517–28.
80. Francis A, Johnson DW, Teixeira-Pinto A, Craig JC, Wong G. Incidence and predictors of post-transplant lymphoproliferative disease after kidney transplantation during adulthood and childhood: a registry study. Nephrol Dial Transplant. 2018;33(5):881–9.
81. Smith JM, Martz K, McDonald RA, Harmon WE. Solid tumors following kidney transplantation in children. Pediatr Transplant. 2013;17(8):726–30.
82. Francis A, Johnson DW, Craig JC, Wong G. Incidence and predictors of cancer following kidney transplantation in childhood. Am J Transplant. 2017;17(10):2650–8.
83. Caillard S, Dharnidharka V, Agodoa L, Bohen E, Abbott K. Posttransplant lymphoproliferative disorders after renal transplantation in the United States in era of modern immunosuppression. Transplantation. 2005;80(9):1233–43.
84. Dharnidharka VR, Sullivan EK, Stablein DM, Tejani AH, Harmon WE, (NAPRTCS) NAPRTCS. Risk factors for posttransplant lymphoproliferative disorder (PTLD) in pediatric kidney transplantation: a report of the North American Pediatric Renal Transplant Cooperative Study (NAPRTCS). Transplantation. 2001;71(8):1065–8.
85. Lustberg ME, Pelletier RP, Porcu P, Martin SI, Quinion CD, Geyer SM, et al. Human leukocyte antigen type and posttransplant lymphoproliferative disorder. Transplantation. 2015;99(6):1220–5.
86. Yadav K, Vock DM, Matas AJ, Robiner WN, Nevins TE. Medication adherence is associated with an increased risk of cancer in kidney transplant recipients: a cohort study. Nephrol Dial Transplant. 2019;34(2):364–70.
87. Vincenti F, Charpentier B, Vanrenterghem Y, Rostaing L, Bresnahan B, Darji P, et al. A phase III study of belatacept-based immunosuppression regimens versus cyclosporine in renal transplant recipients (BENEFIT study). Am J Transplant. 2010;10(3):535–46.
88. Masson P, Henderson L, Chapman JR, Craig JC, Webster AC. Belatacept for kidney transplant recipients. Cochrane Database Syst Rev. 2014;(11):CD010699.
89. Mincham CM, Wong G, Teixeira-Pinto A, Kennedy S, Alexander S, Larkins N, et al. Induction therapy, rejection, and graft outcomes in pediatric and adolescent kidney transplant recipients. Transplantation. 2017;101(9):2146–51.
90. Kirk AD, Cherikh WS, Ring M, Burke G, Kaufman D, Knechtle SJ, et al. Dissociation of depletional induction and posttransplant lymphoproliferative disease in kidney recipients treated with alemtuzumab. Am J Transplant. 2007;7(11):2619–25.
91. Hill P, Cross NB, Barnett AN, Palmer SC, Webster AC. Polyclonal and monoclonal antibodies for induction therapy in kidney transplant recipients. Cochrane Database Syst Rev. 2017;1:CD004759.
92. Ashoor IF, Martz K, Galbiati S, Beyl RA, Dharnidharka VR. Reassessing rabbit antithymocyte globulin induction in kidney transplantation (RETHINK): an analysis of the North American Pediatric Renal Trials and Collaborative Studies (NAPRTCS) registry. Transplant Direct. 2020;6(9):e598.
93. Marks WH, Ilsley JN, Dharnidharka VR. Posttransplantation lymphoproliferative disorder in kidney and heart transplant recipients receiving thymoglobulin: a systematic review. Transplant Proc. 2011;43(5):1395–404.
94. Hertig A, Zuckermann A. Rabbit antithymocyte globulin induction and risk of post-transplant lymphoproliferative disease in adult and pediatric solid organ transplantation: an update. Transpl Immunol. 2015;32(3):179–87.

95. Puliyanda DP, Pizzo H, Rodig N, Somers MJG. Early outcomes comparing induction with antithymocyte globulin vs alemtuzumab in two steroid-avoidance protocols in pediatric renal transplantation. Pediatr Transplant. 2020;24(3):e13685.
96. Dharnidharka VR, Webster AC, Martinez OM, Preiksaitis JK, Leblond V, Choquet S. Post-transplant lymphoproliferative disorders. Nat Rev Dis Primers. 2016;2:15088.
97. Sampaio MS, Cho YW, Shah T, Bunnapradist S, Hutchinson IV. Impact of Epstein-Barr virus donor and recipient serostatus on the incidence of post-transplant lymphoproliferative disorder in kidney transplant recipients. Nephrol Dial Transplant. 2012;27(7):2971–9.
98. Dharnidharka VR, Lamb KE, Gregg JA, Meier-Kriesche HU. Associations between EBV serostatus and organ transplant type in PTLD risk: an analysis of the SRTR National Registry Data in the United States. Am J Transplant. 2012;12(4):976–83.
99. Colombini E, Guzzo I, Morolli F, Longo G, Russo C, Lombardi A, et al. Viral load of EBV DNAemia is a predictor of EBV-related post-transplant lymphoproliferative disorders in pediatric renal transplant recipients. Pediatr Nephrol. 2017;32(8):1433–42.
100. Dharnidharka VR. Peripheral blood Epstein-Barr viral nucleic acid surveillance as a marker for posttransplant cancer risk. Am J Transplant. 2017;17(3):611–6.
101. Ladfors SW, Lindahl JK, Hansson S, Brandström P, Andersson R, Jertborn M, et al. Long-lasting chronic high load carriage of Epstein-Barr virus is more common in young pediatric renal transplant recipients. Pediatr Nephrol. 2020;35(3):427–39.
102. Yamada M, Nguyen C, Fadakar P, Ganoza A, Humar A, Shapiro R, et al. Epidemiology and outcome of chronic high Epstein-Barr viral load carriage in pediatric kidney transplant recipients. Pediatr Transplant. 2018;22(3):e13147.
103. Serrano OK, Bangdiwala AS, Vock DM, Chinnakotla S, Dunn TB, Finger EB, et al. Post-transplant malignancy after pediatric kidney transplantation: retrospective analysis of incidence and risk factors in 884 patients receiving transplants between 1963 and 2015 at the University of Minnesota. J Am Coll Surg. 2017;225(2):181–93.
104. Opelz G, Döhler B. Pediatric kidney transplantation: analysis of donor age, HLA match, and posttransplant non-Hodgkin lymphoma: a collaborative transplant study report. Transplantation. 2010;90(3):292–7.
105. Kinch A, Sundström C, Tufveson G, Glimelius I. Association between HLA-A1 and -A2 types and Epstein-Barr virus status of post-transplant lymphoproliferative disorder. Leuk Lymphoma. 2016;57(10):2351–8.
106. Subklewe M, Marquis R, Choquet S, Leblond V, Garnier JL, Hetzer R, et al. Association of human leukocyte antigen haplotypes with posttransplant lymphoproliferative disease after solid organ transplantation. Transplantation. 2006;82(8):1093–100.
107. Chadban SJ, Ahn C, Axelrod DA, Foster BJ, Kasiske BL, Kher V, et al. KDIGO clinical practice guideline on the evaluation and management of candidates for kidney transplantation. Transplantation. 2020;104(4S1 Suppl 1):S11–S103.
108. Acuna SA, Huang JW, Dossa F, Shah PS, Kim SJ, Baxter NN. Cancer recurrence after solid organ transplantation: a systematic review and meta-analysis. Transplant Rev (Orlando). 2017;31(4):240–8.
109. Serrano OK, Gannon A, Olowofela AS, Reddy A, Berglund D, Matas AJ. Long-term outcomes of pediatric kidney transplant recipients with a pretransplant malignancy. Pediatr Transplant. 2019;23(7):e13557.
110. Dharnidharka VR, Martz KL, Stablein DM, Benfield MR. Improved survival with recent Post-Transplant Lymphoproliferative Disorder (PTLD) in children with kidney transplants. Am J Transplant. 2011;11(4):751–8.
111. Dharnidharka VR, Tejani AH, Ho PL, Harmon WE. Post-transplant lymphoproliferative disorder in the United States: young Caucasian males are at highest risk. Am J Transplant. 2002;2(10):993–8.
112. Smith JM, Corey L, Healey PJ, Davis CL, McDonald RA. Adolescents are more likely to develop posttransplant lymphoproliferative disorder after primary Epstein-Barr virus infection than younger renal transplant recipients. Transplantation. 2007;83(11):1423–8.

113. Nee R, Hurst FP, Dharnidharka VR, Jindal RM, Agodoa LY, Abbott KC. Racial variation in the development of posttransplant lymphoproliferative disorders after renal transplantation. Transplantation. 2011;92(2):190–5.
114. Dharnidharka VR, Talley LI, Martz KL, Stablein DM, Fine RN. Recombinant growth hormone use pretransplant and risk for post-transplant lymphoproliferative disease – a report of the NAPRTCS. Pediatr Transplant. 2008;12(6):689–95.
115. Longmore DK, Conwell LS, Burke JR, McDonald SP, McTaggart SJ. Post-transplant lymphoproliferative disorder: no relationship to recombinant human growth hormone use in Australian and New Zealand pediatric kidney transplant recipients. Pediatr Transplant. 2013;17(8):731–6.
116. Chin-Hong PV. Human papillomavirus in kidney transplant recipients. Semin Nephrol. 2016;36(5):397–404.
117. Nailescu C, Nelson RD, Verghese PS, Twombley KE, Chishti AS, Mills M, et al. Human papillomavirus vaccination in male and female adolescents before and after kidney transplantation: a pediatric nephrology research consortium study. Front Pediatr. 2020;8:46.
118. Ulrich C, Jürgensen JS, Degen A, Hackethal M, Ulrich M, Patel MJ, et al. Prevention of non-melanoma skin cancer in organ transplant patients by regular use of a sunscreen: a 24 months, prospective, case-control study. Br J Dermatol. 2009;161 Suppl 3:78–84.
119. Knoll GA, Kokolo MB, Mallick R, Beck A, Buenaventura CD, Ducharme R, et al. Effect of sirolimus on malignancy and survival after kidney transplantation: systematic review and meta-analysis of individual patient data. BMJ. 2014;349:g6679.
120. Dharnidharka VR, Schnitzler MA, Chen J, Brennan DC, Axelrod D, Segev DL, et al. Differential risks for adverse outcomes 3 years after kidney transplantation based on initial immunosuppression regimen: a national study. Transpl Int. 2016;29(11):1226–36.
121. Savoie A, Perpête C, Carpentier L, Joncas J, Alfieri C. Direct correlation between the load of Epstein-Barr virus-infected lymphocytes in the peripheral blood of pediatric transplant patients and risk of lymphoproliferative disease. Blood. 1994;83(9):2715–22.
122. Martin SI, Dodson B, Wheeler C, Davis J, Pesavento T, Bumgardner GL. Monitoring infection with Epstein-Barr virus among seromismatch adult renal transplant recipients. Am J Transplant. 2011;11(5):1058–63.
123. Dharnidharka VR. Comprehensive review of post-organ transplant hematologic cancers. Am J Transplant. 2018;18(3):537–49.
124. Blaes AH, Peterson BA, Bartlett N, Dunn DL, Morrison VA. Rituximab therapy is effective for posttransplant lymphoproliferative disorders after solid organ transplantation: results of a phase II trial. Cancer. 2005;104(8):1661–7.
125. Orjuela MA, Alobeid B, Liu X, Siebert AL, Kott ER, Addonizio LJ, et al. CD20 expression predicts survival in paediatric post-transplant lymphoproliferative disease (PTLD) following solid organ transplantation. Br J Haematol. 2011;152(6):733–42.
126. Francis A, Johnson DW, Craig J, Teixeira-Pinto A, Wong G. Post-transplant lymphoproliferative disease may be an adverse risk factor for patient survival but not graft loss in kidney transplant recipients. Kidney Int. 2018;94(4):809–17.
127. Maecker B, Jack T, Zimmermann M, Abdul-Khaliq H, Burdelski M, Fuchs A, et al. CNS or bone marrow involvement as risk factors for poor survival in post-transplantation lymphoproliferative disorders in children after solid organ transplantation. J Clin Oncol. 2007;25(31):4902–8.
128. Chiou FK, Beath SV, Wilkie GM, Vickers MA, Morland B, Gupte GL. Cytotoxic T-lymphocyte therapy for post-transplant lymphoproliferative disorder after solid organ transplantation in children. Pediatr Transplant. 2018;22(2).
129. Gupta S, Fricker FJ, González-Peralta RP, Slayton WB, Schuler PM, Dharnidharka VR. Post-transplant lymphoproliferative disorder in children: recent outcomes and response to dual rituximab/low-dose chemotherapy combination. Pediatr Transplant. 2010;14(7):896–902.
130. Rosales BM, De La Mata N, Vajdic CM, Kelly PJ, Wyburn K, Webster AC. Cancer mortality in kidney transplant recipients: an Australian and New Zealand population-based cohort study, 1980-2013. Int J Cancer. 2020;146(10):2703–11.

131. Wagenlehner FME, Bjerklund Johansen TE, Cai T, Koves B, Kranz J, Pilatz A, et al. Epidemiology, definition and treatment of complicated urinary tract infections. Nat Rev Urol. 2020;17(10):586–600.
132. Lofaro D, Vogelzang JL, van Stralen KJ, Jager KJ, Groothoff JW. Infection-related hospitalizations over 30 years of follow-up in patients starting renal replacement therapy at pediatric age. Pediatr Nephrol. 2016;31(2):315–23.
133. Naik AS, Dharnidharka VR, Schnitzler MA, Brennan DC, Segev DL, Axelrod D, et al. Clinical and economic consequences of first-year urinary tract infections, sepsis, and pneumonia in contemporary kidney transplantation practice. Transpl Int. 2016;29(2):241–52.
134. John U, Everding AS, Kuwertz-Bröking E, Bulla M, Müller-Wiefel DE, Misselwitz J, et al. High prevalence of febrile urinary tract infections after paediatric renal transplantation. Nephrol Dial Transplant. 2006;21(11):3269–74.
135. Feber J, Spatenka J, Seeman T, Matousovic K, Zeman L, Dusek J, et al. Urinary tract infections in pediatric renal transplant recipients – a two center risk factors study. Pediatr Transplant. 2009;13(7):881–6.
136. Martín-Peña A, Cordero E, Fijo J, Sánchez-Moreno A, Martín-Govantes J, Torrubia F, et al. Prospective study of infectious complications in a cohort of pediatric renal transplant recipients. Pediatr Transplant. 2009;13(4):457–63.
137. Esezobor CI, Nourse P, Gajjar P. Urinary tract infection following kidney transplantation: frequency, risk factors and graft function. Pediatr Nephrol. 2012;27(4):651–7.
138. Sierralta MC, González G, Nome C, Pinilla C, Correa R, Mansilla J, et al. Kidney transplant in pediatric patients with severe bladder pathology. Pediatr Transplant. 2015;19(7):675–83.
139. Khositseth S, Askiti V, Nevins TE, Matas AJ, Ingulli EG, Najarian JS, et al. Increased urologic complications in children after kidney transplants for obstructive and reflux uropathy. Am J Transplant. 2007;7(9):2152–7.
140. Dharnidharka VR, Araya CE, Wadsworth CS, McKinney MC, Howard RJ. Assessing the value of ureteral stent placement in pediatric kidney transplant recipients. Transplantation. 2008;85(7):986–91.
141. Thompson ER, Hosgood SA, Nicholson ML, Wilson CH. Early versus late ureteric stent removal after kidney transplantation. Cochrane Database Syst Rev. 2018;1:CD011455.
142. Dunn SP, Vinocur CD, Hanevold C, Wagner CW, Weintraub WH. Pyelonephritis following pediatric renal transplant: increased incidence with vesicoureteral reflux. J Pediatr Surg. 1987;22(12):1095–9.
143. Casale P, Grady RW, Mitchell ME, Healey P. Recurrent urinary tract infection in the post-transplant reflux nephropathy patient: is reflux in the native ureter the culprit? Pediatr Transplant. 2005;9(3):324–7
144. Basırı A, Otookesh H, Simforoosh N, Hosseini R, Hosseini-Moghaddam SM, Sharifian M. Does pre-transplantation antireflux surgery eliminate post-renal transplantation pyelonephritis in children? J Urol. 2006;175(4):1490–2.
145. Herthelius M, Oborn H. Bladder dysfunction in children and adolescents after renal transplantation. Pediatr Nephrol. 2006;21(5):725–8.
146. Coussement J, Argudín MA, Heinrichs A, Racapé J, de Mendonça R, Nienhaus L, et al. Host and microbial factors in kidney transplant recipients with Escherichia coli acute pyelonephritis or asymptomatic bacteriuria: a prospective study using whole-genome sequencing. Nephrol Dial Transplant. 2019;34(5):878–85.
147. Magruder M, Sholi AN, Gong C, Zhang L, Edusei E, Huang J, et al. Gut uropathogen abundance is a risk factor for development of bacteriuria and urinary tract infection. Nat Commun. 2019;10(1):5521.
148. Brubaker AL, Wu HY, Lee A, Vuong P, Stoltz DJ, Chaudhuri A, et al. Ureterostomy as an alternative to ileal conduits in pediatric kidney transplantation. Clin Transpl. 2020;34(2):e13777.
149. Williams G, Hodson EM, Craig JC. Interventions for primary vesicoureteric reflux. Cochrane Database Syst Rev. 2019;2:CD001532.
150. Wu HY, Concepcion W, Grimm PC. When does vesicoureteral reflux in pediatric kidney transplant patients need treatment? Pediatr Transplant. 2018;22(8):e13299.

151. Singh R, Bemelman FJ, Hodiamont CJ, Idu MM, Ten Berge IJ, Geerlings SE. The impact of trimethoprim-sulfamethoxazole as Pneumocystis jiroveci pneumonia prophylaxis on the occurrence of asymptomatic bacteriuria and urinary tract infections among renal allograft recipients: a retrospective before-after study. BMC Infect Dis. 2016;16:90.
152. Wojciechowski D, Chandran S. Effect of ciprofloxacin combined with sulfamethoxazole-trimethoprim prophylaxis on the incidence of urinary tract infections after kidney transplantation. Transplantation. 2013;96(4):400–5.
153. Cambareri G, Carpenter C, Stock J, Lewis J, Marietti S. Endoscopic antireflux surgery leading to obstruction in pediatric renal transplant patients. Pediatr Transplant. 2017;21(1).
154. Krishnan A, Swana H, Mathias R, Baskin LS. Redo ureteroneocystostomy using an extravesical approach in pediatric renal transplant patients with reflux: a retrospective analysis and description of technique. J Urol. 2006;176(4 Pt 1):1582–7; discussion 7.
155. John U, Kemper MJ. Urinary tract infections in children after renal transplantation. Pediatr Nephrol. 2009;24(6):1129–36.
156. Nicolle LE, Gupta K, Bradley SF, Colgan R, DeMuri GP, Drekonja D, et al. Clinical practice guideline for the management of asymptomatic bacteriuria: 2019 update by the Infectious Diseases Society of America. Clin Infect Dis. 2019;68(10):e83–e110.
157. Fiorante S, López-Medrano F, Lizasoain M, Lalueza A, Juan RS, Andrés A, et al. Systematic screening and treatment of asymptomatic bacteriuria in renal transplant recipients. Kidney Int. 2010;78(8):774–81.
158. El Amari EB, Hadaya K, Bühler L, Berney T, Rohner P, Martin PY, et al. Outcome of treated and untreated asymptomatic bacteriuria in renal transplant recipients. Nephrol Dial Transplant. 2011;26(12):4109–14.
159. Coussement J, Scemla A, Abramowicz D, Nagler EV, Webster AC. Antibiotics for asymptomatic bacteriuria in kidney transplant recipients. Cochrane Database Syst Rev. 2018;2:CD011357.
160. Origüen J, López-Medrano F, Fernández-Ruiz M, Polanco N, Gutiérrez E, González E, et al. Should asymptomatic bacteriuria be systematically treated in kidney transplant recipients? Results from a randomized controlled trial. Am J Transplant. 2016;16(10):2943–53.
161. Bonnéric S, Maisin A, Kwon T, Deschênes G, Niel O. Asymptomatic bacteriuria in pediatric kidney transplant recipients: to treat or not to treat? A retrospective study. Pediatr Nephrol. 2019;34(6):1141–5.
162. Dharnidharka VR, Agodoa LY, Abbott KC. Effects of urinary tract infection on outcomes after renal transplantation in children. Clin J Am Soc Nephrol. 2007;2(1):100–6.

Part III

Disease Challenges

Urological Considerations for Pediatric Renal Transplantation: CAKUT Challenges

6

Oana Nicoara, Hailey Silverii, and Shumyle Alam

Congenital anomalies of the kidney and urinary tract (CAKUT) represent a spectrum of disease conditions that have a large impact on chronic kidney disease (CKD) and CKD progression in children. Whereas most cases of CKD in adults result from diabetes and hypertension, CAKUT disorders are the most common causes of CKD in pediatric patients. The main diagnoses include obstructive uropathy (21%), renal dysplasia/aplasia (18%), reflux nephropathy (8%), and polycystic kidney disease (4%). This grouping often seen in databases such as US Renal Data System (USRDS) and the North American Pediatric Renal Trials and Collaborative Studies (NAPRTCS) does not necessarily represent unique disease conditions. The main reason is that roughly 30–40% of children with CKD have a concomitant urological issue as the underlying cause. For example, a single child with posterior urethral valves may also have reflux nephropathy, renal dysplasia, and even in some cases carry a diagnosis of cystic kidney disease. This heterogenicity in patient disease condition has made it difficult to track transplant outcomes and progression of disease, given the inherent overlapping conditions (Table 6.1). Use of CAKUT may allow more rationale data collection and help us better understand outcomes. The focus of this chapter will be to explore how CAKUT has significant urologic challenges that can impact transplant, progression of renal disease, and the overall well-being of the child.

The remainder of cases of CKD in children results from glomerular diseases like focal segmental glomerulosclerosis and acquired conditions like hemolytic uremic syndrome and calcineurin inhibitor toxicity [1]. Renal infarction and Wilms' tumor

O. Nicoara
Department of Pediatrics, Division of Pediatric Nephrology, MUSC Shawn Jenkins Children's Hospital/Medical University of South Carolina, Charleston, SC, USA

H. Silverii · S. Alam (✉)
Department of Urology, MUSC Shawn Jenkins Children's Hospital/Medical University of South Carolina, Charleston, SC, USA
e-mail: alams@musc.edu

K. E. Twombley (ed.), *Challenges in Pediatric Kidney Transplantation*,
https://doi.org/10.1007/978-3-030-74783-1_6

Table 6.1 Underlying etiologies for CAKUT

Cloaca	Anorectal Malformations	Exstrophy/Epispadias	Prune Belly Syndrome
OEIS/Cloacal Exstrophy	Spinal Dysraphisms	VUR	PUV
	Ureterocele	Neurogenic Bladder (Often a secondary diagnosis)	

also contribute to ≤1% of cases of end-stage renal disease (ESRD) in children. In one study, cases that progressed to ESRD occurred in 41% of patients with glomerular diseases and 29% with non-glomerular diseases [2]. Predictors of faster CKD progression were proteinuria, hypoalbuminemia, hypertension, dyslipidemia, and anemia. The rate of CKD and ESRD is higher in boys due to increased risk of CAKUT including posterior urethral valves (PUV), renal dysplasia, and prune belly syndrome [1, 3]. Boys account for about 60% of cases of ESRD and subsequent renal transplants. Ultimately, a third of children with CKD who require renal replacement therapy will be found to have a urologic abnormality, and 39% of children on the transplant waiting list carry a CAKUT diagnosis [4].

The high prevalence of urologic pathology in CAKUT children with CKD and ESRD necessitates early urological evaluation and treatment. Abnormal urinary tract function can have a deleterious effect on kidney function, and intervention may be able to delay the need for transplantation. The goals of any pediatric urologist as part of a multidisciplinary team with nephrologists and transplant surgeons should be to optimize the bladder or appropriately reconstruct it prior to transplant and consider appropriate management of the native kidneys [5]. Workup generally involves serum chemistries including a cystatin C, a renal ultrasound, a functional assessment of the bladder, and in some cases a cystoscopy to characterize or treat structural abnormalities.

A main concern in patients with CAKUT relates to the bladder. Bladder dysfunction is relatively poorly understood outside of the patient with neurogenic bladder dysfunction in the patient with a spinal dysraphism. In this group, much is discussed regarding high storage pressures and incomplete bladder emptying. Voiding pressures are not necessarily well understood as it relates to the upper tract. In the CAKUT patient, the bladder dysfunction is not always similar to the patient with neurogenic bladder from a spinal anomaly, and the management is often quite different.

Regarding bladder dysfunction, storage pressures over 40 cm H_2O have been shown to have damaging effects on renal function through increased papillary pressure and intrarenal urine reflux [6], although patients with severe vesicoureteral reflux (VUR) can demonstrate the same deleterious effects to the upper tracts and renal parenchyma as a consequence of voiding (Fig. 6.1). The long-term effects this has on either native or transplant kidneys are poorly understood.

Detrusor sphincter dyssynergia, secondary vesicoureteral reflux (VUR), hydronephrosis, and chronic urinary tract infections (UTI) all contribute to upper tract deterioration. However, in industrialized countries, progressive CKD from neurogenic bladder, especially in spina bifida, has become quite rare due to improvement in management of this patient population.

Despite challenges regarding care standards for bladder dysfunction, the mainstay of management is a high level of suspicion for bladder involvement and early workup in the CAKUT population. Urodynamic studies can be performed in select patients to evaluate bladder compliance, leak point pressure, voiding pressure, and residual volumes. Pending results, these patients might benefit from aggressive bladder management including non-operative interventions such as anticholinergics with clean intermittent self-catheterization (CIC) or operative interventions such as urinary tract diversions, ureteral reimplantation, and/or augmentation cystoplasty to mitigate some of the potential damage from a poorly compliant bladder.

A CAKUT condition requiring transplant that is often discussed is PUVs. PUV patients require a thorough urologic evaluation prior to transplantation. Progression to ESRD develops in up to 50% of patients diagnosed with PUVs [7]. The management of these infants has improved over time which has resulted in more pulmonary-based survival most likely due to early diagnosis and intervention. The rate of

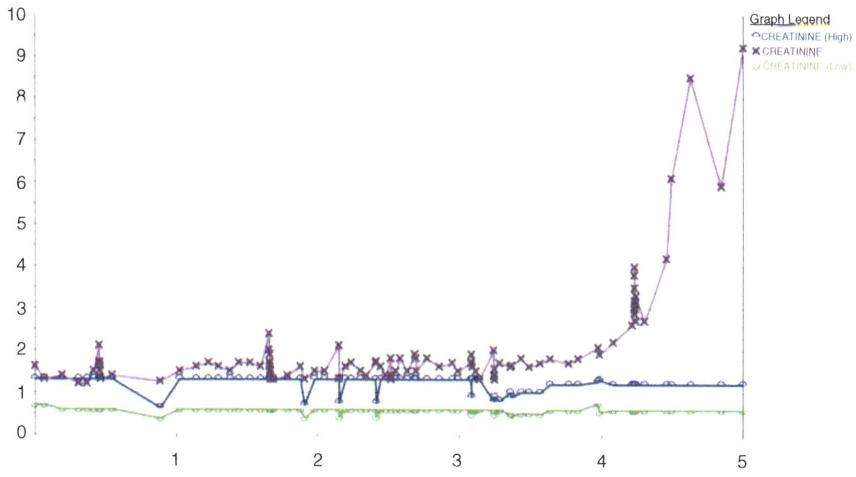

Fig. 6.1 Serum creatinine (sCr) over 13 years after deceased donor transplant. *X*-axis = time (years), *Y*-axis = sCr (mg/dl). We see that the patient's sCr (purple line) was already >1.5 mg/dl immediately post-transplant. Available records indicate that there was never an sCr nadir <1.0.mg/dl. Reference ranges for expected high (blue line) and low (green line) sCr by age are provided

progressive CKD however is not known to have changed. In the last few years, some centers have experienced an uptick in ESRD patients with PUV secondary to the better success rates by our Maternal Fetal Medicine colleages in decreasing pulmonary complications in this patient cohort. Prenatal imaging has allowed a better opportunity for birth planning and the involvement of a multidisciplinary approach to care.

Imaging demonstrating hydronephrosis, VUR, or cystic changes to the kidneys may underline the often subtle changes in loss of bladder compliance and the development of high pressures in the bladder from either storage of urine or voiding. These changes may portend long-term deterioration of renal function without intervention. Pressure in the bladder is transmitted to the kidneys irrespective of VUR. This pressure can result in damage to the kidney and result in an injurious state which can create a concentrating defect. In some cases, infants with PUV have such a profound concentrating defect in the kidney and, therefore, they require a gastrostomy tube for feeds and fluid balance. The resulting cycle is simple fluid mechanics. Increased volume of urine results in filling of the bladder to capacity, at times faster than the child can void, resulting in increased bladder pressures and more damage to the kidney.

This cycle of injury can be seen despite early intervention and valve ablation as patients born with PUV can have life-long bladder dysfunction. As there is no care standard for management of the bladder, especially in the neonatal period, we find that almost a quarter of these patients will still progress to ESRD [8]. Patients exhibiting high voiding pressures and low bladder compliance often necessitate intervention such as urinary diversion with a vesicostomy versus high-dose anticholinergic therapy with CIC [9].

Historically, undiversion was thought to be necessary prior to transplantation to evaluate bladder function and determine if there is a need for augmentation [10]. However, recent series has demonstrated the safety of transplanting a kidney into a diverted system [11]. Older children exhibit low voiding pressures and large bladder capacities, so efforts including timed voiding, CIC, and/or overnight catheterization should focus on maintaining a low post-void residual volume to prevent urinary stasis and infections [12]. Despite recommendations for bladder management, there remains a paucity of evidence regarding the impact of elevated voiding pressures over time to a graft or even native kidneys in the CAKUT patient population. A multidisciplinary approach including pediatric urologists may be of benefit in the care of these patients before, during, and after their transplants.

Interestingly enough, the pathophysiology of the bladder seen in PUV patients can also be seen in many other patients with CAKUT. For example, a female patient with a cloacal anomaly may have high pressure voiding, reflux, and incomplete bladder emptying. All of the diseases shown in Table 6.1 can result in the same pathophysiology as seen in PUV. Utilizing the CAKUT description to group patients may assist us with better data to understand the management of the bladder pre- and post-transplant.

Despite a lack of evidence in CAKUT, bladder management is a big part of the management of the child with spina bifida. Using the principles that are well known in this patient cohort, we can benefit the child with CAKUT. Simple intermittent catheterization and anticholinergic therapy can decrease the need for surgery and stabilize renal function (Figs. 6.2 and 6.3). VUR is often secondary to the bladder condition in children with CAKUT and does not always require surgery for management. In some cases, surgery can actually worsen the progression of renal disease as it does not address the abnormal bladder.

The relationship between high intravesical pressures and transplant graft deterioration is well established, so pre-transplant intervention is aimed at creating a low-pressure reservoir. When medical management fails, augmentation cystoplasty is sometimes necessary to guarantee a low-pressure reservoir [13, 14]. In several small case series, graft survival seems to be equivalent in patients with augmented bladders compared to those who have normal bladders [15–17]. Interestingly enough, graft survival and patient outcomes may not always correlate in the manner that this data is interpreted (Figs. 6.1 and 6.4).

Graft outcomes in CAKUT patients may be affected by the bladder in ways that are not being universally followed. In the case of the patient referenced above, his graft prevented dialysis for 13 years but did not result in any metabolic gain including growth and height. In addition, the child is still functioning at the mental capacity of a fifth grader and had no risk factors for developmental delay except his CAKUT. Despite the specific outcome for the patient, the reported long-term outcome of his graft is favorable.

After transplant, the graft can be impacted by the bladder in the CAKUT population and potentially affect all patients who after transplant have structural

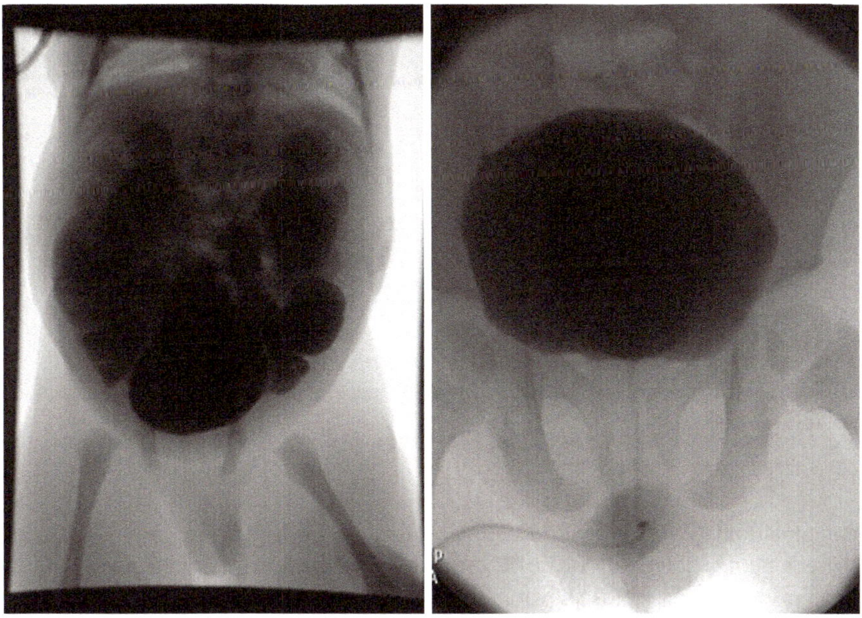

Fig. 6.2 VCUG. A VCUG image showing bilateral grade 5 VUR in a CKD CAKUT patient. The image on the right is without any surgery – simply bladder management with CIC and oxybutynin

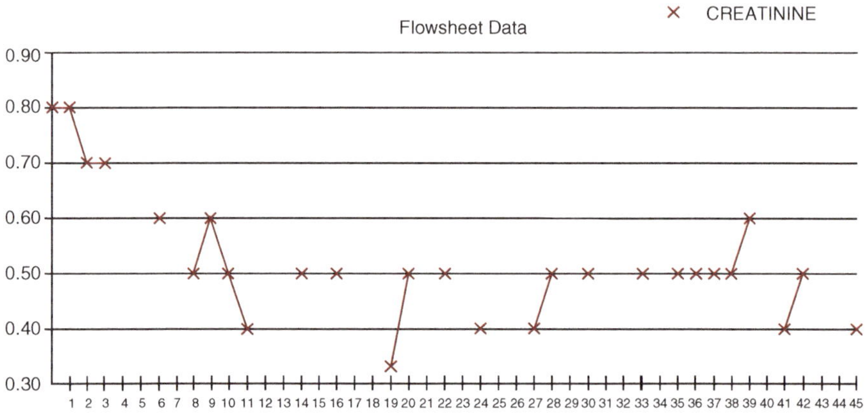

Fig. 6.3 Serum creatinine (sCr) of a patient with CAKUT. *X*-axis = time (years), *Y*-axis = sCr (mg/dl). This is a graph of the same CAKUT patient showing preservation of renal function with bladder management alone. There will likely not be a need for renal transplant in the future, despite the elevated birth sCr. SCr measured in mg/dl

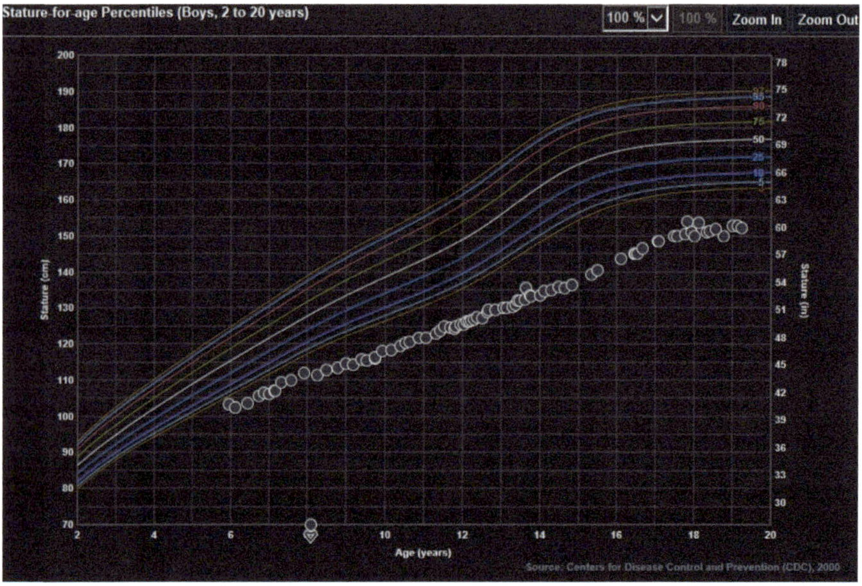

Fig. 6.4 Growth of CAKUT patient. This same child with CAKUT never caught up from a metabolic standpoint after transplant

complications [28]. There are multiple options to mitigate these issues, although there is no real standard of care. The extreme consequence of no bladder management prior to transplant is shown in Figs. 6.5 and 6.6. Options for bladder management vary but range from clean intermittent catherization (CIC), use of

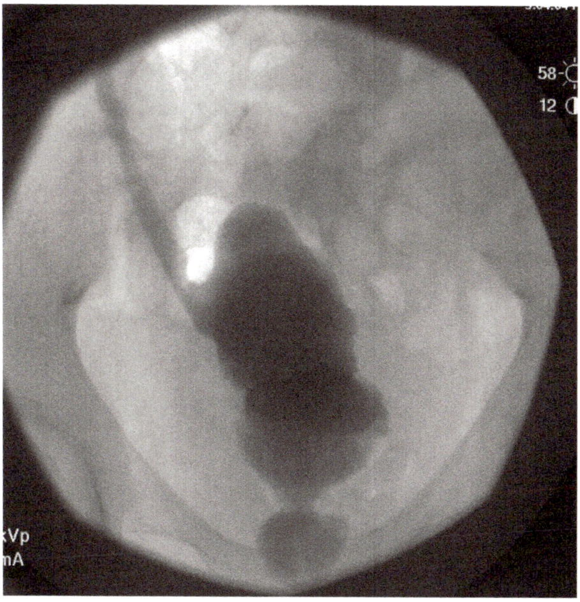

Fig. 6.5 Voiding urodynamics. This is an image from a Voiding Urodynamics study of the same CAKUT patient with unmanaged bladder since transplant

anticholinergics, timed voiding, and bladder surgery. There is not an accepted standard for which management is applicable to the CAKUT patient.

From a surgical standpoint, in the case of a small or poorly compliant bladder, ileocystoplasty is the most common method of bladder augmentation, but risks include mucus production, bladder stones, difficulty emptying, and metabolic acidosis. Acidosis tends to be seen in patients with CKD stage 3–5 and is a result of the absorptive nature of the bowel segments used. In the bowel, sodium and bicarbonate are secreted in exchange for hydrogen and chloride ions. As this absorption is a function of stasis, contact, and time, a well-configured augment is a must. The creation of a sphere after augmentation gives a better chance of complete emptying than a patient with a figure of eight deformity [18].

Alternatively, gastrocystoplasty can obviate some of these problems, but it has distinct disadvantages including hematuria/dysuria syndrome and rare hypochloremic metabolic alkalosis, due to loss of hydrogen and chloride ions, and an increased concern for malignancy. One theory for the etiology of hematuria/dysuria is irritation caused by the production of hydrochloric acid by the gastric segment. However, the symptoms have been seen even with urine acidity in the normal range. An alternative explanation proposed by some was irritation from *Helicobacter pylori* infection, which with treatment showed improvement.

Dysuria is generally only seen is sensate patients, and it is not advisable to use stomach when the urethra is still the conduit for catheterization. Hematuria becomes an issue depending on the segment chosen. Care should be taken to utilize the body

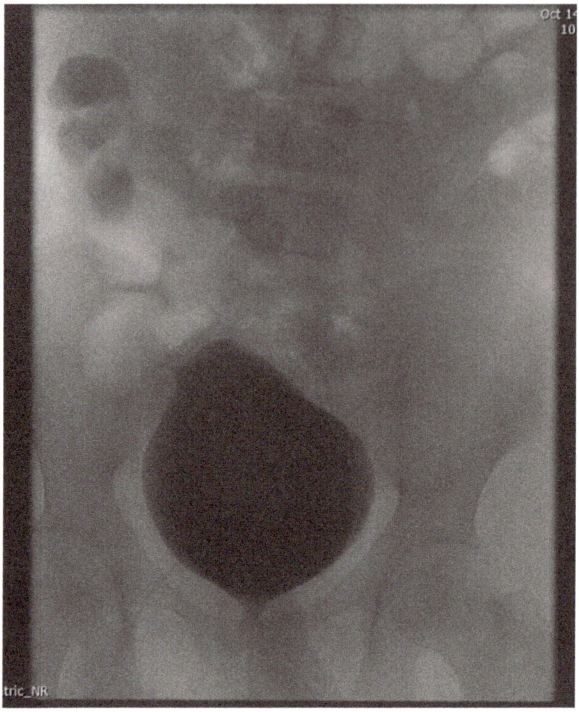

Fig. 6.6 Voiding urodynamics after a trial of intermittent catheterization and anticholinergics. The same patient after a trial of intermittent catheterization and anticholinergics. Patient's bladder ready for re-transplant with simple bladder management

of the stomach away from the cardia and antrum. Although parietal cells are found throughout the stomach, this section reconfigures nicely and has a lower tendency to secrete acid.

The risk of malignancy is a concern for some, but it is estimated to occur in <5% of cases [19]. Regardless, surveillance with cystoscopy and ultrasound is recommended beginning 10 years after augmentation [20]. Autoaugmentation and ureterocystoplasty were performed historically, but both techniques have fallen out of favor [21]. Autoaugmentation, which is basically the creation of a diverticulum, did not hold up over time and patients did not reliably experience an improvement in compliance and capacity. Ureterocystoplasy is a simple operation and can be performed without opening the peritoneal cavity, but it has the tendency to create a diverticulum or a deformity that impairs drainage and can promote stasis and UTI. Utilizing the dilated ureter also sacrifices the kidney, and when performed on the lateral wall of the bladder, it can impact the reimplant of the transplant kidney [22].

Augmentation can be performed either when the patient is ready for transplant listing or 6 to 12 weeks before a scheduled living donor transplant, prior to starting immunosuppression. For patients on peritoneal dialysis, it is important to realize that any transperitoneal surgery can compromise this approach by creating serosal disruptions and adhesions which will interfere with ultrafiltration.

The management of retained native renal units can also be a concern for urologists. Residual excretory capacity and erythropoietin production can provide physiologic benefit; however, issues like reflux and infection can present challenges [23]. Some studies have suggested an increased incidence of bacteriuria in patients with VUR [24]. The management of VUR in this setting is controversial with options including observation, endoscopic bulking injection, ureteral reimplantation, and native nephrectomy. One study showed no difference in infection rates between observation and native nephrectomy but showed decreased infections with reimplantation [25]. For high-grade reflux, reimplantation is preferred because it maintains the native ureters in case they are needed for future complication management with ureteroureterostomy or ureteropyelostomy.

Native nephrectomy is indicated for patients with persistent high-grade reflux, chronic renal infections (i.e., xanthogranulomatous pyelonephritis), infected renal stones, large cystic kidneys, or refractory hypertension. Heavy proteinuria (>40 mg/ m^2/hour) can also merit native nephrectomy to eliminate protein loss and potentially decrease risk of thrombotic events [23, 26, 27]. Nephrectomy can be performed early, several weeks before transplant, or simultaneously with transplant. However, some conditions like xanthogranulomatous pyelonephritis or polycystic kidney disease may make nephrectomy at the time of transplant too difficult or risky. Widespread use of minimally invasive techniques for nephrectomy has decreased some of the concerns regarding timing and impact on dialysis [28]. Finally, nephrectomy may reduce the risk of graft hypoperfusion by reducing organ steal and volume depletion from large native urine output [23]. The decision to perform native nephrectomy should be individualized with a discussion of potential risks and benefits of this strategy.

Urological Complications Post-transplant

Acute urological complications occur in 5–22% of pediatric transplants [29, 30]. Postoperative urinary obstruction and urine extravasation are the most common complications. Extravasation results from anastomotic leak, ureteral necrosis, or bladder injury and is managed conservatively with stenting and bladder drainage or surgically with nephrostomy drainage, dilation, or reimplantation. Case series have shown that urological complications are not associated with donor type, preexisting urological pathology, surgical technique, or patient age [29]. Ureteral obstruction is more common in boys with PUV, but it can also result from transient ureteral edema, anastomotic stricture, or hematuria with clots. In one case series, half of the patients with ureteral obstruction presented within 100 days of transplant and 79% were found to have obstruction at the level of the ureterovesical junction [31].

Urolithiasis can also affect transplant recipients. Stones are formed in 6% of adults and 1% of pediatric patients after transplant [32]. Diagnosis and treatment can be challenging since obstruction will not cause typical renal colic, and endoscopic access to a transplant kidney can be problematic. In the largest series of 20 patients, presenting signs/symptoms were UTI (40%), hematuria (35%), dysuria or straining (45%), and asymptomatic (10%) [33]. Risk factors identified included retained suture material, hypercalciuria, recurrent UTI, and urinary stasis. Other factors that contribute to stone formation in transplant patients are low urine output, alkaline urinary pH, hypomagnesuria, hypocitraturia, and hyperparathyroidism [34]. Stones can be treated with extracorporeal shock wave lithotripsy, retrograde ureteroscopy, or percutaneous nephrolithotomy, but comparative effectiveness data between these techniques are scant.

Postoperative VUR is noted in up to 58% of transplants [35]. If incidentally detected during screening or imaging, there appears to be no effect on graft survival [29, 36]. However, if hydronephrosis and/or pyelonephritis develop, outcomes are worse [37, 38]. As discussed, earlier graft survival is not the only metric that can be assessed when it comes to the health and well-being of a pediatric transplant recipient.

Urologic disorders that predispose patients to transplant VUR include noncompliant bladder, detrusor overactivity, posterior urethral valves, or urethral stricture [39]. In certain cases with incompletely controlled bladder dysfunction, aggressive bladder management with anticholinergic pharmacotherapy and CIC can be enough to decrease urinary stasis and prevent renal damage. Ideally this should all be addressed prior to transplant. In a few patients, endoscopic management with injection of collagen bulking agents has been attempted in transplanted kidneys with limited success [40, 41]. Ureteral reimplant and/or submucosal tunnel lengthening has been shown to have success rates of almost 100% [39]. This procedure is performed in a small fraction (2%) of pediatric transplant recipients nationally [42].

The management of the CAKUT patient with CKD and ESRD is not standardized. Although the focus of this chapter was to educate the reader about successful ESRD management and ensuring graft survival, there exist multiple opportunities to utilize these lessons to improve native kidney function and potentially delay the progression of CKD. Many of the principles mentioned in this chapter can be applied earlier in the patient's life to preserve renal function. We are hopeful that a broader understanding of the CAKUT patient will help the medical community continue to improve care and treatment of this condition as time progresses.

1. Conditions that comprise congenital anomalies of kidney and urinary tract (CAKUT) include all of the following except:
   (a) Posterior urethral valves
   (b) Ureteropelvic obstruction
   (c) Autosomal recessive polycystic kidney disease
   (d) Megaureter
   (e) Renal scarring

Congenital anomalies of the kidney and urinary tract (CAKUT)

Kidney anomalies	Urinary tract anomalies
Renal agenesis	Posterior urethral valves
Renal hypoplasia	Bladder malformations
Renal dysplasia	Prune-Belly syndrome
Multicystic dysplastic kidney	Vesicoureteral reflux

Kidney anomalies	Urinary tract anomalies
Autosomal recessive polycystic kidney disease	Megaureter
Ureteropelvic junction (UPJ) obstruction	Ureterovesical junction (UVJ) obstruction
Duplex renal collecting system	

Answer: (e)

2. Native nephrectomy prior to kidney transplant is indicated in the following situations except:
   (a) High-grade urinary reflux
   (b) Chronic urinary infections
   (c) Renal dysplasia
   (d) Large proteinuria
   (e) Refractory hypertension

   Native nephrectomy is indicated for patients with persistent high-grade reflux, chronic renal infections (i.e., xanthogranulomatous pyelonephritis), infected renal stones, large cystic kidneys, or refractory hypertension. Heavy proteinuria (>40 mg/m^2/hour) can also merit native nephrectomy to eliminate protein loss and potentially decrease the risk of thrombotic events.

   Answer: (c)
3. Which of the following is true regarding bladder dysfunction:

(a) Storage pressures over 40 cm H_2O have been shown to have damaging effects on renal function.

(b) Children with large volume urine output CAKUT do not need to have their bladder evaluated pre-transplant.

(c) Patients exhibiting low voiding pressures and high bladder compliance often necessitate intervention such as urinary diversion with a vesicostomy versus high-dose anticholinergic therapy with CIC.

(d) VUR is often secondary to the bladder condition in children with CAKUT and does require surgery for management.

The correct answer is that storage pressures over 40 cm H_2O have been shown to have damaging effects on renal function. The amount of urine does not correlate to the degree of bladder dysfunction. It can be an effect of the damage on the kidney and loss of concentrating ability. Patients exhibiting high voiding pressures and low bladder compliance often necessitate intervention such as urinary diversion with a vesicostomy versus high-dose anticholinergic therapy with CIC. VUR is often secondary to the bladder condition in children with CAKUT and does not always require surgery for management. In some cases, surgery can actually worsen the progression of renal disease as it does not address the abnormal bladder. VUR is often secondary to the bladder condition in children with CAKUT and does not always require surgery for management.

Answer: (a)

References

1. NAPRTCS 2014 Annual Transplant Report. 2014. Section 1, p1–10. Accessed 11/20/2020. https://naprtcs.org/system/files/2014_Annual_Transplant_Report.pdf.
2. Warady BA, et al. Predictors of rapid progression of glomerular and nonglomerular kidney disease in children and adolescents: the chronic kidney disease in children (CKiD) cohort. Am J Kidney Dis. 2015;65(6):878–88.
3. Wong CJ, et al. CKiD (CKD in children) prospective cohort study: a review of current findings. Am J Kidney Dis. 2012;60(6):1002–11.
4. Hart A, et al. OPTN/SRTR 2015 annual data report: kidney. Am J Transplant. 2017;17(Suppl 1):21–116.
5. Penna FJ, Elder JS. CKD and bladder problems in children. Adv Chronic Kidney Dis. 2011;18(5):362–9.
6. McGuire EJ, et al. Prognostic value of urodynamic testing in myelodysplastic patients. J Urol. 1981;126(2):205–9.
7. Casella DP, Tomaszewski JJ, Ost MC. Posterior urethral valves: renal failure and prenatal treatment. Int J Nephrol. 2012;2012:351067.
8. Bryant JE, et al. Renal transplantation in children with posterior urethral valves. J Urol. 1991;146(6):1585–7.
9. Lyon RP, Marshall S, Baskin LS. Normal growth with renal insufficiency owing to posterior urethral valves: value of long-term diversion. Urol Int. 1992;48(2):125–9.
10. Macedo P, Romero F, Silva F. Metástases penianas: relato de dois casos e revisão da literatura. Urominas. 2019;7:52–4.
11. Viswanathan A, et al. Early transplantation into a vesicostomy: a safe approach for managing patients with severe obstructive lesions who are not candidates for bladder augmentation. J Pediatr Urol. 2018;14(4):332.e1–6.
12. Nguyen MT, et al. Overnight catheter drainage in children with poorly compliant bladders improves post-obstructive diuresis and urinary incontinence. J Urol. 2005;174(4 Pt 2):1633–6; discussion 1636.
13. Riley P, et al. Challenges facing renal transplantation in pediatric patients with lower urinary tract dysfunction. Transplantation. 2010;89(11):1299–307.
14. Salomon L, et al. Posterior urethral valves: long-term renal function consequences after transplantation. J Urol. 1997;157(3):992–5.
15. López Pereira P, et al. Does bladder augmentation negatively affect renal transplant outcome in posterior urethral valve patients? J Pediatr Urol. 2014;10(5):892–7.
16. Luke PPW, et al. Long-term results of pediatric renal transplantation into a dysfunctional lower urinary tract. Transplantation. 2003;76(11):1578–82.
17. Djakovic N, et al. Intestinal reconstruction of the lower urinary tract as a prerequisite for renal transplantation. BJU Int. 2009;103(11):1555–60.
18. Stein R, Rubenwolf P. Metabolic consequences after urinary diversion. Front Pediatr. 2014;2:15.
19. Higuchi TT, et al. Augmentation cystoplasty and risk of neoplasia: fact, fiction and controversy. J Urol. 2010;184(6):2492–6.
20. Soergel Trevor M, et al. Transitional cell carcinoma of the bladder following augmentation cystoplasty for the neuropathic bladder. J Urol. 2004;172(4 Part 2):1649–52.
21. González R, Ludwikowski BM. Alternatives to conventional enterocystoplasty in children: a critical review of urodynamic outcomes. Front Pediatr. 2013;1:25.
22. Alexopoulos S, et al. Pediatric kidney recipients with small capacity, defunctionalized urinary bladders receiving adult-sized kidney without prior bladder augmentation. Transplantation. 2011;91(4):452–6.
23. Ghane Sharbaf F, et al. Native nephrectomy prior to pediatric kidney transplantation: biological and clinical aspects. Pediatr Nephrol (Berlin, Germany). 2012;27(7):1179–88.

24. Sharifian M, Rees L, Trompeter RS. High incidence of bacteriuria following renal transplantation in children. Nephrol Dial Transplant. 1998;13(2):432–5.
25. Erturk E, et al. Outcome of patients with vesicoureteral reflux after renal transplantation: the effect of pretransplantation surgery on posttransplant urinary tract infections. Urology. 1998;51(5A Suppl):27–30.
26. Slaughenhoupt BL, et al. Urologic management of congenital nephrotic syndrome of the Finnish type. Urology. 1998;51(3):492–4.
27. Wang C-S, et al. Renal allograft loss due to renal vascular thrombosis in the US pediatric renal transplantation. Pediatr Nephrol. 2019;34(9):1545–55.
28. Szymanski KM, Bitzan M, Capolicchio JP. Is retroperitoneoscopy the gold standard for endoscopic nephrectomy in children on peritoneal dialysis? J Urol. 2010;184(4 Suppl):1631–7.
29. Routh JC, et al. Urological complications and vesicoureteral reflux following pediatric kidney transplantation. J Urol. 2013;189(3):1071–6.
30. Irtan S, et al. Renal transplantation in children: critical analysis of age related surgical complications. Pediatr Transplant. 2010;14(4):512–9.
31. Smith KM, et al. Risk factors and treatment success for ureteral obstruction after pediatric renal transplantation. J Urol. 2010;183(1):317–22.
32. Cheungpasitporn W, et al. Incidence of kidney stones in kidney transplant recipients: a systematic review and meta-analysis. World J Transplant. 2016;6(4):790–7.
33. Khositseth S, et al. Urolithiasis after kidney transplantation in pediatric recipients: a single center report. Transplantation. 2004;78(9):1319–23.
34. Harper JM, et al. Risk factors for calculus formation in patients with renal transplants. Br J Urol. 1994;74(2):147–50.
35. Ranchin B, et al. Vesicoureteral reflux after kidney transplantation in children. Nephrol Dial Transplant. 2000;15(11):1852–8.
36. Fontana I, et al. Vesico-ureteral reflux in pediatric kidney transplants: clinical relevance to graft and patient outcome. Pediatr Transplant. 1999;3(3):206–9.
37. Chu L, et al. Hydronephrosis in pediatric kidney transplant: clinical relevance to graft outcome. J Pediatr Urol. 2013;9(2):217–22.
38. Ohba K, et al. Clinicopathological study of vesicoureteral reflux (VUR)-associated pyelonephritis in renal transplantation. Clin Transpl. 2004;18(Suppl 11):34–8.
39. Barrero R, et al. Vesicoureteral reflux after kidney transplantation in children. Pediatr Transplant. 2007;11(5):498–503.
40. Latchamsetty KC, et al. Use of collagen injections for vesicoureteral reflux in transplanted kidneys. Transplant Proc. 2003;35(4):1378–80.
41. Alkan M, et al. Endoscopic treatment of vesicoureteral reflux in children: our experience and analysis of factors affecting success rate. Urol Int. 2008;81(1):41–6.
42. Van Arendonk KJ, et al. National trends over 25 years in pediatric kidney transplant outcomes. Pediatrics. 2014;133(4):594–601.

Rheumatologic Challenges

7

Sonia I. Savani and Mileka Gilbert

Systemic Lupus Erythematosus

Introduction

Systemic lupus erythematosus (SLE) is a rare, chronic autoimmune disease that can result in multi-organ damage and is known for its waxing and waning disease course [1–3]. SLE is characterized by the abnormal immune dysregulation of both the innate and adaptive immune processes, leading to the breakdown of self-tolerance and the development of autoantibodies directed against self-antigens (most notably against endogenous nuclear antigens) [4]. Autoantibody and self-antigen immune complexes deposit in various tissues and organs, causing localized inflammation [4] and triggering activation of complement and accrual of neutrophils, monocytes, and self-reactive lymphocytes [4]. While genetic, environmental, and hormonal elements all are believed to contribute to the development of SLE, the exact pathogenesis is exceedingly complex and remains largely unknown [4].

The American College of Rheumatology (ACR), in conjunction with the European League Against Rheumatism, has developed an updated set of classification criteria for SLE (revised in 2019) based on presence of a positive antinuclear antibody (ANA) at titer of ≥1:80 with additive clinical and immunologic criteria [5]. The clinical criteria include the domains of constitutional, hematologic, neuropsychiatric, mucocutaneous, serosal, musculoskeletal, and renal manifestations. The immunological criteria include presence of antiphospholipid antibodies,

S. I. Savani (✉)
Department of Medicine and Department of Pediatrics, Medical University of South Carolina, Charleston, SC, USA
e-mail: savani@musc.edu

M. Gilbert
Department of Pediatrics, Division of Pediatric Rheumatology, MUSC Shawn Jenkins Children's Hospital/Medical University of South Carolina, Charleston, SC, USA
e-mail: gilbertm@musc.edu

K. E. Twombley (ed.), *Challenges in Pediatric Kidney Transplantation*,
https://doi.org/10.1007/978-3-030-74783-1_7

hypocomplementemia, and presence of SLE-specific antibodies [5]. The Systemic Lupus International Collaborating Clinics (SLICC) has also published a new set of classification criteria in 2012, which includes 11 clinical and 6 immunologic items [6]. These sets of classification criteria serve as guides for identifying SLE; however, diagnosis is largely clinical and does not depend on meeting criteria for either ACR or SLICC.

SLE predominantly affects young, non-white women [1, 2] with a 3:1 female-to-male ratio in children and a 10:1 female-to-male ratio in the reproductive years [7]. Between 10 and 20% of SLE cases are diagnosed in the pediatric population prior to 18 years of age [1–3, 8]. There is wide variability in upper limit of ages in the literature used to define childhood-onset SLE (cSLE), ranging from 14 years to 21 years of age [1]. The mean age of onset is between 11 and 12 years [3]. In the United Sates, studies have suggested an annual incidence of cSLE of 0.6 per 100,000 population [9]. Others suggest an annual incidence of 0.3–2 cases per 100,000 patient-years and a prevalence of 1.89–25.7 per 100,000 children worldwide [2, 3]. Patients with cSLE typically have a more severe disease course when compared to adult counterparts [10], and mortality can approach 95% if the disease is left untreated [11].

Although mortality for cSLE has improved over the years with some advancements in treatment, there continues to be significant associated morbidity depending on the extent of organ involvement. Comorbidities, such as progression to end-stage renal disease (ESRD), have become more prominent as the overall survival of patients with SLE increases. Lupus nephritis (LN) is one of the most severe complications of SLE and serves as a strong predictor of poor outcome and increased mortality rates in SLE [2, 12], often occurring in the first years of disease [13]. It is reported that as many as 40–80% of patients with cSLE will develop kidney involvement in the form of LN during their disease course [1, 2, 7, 12, 14], with approximately 80% of childhood LN occurring at or within the first year of diagnosis [15]. cSLE characteristically presents with a more aggressive disease course with a reported 10–30% higher prevalence of LN when compared to adults [1].

Clinical Course of Renal Involvement and Outcomes

Renal involvement significantly contributes to increased morbidity and mortality in SLE. In the literature, kidney disease as a predictor of death in adults and children is consistently reported [2]. Prior to use of corticosteroids, patients with LN did not survive greater than 5 years [1]. Outcomes improved by the 1990s in children with LN with 10-year patient survival of 92–95% and 10-year renal survival 89–90% after diagnosis, but these numbers have since plateaued [1]. Yet, mortality rates can be as high as 20% in cSLE in some parts of the world [2, 16].

Renal involvement in SLE can range broadly from mild hematuria and/or proteinuria to progression to acute or chronic kidney disease (CKD) and ESRD [17]. Per the 2012 "Kidney Disease: Improving Global Outcomes (KDIGO) Clinical Practice Guidelines for Glomerulonephritis," renal involvement should be considered in any patient with lupus with new impairment of kidney function or presence of proteinuria, active urine sediment, or elevated blood pressures. LN is most often due to deposition of immune complexes in the glomerulus leading to inflammation. The gold standard for diagnosis of LN is kidney biopsy [1]. Histological classification of renal pathology is graded according to the 2003 International Society of Nephrology and Renal Pathology Society (ISN/RPS) classification system [Table 7.1] and can range from minimal mesangial involvement (class I LN) to proliferative glomerulonephritis (GN) (class III and IV LN) to advanced sclerosing LN (class VI LN) [17]. Class V LN represents a membranous form of LN and can occur in combination with class III or IV LN. ISN/RPS class IV LN, the most common of the histological classifications, is the most active disease class and is associated with worse prognosis [2, 18]. Extent of kidney involvement, including features of activity and chronicity seen histologically, often predicts kidney outcomes and guides treatment decisions [2].

While a full discussion of treatment protocols for cSLE and LN are outside the scope of this text, it should be noted that several international groups have produced protocols that are based on an intensive period of induction therapy, often with high doses of corticosteroids and either mycophenolate mofetil (MMF) or IV cyclophosphamide (CYC), followed by maintenance immunosuppressive therapy for LN with close monitoring of disease activity to ensure disease remission [2]. However,

Table 7.1 ISN/RPS 2003 classification of lupus nephritis [17]

Class	Definition	Description
I	Minimal mesangial LN	Light microscopy – normal IF – mesangial immune deposits
II	Mesangial proliferative LN	Light microscopy – purely mesangial hypercellularity and matrix expansion with mesangial immune deposits IF and EM – few isolated subepithelial or subendothelial deposits
III	Focal LN	Active or inactive focal, segmental, or global endo- or extracapillary glomerulonephritis involving <50% of all glomeruli Focal subendothelial immune deposits with or without mesangial alterations Proportion of glomeruli with active and chronic lesions indicated
IV	Diffuse LN	Active or inactive focal, segmental, or global endo- or extracapillary glomerulonephritis involving ≥50% of all glomeruli Diffuse subendothelial immune deposits with or without mesangial alterations Further divided into diffuse segmental or diffuse global Proportion of glomeruli with active and chronic lesions indicated Proportion of glomeruli with fibrinoid necrosis and/or cellular crescents indicated
V	Membranous LN	Global or segmental subepithelial deposits by light microscopy, IF, or EM with or without mesangial alterations May occur in combination with class III or IV
VI	Advanced sclerosis LN	≥90% of glomeruli globally sclerosed without residual activity
		Indicate and grade (mild, moderate, severe) tubular atrophy, interstitial inflammation and fibrosis, severity of arteriosclerosis or other vascular lesions

despite advancements in immunosuppressive treatment protocols, rates of LN flare or remain between 25 and 50% [1]. Only approximately 55% of cSLE with proliferative LN are able to achieve remission of renal disease [1]. Additionally, 90% of patients with membranous LN are able to reach renal remission; however, only 76% are able to maintain remission despite immunosuppression [1]. Renal relapse rate in a cohort of 73 patients with cSLE was reported as occurring in 35% of those with cumulative partial or complete response to induction therapy within 1 year of treatment, which is comparable to data published in the adult population [19]. Those patients who fail to achieve a complete response are at risk of progressing to ESRD [19]. Even with optimal treatment, 10–30% of adult patients that develop clinically significant LN will progress to ESRD and ultimately require consideration of renal replacement therapy (RRT), oftentimes within 10 years of lupus diagnosis [13, 20–22]. A similar trend is seen in the pediatric population, with the risk of progressing to ESRD in children with LN ranging from 18 to 50% [9, 12, 18, 19], oftentimes within 5 to 6 years of diagnosis [7, 18].

Risk factors for progression to ESRD include demographic factors (male gender and African American race), clinical features (presence of hypertension, nephrotic syndrome, antiphospholipid antibodies, low C3 in conjunction with an elevated serum creatinine, poor response to induction therapy, and occurrence of renal flare), and histologic features on renal biopsy (class IV LN, chronicity, and high glomerular staining for monocyte chemoattractant protein-1) [1, 9, 18, 19, 21]. In a cohort of 72 children with LN, risk factors for developing ESRD included failure to reach complete remission, higher serum creatinine at beginning of therapy, and not receiving CYC pulse treatment [12]. Predictors for achieving complete remission in this cohort included younger age of diagnosis of LN, lower serum creatinine and C3 at treatment, and receiving CYC pulse treatment [12]. Additionally, *Freedman* et al. demonstrated through genotyping studies that African American adults with LN were more likely to progress to ESRD if they had two of the APOL1 risk alleles (G1/G1, G1/G2, or G2/G2) [21, 23]. APOL1 G1/G2 alleles are more common in the African American population and are felt to strongly impact the risk of developing LN and ESRD and to influence the time of progression to ESRD in this population [21, 23].

In both adults and children with LN, there is increased mortality on dialysis, more commonly related to cardiovascular causes and infections, when compared to patients that have ESRD from other causes [17]. There is limited data on the outcomes of children with ESRD secondary to LN. One review reports the mortality rate on dialysis for cSLE is 22% at 5 years, similar to the mortality rate reported in other causes of pediatric ESRD [1, 8]. However, a survival analysis using retrospective data from the US Renal Data System (USRDS) that included 171 children demonstrated that pediatric patients with LN and ESRD on dialysis have a twofold increased risk of death when compared to other pediatric patients with ESRD, even after adjusting for gender, race, and age at death [17]. Upon progression of LN to ESRD, it is generally believed that lupus activity decreases in the majority of patients through an unclear mechanism [21], including extra-renal manifestations [24]. However, this is not always the case. Higher risk of disease flare in ESRD occurred in those that had a history of hematologic disease activity, positive anti-cardiolipin IgM antibody, lower C4 levels, and a younger age of beginning RRT [22].

Renal Transplantation in Lupus Nephritis

Prior to 1975, patients with SLE with renal failure had poor prognosis with significant mortality after hemodialysis was initiated [9]. For many years, the concerns of poor long-term outcomes and risk of development of recurrent disease in the allograft precluded these patients from receiving renal transplants [25–27]. This changed in 1975 when the Advisory Committee to the Renal Transplant Registry reported reassuring results of renal transplantation in 56 lupus patients at 1 and 2 years of follow-up [9, 28]. Since that time, most published articles involving renal transplant outcomes in the adult lupus population have generally been encouraging, though graft survival is variable and has not been equivalent across all studies [9]. Pediatric data remain sparse in this regard; however, it is now reported that one third of children with LN who progress to ESRD receive a kidney transplant within 5 years [1, 8].

Achieving remission of SLE and clinical control of disease prior to transplant is felt to be important in preventing post-transplant complications [21], as there are risks involved in transplanting patients with active systemic inflammatory disease processes associated with cytopenias, hemolysis, and pro-coagulation antibodies as an example [2]. It should be noted that at time of listing for transplant, serological activity (such as the level of anti-double stranded DNA antibody elevation) does not always correlate with clinical disease activity [21]. Historically, a "waiting period" of 1–2 years of pre-transplant dialysis was advised for LN patients to allow a period of time for the disease to become quiescent; however, there are presently no standardized recommendations regarding the length of time a patient with LN-related ESRD should wait prior to receiving a kidney transplant [21]. Additionally, no pediatric studies exist to help clarify this question in children with LN. When investigated in the adult population, there does not appear to be a significant advantage of longer intervals of dialysis pre-transplant in graft survival or recurrence of lupus in the graft [26]. In fact, in the adult population, it has been suggested that an increased wait time on dialysis could be associated with an increased risk of graft failure post-transplantation [21, 29]. In a study of 40 adult patients with LN, it was demonstrated that mortality worsened by 1.3% for every additional month of dialysis, and in those that exceeded 24 months on dialysis, there was almost a threefold increase in mortality [21, 30]. The adult literature also suggests in some reports superior graft survival and patient survival in patients with ESRD due to LN who received pre-emptive kidney transplantation [31]. However, data is conflicting in some reports. For example, *Wu* et al. reported that outcomes of patient and graft survival in LN patients undergoing renal transplantation with 1 year of ESRD were not worse than those receiving transplant 1 year later [32]. Thus, the decision of when best to transplant LN patients has to be carefully weighed against the risks of long-term dialysis [2]. Additional factors found to be associated with worse renal transplant outcomes in

LN include the number of pre-transplant pregnancies, prior transplantation, and both non-use of calcineurin inhibitors and the use of both tacrolimus and cyclosporine post-transplant (the latter possibly indicating the need to switch to a second agent in the setting of poor response) [21, 33].

Studies evaluating the outcomes of renal transplantation in pediatric patients with LN are sparse with small sample sizes, and information of predictors and outcomes of LN in cSLE is often extrapolated from adult data. Pediatric-specific data on the ideal timing of performing a renal transplant is not available and thus remains uncertain [2]. Pediatric-specific studies relating to renal transplantation outcomes are summarized here.

One pediatric study (*Gipson et al.*) retrospectively investigated 254 patients with LN receiving renal transplant for ESRD in the United Network for Organ Sharing (UNOS) registry in the United States between 1987 and 1997 [7]. Pediatric LN patients were more commonly older (median age 19), female, and African American when compared to pediatric patients without LN. After a median follow-up of 4.2 years, mortality was almost 1.8 times higher in those with LN when compared to those patients without LN in a multivariate analysis after adjusting for sex, race, age, and allograft source (95% CI 1.14–2.74, $p = 0.01$) [7]. Univariate survival rates in patients with LN were 98%, 92%, and 91% at 1, 3, and 5 years, respectively (compared to 98%, 96%, and 95% at 1, 3, and 5 years in those without lupus) [7]. African American race, deceased donor kidney transplant (DDKT), and receiving renal transplant before 1993 were associated with increased risk of mortality in this study [7].

In regard to allograft function, *Gipson* et al. showed that 33% of patients with LN compared to 27% of patients without LN lost allograft function ($p = 0.04$), and univariate graft survival among patients with LN was 90%, 80%, and 71% at 1, 3, and 5 years, respectively, compared to 93%, 86%, and 77% in those without LN [7]. However, there was no difference between the two groups with regard to long-term renal allograft survival after adjusting for sex, race, age, and use of DDKT ($p = 0.98$) [7]. There was also no difference in number of allograft rejection episodes [7]. This study also showed that LN patients with DDKT were 1.9 times more likely to lose their graft compared to living donor transplants (95% CI 1.1–3.3, $p = 0.02$) after controlling for sex, age, race, and type of graft received [7]. The 5-year graft survival rate was 56% with DDKT allografts compared to 85% with living donor grafts in LN patients [7]. This was also observed, though to a lesser degree, in patients without LN (5-year allograft survival for DDKT 70% compared to 83% for living donor grafts). The same study showed that LN-ESRD patients receiving DDKT had a longer duration of pre-transplant dialysis, which in adults has been linked with increased risk of DDKT allograft failure [7].

Another prominent pediatric study (*Bartosh* et al.) retrospectively investigated 100 kidney transplant recipients in 95 patients with lupus using the North American Pediatric Renal Transplant Cooperative Study registry in the United States between 1987 and 1998 as part of a case-control study comparing patient and allograft outcomes of cSLE renal transplant recipients against an age, race, and gender matched control group (consisting of 470 children with 501 renal transplants) [9].

Immunosuppressive medications were also reportedly similar between the two groups. At baseline the LN cohort was less likely to be pre-emptively transplanted, received longer pre-transplant dialysis, and was more likely to have received five pre-transplant transfusions [9]. After transplant, there was no significant difference in 3-year patient survival (89% vs. 95%) or in overall graft failure rates (31% vs. 29%) between the LN and non-LN groups, respectively, although graft survival was uniformly better in all patients receiving living donor grafts versus DDKT [9]. The authors did not find significant differences in graft failure related to race, though they noted a trend toward worse graft survival in non-white LN patients compared to white LN patients receiving living donor grafts (33% vs. 6% graft failure, respectively, $p = 0.05$) [9]. There was no difference in graft failure rate related dialysis mechanism in living donor transplants, but there was an unexplained increased graft failure rate in patients with SLE who received PD prior to DDKT when compared to controls and compared to patients with SLE receiving HD [9]. There was no difference seen in the overall incidence of acute rejection and graft loss due to chronic rejection; however, there was an unexplained increase in incidence of recurrent rejections (>4 episodes) in cSLE with living donor grafts [9]. Overall *Bartosh* et al. concluded that the outcomes of renal transplantation in patients with cSLE were comparable to an age, race, and gender-matched control group with similar overall patient and graft survival. The authors also note that the trends of increased graft failures in non-white patients with SLE receiving living donor transplants need further investigation [9].

Finally, a retrospective analysis using data from the European Society for Pediatric Nephrology (ESPN) and the European Renal Association-European Dialysis and Transplant Association (ERA-EDTA) registry investigated 1955 children from 33 countries who underwent renal transplantation before age 20 years old between 1990 and 2009 [34]. In this analysis, patients transplanted specifically for LN had no significant increase in one and five-year risk of graft loss when compared to the 1048 patients transplanted for congenital abnormalities of the kidney and urinary tract (CAKUT) (20.3% increased risk of graft loss in LN patients compared to 14.4% in CAKUT patients, NS). However, LN patients underwent pre-emptive transplantation significantly less often than CAKUT patients (even after adjusting for age, gender, and time period) and had lower rates of living donor transplant (OR 3.5, 95% CI 1.14–10.8). Without adjusting for variables, there was no difference in graft loss between SLE and CAKUT patients, but after adjusting for this pre-emptive and donor type, along with age at start of RRT, age at transplant, gender, and era of transplantation, the differences between cSLE and CAKUT patients significantly demonstrated a threefold increased risk of graft loss for patients with LN compared to CAKUT patients (HR 3.21 with CI 1.19–8.69) [34]. The authors did not provide information on whether increased risk of graft loss was related to recurrence of disease.

While these three studies show similar rates of graft survival in pediatric patients with LN compared to those without LN [7, 9, 34], only one of the two studies that report mortality data suggests an increased mortality rate in cSLE after renal transplantation [7]. These studies and other small studies [8, 35] suggest a benefit in receiving a living donor graft over DDKT in pediatric patients with LN. It is unclear if this is secondary to increased immunosuppression that is sometimes needed with DDKT patients or if there is a direct effect from the graft itself. Given that the type of renal transplant appears to have implications for survival of the transplanted kidney, additional updated pediatric studies in this area are needed.

Taking existing data into account, renal transplantation is the treatment of choice for most patients with LN-related ESRD [21]. There is no absolute contraindication for renal transplantation in this patient population aside from the typical contraindications applicable to all patients undergoing consideration of renal transplantation (such as presence of infection, ongoing cancer therapies, and substance abuse) [21]. While active lupus may be a relative contraindication, there are no currently existing guidelines regarding recommended wait periods till transplant [21], though a reasonable approach may be to wait a period of 6–12 months of disease remission to ensure no chance of native renal recovery [2]. Others feel that with advanced CKD or ESRD due to LN without evidence of clinically active SLE, pre-emptive kidney transplant should be considered without a wait period [21]. In the adult and pediatric populations, the recommendation is that patients with SLE should be referred for transplant evaluation when glomerular filtration rate (GFR) is 20 mL/min or less [21]. Finally, from available pediatric data, overall allograft survival is not different for children with lupus with ESRD requiring renal transplant compared to those without lupus [7].

Recurrence of Lupus Nephritis Post-transplantation

Recurrence of LN after renal transplantation can present as decline in renal function, new proteinuria, and/or new hematuria [21]. Despite the underlying immunologic characteristics of SLE, clinically significant recurrence of disease in renal transplant patients is felt to be relatively rare [9]. However, the true incidence has been difficult to establish, and there is little consensus among studies. This may be attributable to widespread use of immunosuppression post-transplant with regimens that are often felt to be appropriate therapies for SLE as well [36].

Again, the pediatric data on this topic are limited. In adults, the risk of recurrence of LN in transplanted kidney may be higher than previously considered, ranging between 1 and 13% [7, 9, 20, 27, 36, 37], though some series report higher numbers ranging between 10 and 50% of transplanted patients having histologically confirmed recurrence of LN [38–40]. In a cross-sectional study using surveillance biopsies to assess incidence of LN recurrence post-transplant, *Norby* et al. reported 54% biopsy-proven recurrence of LN (22 out of 41 adult patients), the majority of which were subclinical cases characterized as Class I and Class II LN [40]. Those that had recurrence of LN had increased proteinuria, more frequent presence of lupus anticoagulant, and had more often received the kidney transplant from a living donor [40]. Of note, when analysis was corrected for non-related living donors, the statistical association of the latter became marginal [40]. Classic indicators of lupus activity, however, such as Systemic Lupus Erythematosus Disease Activity Index (SLEDAI) and SLICC indices, were low and did not differentiate between the two groups with regard to LN recurrence [40]. Importantly, there was also no difference in primary immunosuppressive regimen between the two groups [40]. The authors commented that the higher recurrence rate than previously reported may be due to the fact that the majority of biopsies assessing for recurrent LN are performed for clear clinical indications (i.e., increasing serum creatinine or active urinary sediment on urine), whereas this study demonstrated that silent recurrence of LN may be more frequent than originally thought [40]. There was no longitudinal data on this cohort of patients.

In another study, Stone and colleagues, in a large single medical center retrospective analysis of LN patients that underwent renal transplant (with disease quiescent at time of transplant), demonstrated that 8.5% (9 out of 106 patients) had pathologic recurrence of LN following first renal biopsy during a mean follow-up period of 250.4 weeks [25]. In this cohort of lupus patients, recurrent LN contributed to 7.7% of all allograft losses during study duration [25]. The patients with recurrence of disease were slightly younger at time of transplant (29.9 years compared to 35.1 years, $p = 0.12$) but otherwise were similar in terms of demographics (such as sex and race), pre-treatment disease activity, immunosuppression, HLA matching, and episodes of acute rejection [25]. The authors also note that recurrent LN was oftentimes noted even without clinical and serological evidence of active disease [25]; thus, it is important to detect presence of LN recurrence by histologic exam of renal biopsies with use of light microscopy, immunofluorescence (IF), and electron microscopy for diagnosis [21]. The histologic patterns of recurrent LN are typically identical to the original glomerulonephritis process [26], though this is not always the case. A study of 177 patients with ESRD due to LN had recurrence of mostly Class II lesions in transplanted kidneys as opposed to having previously class III, IV, or V LN in native kidneys [21, 39].

In a review by *Wong* et al., LN recurrence was reported anywhere from 5 days to 16 years after transplant (median time of 4.3 years) [21]. While primary disease recurrence after transplant has been associated with allograft failure in the literature, it appears to only constitute approximately 7–8% of graft loss in this population [38]. We again emphasize that the overall survival of allografts in adults with lupus-induced ESRD has not been shown to be different than allograft survival in other causes of ESRD [7]. Additionally, the recurrence of LN post-transplant has not been shown to impact patient survival in adults, despite having an association with allograft loss [20, 39]. The features in adults that have been associated with an increased risk for LN recurrence in a transplant include non-Hispanic black race (1.88-fold increased risk), female gender (1.70-fold increased risk), and younger age less than 33 years old (1.69-fold increased risk) [21, 41]. There is also a suggestion of lupus anticoagulant being found more frequently in patients that experienced recurrence of LN post-transplantation [40]. However, while there are not many studies investigating baseline clinical or serological features that increase risk of recurrent LN post-transplant, other serologic parameters do not seem to be reliable predictors of LN recurrence [21]. *Goss* et al., in a 1991 study, found a relationship between presence of a positive ANA and an elevated anti-double stranded DNA antibody pre- and post-transplant with recurrence of SLE. The authors suggested that seropositive patients who remain seropositive post-transplant should be monitored closely for recurrence of disease. However, this study had a very small sample size (a review of seven cases of recurrent LN post-transplantation in a single center) [26].

Interestingly, in the adult population of patients with ESRD due to LN receiving living-related kidney transplants, increasing haplotype match was associated with lower rates of allograft loss due to recurrence of LN [42]. Additionally, one retrospective adult study (n = 7826) compared use of cyclosporine and azathioprine (AZA) post-transplant with the use of cyclosporine and mycophenolate mofetil (MMF) in patients with deceased donor and living donor kidney transplants and showed no difference in renal allograft loss due to recurrence of LN with either form of therapy after follow-up for 10 years [21, 43]. As it stands, there are no existing evidence-based guidelines on which immunosuppressant to choose to treat recurrent LN after transplantation, although *Wong* et al. suggest that MMF is likely the easiest choice, given its regular use in kidney transplant regimens and current recommendations for use in the treatment of native LN [21].

In the limited pediatric data, LN recurrence post-transplantation is reported to be as low as <3% of patients having symptomatic disease and only 3–7% of graft failures attributable to recurrent LN [1, 9]. *Bacchetta* et al., in a comprehensive review investigating disease recurrence after pediatric renal transplantation, noted 0–30% recurrence rate of LN after first renal transplant with 0–5% graft loss due to recurrence [38]. However, other reviews are contradictory, indicating that if recurrent LN does occur, there is a fourfold increased risk of graft failure [1]. Interestingly, there have been isolated case reports in the pediatric literature of de novo LN developing in pediatric patients post-renal transplant, including a case report in a patient with prune belly syndrome [37]. While this phenomenon is exceedingly rare, the presence of new-onset nephritic syndrome post-renal transplantation should encourage consideration of de novo LN, even without the presence of other clinical manifestations of SLE [37].

In summary, given limited reports overall of recurrence of LN in the kidney allograft, concerns about recurrent LN should not impede consideration of pursuing renal transplantation in patients with ESRD secondary to SLE in either pediatric or adult populations [25], but should be taken into consideration when picking immunosuppression protocols. Recurrence, when it occurs, generally appears to be mild in severity without significant association with decreased patient survival (though there is some association with a higher rate of allograft loss as noted above). Prediction of patients that are at higher risk of LN recurrence after kidney transplant remains challenging and deserves dedicated investigation in the pediatric lupus population.

Health Disparities in Systemic Lupus Erythematosus and Lupus Nephritis

It is essential in discussion of renal outcomes in SLE to discuss the significant disparities that exist in LN outcomes in African Americans. In the Hopkins Lupus Cohort with over 1500 adult patients with lupus, it was shown that 75% of African Americans with SLE develop LN compared to 30–40% of whites [44]. African Americans have a threefold increase in incidence of SLE with development of lupus at younger ages (presenting at 12.6 years compared to 14.6 years in white patients) and more frequent development of LN compared to other races (62% vs. 45% in white patients), along with more rapid progression to ESRD despite similar treatments [7, 45]. These results are statistically significant independent of age, disease duration, presence of hypertension, or activity/chronicity indices on renal biopsy [7]. *Sule* et al. found that both African American children and African American adults with ESRD due to SLE in the United States Renal Data System (USRDS) have increased mortality when compared to white patients with ESRD due to SLE and when compared to African Americans with ESRD due to other etiologies [14]. African American children with ESRD due to SLE had a twofold increase in risk of death compared to African American children with other causes of ESRD [14], and mortality is almost doubled for African American children when compared to white children with ESRD from LN [1, 8]. African American children with LN have also been found to have more treatment resistance when compared to other populations [19].

These disparities were further highlighted by *Hiraki* et al., who investigated pediatric patients in the USRDS between 1995 and 2006 with regard to identifying predictors for being listed for renal transplantation. It was demonstrated that significantly fewer kidney transplants were done among children that had Medicaid (vs. private insurance) and who were older (vs. younger), African American (vs. white), and Hispanic (vs. non-Hispanic) [1, 8]. In a recent 2020 review by *Rubinstein* et al., it was suggested that African American children with ESRD from SLE are half as likely to receive renal transplants when compared to white children and are almost twice as likely to die [46]. More studies are needed in investigating these health disparities in the pediatric lupus and LN population to better understand and serve this vulnerable population. These reports highlight the need for aggressive monitoring of African American patients (adults and children) with ESRD secondary to lupus.

Conclusion

Despite advancements in immunosuppressive treatment regimens, 18–50% of children with SLE and LN will progress to ERSD [7, 18]. Renal transplantation is the preferred choice of RRT in these patients with overall reassuring results related to long-term patient survival, graft survival and function, and generally low rates of recurrent LN in the allograft. Renal transplant outcomes in LN-ESRD have been

Box 7.1 Key Points for Lupus Nephritis

- cSLE has a more aggressive disease course compared to adults.
- LN is a strong predictor of poor outcome and mortality in SLE.
- LN develops in 40–80% of children with SLE (often within first year of diagnosis) with 18–50% progressing to ESRD despite optimal treatment.
- Class IV LN is the most active disease class and carries worst prognosis.
- Renal transplantation is the recommended treatment of choice for most patients with LN-related ESRD.
- Allograft survival is similar for children with ESRD from lupus compared to those with other causes of ESRD.
- Clinically significant recurrence of LN in renal allograft is relatively rare, and concerns about this should not discourage consideration of renal transplant.
- No current guidelines exist regarding appropriate wait time prior to receiving renal transplant in the pediatric population.
- Significant health disparities exist in SLE and LN with African American children having increased risk of LN, increased treatment resistance, more rapid progression to ESRD, and a twofold increased risk of mortality compared to white children with ESRD from LN.

shown to be similar to those receiving transplant for other causes of ESRD. Timely consideration of renal transplant should be part of the routine care for patients with SLE with ESRD from LN, and efforts should be made to improve access to renal transplant in this vulnerable population (with special attention given to the healthcare disparities that exist in this regard) in hopes of improving long-term outcomes (Box 7.1).

IgA Vasculitis

Introduction

Immunoglobulin A vasculitis (IgAV) (formerly Henoch-Schonlein Purpura, HSP) is a systemic vasculitis involving small vessels. IgA nephropathy (IgAN) will be discussed in a separate chapter. HSP was renamed IgAV by the International Chapel Hill Consensus Conference in 2012 [47]. It is the most common vasculitis of childhood with an incidence of 3–27 cases per 100,000 children and a slight male predominance of 1.5:1. It can occur at any age but peaks around 4 to 6 years old with 90% of cases occurring before 10 years of age. There appears to be a genetic predisposition as evidenced by its geographical variation in incidence and is more common in the Asian population. The pathophysiology is still being investigated but appears to involve abnormal IgA1 glycosylation [48]. The most sensitive and specific classification criteria for IgAV were proposed by the European League Against

Rheumatism (EULAR) and the Pediatric Rheumatology European Society (PRES) in 2005 and validated by the Pediatric Rheumatology International Trials Organization (PRINTO) in 2010. It is classified by the presence of a palpable purpuric rash in dependent areas in addition to at least one of the following at diagnosis: abdominal pain, arthritis or arthralgia, renal involvement, or histopathology showing IgA deposition [49, 50]. IgAV without renal involvement has a very good prognosis with resolution of symptoms by 1 month in the majority of children, although it may take on a persistent or refractory course with complete recovery in 94% of cases by 2 years. Recurrence of disease can occur usually within the first 2 years in 25% of cases [48].

Clinical Course of Renal Involvement and Outcomes

Renal involvement varies from mild proteinuria or hematuria to nephritis with CKD and ESRD and is a major contributor to poor outcomes of IgAV. Any renal involvement occurs in about one third to half of children with IgAV with the majority of children developing renal involvement in the first month of disease activity [48, 51]. In a study of 1133 children with IgAV without renal involvement at diagnosis in 2005, 34% subsequently developed proteinuria and/or hematuria: 85% of these cases occurred within 4 weeks of diagnosis, in 91% within 6 weeks of diagnosis, and in 97% within 6 months of diagnosis [52]. Of those children with renal involvement, 20% of cases developed nephritic or nephrotic syndrome [52]. Given the risk of development of nephritis and ESRD, there is consensus agreement that all patients with IgAV should undergo renal monitoring with urinalysis and blood pressure checks for at least 6 months with more frequent monitoring in the first 1–3 months as onset of renal disease is usually asymptomatic [48, 53, 54]. Published review of the literature in 2009 found that the most significant risk factors for later developing IgAV nephritis were persistent or recurrent purpura, severe abdominal symptoms, and older age [51].

Corticosteroid is helpful in treatment of severe gastrointestinal (GI) and joint involvement, but the literature does not support early use of prednisone to prevent subsequent development of renal involvement in IgAV. Several retrospective studies and a few randomized controlled trials (RCT) have mostly found little to no benefit with prednisone [51]. Two more recent Cochrane Systematic Reviews (one published by the KDIGO group) have confirmed the lack of benefit in use of early short-term prednisone to prevent persistent kidney disease in IgAV with relative risk (RR) 0.74, 95% confidence interval (CI) 0.42–1.32 [55, 56].

Renal involvement is the only organ linked to long-term morbidity and mortality in IgAV. Progression to ESRD occurs in 5–15% of children with IgAV nephritis [38], and IgAV nephritis comprises ~1–2% of all ESRD in children [48]. Some tertiary care centers report numbers as high as 5–18% CKD or ESRD at 5 years, 10–20% at 10 years, and 20–32% at 20 years [51]. Over time, progression to CKD and ESRD is increased in children with persistent or refractory IgAV nephritis. Progression to CKD occurs in 41% of children when low GFR or nephritic or nephrotic syndrome is present in the acute period versus 15% of children when only microscopic urine abnormalities occur [57, 58]. A more recent meta-analysis of nine case-control studies of children with IgAV nephritis published in 2019 confirmed these risk factors, in addition to older age at onset and renal biopsy with crescentic nephritis, for progression to CKD [59]. However, *Coppo* et al. reported somewhat different risk factors for poor renal outcomes in a study that included both children and adults [60]. Multivariate analysis of patients with IgAV nephritis in 2006 showed poor renal outcomes, including renal survival, doubling of baseline serum creatinine level, and dialysis therapy, and were significantly worse in adults (compared to children), in females, and in patients with high mean follow-up proteinuria values, whereas proteinuria values at baseline, presence of crescents on renal biopsy, histologic class, and therapy were not predictive of poor renal outcomes [60].

Groups in Europe have recommended that a renal biopsy should be performed if there is severe proteinuria (>250 mg/mmol for at least 4 weeks), persistent moderate proteinuria (100–250 mg/mmol), or impaired glomerular filtration rate [48, 53]. Nephritis from IgAV is graded histologically according to the International Study on Kidney Diseases in Children (ISKDC) classification: grade I, minimal glomerular abnormalities; grade II, mesangial proliferation without crescents; grade III, focal (IIIa) or diffuse (IIIb) mesangial proliferation with <50% crescents; grade IV, mesangial proliferation with 50–70% crescents; grade V, mesangial proliferation with >75% crescents; grade VI, membranoproliferative-like lesions [61] [Table 7.2]. Glomerular sclerosis, tubular loss, interstitial fibrosis, and hyaline arteriolosclerosis may be present and indicate chronic damage. IgA deposition in the mesangium is seen on IF with variable IgG, IgM, and C3 staining. Electron microscopy shows mesangial and subendothelial deposits and may show subepithelial deposits. A scoring system for activity, chronicity, and tubulointerstitial indices has also been proposed [48]. One study showed IgAV in children with nephrotic syndrome, acute nephritic syndrome, and creatinine clearance less than 30 mL/min/1.73 m^2 were at increased risk of developing higher grades (IV and V) of IgAV nephritis on biopsy [62]. Furthermore, the risk of long-term renal impairment is increased in children with higher grades of IgAV nephritis on biopsy, particularly in children with nephritic or nephrotic syndrome at presentation and/or had >50% crescents or sclerosing lesions in glomeruli or interstitial fibrosis on biopsy [51, 63–65].

Table 7.2 ISKDC classification of nephritis in IgA vasculitis [60]

Grade	Definition
I	Minimal glomerular abnormalities
II	Mesangial proliferation without crescents
III	Focal segmental (IIIa) or diffuse (IIIb) mesangial proliferation with <50% crescents
IV	Mesangial proliferation with 50–75% crescents
V	Mesangial proliferation with >75% crescents
VI	Membranoproliferative-like lesions

Treatment of IgAV nephritis is highly variable, and there is a lack of evidence in the literature to support a specific therapy in mild, moderate, or severe nephritis. Therapy options have been reported in several retrospective case series, uncontrolled studies, and RCTs, including prednisolone, IV pulse methylprednisolone, angiotensin converting enzyme (ACE) inhibitor, fish oil, AZA, cyclosporine, MMF, cyclophosphamide (CYC), rituximab (RTX), and plasmapheresis, alone or in combination [48, 51, 65]. There are also reports of use of antiplatelet and/or anticoagulant agents. Additionally, tonsillectomy and improving dental hygiene to eradicate infection have been employed with or without drug therapy [48, 51, 53]. New international consensus guidelines proposed treatment recommendations for renal disease in IgAV based on best available evidence that include oral prednisolone in mild nephritis (grade II or IIIa), IV prednisolone in combination with AZA, MMF, or IV CYC in moderate nephritis (grade IIIb), or intravenous (IV) corticosteroids and IV CYC in severe nephritis (grade IV–V) to induce remission followed by a period of maintenance therapy. In addition, consensus guidelines recommend that all patients should receive adjunctive ACE inhibitor or angiotensin receptor blocker (ARB) for persistent proteinuria. Use of calcineurin inhibitors or oral CYC was not recommended [53].

Adults with IgAV nephritis may have worse outcomes compared to children. In a study of 57 children and 95 adults with IgAV nephritis who had renal biopsy with IgA deposits, 25% of children and 32% of adults had renal function impairment. These patients were treated with variable regimens and had follow-up for 1 to 20 years. Rates of remission defined as normal renal function and proteinuria <4 mg/kg/day in children and <200 mg/day in adults were similar in children (25%) and adults (33%). ESRD developed in 7% of children compared to 16% of adults [66].

In another study of 83 children and 136 adults with biopsy-proven IgAV nephritis in Italy [60], most patients had mesangial proliferation with or without endocapillary or extracapillary proliferation and less than 50% crescents on biopsy; 25% of children and 15% of adults had nephrotic syndrome; close to 30% of children and adults had renal function impairment and hypertension at onset; gross hematuria was uncommon. Treatment varied widely but included steroid therapy in 60% of children and 72% of adults alone or in addition to various regimens of immunosuppressants, antiplatelet drugs, plasma exchange, and ACE inhibitors. No treatment was given to 29% of children and 21% of adults. Mean follow-up was 6.7 years in children and 5.5 years in adults. There were zero deaths in children; however 15% doubled baseline creatinine level, and 7% developed ESRD requiring dialysis. In adults, 5% died of neoplasia or cerebrovascular accidents, 25% doubled baseline creatinine level, and 13% reached ESRD and required dialysis. Renal survival rates at 10 years were 90% in children and 76% in adults. Eight patients (three children) underwent renal transplantation, and none developed IgAV recurrence in the graft [60].

Renal Transplantation in IgAV Nephritis and Outcomes

Pediatric patients with IgAV nephritis who undergo renal transplantation have good outcomes. A pediatric registry of IgAV nephritis and IgAN found no increased risk of graft loss at 5 years in comparison to patients with CAKUT [34]. Additional case series that include children and adults also report good outcomes. In the United Network of Organ Sharing database from 1987 to 2005, 0.18% of 189,211 patients with renal allografts had a primary diagnosis of IgAV. A retrospective matched cohort study was done with 333 IgAV patients with renal transplantation. Average age of IgAV patients at time of transplant was 25 years old, and 47% were women and 77% Caucasian. Renal graft survival in IgAV was 80% at 5 years and 59% at 10 years similar to IgAN and the rest of the population. However, there was increased graft loss from disease recurrence in IgAV with 14% compared to 7% in non-IgAV patients [67].

In a 1994 study of pooled data of 78 total renal transplants in adults and children with IgAV, the risk of recurrence of IgAV nephritis in the graft was 35%, and risk of graft loss was 11% at 5 years post-transplant. The report suggested that shorter duration of the original disease was associated with recurrence of IgAV nephritis. In addition, recurrence can occur despite 1 year of disease remission and on immunosuppressive therapy [68].

In a study in Korea, ~2% of 1139 patients between 1972 and 2007 who received kidney transplants were diagnosed with nephritis from IgAV. Twenty patients with IgAV nephritis (15 men, average age 22 years at transplant) were retrospectively reviewed and outcomes compared to 40 patients with IgAN and 40 patients with other diseases matched for age, sex, and donor source who required kidney transplant. IgAV nephritis was treated with steroids, calcineurin inhibitors, and inhibitors of purine synthesis, and patients were on dialysis for an average of 8 months prior to transplant. Source of graft in 90% of IgAV patients was living donor. The incidence of acute and chronic rejection in IgAV was 21% and 26%, respectively, and recurrence of IgAV occurred in three patients (15%) at 10 year follow-up, not statistically different compared to IgAN and other diseases. All patients with recurrence of IgAV had transplantations from a related donor. Cumulative 5-year and 10-year graft survival rates were 95% and 88%, respectively [69].

In a cohort of 43 patients with IgAV nephritis who received renal transplant in Belgium and France, rate of disease recurrence was 12%. Three patients lost their first graft due to IgAV. Overall risk of graft loss was 3% at 5 years and 8% at 10 years. The authors note that severity of disease at presentation and type of immunosuppression used after transplantation did not affect recurrence [70].

In a pooled data from 12 published international case series, the rate of incidence of recurrent IgAV ranged from 0% to 62%, and rate of graft loss due to recurrent IgAV ranged from 0% to 25%. Related donor transplants showed a trend to higher risk of cumulative recurrence as compared to unrelated donor transplants [69]. Despite the small but significant risk of graft loss, the long-term graft outcomes are similar to transplanted patients with other diseases [67].

Box 7.2 Key Points for IgA Vasculitis (IgAV) Nephritis

- Renal involvement occurs in one third to half of children with IgAV.
- Treatment of IgAV nephritis is highly variable, as there is no good evidence for specific therapy regimens in IgAV nephritis.
- Risk factors for CKD include the older age at onset, presence of low GFR, nephritic or nephrotic syndrome in the acute period of disease, and crescentic nephritis on renal biopsy.
- Progression to ESRD occurs in 5–15% of children with IgAV nephritis.
- Renal graft survival ranges 80–95% at 5 years and 59–88% at 10 years.
- Recurrence of IgAV nephritis in renal graft ranges from 0% to 62%, with rate of graft loss from disease recurrence ranging 0–25%.
- Despite the small but significant risk of graft loss, the long-term graft outcomes are similar to transplanted patients with other diseases.

There is no clear data to provide guidance to recommend a particular immunosuppressant therapy regimen to protect against or treat recurrence of IgAV in renal graft [68, 71, 72]. Successful use of plasmapheresis [73] and tonsillectomy [74] have also been reported in young adults with recurrent IgAV nephritis.

In summary (Box 7.2), renal involvement occurs in a significant proportion of children with IgAV, and about 15% will progress to ESRD. Outcomes of renal transplantation in these patients based on available evidence are comparable to children with other diseases, although there may be increased risk of graft loss from recurrence of disease. More pediatric studies are needed to provide better evidence for appropriate immunosuppressant therapies in children with nephritis from IgAV and to better inform outcomes of renal transplantation.

ANCA-Associated Vasculitis

Introduction

Antineutrophil cytoplasmic antibody (ANCA)-associated vasculitis (AAV) is a small-vessel vasculitis that includes granulomatosis with polyangiitis (GPA), microscopic polyangiitis (MPA), and eosinophilic GPA (EGPA). The definitions of these separate entities of AAV have been proposed by the 2012 Chapel Hill Consensus Conference [47]. Development of diagnostic and classification criteria for AAV is underway [75]. GPA is more commonly associated with ANCA targeting proteinase 3 (PR3), whereas myeloperoxidase antibody (MPO) is more commonly associated with MPA and EGPA, although they all can be ANCA negative. The pathogenesis of AAV is under investigation but appears to involve a necrotizing vasculitis induced by loss of T cell and B cell tolerance to self PR3 or MPO neutrophil proteins. PR3-ANCA and MPO-ANCA activate neutrophils which cause microvascular endothelial inflammation leading to extravascular inflammation, progressive injury, tissue destruction, fibrosis, and loss of function [76].

There is evidence that genetics, environmental factors, and infection contribute to the onset of disease, and infection influences disease chronicity and relapse [76]. GPA and MPA typically involve small vessels in the upper and lower respiratory tract and the kidneys but can affect any organ, although GPA may be limited to the upper airway. EGPA is characterized by asthma, eosinophilia, and in many cases vasculitis [76]. The hallmark of AAV pathology is fibrinoid necrosis and inflammation of small vessels. In addition, granulomas are defining features in GPA, whereas EGPA has prominent eosinophilic infiltrates [76]. In the kidney, AAV is characterized by segmental necrosis of glomerular loops with little to no immune deposits, "pauci-immune," focal necrotizing and crescentic GN [76]. Histopathological classification system proposed for ANCA-associated GN [77] has been validated in a pediatric population [78]. Glomerular lesions are used to stage renal disease based on this classification system to help with prognostication: sclerotic lesions (≥50% global sclerosis, worst outcomes), focal lesions (≥50% normal glomeruli, best outcomes), crescentic lesions (≥50% cellular crescents, intermediate outcomes), and mixed (no single dominant type lesion, outcomes between crescentic and sclerotic classes) [77] [Table 7.3].

AAV is very rare in the pediatric population and few studies exist in children. The annual incidence of AAV in children is unknown, but a few studies report anywhere from 0.22 to 6.39 per million children in two studies with median age at diagnosis of 11 to 14 years [79, 80]. One study reported an estimated prevalence of 3.41 to 4.28 per million children [81]. Additionally, one study reported that only 2% of all the pediatric patients with GN at their center were ANCA-positive GN [82]. The European League Against Rheumatism (EULAR), Paediatric Rheumatology International Trials Organisation (PRINTO), and Pediatric Rheumatology European Society (PRES) proposed classification criteria specifically for children with GPA in 2008 that includes the presence of at least three of the following criteria: granulomatous inflammation on histopathology, upper airway involvement, laryngo-tracheo-bronchial stenosis, pulmonary involvement, ANCA positivity, and renal involvement [50]. Children with GPA can present with constitutional symptoms, pulmonary, renal, ear, nose, throat (ENT), musculoskeletal, mucocutaneous, ocular, cardiovascular, gastrointestinal, and nervous system involvement, and greater than 50% have renal involvement with hematuria and proteinuria similar to adults [82,

Table 7.3 Classification of ANCA-associated glomerulonephritis

Required	Light microscopy: ≥1 glomerulus with necrotizing crescentic GN and Immunofluorescence microscopy: pauci-immune staining pattern
Focal class	≥50% normal glomeruli
Crescentic class	≥50% glomeruli with cellular crescents
Mixed class	No single dominant type lesion <50% normal, <50% crescentic, <50% globally sclerotic glomeruli
Sclerotic class	≥50% globally sclerotic glomeruli

Adapted from [76]

83]. However, female involvement, constitutional, ENT, respiratory symptoms, and conductive hearing loss are more frequent than in adults [83]. MPA in children more predominantly presents with hematuria, proteinuria, and purpura, but may also have a pulmonary-renal syndrome [82, 84]. The Pediatric Vasculitis Activity Score (PVAS) [85], based on modification of the Birmingham Vasculitis Activity Score (BVAS) in adults [86], was developed and preliminarily validated to assess disease activity in children with vasculitis. While 21% of the 63 patients in this study were diagnosed with GPA, only 8% had renal involvement at initial assessment [85].

There are no RCTs for the treatment of AAV in children, and thus recommendations for treatment in children have been extrapolated from primarily adult data [79, 87]. A combination of glucocorticoids and either CYC or RTX is recommended for induction therapy in adults and children with organ- or life-threatening AAV disease [88–90]. RTX has been found to be non-inferior to CYC in remission induction in adults [91, 92]. Despite the lack of RCTs in children, there has been an increasing trend in use RTX over CYC in children hospitalized for AAV in the United States between 2004 and 2014 [93]. The lack of adverse effect on fertility and apparent lower risk of malignancy likely contribute to increased use of RTX in the pediatric population. MMF was recently found to be non-inferior to CYC in inducing remission in AAV but resulted in higher relapse rate [94]. The use of plasmapheresis to reduce risk of ESRD is controversial [95, 96]. AZA, methotrexate, MMF, RTX, and belimumab have been studied primarily in adults for maintenance therapy with varying rates of disease relapse [80, 87]. Pediatric-specific studies of AAV report 92–100% with disease remission and relapse rate of 41–75% [80].

Clinical Course of Renal Involvement and Outcomes

The majority of patients with AAV present with renal involvement, although the clinical spectrum in children ranges from isolated proteinuria, microscopic hematuria, and/or red blood cell casts to rapidly progressive glomerulonephritis (GN) with acute kidney injury [80]. Studies in children with AAV have shown 33–88% renal involvement in GPA, 75–100% in MPA, and 0–16% in EGPA [80]. The risk of ESRD is 20–40% in patients with GN caused by AAV, and thus is a significant contributor to morbidity and mortality in AAV [38, 97].

The Pediatric Vasculitis (PedVas) Initiative study evaluated early outcomes of children with AAV in the ARChiVe registry from 22 international sites [98]. In 105 children with AAV (81% GPA, 13% MPA, and 6% EGPA), 78% had renal involvement at diagnosis: 73% had hematuria, 70% had proteinuria defined as >0.3 gm/24 hours, 35% had rise in serum creatinine >10% or fall in creatinine clearance >25%, and renal failure requiring dialysis in 16% with ESRD in 5%. After 12 months of induction and maintenance therapy, a third of children with AAV had evidence of renal damage: proteinuria remained in 20%, GFR ≤50% of normal was found in 18%, and ESRD had increased to 12% of children. Two patients had received renal transplants and there were zero deaths [98]. Analysis of predictors of worse renal outcomes in children with AAV was not performed in the PedVas study. Predictors for worse renal outcome and overall survival in adults include older age, female gender, higher serum creatinine, and chronic histologic lesions [99].

Cabral et al. also published a description of pediatric patients with GPA and MPA from the ARChiVe registry whose diagnosis was reclassified according to an algorithm proposed by the European Medicines Agency to distinguish all types of AAV and polyarteritis nodosa [100]. In this cohort of 183 children with GPA and 48 children with MPA, 83% of GPA and 75% of MPA presented with renal involvement similar to the numbers in the PedVas study: 72% of GPA and 60% of MPA presented with hematuria or red blood cell casts, 72% and 69% had proteinuria (nephrotic syndrome in 11% and 23%), 54% and 58% had fall in creatinine clearance >25% or abnormal urine protein/creatinine ratio, and renal failure requiring dialysis in 13% and 25% with ESRD of 7% and 10% in GPA and MPA, respectively [100]. Thus, more children with MPA had severe renal disease at presentation compared to GPA. Data on outcomes following treatment were not presented in this study.

Outcomes of a series of 22 pediatric patients specifically with AAV GN at a single center in the United States from 1991 to 2013 were published [82]. These patients presented with a median serum creatinine of 2.7 mg/dL, and median urine protein/creatinine ratio of 1.5. 41% had cytoplasmic-ANCA with PR3 antibody, and another 41% were positive for perinuclear-ANCA/MPO. Renal pathology on biopsy found 53% of patients with crescentic histological classification, 21% mixed focal and crescentic, and 26% sclerotic. Thirty-six percent of patients required RRT at presentation, and half of those discontinued dialysis after sufficient recovery of renal function. Plasmapheresis was performed in 23% of patients. Induction therapy included pulse dose methylprednisolone followed by prednisone in all patients, and 80% were treated with oral or IV CYC. Maintenance immunosuppression therapies included MMF, AZA, hydroxychloroquine, or etanercept. Two patients were refractory to induction therapy. Serologic or clinical relapse occurred in 55% of patients. ESRD occurred in 32% of patients [82].

Renal Transplantation in Childhood AAV and Outcomes

There are several studies in the literature that include children in their analyses of outcomes in AAV, ESRD, and renal transplantation, but only a few case reports and series exist that describe renal transplant outcomes in AAV specifically in pediatric populations [38, 82]. Renal transplantation before 1 year of vasculitis remission was the strongest predictor of death post-renal transplant in univariate and multivariate analyses of 107 patients with AAV that included children [101]. Thus, the KDIGO 2012 Guidelines and other experts recommend performing transplantation after at least 12 months of disease remission [101, 102].

In the series of 22 pediatric patients with AAV GN, ESRD occurred in 32% of patients, and renal transplantation occurred at a median time of 3.5 years after presentation. Additionally, 63% of those that required RRT at presentation ultimately required renal transplant. None of the patients had recurrence of disease in the renal graft or died post-transplantation. One patient died during the acute illness [82].

A cohort of seven pediatric patients with AAV and ESRD were transplanted in Canada between 2000 and 2014, accounting for 2.5% of all renal transplants at a single center [103]. Four patients were diagnosed with MPA and three had GPA. Renal biopsy category was crescentic in three and sclerotic in four. All patients were treated with pulse dose methylprednisolone and CYC, and three patients additionally received plasmapheresis due to pulmonary hemorrhage and severe rapidly progressive GN. Six of the patients required dialysis by 6 months. Mean time to renal transplantation was 30 months, and six patients received a deceased donor graft. All patients had quiescent disease by at least 12 months and were ANCA negative by the time of transplant. After a median follow-up of 27 months, there was no recurrence of AAV in the graft, and only one graft loss due to severe acute cellular rejection secondary to poor medication adherence [103].

Additional case studies report no recurrence of disease in the renal graft of children with AAV 3–4 years after transplantation [104, 105], although there is one report of a pediatric patient thought to likely have AAV as their primary disease who had recurrence of disease shortly after renal transplantation [106]. Thus, there is low risk of disease recurrence and renal graft loss in children with AAV.

In adult patients, the risk of relapse of AAV is lower in patients who have been transplanted than in those with chronic kidney disease or on dialysis [107–109]. Disease recurrence was 5% in a cohort of 107 patients with AAV who had renal transplant, and overall graft survival was 70% after 10 years [101]. However, the evidence is less clear regarding the risk of relapse associated with the persistence of ANCA positivity [102]. *Marco* et al. found increased relapse rates for adults with positive ANCA titers [110], whereas another study found no association of relapse rate with ANCA positivity [111]. Relapse of AAV can occur even with a negative ANCA [111, 112] and within the first month of transplantation [106, 113–115]. In addition, those who relapse after transplantation may be at increased risk of graft loss as one study reported 36% of adult patients with recurrence of AAV experienced graft loss within 5 years of transplantation [111], although older studies report few to no cases of graft loss due to recurrence of AAV [112, 116].

There is no pediatric data available regarding risk of graft loss after recurrence of AAV, although risk of graft loss after recurrence of other rheumatologic diseases in children is low [38]. Thus, close monitoring of recurrence of symptoms of systemic vasculitis and evidence of GN after renal transplantation is warranted. KDIGO suggests screening for hematuria and proteinuria in AAV after transplant once in the first month as a baseline, then every 3 months during the first year, and annually thereafter, in addition to monitoring serum creatinine [117].

In summary (Box 7.3), the majority of children with AAV present with renal involvement and a significant proportion progress to ESRD. Renal outcomes post-transplantation are very good with low risk of disease recurrence in renal graft and loss of graft in children with AAV.

Box 7.3 Key Points for Glomerulonephritis in ANCA-Associated Vasculitis

- Studies in children with AAV have shown 33–88% renal involvement in GPA, 75–100% in MPA, and 0–16% in EGPA.
- More children with MPA have severe renal disease at presentation compared to GPA.
- Treatment guidelines for glomerulonephritis in children with AAV are extrapolated from adult data.
- The risk of ESRD is 20–40% in patients with GN caused by AAV.
- Expert guidelines recommend performing renal transplantation after at least 12 months of disease remission due to increased risk of death post-transplantation with shorter disease-free intervals.
- There is low risk of disease recurrence in renal graft and loss of graft in children with AAV.

Conclusion

Progression of renal involvement to ESRD in children with LN, IgAV, and AAV continues to cause significant morbidity and mortality despite advancements in medical therapy for these diseases. Pediatric specific data to guide management of ESRD and describe outcomes of renal transplantation are sparse. However, available studies suggest good outcomes and improved patient survival in pediatric patients with rheumatic diseases. Recurrence of pediatric rheumatic diseases like LN, IgAV, and AAV is associated with limited risk of graft loss compared to other primary diseases of the kidney in children. As a result, rheumatologic disease alone should not exclude pediatric patients from renal transplantation. Despite the many challenges that exist for managing children with ESRD from rheumatic diseases, renal transplantation should be pursued under good disease control in a multidisciplinary team approach.

Questions

1. Approximately 80% of lupus nephritis occurs ____________ of childhood SLE?
   (a) At time of diagnosis or within first year of diagnosis
   (b) 3–5 years after diagnosis
   (c) 6–9 years after diagnosis
   (d) >10 years after diagnosis

   Correct Answer: (a)

   Explanation: Approximately 40–80% of patients with cSLE will develop kidney involvement at some point during their disease [1, 2, 7, 12, 14], with *approximately 80% of childhood LN occurring at or within the first year of diagnosis* [15]. cSLE characteristically presents with a more aggressive disease course with 10–30% higher prevalence of LN when compared to adults [1].

2. A 15yo Caucasian female presents to clinic with her mother for follow-up of newly diagnosed SLE with Class IV lupus nephritis on recent renal biopsy. Which of the following are risk factors for progression to ESRD in this particular patient?
   (a) Class IV lupus nephritis
   (b) Female gender
   (c) Caucasian race
   (d) Choices a and b
   (e) Choices b and c
   (f) All of the above

   Correct Answer: (a)

   Explanation: Risk factors for progression to ESRD include demographic factors (*male gender, African American race*), clinical features (hypertension, nephrotic syndrome, antiphospholipid antibodies, low C3 with an elevated serum creatinine, poor response to induction therapy, and occurrence of renal flare), and histologic features on renal biopsy (*class IV LN*, chronicity, and high glomerular staining for monocyte chemoattractant protein-1) [1, 9, 18, 19, 21].
3. Per the 2012 KDIGO guidelines, how long should disease be in remission in childhood ANCA associated vasculitis prior to performing renal transplant?
   (a) At least 3 months
   (b) At least 6 months
   (c) At least 12 months
   (d) At least 18 months
   (e) At least 24 months

   Correct Answer: (c)

   Explanation: In this cohort, renal transplant before 1 year of vasculitis remission was the strongest predictor of death post-renal transplant in univariate and multivariate analysis of 107 patients with AAV (that included pediatric patients) [101]. Thus, *the KDIGO 2012 Guidelines and other experts recommend performing transplantation after at least 12 months of disease remission in ANCA associated vasculitis* [101, 102].
4. A 5yo male presents to clinic with newly diagnosed IgA vasculitis, diagnosed with features of purpuric rash, arthritis, and abdominal pain. Initial urine studies have been unremarkable. His blood pressure is normal during the clinic visit. How long should this patient undergo monitoring for the development of kidney disease with urinalysis and blood pressure checks?
   (a) At least 3 months with more frequent monitoring in the first 1 month
   (b) At least 6 months with more frequent monitoring in the first 1–3 months
   (c) At least 9 months with more frequent monitoring in the first 1–6 months
   (d) At least 1 year with more frequent monitoring in the first 1–6 months
   (e) Only if he becomes symptomatic

   Correct Answer: (b)

   Explanation: In a 2005 study of 1133 children with IgAV without renal involvement at diagnosis, 34% developed proteinuria and/or hematuria: 85% occurred within 4 weeks of diagnosis, 91% within 6 weeks of diagnosis, and

97% within 6 months of diagnosis [52]. Given the risk of development of nephritis and ESRD, *there is consensus agreement that all patients with IgAV should undergo renal monitoring with urinalysis and blood pressure checks for at least 6 months with more frequent monitoring in the first 1–3 months as onset of renal disease is usually asymptomatic* [48, 53, 54]. The most significant risk factors for later developing IgAV nephritis have been shown to be persistent or recurrent purpura, severe abdominal symptoms, and older age [51].

References

1. Wenderfer SE, Ruth NM, Brunner HI. Advances in the care of children with lupus nephritis. Pediatr Res. 2017;81(3):406–14. https://doi.org/10.1038/pr.2016.247.
2. Oni L, Wright RD, Marks S, Beresford MW, Tullus K. Kidney outcomes for children with lupus nephritis. Pediatr Nephrol. 2020; https://doi.org/10.1007/s00467-020-04686-1.
3. Groot N, Shaikhani D, Teng YKO, de Leeuw K, Bijl M, Dolhain R, et al. Long-term clinical outcomes in a cohort of adults with childhood-onset systemic lupus erythematosus. Arthritis Rheumatol. 2019;71(2):290–301. https://doi.org/10.1002/art.40697.
4. Pan L, Lu MP, Wang JH, Xu M, Yang SR. Immunological pathogenesis and treatment of systemic lupus erythematosus. World J Pediatr. 2020;16(1):19–30. https://doi.org/10.1007/s12519-019-00229-3.
5. Aringer M, Costenbader K, Daikh D, Brinks R, Mosca M, Ramsey-Goldman R, et al. 2019 European league against rheumatism/American College of Rheumatology classification criteria for systemic lupus erythematosus. Arthritis Rheumatol. 2019;71(9):1400–12. https://doi.org/10.1002/art.40930.
6. Petri M, Orbai AM, Alarcon GS, Gordon C, Merrill JT, Fortin PR, et al. Derivation and validation of the Systemic Lupus International Collaborating Clinics classification criteria for systemic lupus erythematosus. Arthritis Rheum. 2012;64(8):2677–86. https://doi.org/10.1002/art.34473.
7. Gipson DS, Ferris ME, Dooley MA, Huang K, Hogan SL. Renal transplantation in children with lupus nephritis. Am J Kidney Dis. 2003;41(2):455–63. https://doi.org/10.1053/ajkd.2003.50056.
8. Hiraki LT, Lu B, Alexander SR, Shaykevich T, Alarcon GS, Solomon DH, et al. End-stage renal disease due to lupus nephritis among children in the US, 1995-2006. Arthritis Rheum. 2011;63(7):1988–97. https://doi.org/10.1002/art.30350.
9. Bartosh SM, Fine RN, Sullivan EK. Outcome after transplantation of young patients with systemic lupus erythematosus: a report of the North American pediatric renal transplant cooperative study. Transplantation. 2001;72(5):973–8. https://doi.org/10.1097/00007890-200109150-00047.
10. Tucker LB, Uribe AG, Fernandez M, Vila LM, McGwin G, Apte M, et al. Adolescent onset of lupus results in more aggressive disease and worse outcomes: results of a nested matched case-control study within LUMINA, a multiethnic US cohort (LUMINA LVII). Lupus. 2008;17(4):314–22. https://doi.org/10.1177/0961203307087875.
11. Klein-Gitelman MLJB. Systemic lupus erythematosus. Textbook Pediatr Rheumatol. 2016;23:285–317.e14.
12. Wang LC, Yang YH, Lu MY, Chiang BL. Retrospective analysis of the renal outcome of pediatric lupus nephritis. Clin Rheumatol. 2004;23(4):318–23. https://doi.org/10.1007/s10067-004-0919-2.
13. Mattos P, Santiago MB. Disease activity in systemic lupus erythematosus patients with end-stage renal disease: systematic review of the literature. Clin Rheumatol. 2012;31(6):897–905. https://doi.org/10.1007/s10067-012-1957-9.

14. Sule S, Fivush B, Neu A, Furth S. Increased risk of death in African American patients with end-stage renal disease secondary to lupus. Clin Kidney J. 2014;7(1):40–4. https://doi.org/10.1093/ckj/sft157.
15. Hiraki LT, Benseler SM, Tyrrell PN, Hebert D, Harvey E, Silverman ED. Clinical and laboratory characteristics and long-term outcome of pediatric systemic lupus erythematosus: a longitudinal study. J Pediatr. 2008;152(4):550–6. https://doi.org/10.1016/j.jpeds.2007.09.019.
16. Abujam B, Gupta A, Suri D, Rawat A, Singh S. Trends and predictors of mortality in childhood onset lupus in a single North-Indian centre over 23 years: a retrospective study. Clin Exp Rheumatol. 2016;34(3):554–9.
17. Sule S, Fivush B, Neu A, Furth S. Increased risk of death in pediatric and adult patients with ESRD secondary to lupus. Pediatr Nephrol. 2011;26(1):93–8. https://doi.org/10.1007/s00467-010-1640-9.
18. Baqi N, Moazami S, Singh A, Ahmad H, Balachandra S, Tejani A. Lupus nephritis in children: a longitudinal study of prognostic factors and therapy. J Am Soc Nephrol. 1996;7(6):924–9.
19. Gibson KL, Gipson DS, Massengill SA, Dooley MA, Primack WA, Ferris MA, et al. Predictors of relapse and end stage kidney disease in proliferative lupus nephritis: focus on children, adolescents, and young adults. Clin J Am Soc Nephrol. 2009;4(12):1962–7. https://doi.org/10.2215/CJN.00490109.
20. Tsai WT, Chang HC, Wang CT, Chiang BL, Lin YT. Long-term outcomes in lupus patients receiving different renal replacement therapy. J Microbiol Immunol Infect. 2019;52(4):648–53. https://doi.org/10.1016/j.jmii.2018.12.010.
21. Wong T, Goral S. Lupus nephritis and kidney transplantation: where are we today? Adv Chronic Kidney Dis. 2019;26(5):313–22. https://doi.org/10.1053/j.ackd.2019.08.007.
22. Barrera-Vargas A, Quintanar-Martinez M, Merayo-Chalico J, Alcocer-Varela J, Gomez-Martin D. Risk factors for systemic lupus erythematosus flares in patients with end-stage renal disease: a case-control study. Rheumatology (Oxford). 2016;55(3):429–35. https://doi.org/10.1093/rheumatology/kev349.
23. Freedman BI, Langefeld CD, Andringa KK, Croker JA, Williams AH, Garner NE, et al. End-stage renal disease in African Americans with lupus nephritis is associated with APOL1. Arthritis Rheumatol. 2014;66(2):390–6. https://doi.org/10.1002/art.38220.
24. Mojcik CF, Klippel JH. End-stage renal disease and systemic lupus erythematosus. Am J Med. 1996;101(1):100–7. https://doi.org/10.1016/s0002-9343(96)00074-5.
25. Stone JH, Millward CL, Olson JL, Amend WJ, Criswell LA. Frequency of recurrent lupus nephritis among ninety-seven renal transplant patients during the cyclosporine era. Arthritis Rheum. 1998;41(4):678–86. https://doi.org/10.1002/1529-0131(199804)41:4<678::AID-ART15>3.0.CO;2-7.
26. Goss JA, Cole BR, Jendrisak MD, McCullough CS, So SK, Windus DW, et al. Renal transplantation for systemic lupus erythematosus and recurrent lupus nephritis. A single-center experience and a review of the literature. Transplantation. 1991;52(5):805–10. https://doi.org/10.1097/00007890-199111000-00009.
27. Moroni G, Tantardini F, Gallelli B, Quaglini S, Banfi G, Poli F, et al. The long-term prognosis of renal transplantation in patients with lupus nephritis. Am J Kidney Dis. 2005;45(5):903–11. https://doi.org/10.1053/j.ajkd.2005.01.038.
28. Renal transplantation in congenital and metabolic diseases. A report from the ASC/NIH renal transplant registry. JAMA. 1975;232(2):148–53. https://doi.org/10.1001/jama.1975.03250020022018.
29. Plantinga LC, Patzer RE, Drenkard C, Kramer MR, Klein M, Lim SS, et al. Association of time to kidney transplantation with graft failure among U.S. patients with end-stage renal disease due to lupus nephritis. Arthritis Care Res (Hoboken). 2015;67(4):571–81. https://doi.org/10.1002/acr.22482.
30. Ntatsaki E, Velo-Garcia A, Vassiliou VS, Salama AD, Isenberg DA. Impact of pre-transplant time on dialysis on survival in patients with lupus nephritis. Clin Rheumatol. 2018;37(9):2399–404. https://doi.org/10.1007/s10067-018-4115-1.

31. Naveed A, Nilubol C, Melancon JK, Girlanda R, Johnson L, Javaid B. Preemptive kidney transplantation in systemic lupus erythematosus. Transplant Proc. 2011;43(10):3713–4. https://doi.org/10.1016/j.transproceed.2011.08.092.
32. Wu MJ, Lo YC, Lan JL, Yu TM, Shu KH, Chen DY, et al. Outcome of lupus nephritis after entering into end-stage renal disease and comparison between different treatment modalities: a nationwide population-based cohort study in Taiwan. Transplant Proc. 2014;46(2):339–41. https://doi.org/10.1016/j.transproceed.2013.11.080.
33. Tang H, Chelamcharla M, Baird BC, Shihab FS, Koford JK, Goldfarb-Rumyantzev AS. Factors affecting kidney-transplant outcome in recipients with lupus nephritis. Clin Transpl. 2008;22(3):263–72. https://doi.org/10.1111/j.1399-0012.2007.00781.x.
34. Van Stralen KJ, Verrina E, Belingheri M, Dudley J, Dusek J, Grenda R, et al. Impact of graft loss among kidney diseases with a high risk of post-transplant recurrence in the paediatric population. Nephrol Dial Transplant. 2013;28(4):1031–8. https://doi.org/10.1093/ndt/gfs549.
35. Ishitani M, Isaacs R, Norwood V, Nock S, Lobo P. Predictors of graft survival in pediatric living-related kidney transplant recipients. Transplantation. 2000;70(2):288–92. https://doi.org/10.1097/00007890-200007270-00008.
36. Sanchez C, Rebolledo A, Gahona J, Rojas M, Jimenez R, Bojorquez A. Post-transplant immune complex nephritis in a patient with systemic lupus erythematosus associated with ANCA vasculitis. Pediatr Transplant. 2017;21(3) https://doi.org/10.1111/petr.12895.
37. Wisanuyotin S, Jiravuttipong A, Puapairoj A. De novo lupus nephritis in a renal transplanted child: a case report. Transplant Proc. 2014;46(2):648–50. https://doi.org/10.1016/j.transproceed.2013.12.023.
38. Bacchetta J, Cochat P. Primary disease recurrence-effects on paediatric renal transplantation outcomes. Nat Rev Nephrol. 2015;11(6):371–84. https://doi.org/10.1038/nrneph.2015.54.
39. Burgos PI, Perkins EL, Pons-Estel GJ, Kendrick SA, Liu JM, Kendrick WT, et al. Risk factors and impact of recurrent lupus nephritis in patients with systemic lupus erythematosus undergoing renal transplantation: data from a single US institution. Arthritis Rheum. 2009;60(9):2757–66. https://doi.org/10.1002/art.24776.
40. Norby GE, Strom EH, Midtvedt K, Hartmann A, Gilboe IM, Leivestad T, et al. Recurrent lupus nephritis after kidney transplantation: a surveillance biopsy study. Ann Rheum Dis. 2010;69(8):1484–7. https://doi.org/10.1136/ard.2009.122796.
41. Contreras G, Mattiazzi A, Guerra G, Ortega LM, Tozman EC, Li H, et al. Recurrence of lupus nephritis after kidney transplantation. J Am Soc Nephrol. 2010;21(7):1200–7. https://doi.org/10.1681/ASN.2009101093.
42. Pham PT, Pham PC. Graft loss due to recurrent lupus nephritis in living-related kidney donation. Clin J Am Soc Nephrol. 2011;6(9):2296–9. https://doi.org/10.2215/CJN.00190111.
43. Pham PT, Pham PC. The impact of mycophenolate mofetil versus azathioprine as adjunctive therapy to cyclosporine on the rates of renal allograft loss due to glomerular disease recurrence. Nephrol Dial Transplant. 2012;27(7):2965–71. https://doi.org/10.1093/ndt/gfr731.
44. Petri M. Lupus in Baltimore: evidence-based 'clinical pearls' from the Hopkins Lupus Cohort. Lupus. 2005;14(12):970–3. https://doi.org/10.1191/0961203305lu2230xx.
45. Hiraki LT, Benseler SM, Tyrrell PN, Harvey E, Hebert D, Silverman ED. Ethnic differences in pediatric systemic lupus erythematosus. J Rheumatol. 2009;36(11):2539–46. https://doi.org/10.3899/jrheum.081141.
46. Rubinstein TB, Knight AM. Disparities in childhood-onset lupus. Rheum Dis Clin N Am. 2020;46(4):661–72. https://doi.org/10.1016/j.rdc.2020.07.007.
47. Jennette JC, Falk RJ, Bacon PA, Basu N, Cid MC, Ferrario F, et al. 2012 revised international Chapel Hill consensus conference nomenclature of vasculitides. Arthritis Rheum. 2013;65(1):1–11. https://doi.org/10.1002/art.37715.
48. Oni L, Sampath S. Childhood IgA vasculitis (Henoch Schonlein Purpura)-advances and knowledge gaps. Front Pediatr. 2019;7:257. https://doi.org/10.3389/fped.2019.00257.
49. Ozen S, Ruperto N, Dillon MJ, Bagga A, Barron K, Davin JC, et al. EULAR/PReS endorsed consensus criteria for the classification of childhood vasculitides. Ann Rheum Dis. 2006;65(7):936–41. https://doi.org/10.1136/ard.2005.046300.

50. Ozen S, Pistorio A, Iusan SM, Bakkaloglu A, Herlin T, Brik R, et al. EULAR/PRINTO/PRES criteria for Henoch-Schönlein purpura, childhood polyarteritis nodosa, childhood Wegener granulomatosis and childhood Takayasu arteritis: Ankara 2008. Part II: final classification criteria. Ann Rheum Dis. 2010;69(5):798–806. https://doi.org/10.1136/ard.2009.116657.
51. Bogdanović R. Henoch-Schönlein purpura nephritis in children: risk factors, prevention and treatment. Acta Paediatr. 2009;98(12):1882–9. https://doi.org/10.1111/j.1651-2227.2009.01445.x.
52. Narchi H. Risk of long term renal impairment and duration of follow up recommended for Henoch-Schonlein purpura with normal or minimal urinary findings: a systematic review. Arch Dis Child. 2005;90(9):916–20. https://doi.org/10.1136/adc.2005.074641.
53. Ozen S, Marks SD, Brogan P, Groot N, de Graeff N, Avcin T, et al. European consensus-based recommendations for diagnosis and treatment of immunoglobulin A vasculitis-the SHARE initiative. Rheumatology (Oxford). 2019;58(9):1607–16. https://doi.org/10.1093/rheumatology/kez041.
54. Nicoara O, Twombley K. Immunoglobulin a nephropathy and immunoglobulin a vasculitis. Pediatr Clin N Am. 2019;66(1):101–10. https://doi.org/10.1016/j.pcl.2018.08.008.
55. Chartapisak W, Opastirakul S, Hodson EM, Willis NS, Craig JC. Interventions for preventing and treating kidney disease in Henoch-Schönlein Purpura (HSP). Cochrane Database Syst Rev. 2009;(3):CD005128. https://doi.org/10.1002/14651858.CD005128.pub2.
56. Hahn D, Hodson EM, Willis NS, Craig JC. Interventions for preventing and treating kidney disease in Henoch-Schönlein Purpura (HSP). Cochrane Database Syst Rev. 2015;(8):CD005128. https://doi.org/10.1002/14651858.CD005128.pub3.
57. Edström Halling S, Söderberg MP, Berg UB. Predictors of outcome in Henoch-Schönlein nephritis. Pediatr Nephrol. 2010;25(6):1101–8. https://doi.org/10.1007/s00467-010-1444-y.
58. Mir S, Yavascan O, Mutlubas F, Yeniay B, Sonmez F. Clinical outcome in children with Henoch-Schönlein nephritis. Pediatr Nephrol. 2007;22(1):64–70. https://doi.org/10.1007/s00467-006-0278-0.
59. Shi D, Chan H, Yang X, Zhang G, Yang H, Wang M, et al. Risk factors associated with IgA vasculitis with nephritis (Henoch-Schönlein purpura nephritis) progressing to unfavorable outcomes: a meta-analysis. PLoS One. 2019;14(10):e0223218. https://doi.org/10.1371/journal.pone.0223218.
60. Coppo R, Andrulli S, Amore A, Gianoglio B, Conti G, Peruzzi L, et al. Predictors of outcome in Henoch-Schönlein nephritis in children and adults. Am J Kidney Dis. 2006;47(6):993–1003. https://doi.org/10.1053/j.ajkd.2006.02.178.
61. Counahan R, Winterborn MH, White RH, Heaton JM, Meadow SR, Bluett NH, et al. Prognosis of Henoch Schönlein nephritis in children. Br Med J. 1977;2(6078):11–4. https://doi.org/10.1136/bmj.2.6078.11.
62. Assadi F. Childhood Henoch-Schonlein nephritis: a multivariate analysis of clinical features and renal morphology at disease onset. Iran J Kidney Dis. 2009;3(1):17–21.
63. Shenoy M, Bradbury MG, Lewis MA, Webb NJ. Outcome of Henoch-Schönlein purpura nephritis treated with long-term immunosuppression. Pediatr Nephrol. 2007;22(10):1717–22. https://doi.org/10.1007/s00467-007-0557-4.
64. Xia Y, Mao J, Chen Y, Wang D, Cao L, Yao S, et al. Clinical outcomes in children with Henoch-Schönlein purpura nephritis grade IIIa or IIIb. Pediatr Nephrol. 2011;26(7):1083–8. https://doi.org/10.1007/s00467-011-1834-9.
65. Delbet JD, Hogan J, Aoun B, Stoica I, Salomon R, Decramer S, et al. Clinical outcomes in children with Henoch-Schönlein purpura nephritis without crescents. Pediatr Nephrol. 2017;32(7):1193–9. https://doi.org/10.1007/s00467-017-3604-9.
66. Coppo R, Mazzucco G, Cagnoli L, Lupo A, Schena FP. Long-term prognosis of Henoch-Schönlein nephritis in adults and children. Italian Group of Renal Immunopathology Collaborative Study on Henoch-Schönlein purpura. Nephrol Dial Transplant. 1997;12(11):2277–83. https://doi.org/10.1093/ndt/12.11.2277.

67. Samuel JP, Bell CS, Molony DA, Braun MC. Long-term outcome of renal transplantation patients with Henoch-Schonlein purpura. Clin J Am Soc Nephrol. 2011;6(8):2034–40. https://doi.org/10.2215/cjn.01410211.
68. Meulders Q, Pirson Y, Cosyns JP, Squifflet JP, van Ypersele de Strihou C. Course of Henoch-Schönlein nephritis after renal transplantation. Report on ten patients and review of the literature. Transplantation. 1994;58(11):1179–86.
69. Han SS, Sun HK, Lee JP, Ha JW, Kim SJ, Kim YS. Outcome of renal allograft in patients with Henoch-Schönlein nephritis: single-center experience and systematic review. Transplantation. 2010;89(6):721–6. https://doi.org/10.1097/TP.0b013e3181c9cc4a.
70. Kanaan N, Mourad G, Thervet E, Peeters P, Hourmant M, Vanrenterghem Y, et al. Recurrence and graft loss after kidney transplantation for henoch-schonlein purpura nephritis: a multicenter analysis. Clin J Am Soc Nephrol. 2011;6(7):1768–72. https://doi.org/10.2215/cjn.00520111.
71. Moroni G, Gallelli B, Diana A, Carminati A, Banfi G, Poli F, et al. Renal transplantation in adults with Henoch-Schonlein purpura: long-term outcome. Nephrol Dial Transplant. 2008;23(9):3010–6. https://doi.org/10.1093/ndt/gfn209.
72. Hasegawa A, Kawamura T, Ito H, Hasegawa O, Ogawa O, Honda M, et al. Fate of renal grafts with recurrent Henoch-Schönlein purpura nephritis in children. Transplant Proc. 1989;21(1 Pt 2):2130–3.
73. Lee J, Clayton F, Shihab F, Goldfarb-Rumyantzev A. Successful treatment of recurrent Henoch-Schönlein purpura in a renal allograft with plasmapheresis. Am J Transplant. 2008;8(1):228–31. https://doi.org/10.1111/j.1600-6143.2007.02022.x.
74. Yamakawa T, Yamamoto I, Komatsuzaki Y, Niikura T, Okabayashi Y, Katsumata H, et al. Successful treatment of recurrent Henoch-Schönlein purpura nephritis in a renal allograft with tonsillectomy and steroid pulse therapy. Nephrology (Carlton). 2016;21(Suppl 1):53–6. https://doi.org/10.1111/nep.12770.
75. Craven A, Robson J, Ponte C, Grayson PC, Suppiah R, Judge A, et al. ACR/EULAR-endorsed study to develop Diagnostic and Classification Criteria for Vasculitis (DCVAS). Clin Exp Nephrol. 2013;17(5):619–21. https://doi.org/10.1007/s10157-013-0854-0.
76. Kitching AR, Anders HJ, Basu N, Brouwer E, Gordon J, Jayne DR, et al. ANCA-associated vasculitis. Nat Rev Dis Primers. 2020;6(1):71. https://doi.org/10.1038/s41572-020-0204-y.
77. Berden AE, Ferrario F, Hagen EC, Jayne DR, Jennette JC, Joh K, et al. Histopathologic classification of ANCA-associated glomerulonephritis. J Am Soc Nephrol. 2010;21(10):1628–36. https://doi.org/10.1681/asn.2010050477.
78. Noone DG, Twilt M, Hayes WN, Thorner PS, Benseler S, Laxer RM, et al. The new histopathologic classification of ANCA-associated GN and its association with renal outcomes in childhood. Clin J Am Soc Nephrol. 2014;9(10):1684–91. https://doi.org/10.2215/cjn.01210214.
79. Calatroni M, Oliva E, Gianfreda D, Gregorini G, Allinovi M, Ramirez GA, et al. ANCA-associated vasculitis in childhood: recent advances. Ital J Pediatr. 2017;43(1):46. https://doi.org/10.1186/s13052-017-0364-x.
80. Jariwala M, Laxer RM. Childhood GPA, EGPA, and MPA. Clin Immunol. 2020;211:108325. https://doi.org/10.1016/j.clim.2019.108325.
81. Hirano D, Ishikawa T, Inaba A, Sato M, Shinozaki T, Iijima K, et al. Epidemiology and clinical features of childhood-onset anti-neutrophil cytoplasmic antibody-associated vasculitis: a clinicopathological analysis. Pediatr Nephrol. 2019;34(8):1425–33. https://doi.org/10.1007/s00467-019-04228-4.
82. Kouri AM, Andreoli SP. Clinical presentation and outcome of pediatric ANCA-associated glomerulonephritis. Pediatr Nephrol. 2017;32(3):449–55. https://doi.org/10.1007/s00467-016-3490-6.
83. Bohm M, Gonzalez Fernandez MI, Ozen S, Pistorio A, Dolezalova P, Brogan P, et al. Clinical features of childhood granulomatosis with polyangiitis (wegener's granulomatosis). Pediatr Rheumatol Online J. 2014;12:18. https://doi.org/10.1186/1546-0096-12-18.

84. Peco-Antic A, Bonaci-Nikolic B, Basta-Jovanovic G, Kostic M, Markovic-Lipkovski J, Nikolic M, et al. Childhood microscopic polyangiitis associated with MPO-ANCA. Pediatr Nephrol. 2006;21(1):46–53. https://doi.org/10.1007/s00467-005-2063-x.
85. Dolezalova P, Price-Kuehne FE, Özen S, Benseler SM, Cabral DA, Anton J, et al. Disease activity assessment in childhood vasculitis: development and preliminary validation of the Paediatric Vasculitis Activity Score (PVAS). Ann Rheum Dis. 2013;72(10):1628–33. https://doi.org/10.1136/annrheumdis-2012-202111.
86. Mukhtyar C, Lee R, Brown D, Carruthers D, Dasgupta B, Dubey S, et al. Modification and validation of the Birmingham Vasculitis Activity Score (version 3). Ann Rheum Dis. 2009;68(12):1827–32. https://doi.org/10.1136/ard.2008.101279.
87. Lee JJY, Alsaleem A, Chiang GPK, Limenis E, Sontichai W, Yeung RSM, et al. Hallmark trials in ANCA-associated vasculitis (AAV) for the pediatric rheumatologist. Pediatr Rheumatol Online J. 2019;17(1):31. https://doi.org/10.1186/s12969-019-0343-4.
88. Yates M, Watts RA, Bajema IM, Cid MC, Crestani B, Hauser T, et al. EULAR/ERA-EDTA recommendations for the management of ANCA-associated vasculitis. Ann Rheum Dis. 2016;75(9):1583–94. https://doi.org/10.1136/annrheumdis-2016-209133.
89. Guerry MJ, Brogan P, Bruce IN, D'Cruz DP, Harper L, Luqmani R, et al. Recommendations for the use of rituximab in anti-neutrophil cytoplasm antibody-associated vasculitis. Rheumatology (Oxford). 2012;51(4):634–43. https://doi.org/10.1093/rheumatology/ker150.
90. de Graeff N, Groot N, Brogan P, Ozen S, Avcin T, Bader-Meunier B, et al. European consensus-based recommendations for the diagnosis and treatment of rare paediatric vasculitides - the SHARE initiative. Rheumatology (Oxford). 2019;58(4):656–71. https://doi.org/10.1093/rheumatology/key322.
91. Stone JH, Merkel PA, Spiera R, Seo P, Langford CA, Hoffman GS, et al. Rituximab versus cyclophosphamide for ANCA-associated vasculitis. N Engl J Med. 2010;363(3):221–32. https://doi.org/10.1056/NEJMoa0909905.
92. Jones RB, Tervaert JW, Hauser T, Luqmani R, Morgan MD, Peh CA, et al. Rituximab versus cyclophosphamide in ANCA-associated renal vasculitis. N Engl J Med. 2010;363(3):211–20. https://doi.org/10.1056/NEJMoa0909169.
93. James KE, Xiao R, Merkel PA, Weiss PF. Variation in the treatment of children hospitalized with antineutrophil cytoplasmic antibody-associated vasculitis in the US. Arthritis Care Res (Hoboken). 2017;69(9):1377–83. https://doi.org/10.1002/acr.23142.
94. Jones RB, Hiemstra TF, Ballarin J, Blockmans DE, Brogan P, Bruchfeld A, et al. Mycophenolate mofetil versus cyclophosphamide for remission induction in ANCA-associated vasculitis: a randomised, non-inferiority trial. Ann Rheum Dis. 2019;78(3):399–405. https://doi.org/10.1136/annrheumdis-2018-214245.
95. Walsh M, Merkel PA, Peh CA, Szpirt WM, Puéchal X, Fujimoto S, et al. Plasma exchange and glucocorticoids in severe ANCA-associated vasculitis. N Engl J Med. 2020;382(7):622–31. https://doi.org/10.1056/NEJMoa1803537.
96. Jayne DR, Gaskin G, Rasmussen N, Abramowicz D, Ferrario F, Guillevin L, et al. Randomized trial of plasma exchange or high-dosage methylprednisolone as adjunctive therapy for severe renal vasculitis. J Am Soc Nephrol. 2007;18(7):2180–8. https://doi.org/10.1681/asn.2007010090.
97. Phillip R, Luqmani R. Mortality in systemic vasculitis: a systematic review. Clin Exp Rheumatol. 2008;26(5 Suppl 51):S94–104.
98. Morishita KA, Moorthy LN, Lubieniecka JM, Twilt M, Yeung RSM, Toth MB, et al. Early outcomes in children with antineutrophil cytoplasmic antibody-associated vasculitis. Arthritis Rheumatol. 2017;69(7):1470–9. https://doi.org/10.1002/art.40112.
99. Sinico RA, Di Toma L, Radice A. Renal involvement in anti-neutrophil cytoplasmic autoantibody associated vasculitis. Autoimmun Rev. 2013;12(4):477–82. https://doi.org/10.1016/j.autrev.2012.08.006.
100. Cabral DA, Canter DL, Muscal E, Nanda K, Wahezi DM, Spalding SJ, et al. Comparing presenting clinical features in 48 children with microscopic polyangiitis to 183 children

who have granulomatosis with polyangiitis (Wegener's): an ARChiVe cohort study. Arthritis Rheumatol. 2016;68(10):2514–26. https://doi.org/10.1002/art.39729.
101. Little MA, Hassan B, Jacques S, Game D, Salisbury E, Courtney AE, et al. Renal transplantation in systemic vasculitis: when is it safe? Nephrol Dial Transplant. 2009;24(10):3219–25. https://doi.org/10.1093/ndt/gfp347.
102. Hruskova Z, Geetha D, Tesar V. Renal transplantation in anti-neutrophil cytoplasmic antibody-associated vasculitis. Nephrol Dial Transplant. 2015;30(Suppl 1):i159–63. https://doi.org/10.1093/ndt/gfu328.
103. Noone D, Yeung RSM, Hebert D. Outcome of kidney transplantation in pediatric patients with ANCA-associated glomerulonephritis: a single-center experience. Pediatr Nephrol. 2017;32(12):2343–50. https://doi.org/10.1007/s00467-017-3749-6.
104. Besbas N, Ozaltin F, Tinaztepe K, Güçer S, Ozen S, Bakkaloglu M, et al. Successful renal transplantation in a child with ANCA-associated microscopic polyangiitis. Pediatr Nephrol. 2003;18(7):696–9. https://doi.org/10.1007/s00467-003-1114-4.
105. Kaseda K, Marui Y, Suwabe T, Hoshino J, Sumida K, Hayami N, et al. Kidney transplantation for a patient with refractory childhood-onset ANCA-associated vasculitis. Mod Rheumatol. 2016;26(2):307–9. https://doi.org/10.3109/14397595.2013.877327.
106. Hasegawa J, Wakai S, Shirakawa H. Juvenile slow progressive antineutrophil cytoplasmic antibody-associated vasculitis diagnosed after kidney transplantation: a case report. Ther Apher Dial. 2015;19(3):303–4. https://doi.org/10.1111/1744-9987.12249.
107. Segelmark M. L23. Renal transplantation in ANCA-associated vasculitis. Presse Med. 2013;42(4 Pt 2):568–71. https://doi.org/10.1016/j.lpm.2013.01.023.
108. Lionaki S, Hogan SL, Jennette CE, Hu Y, Hamra JB, Jennette JC, et al. The clinical course of ANCA small-vessel vasculitis on chronic dialysis. Kidney Int. 2009;76(6):644–51. https://doi.org/10.1038/ki.2009.218.
109. Geetha D, Eirin A, True K, Valentina Irazabal M, Specks U, Seo P, et al. Renal transplantation in antineutrophil cytoplasmic antibody-associated vasculitis: a multicenter experience. Transplantation. 2011;91(12):1370–5. https://doi.org/10.1097/TP.0b013e31821ab9aa.
110. Marco H, Mirapeix E, Arcos E, Comas J, Ara J, Gil-Vernet S, et al. Long-term outcome of antineutrophil cytoplasmic antibody-associated small vessel vasculitis after renal transplantation. Clin Transpl. 2013;27(3):338–47. https://doi.org/10.1111/ctr.12084.
111. Göçeroğlu A, Rahmattulla C, Berden AE, Reinders ME, Wolterbeek R, Steenbergen EJ, et al. The Dutch transplantation in vasculitis (DUTRAVAS) study: outcome of renal transplantation in antineutrophil cytoplasmic antibody-associated glomerulonephritis. Transplantation. 2016;100(4):916–24. https://doi.org/10.1097/tp.0000000000000910.
112. Elmedhem A, Adu D, Savage CO. Relapse rate and outcome of ANCA-associated small vessel vasculitis after transplantation. Nephrol Dial Transplant. 2003;18(5):1001–4. https://doi.org/10.1093/ndt/gfg087.
113. Chow KM, Wang AY, Mac-Moune Lai F, Wong TY, Li PK. Rapid recurrence of ANCA-negative pauci-immune vasculitis after cadaveric renal transplantation. Am J Kidney Dis. 2001;38(1):E3. https://doi.org/10.1053/ajkd.2001.25217.
114. Lobbedez T, Comoz F, Renaudineau E, Pujo M, Ryckelynck JP, Hurault de Ligny B. Recurrence of ANCA-positive glomerulonephritis immediately after renal transplantation. Am J Kidney Dis. 2003;42(4):E2–6. https://doi.org/10.1016/s0272-6386(03)00917-x.
115. Le Berre L, Dufay A, Cantarovich D, Meurette A, Audrain M, Giral M, et al. Early and irreversible recurrence MPO-ANCA-positive glomerulonephritis after renal transplantation. Clin Nephrol. 2015;83(6):357–62. https://doi.org/10.5414/cn108303.
116. Briggs JD, Jones E. Renal transplantation for uncommon diseases. Scientific Advisory Board of the ERA-EDTA Registry. European Renal Association-European Dialysis and Transplant Association. Nephrol Dial Transplant. 1999;14(3):570–5. https://doi.org/10.1093/ndt/14.3.570.
117. KDIGO clinical practice guideline for the care of kidney transplant recipients. Am J Transplant. 2009;9(Suppl 3):S1–155. https://doi.org/10.1111/j.1600-6143.2009.02834.x.

8 Recurrent Disease Challenges in Pediatric Kidney Transplantation

Lyndsay A. Harshman and Sharon M. Bartosh

Introduction

For some pediatric transplant recipients, the risk for native disease recurrence following successful kidney transplantation remains a worrisome and stark reality. Overall recurrence of disease accounts for 7–8% of graft losses in pediatric kidney transplant recipients and is the fourth most common cause of graft loss after chronic rejection, acute rejection, and death with a functioning graft [1]. Recurrent diseases leading to graft loss are most commonly glomerulonephritis (70–80%) and inherited metabolic diseases (Table 8.1) [1].

Disease recurrence within the graft may render the graft unsalvageable and/or lead to years of patient and graft life lost. General features of disease recurrence may include elevated creatinine, hematuria, and/or proteinuria. Recurrence may occur at variable time points post-transplant with some diseases such as focal segmental glomerulosclerosis (FSGS) having the potential to recur within hours to days after transplant.

In a report from the European Society of Pediatric Nephrology/European Renal Association – European Dialysis and Transplant Association registry, a competing risk analysis of 1955 European children transplanted before age 20 from 33 European countries demonstrated that the highest rates of graft failure were seen in those children with FSGS, membranoproliferative glomerulonephritis (MPGN), and systemic lupus erythematosus compared to children with end-stage kidney disease (ESKD) secondary to congenital anomalies of the kidney and urinary tract

L. A. Harshman (✉)
University of Iowa Organ Transplant Center, Iowa City, IA, USA
e-mail: Lyndsay-harshman@uiowa.edu

S. M. Bartosh
University of Wisconsin, Division of Pediatric Nephrology, Pediatric Kidney Transplantation, Madison, WI, USA
e-mail: smbartosh@wisc.edu

K. E. Twombley (ed.), *Challenges in Pediatric Kidney Transplantation*,
https://doi.org/10.1007/978-3-030-74783-1_8

Table 8.1 Rates of primary disease recurrence after kidney transplantation

Primary disease	Recurrence rate	Graft loss to recurrence
FSGS	14–50%	40–60%
Atypical HUS	20–80%	10–83%
Typical HUS	0–1%	0–1%
MPGN type 1	30–77%	17–50%
MPGN type 2	66–100%	25–61%
SLE nephritis	0–30%	0–5%
IgA nephritis (Berger disease)	35–60%	7–10%
Henoch-Schonlein nephritis	31–100%	8–22%
Primary hyperoxaluria type 1	90–100%	80–100%

FSGS focal segmental glomerulosclerosis, HUS hemolytic uremic syndrome, IgA immunoglobulin A, MPGN membranoproliferative glomerulonephritis, SLE systemic lupus erythematosus. Reproduced with permission from Cochat et al. [1]

[2]. Statistically significant differences in 5-year graft losses were seen for children with FSGS (25.7%) and MPGN (32.4%) compared to transplant recipients with congenital anomalies (14.4%) as the cause of ESKD [2].

The percentage of children listed as having either FSGS or other glomerular disease as the cause of their ESKD has been decreasing over the past decade, perhaps related to improved therapeutics and success in treating glomerulonephritis in children. Despite improvements, glomerulonephritis (non-FSGS) is the identified cause of ESKD in 6.5% of children undergoing kidney transplant in the USA [3]. This chapter will review what is known regarding the nature and frequency of kidney diseases at high risk for recurrence post-transplantation. FSGS will be discussed separately in another chapter. We will discuss the genetic and/or immune-mediated risk factors that drive disease recurrence, considerations for transplant planning (e.g., donor type and induction agents), and available evidence-based options for management of disease recurrence post-transplantation.

Case A 10-year-old male with a history of biopsy-documented crescentic C3 glomerulopathy (C3G) was referred for transplant evaluation. He is C3 nephritic factor positive. In the months prior to transplant evaluation, his laboratory studies continued to demonstrate nephrotic range proteinuria (urine protein to creatinine ratio – 15 g/g), significant microscopic hematuria, and C3 of 35 mg/dL (normal 90–180 mg/dL). His immune workup was otherwise negative/normal. He remains hypertensive on three agents despite appropriate fluid balance. His prior therapies had included plasma exchange, eculizumab, and mycophenolate mofetil; however, none led to disease remission and the patient has progressed to end-stage kidney disease.

- How do you counsel the family regarding chance/risk for C3G recurrence? What clinical variables do you include in your counseling and risk assessment?
- Is it safe for a parent/family member to donate a kidney to this child or do they risk development of disease as well?

Atypical Hemolytic Uremic Syndrome (aHUS)

Nature and Frequency of Primary Disease

The prevalence of aHUS in patients less than 20 years of age is estimated at 2.21 and 9.4 per million people [4] with the highest disease prevalence occurring in children between 0 and 4 years of age [5]. Uncontrolled overactivation of the alternative complement pathway (ACP) at the level of the endothelium is a primary immunological feature of aHUS [6]. There are known genetic abnormalities within the ACP which predispose to aHUS, including complement factor H (CFH), complement factor I (CFI), complement component C (C3), complement factor B (CFB), and membrane cofactor protein (MCP). The clinical hallmark of aHUS is a thrombotic microangiopathy (TMA) with associated intravascular hemolysis, anemia, and thrombocytopenia. Direct kidney injury is largely driven by damage to the glomerular endothelium from the complement-associated membrane attack complex (MAC) composed of complement components (C) C5b-9 [7]. Kidney injury results in acute kidney injury, difficult-to-control hypertension, microscopic hematuria, and proteinuria.

Considerations for Transplant Planning

Kidney transplantation should be delayed at least 6 months after starting rescue therapy with eculizumab (a recombinant, humanized monoclonal antibody against complement protein, C5 [8]) as there may be limited recovery of kidney function that occurs within the first several months of eculizumab initiation [9–11]. Furthermore, aHUS-associated hematological features/extra-renal manifestations should be resolved prior to transplantation [9].

The risk for aHUS recurrence post-transplant is strongly linked with several pathogenic complement-based mutations. Factor H (FH), factor I (FI), and C3 mutations have the highest risk for aHUS recurrence (68–90%, 70–80%, and 40–50%, respectively) [12]. It is important to note that approximately 30–50% of patients with aHUS have no identifiable genetic mutation or autoantibody using currently available testing platforms [13, 14]. Pediatric patients and families should meet with a genetic counselor having expertise in complement-mediated genetic abnormalities. When counseling families with a gene/autoantibody negative child, it should be emphasized that the absence of an identifiable genetic mutation does not rule out an underlying genetic contribution to aHUS that could confer recurrence risk post-kidney transplant.

The diagnosis of aHUS has implications for evaluation of potential living donors. For example, kidney donation from a living-related donor has historically not been advised, given the potential for the related donor who may have genetic susceptibility factor(s) in parallel to the recipient [15]. As noted, if there is no identifiable complement genetic mutation for the patient, then living-related donation is contraindicated, given the risk for an unidentified, underlying genetic mutation which could adversely impact the donor [16]. Conversely if an identifiable pathogenic gene variant is identified in the recipient and negative for a potential living-related donor (and the donor has no other evidence of abnormal complement activation), then living-related donation may be feasible [15]. Living donation may, in fact, confer a decreased risk for complement activation secondary to increased ischemia-reperfusion injury typically encountered with deceased donation [17].

Risk Factors for Recurrence and Treatment of Recurrence

Most aHUS recurrences will occur within the first year following kidney transplant. The strongest risk factor for aHUS recurrence is the presence of known genetic complement abnormalities [14, 15, 18]. Feitz et al. [12] provide an excellent review of the estimated risk for aHUS recurrence based on complement gene mutation. The development and availability of eculizumab have drastically changed how transplant nephrologists approach prevention of aHUS recurrence for kidney transplant recipients. For patients with a known genetic mutation conferring risk for recurrence, eculizumab should be initiated within 24 hours prior to transplantation with an additional dose on post-operative day 1 [15].

Current guidelines from the Kidney Disease Improving Global Outcomes (KDIGO) consensus report provide expert opinion regarding prophylaxis strategies against aHUS recurrence post-transplant based on a risk-assessment strategy (Fig. 8.1); for example, patients with persistently negative factor H autoantibody and/or isolated MCP mutations can potentially be transplanted without prophylactic eculizumab [9, 19]. In this situation, the child should be followed closely post-transplant for disease recurrence with a low threshold to initiate eculizumab. Markers of disease recurrence might include dropping C3, anemia, thrombocytopenia, low haptoglobin, elevated lactate dehydrogenase, new onset hypertension, microscopic hematuria, and/or proteinuria.

There is no data to support that nephrectomy prior to or coincident with transplant decreases risk for recurrence. Available, limited data suggest that targeted transplant protocols attempting to minimize endothelial damage may decrease risk for aHUS recurrence in patients not receiving prophylactic eculizumab – for example, induction therapy with basiliximab (interleukin-2 receptor blocker) may be preferable to use of lymphocyte depleting agents [20] in addition to decreasing the target troughs for calcineurin inhibitors [21]. A case series by Duinevald et al. [22] demonstrated excellent patient and graft outcomes using an induction regimen with basiliximab, reduced-dose tacrolimus, and high-dose mycophenolate mofetil in conjunction with early strict blood pressure control, statin therapy, and angiotensin-converting enzyme inhibition to diminish the risk for endothelial injury that might upregulate complement activation within the graft. Acute rejection is an additional risk factor for aHUS recurrence; thus, intensified monitoring may be required during rejection episodes [23].

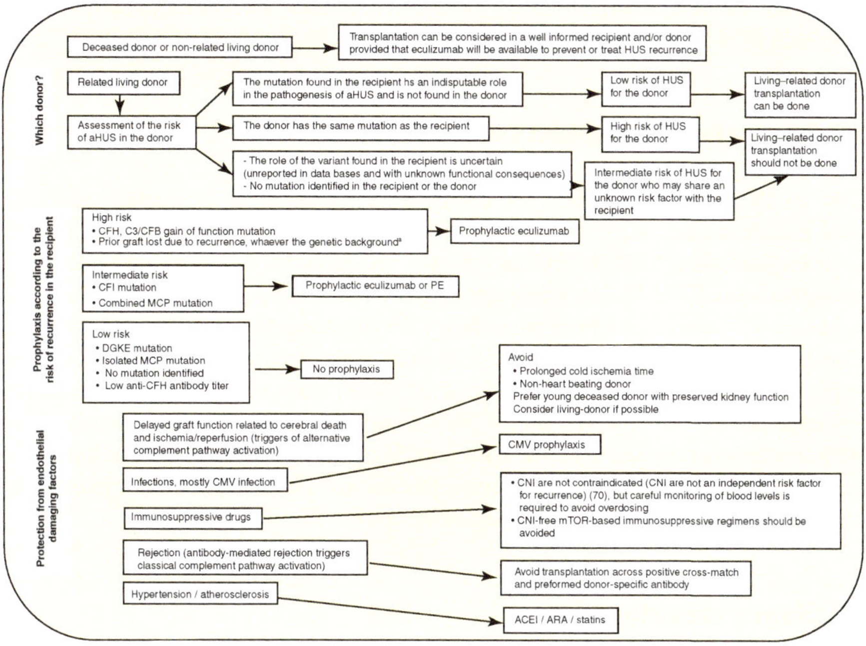

Fig. 8.1 Expert opinion regarding prophylaxis strategies against aHUS recurrence post-transplant based on a risk-assessment strategy. (*ACEI* angiotensin-converting enzyme inhibitor, *ARA* angiotensin receptor antagonists, *CFB* complement factor B, *CFH* complement factor H, *CFI* complement factor I, *CNI* calcineurin inhibitors, *DGKE* diacylglycerol kinase, *MCP* membrane cofactor protein, *PE* plasma exchange. Reproduced with permission from Loirat et al. [19])

Risk of Disease Recurrence in the Era of Eculizumab

Prior to the widespread use of eculizumab, kidney transplantation was not a viable option for many aHUS patients, given the substantial risk for morbidity/mortality associated with disease recurrence. Without eculizumab, the risk of recurrent disease after kidney transplantation was estimated to be 50 to 80%, with an overall 5-year graft survival of 36 ± 7% in patients with a recurrence compared with 70 ± 8% in patients without a recurrence [24, 25]. In the absence of effective anti-complement treatment, nearly 30% of the pediatric patients and half of adult patients with aHUS who survived in the acute phase of disease recurrence required, often permanent, renal replacement therapy [13, 24]. The 2016 KDIGO consensus report on aHUS suggests that withdrawal of eculizumab should not be considered in patients treated for post-transplant recurrence of aHUS, pending additional future data to support safety in doing so [19]. Limited case-series data provide the opinion that cessation of eculizumab after the first-year post-transplant may be a viable, safe option for the recipient [26]; however, there is limited consensus to support this approach at current.

Additional Post-transplant Considerations

Due to the risk for sepsis from encapsulated organisms, recipients receiving eculizumab should receive full meningococcal and pneumococcal vaccination prior to transplantation with additional booster vaccinations as necessary following transplantation [27]. The recipient additionally requires prophylactic antimicrobial coverage with ciprofloxacin or penicillin-V for the duration of eculizumab use [27]. The use of eculizumab, mycophenolate mofetil, and calcineurin inhibitor constitutes triple immunosuppression; thus, terminal calcineurin inhibitor levels can potentially be targeted at the lowest end of the clinician's goal range to avoid over-immunosuppression and risk for infection. For example, this may correlate with targeting tacrolimus levels to 3–5 ng/mL after the first 12-month post-transplantation and in the absence of rejection (expert opinion).

C3 Glomerulopathy (C3G)

Nature and Frequency of C3G

The term C3G is an umbrella term that encompasses both C3 glomerulonephritis (C3GN) and dense deposit disease (DDD). C3G is caused by overactivation of the alternative complement pathway. Abnormal complement activation typically results either from loss of function of one of the complement regulatory proteins (factor H or factor I) or from gain-of-function mutations in C3 that lead to resistance to regulation by factor H [28] (see Fig. 8.2). Overactivation of the complement pathway can also be secondary to generation of a C3 convertase-stabilizing autoantibody, C3 nephritic factor (C3NeF), or production of an autoantibody to factor H. Ultimately, these abnormalities result in overactivity of the C3 convertase and consumption of complement. Thus, depressed C3 is a feature of C3G in approximately 75% of cases [6, 29].

C3GN and DDD have an overlapping spectrum of pathological and clinical features. Clinical features are consistent with active glomerulonephritis: nephrotic range proteinuria, microscopic hematuria, hypertension, and elevated creatinine. The diagnosis of C3G requires a kidney biopsy demonstrating significant C3 deposition within the kidney, specifically the glomerulus. C3 deposition occurs in the absence of immunoglobulin deposition on pathological examination (e.g., negative/near-absent immunoglobulin G [IgG], immunoglobulin A [IgA], and immunoglobulin M [IgM]) [30, 31]. Electron microscopy findings of electron-dense, "sausage-shaped" deposits within the glomerular basement membrane are pathognomonic of DDD, whereas in C3G, the deposits are less dense and primarily located within the mesangium.

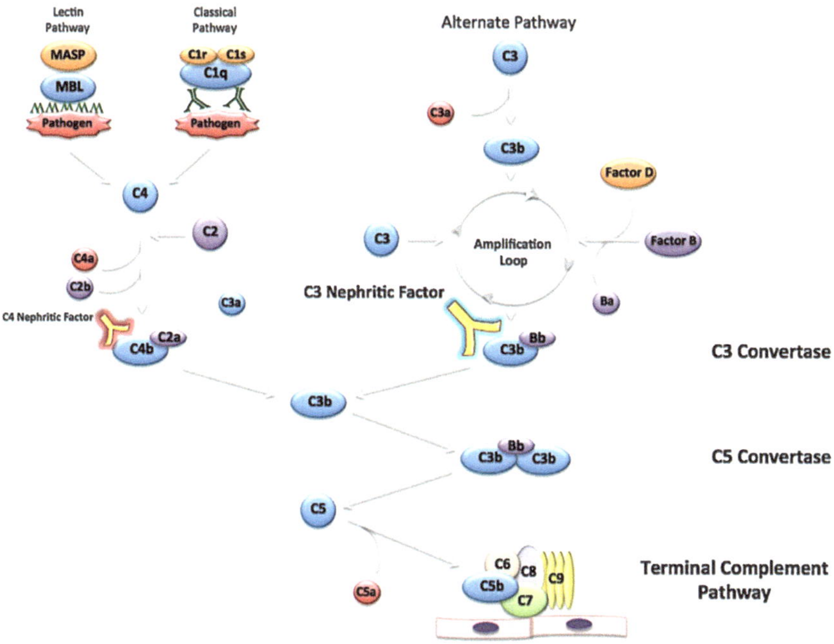

Fig. 8.2 The complement system has three interrelated initiating pathways – the classical, lectin, and alternative – that lead to formation of two C3 convertases, C4b2a, the C3 convertase of the classical and lectin pathways, and C3bBb, the C3 convertase of the alternative pathway. Autoantibodies to both convertases occur in C3G and are known as C4 nephritic factors (C4Nefs) and C3 nephritic factors (C3Nefs), respectively. Autoantibodies to factor B and factor H are also occasionally identified. C3bBb is the foundational convertase from which C5 convertase (C3bBbC3b) forms to cleave C5 into C5a, a potent anaphylatoxin, and C5b, triggering the terminal complement pathway. In C3G, dysregulation of both the initiating pathway at the level of C3bBb and the terminal pathway at the level of C3bBbC3b occurs, although dysregulation of the C3 convertase is typically greater. The site of complement dysregulation can be utilized to inform therapeutic intervention in patients with recurrent C3G following transplantation. (Figure reproduced with permissions from Nester and Smith [28])

C3G can be considered an ultra-rare disease with an incidence of ~0.2–1 in 1,000,000 people [32, 33]. The diagnosis of C3G is strongly associated with a 10-year kidney survival of 50% leading to eventual need for renal replacement therapy (e.g., transplantation) [6].

Considerations for Transplant Planning

As with aHUS, planning for transplant in the setting of C3G should include an evaluation with a team experienced in the genetics of complement-mediated kidney disease. This evaluation should include genetic testing of complement genes, measurement/assessment of complement function, and screening for complement autoantibodies. Genetic screening of complement regulatory genes (e.g., CFH and CFI), activation protein genes (C3, CFB), autoantibodies (C3 nephritic factor [C3nef] and FH autoantibodies), and assessment of copy number variation across the CFH-CFHR locus should be done on a case-by-case basis given the need for expert interpretation and clinical validation [9, 30]. Genetic and functional studies may provide insight regarding utility and efficacy of targeted anti-complement therapy (e.g., eculizumab or novel anti-complement therapies in development) should C3G recur following transplant.

Living-related donor kidney transplantation should be approached with caution for both the presumed healthy donor and recipient with C3G. Current international recommendations are that all potential recipients of a living-related kidney be screened for genetic abnormalities within the complement system [9]. If a genetic abnormality is found, the donor should subsequently be tested. The presence of an identical genetic abnormality may not constitute an absolute contraindication to donation; however, the individual case be evaluated in conjunction with persons having expertise in complement genetics/C3G. Furthermore, for donors with identified complement genetic abnormalities, the donor team must disclose the theoretical risks that donation may trigger new disease onset.

There are no published data supporting any single induction modality for transplant; thus, induction agent at the time of transplant is based on center preference. There is no data to support pre-/peri-transplant nephrectomy to prevent disease recurrence. The presence of active disease, specifically heavy proteinuria, is a relative contraindication to transplantation and all efforts should be made to delay transplantation until there is consistent resolution of nephrotic range proteinuria [9].

Risk Factors for Recurrence and Treatment of C3G Recurrence

C3G recurs at a high rate in transplant allografts with graft loss due to C3G in approximately 50% of those patients [9]. Patients/families should be clearly counseled on the high risk for disease recurrence with C3G. The reported recurrence rate of C3GN is typically estimated as greater than 50% [34, 35]. The recurrence rate of dense deposit disease (DDD) is much higher and approaches approximately 80 to 100% [36, 37].

Age at transplantation may be a risk factor for poorer graft survival, with pediatric patients experiencing lower long-term graft survival. It has been hypothesized that this may be due to more significant complement disruption and aggressive disease in pediatric patients as compared to the adult population. One case series demonstrated a 10-year graft survival in only 8 of 72 (11%) pediatric allograft recipients, in contrast to 22 of 107 (20.6%) adult recipients [38].

Pretransplant C3 levels may also predict graft outcomes. In one small case series, six of eight patients with recurrent C3GN had very low pre-transplantation C3 levels (median 1.65 µmol/l; normal range 3.75–8.75 µmol/l) compared to those with low or near-normal C3 levels [39]. Other factors associated with an increased risk of C3G recurrence include high levels of circulating autoantibodies (C3 nephritic factor and factor H autoantibody), rapid progression to ESKD in the native kidneys (crescentic disease), and living-related kidney transplantation [40].

Diagnosis of C3G recurrence requires pathological features of the disease and should be supported by clinical history. Following transplant, patients with a history of C3G should be closely followed for signs of recurrence including proteinuria, hematuria, dropping C3, and/or elevated creatinine. Up to 90% of C3G allograft recipients will show histological C3 deposition [37, 41]. Data support that protocol biopsies from C3G transplant recipients can show deposition of C3 as early as the first month post-transplant in the absence of clinical disease [41, 42]. Furthermore, glomerular C3 deposition in the absence of other clinicopathological findings is independently associated with a higher risk of allograft failure [42].

Unfortunately, even when recurrence is diagnosed early, therapeutic options in the setting of recurrence are very limited. The decision to utilize any therapy for C3G recurrence should be done in parallel with clinical and pathological data as well as comprehensive complement biomarker assessment. There is insufficient data to recommend routine use of plasma exchange for C3G recurrence unless there is an identified complement factor deficiency or autoantibody, such as complement factor H [9, 30]. Insufficient data exist to support routine use of eculizumab for C3G recurrence [9, 30]. One study [43, 44] suggests that the lowest incidence of allograft loss (33%) among patients with recurrent C3G is found among those who were treated with eculizumab. Among those who received no treatment for C3G due to stable allograft function, there is a high incidence of allograft loss of 32% in C3GN and 53% in DDD [43]. Consideration to plasma exchange and/or eculizumab should incorporate assessment of patient complement biomarkers [43]. For example, soluble membrane attack complex (sMAC) levels may help to select good responders to eculizumab.

Due to the mechanistic complexity of C3G, there may not be a single therapeutic option, such as eculizumab for aHUS, that provides comprehensive treatment for C3G recurrence. More promising, perhaps, is the development of complement inhibitors (e.g., inhibition of C3 or complement factor B) which could provide targeted therapy for recurrence of C3G following transplant. Early clinical trial (phase II) data for the novel complement factor B agent, LNP023, demonstrate resolution of proteinuria and stability of kidney function in native kidneys [45]. Data from allograft recipients with C3G recurrence have not been published at the time of this chapter. With the current lack of treatment options for C3G recurrence post-transplant, loss of a prior graft due to recurrent C3G indicates a high risk of recurrence upon subsequent transplantation, and this factor should be a major consideration in determining candidacy for retransplant [40].

IgA Nephropathy

Nature and Frequency of IgA Nephropathy (IgAN)

IgAN is characterized by a highly variable course ranging from a benign condition to rapidly progressive renal failure. IgAN affects 10–20% of the world population, rendering IgAN the most prevalent primary chronic glomerular disease worldwide [46]. Prevalence of IgAN differs among populations of different ancestries, being most frequent among persons of Asian descent, rare in those of African descent, and with an intermediate prevalence among those with European descent.

IgAN is thought to occur due to a primary, inherited defect leading to preferential production of IgA with galactose-deficient O-glycans in the hinge region. IgA deficient in galactose elicits the production of antiglycan autoantibodies that lead to the formation and subsequent glomerular deposition of immune complexes. IgA-based activation of alternative complement pathway plays a critical role in the pathogenesis of IgAN; for example, C3 is frequently involved in the formation of circulating immune deposits inducing mesangial stress, podocyte damage, and progressive deterioration of kidney function. On this basis, IgAN can be classified as an autoimmune glomerular disease. While the pathogenesis of the disease resulting in IgA1 subclass deficient in galactose is not completely clarified, genome-wide association studies have identified multiple susceptibility loci for IgAN implicating independent defects in adaptive and innate immunity and alternative complement pathways that potentially influence the different pathogenetic steps toward the development of disease [47].

IgAN generally runs an indolent course with a 10-year native kidney survival rate of 90% in adults and children with normal renal function at diagnosis; however, 71% of patients will develop hematuria or proteinuria in upwards of 20 years follow-up [48]. Clinical risk factors for progression to ESKD include heavy proteinuria, decreased eGFR at diagnosis, and uncontrolled hypertension, although the ability to accurately predict individual patient-level risk remains limited [49].

Risk Factors for Recurrence

The reported frequency of histologic or clinically significant recurrence of IgAN post-transplantation varies in the literature. An excellent review of recurrence rates can be found by Moroni et al. (2019) [50]. The recurrence rate reported in 2393 patients with IgAN in the large registry study of Australia and New Zealand (ANZDATA) was 5.4% and 10.8% at 5 and 10 years, respectively, with a median time to recurrence of 4.63 (IQR, 2.12–8.66) years [51]. The same ANZDATA registry showed no increased risk of recurrence in a second graft after loss of a first graft to recurrence despite prior reports of increased risk.

Recurrence of IgAN can be "histologic only" when diagnosed on protocol biopsies in asymptomatic patients or "clinical" when associated with urinary abnormalities and/or graft dysfunction. Histologic recurrence in protocol biopsies in adults, with or without evidence of clinical disease, is common with IgA mesangial deposition being found in up to 32 to 58% of grafts [52, 53]. In children with IgAN, the recurrence of IgA deposits in the graft following transplantation is very common, but clinically relevant recurrent disease has been reported to be infrequent [54]. Hematuria, the hallmark of IgAN in the native kidney, is not a reliable manifestation of recurrence being absent in 52% of cases diagnosed by protocol biopsy [52]. Given the lack of a prospective study involving allograft protocol biopsies in pediatric transplant recipients, the true risk of significant graft dysfunction and/or graft loss from recurrent disease in the pediatric population remains unclear.

No single parameter including age, gender, race, donor source, HLA typing, pre-transplant course, or biochemical characteristics of serum IgA has been shown to reliably predict recurrence. Risk factors for recurrence in IgAN have been suggested to be younger age at transplant, male gender, and rapidly progressive course of original disease, but there is no consensus. Furthermore, one study of native kidney biopsies in adults with IgAN showed that younger age at onset of IgAN and greater burden of crescents in the native kidney biopsy predicted recurrence after transplant [55]. Longer time following transplantation may also be a risk factor for disease recurrence and supports the suggestion that recurrence may be a time-dependent event; the longer the follow-up, the higher the probability of recurrence [53]. The relationship between donor type and recurrence of disease is discussed below.

Considerations for Transplant Planning

The relationship between the risk of recurrence and the donor type remains controversial with conflicting reports in the literature [56–61]. There have been no large, prospective studies defining the risk of recurrence in patients with IgAN who receive either living donor or deceased donor renal allograft, although there are large registry reports. In transplants performed in 1354 recipients with IgAN (488 living donors), the ANZDAT registry found that recurrence was significantly more frequent in the 108 zero HLA-mismatched living donors at 17% vs 7% in the cohort overall. In this report, graft survival did not differ compared to those with one or more HLA mismatches (and no recurrence) suggesting loss of the survival advantage expected with zero HLA-mismatched transplants [62]. The authors concluded that despite increased recurrence risk, since graft survivals were similar, there is no reason to avoid living donor-recipient pairs with zero HLA-mismatches in IgAN. In the same study by Mc Donald et al., no differences were seen in recurrence rates in those with HLA B12, B35, or DR4. A more recent report from the same registry, spanning 28 years and including 2393 patients with IgAN, showed a 10-year recurrence rate of 16.7% in living donors compared to 7.1% in living unrelated donors and 9.2% with deceased donors with a HR of 1.7 for living related vs deceased donors ($p = 0.0005$) [63].

Genome-wide association studies (GWAS) have identified abnormalities in the complement factor H (CFH) and CFH-related (CFHR) genes in patients with IgAN

[47, 64, 65]. Although it is unclear whether these variants increase the risk of recurrence following transplant, familial IgAN should be rigorously excluded in potential living-related donors since familial IgAN is associated with a high risk of development of renal failure in affected members [66].

The effect of immunosuppression regimen on IgAN recurrence risk is unclear. Despite initial enthusiasm, newer immunosuppressants seem ineffective in preventing recurrence [67]. Retrospective data suggest that induction with anti-thymocyte or anti-lymphocyte globulin is associated with a lower risk of recurrence compared to interleukin receptor-2 blockade [68–70].

In children, steroid avoidance has become a major goal in pediatric kidney transplantation and has been safely practiced in select transplant recipients [71, 72]. There are conflicting reports relating to the effect of rapid steroid withdrawal or steroid avoidance on recurrence risk and graft survival. In a retrospective analysis of adults with IgAN in the Organ Procurement and Transplantation Network/United Network for Organ Sharing (OPTN/UNOS) database, early steroid withdrawal was associated with statistically increased risk of recurrence compared to patients in the steroid continuation group. Patient survival and death-censored graft survival were not different [73]. Similarly, in a report from the analysis of the ANZDATA registry of adult recipients of a primary transplant with IgAN, steroid use was strongly associated with a reduced risk of recurrence, after adjusting for age, sex, HLA mismatch, dialysis duration, and transplant era [74]. In this report, 12.6% of graft loss was attributed to recurrence. A study of pediatric patients within the OPTN database conversely reported that children with a pre-transplant diagnosis of glomerular kidney disease receiving a steroid avoidance regimen did not experience an increased risk of graft failure, although this study of children in the OPTN database was unable to differentiate recurrence rates in the varying disease cohorts [75].

Treatment of IgAN Recurrence

Just as with native kidney IgAN, no clear course of therapy for recurrent IgAN following transplantation has been shown to be effective. In the setting of disease recurrence, KDIGO guidelines for the care of transplant recipients recommend treatment strategies to reduce proteinuria and optimize blood pressure as well as to reduce inflammation [76].

Use of corticosteroids as well as rituximab to treat recurrence in small numbers of patients has been described [77–79]. Data from Japan have reported favorable outcomes after tonsillectomy in patients with recurrent IgAN, but these results have not been confirmed in other ethnicities [80–82]. The effect of fish oil on recurrent IgAN has not been systematically examined for risk reduction or treatment of IgAN. Fellstrom et al. reported a reduction in proteinuria and stabilization of kidney function after budesonide administration in native kidney IgAN patients, possibly by targeting the intestinal mucosa directly, suggesting a possible role in patients with recurrence post-transplant [83].

Impact of IgAN on Graft Function and Survival

Recurrent disease was thought to have little impact on graft outcomes; however, recent studies with longer duration of follow-up suggest that recurrent disease may contribute substantially to allograft injury. The rate of graft loss due to recurrence of IgAN varies based on time from transplant with less early graft loss attributed to IgAN and significantly more at 10-year post-transplant [52, 54]. True estimates of graft loss purely attributable to disease recurrence are difficult, given the interplay of acute or chronic rejection or calcineurin toxicity particularly if histology close to the time of graft loss is not available [53, 84, 85].

IgA Vasculitis (Henoch-Schonlein Purpura)

Current available data suggest that the recurrence rate of IgA vasculitis (IgAV) after transplantation is similar to that of IgAN, although data are limited. A matched retrospective cohort study of 339 patients with the diagnosis of IgAV/Henoch-Schonlein purpura (HSP) in the UNOS/OPTN data base reported graft failure from recurrent disease in 13.6% but no difference in 10-year allograft survival compared to the matched cohort [86].

In a study from six European transplant centers [87], overall graft survival rates were 84%, 66%, and 56% at 5, 10, and 15 years, respectively. Histologic recurrence occurred in 33% on for-cause biopsies. Clinical recurrence occurred in five patients at a median time of 96 months post-transplant. Graft loss occurred in three patients resulting in an actuarial risk of graft loss from recurrence in a first graft of 7.5% at 10-year post-transplant. Severity of disease at presentation and type of immunosuppression post-transplant did not affect recurrence. Although not reaching significance, 60% of those with clinically significant recurrence had living donors compared to 16% of living donors in the cohort who did not experience recurrence.

Lupus Nephritis

Nature and Frequency of Disease

Systemic lupus erythematosus (SLE) is an autoimmune inflammatory disease that is characterized by antibodies directed against self-antigens, resulting in multi-organ damage. Involvement of lupus within the kidney is termed lupus nephritis (LN). Systemic lupus erythematosus (SLE) in children is usually more severe than it is in adults and there is a higher incidence of kidney involvement [88, 89]. Lupus nephritis is responsible for approximately 3% of ESKD leading to transplant in North America [90].

The presence of lupus nephritis increases patient morbidity due to the effects of high-dose immunosuppression, renal dysfunction, and hypertension on the brain, cardiovascular system, and the bones during growth and development [91]. Despite immunosuppression, only 55% of childhood SLE patients with proliferative LN (class III and IV) will achieve remission of lupus nephritis [92–94]. Furthermore, while the vast majority of childhood SLE patients with class V LN achieve renal remission, only 76% can maintain remission despite low-dose oral corticosteroids and/or maintenance immunosuppression such as azathioprine or mycophenolate mofetil [95, 96]. Risk factors for development of ESKD due to LN include class IV LN, male gender, black race, hypertension, nephrotic syndrome, anti-phospholipid antibodies, high glomerular staining for monocyte chemoattractant protein-1 (MCP-1), chronicity on biopsy, poor response to induction therapy, and occurrence of nephritic kidney flare [94, 97].

Risk for Disease Recurrence

The reported risk for recurrent lupus nephritis (RLN) after renal transplantation has been quite variable, ranging from very low (<5% [40]) to between 30 and 50% [98] in studies implementing protocol biopsies to evaluate prospectively for recurrence. The variability in reported recurrence rates has been attributed to varying indications for renal allograft biopsy across transplant centers, single-center versus registry-based study design, follow-up duration, and varying ethnicities represented in study samples [99].

Large-scale data derived from UNOS between 1987 and 2006 estimated period prevalence as well as predictors of RLN and assessed the effects of RLN on both allograft failure and recipient survival [100]. The period prevalence of RLN within the cohort was 2.44% with 167 out of 6850 recipients experiencing RLN. Non-Hispanic black race, female gender, and age < 33 years were each independent risk factors for RLN. Moroni et al. suggest that pre-transplant antiphospholipid autoantibodies confer a higher risk for RLN [101].

Considerations for Transplant Planning

Data are mixed regarding the impact of donor type on RLN. Historical data from over thirty years ago suggest that grafts from deceased donors are a better option for transplantation patients with lupus nephritis than grafts from living-related donors with lower 1-year survival in those with living donation – thought presumably due to the possibility of familial inheritance through the HLA system [102, 103]. In contrast, more recent large-scale data show no difference in graft loss observed between the two types of donors [104].

Pre-transplant clinical condition and past immunosuppressive history may be more considerable factors in transplant planning. KDIGO guidelines recommend that lupus activity should be clinically quiescent and/or that the patient is receiving minimal (no) immunosuppression prior to transplantation [40]. Transplant nephrologists may need to delay time to transplantation for those patients who have received pre-transplant immunosuppression or long-term glucocorticoid therapy to minimize the cumulative risk of prior therapy on top of the need for potent induction of immunosuppression at the time of transplant [105]. As noted previously, the presence of antiphospholipid autoantibodies should be carefully considered in transplant planning due to the risk of vascular thrombosis and early graft failure [106, 107]. Anticoagulation in the peri- and post-transplant period should be considered to reduce the risk of vascular thrombosis [40, 108]; however, this risk should be weighed in the context of complications due to bleeding in the immediate post-transplant period [107].

The basic post-transplant immunosuppression for LN patients does not differ from that normally used in management. Data from the OPTN/UNOS database were utilized to compare the rates of graft loss due to disease recurrence between transplant patients receiving cyclosporine plus azathioprine (CSA + AZA) and those receiving cyclosporine plus mycophenolate mofetil (CSA + MMF) [109]. There was no difference in the rates of allograft loss due to RLN among recipients receiving either CSA + AZA or CSA + MMF maintenance immunosuppressive therapy at 10-year follow-up. In patients with LN recurrence, an intensification of immunosuppression should be reserved for the exceptional cases showing a severe (life threatening) lupus flare due to the potential risks of serious or lethal infection post-transplant [99].

Impact of RLN on Graft Function and Survival

Retrospective multi-center data from the North American Pediatric Renal Transplant Cooperative Study (NAPRTCS) database demonstrated that kidney transplant outcomes in young patients with LN were comparable to those seen in an age-, ancestry-, and gender-matched control group, in spite of an unexplained increase in recurrent rejections in the living donor LN patients [110].Contreras et al. (2010) evaluated the rates of graft failure using an analysis of UNOS data [100]. Graft failure occurred in 156 (93%) of those with RLN, 1517 (86%) of those with rejection, and 923 (19%) of control subjects without rejection. Although recipients with RLN had a fourfold greater risk for graft failure compared with control subjects without rejection, only 7% of graft failure episodes were attributable to RLN compared and 43% to rejection. Mortality was similar (11–18%) between those with RLN, rejection, and controls.

Other Diseases

Primary Hyperoxaluria Type 1 (Oxalosis)

Primary hyperoxaluria type 1 (PH1) is an autosomal recessive disease caused by a deficiency of hepatic alanine glyoxylate aminotransferase (AGT) [111, 112]. The enzyme AGT catalyzes the conversion of glyoxylate to glycine such that deficiency of AGT leads to significant overproduction of oxalate. This results in extremely elevated urinary excretion of monohydrated calcium oxalate leading to urolithiasis and nephrocalcinosis, insoluble oxalates deposition throughout the body (particularly blood vessels and skeleton), and development of CKD/ESKD [113, 114]. Since the metabolic defect in PH1 involves deficiency of a hepatic enzyme, liver transplant will reverse the metabolic abnormality responsible for PH1 and lessen the risk of PH1 within the transplanted kidney. Liver transplant can be performed synchronously or asynchronously with kidney transplant. Synchronous liver-kidney transplant provides improved death-censored graft survival compared with kidney transplant alone [113, 115]; however, sequential (asynchronous) liver-kidney transplant can be performed, whereby the patient receives a liver transplant followed by a prolonged period of hemodialysis to fully clear extra-systemic oxalate before kidney transplantation [116–118]. Without liver transplantation prior to kidney transplant, graft (kidney) survival is less than 50% at 5 years [113, 119].

Membranous Nephropathy

The clinical phenotype of recurrent membranous nephropathy (MN) may vary widely in severity from a subclinical finding on biopsy, proteinuric nephrotic syndrome associated with features of MN on biopsy, and/or graft loss due to autoantibody-mediated injury. Recommendations from KDIGO support that patients with membranous nephropathy should not be excluded from transplant evaluation; however, the risk for recurrence should be considered and reviewed with the patient [40]. MN is estimated to recur in anywhere between 10% and 50% of patients transplanted with primary MN [120–122]. Recurrence of MN is thought to be, most frequently, caused by the recurrence of autoantibody that catalyzed primary MN within the native kidneys (e.g., anti-phospholipase A2 receptor (anti-PLA2R)) leading to subsequent post-transplant injury within the transplanted kidney [123].

PLA2R autoantibodies should be measured prior to transplant to inform the risk for MN recurrence [40]. Patients with high anti-PLA2R levels or severe proteinuria in the pre-transplant period should be closely monitored for disease recurrence after transplant [121, 124, 125]. Following transplant, proteinuria and anti-PLA2R titers should be followed closely. Consideration should be given to surveillance biopsy for patients with MN necessitating transplant. Adult data suggest that centers performing surveillance transplant biopsies are more likely to detect asymptomatic, recurrent MN earlier compared to centers that do not perform surveillance biopsies [126–128]. Electron microscopy is necessary to confirm the diagnosis of recurrent MN as light microscopy abnormalities, such as membrane spikes, may not be observed in early disease relapse.

Prophylactic therapy with rituximab or alkylating agents is not recommended to prevent disease [40]; however, rituximab has utility in treating biopsy-proven, recurrent disease [121, 123].

Conclusion

Transplant planning and care require a thorough understanding of the underlying cause of ESKD. In most instances, the risk of disease recurrence is low; however, exceptions are notable in the case of complement-mediated kidney disease where risk for disease recurrence may be greater than 50%. As reviewed here, the majority of patients with recurrent disease due to glomerulonephritis still have generally equivalent graft and patient survival compared to those with non-recurrent etiologies, such as congenital anomalies of the kidney and urinary tract. With rare exceptions, living-related kidney donation can and should still be encouraged in carefully selected patients and donors.

Certainly, the management of disease recurrence after pediatric kidney transplant remains challenging; however, emerging therapies for high-risk diseases, such as aHUS and C3G, provide hope for improved graft survival among these pediatric kidney diseases at highest risk for recurrence following transplantation. Our understanding of recurrent disease risk and treatment(s) is limited by the lack of systematic, randomized studies – particularly in pediatric patients. Thus, systematic use of international registries and prospective multi-center collaborative studies is absolutely necessary to allow improvement in pre-transplantation risk evaluation and facilitate data-driven yet individualized post-transplantation management.

References

1. Cochat P, et al. Disease recurrence in paediatric renal transplantation. Pediatr Nephrol. 2009;24(11):2297–108.
2. Van Stralen KJ, et al. Impact of graft loss among kidney diseases with a high risk of post-transplant recurrence in the paediatric population. Nephrology Dialysis Transplantation. 2013;28(4):1031–8.
3. Hart A, et al. OPTN/SRTR 2018 Annual Data Report: Kidney. Am J Transplant. 2020;20(Suppl s1):20 130.
4. Yan K, et al. Epidemiology of atypical Hemolytic uremic syndrome: a systematic literature review. Clin Epidemiol. 2020;12:295–305.
5. Jenssen GR, et al. Incidence and etiology of hemolytic-uremic syndrome in children in Norway, 1999-2008--a retrospective study of hospital records to assess the sensitivity of surveillance. BMC Infect Dis. 2014;14:265.
6. Servais A, et al. Acquired and genetic complement abnormalities play a critical role in dense deposit disease and other C3 glomerulopathies. Kidney Int. 2012;82(4):454–64.
7. Thurman JM, Nester CM. All things complement. Clin J Am Soc Nephrol. 2016;11(10):1856–66.
8. Rother RP, et al. Discovery and development of the complement inhibitor eculizumab for the treatment of paroxysmal nocturnal hemoglobinuria. Nat Biotechnol. 2007;25(11):1256–64.
9. Goodship TH, et al. Atypical hemolytic uremic syndrome and C3 glomerulopathy: conclusions from a "kidney disease: improving global outcomes" (KDIGO) controversies conference. Kidney Int. 2017;91(3):539–51.
10. Povey H, et al. Renal recovery with eculizumab in atypical hemolytic uremic syndrome following prolonged dialysis. Clin Nephrol. 2014;82(5):326–31.
11. Licht C, et al. Efficacy and safety of eculizumab in atypical hemolytic uremic syndrome from 2-year extensions of phase 2 studies. Kidney Int. 2015;87(5):1061–73.

12. Feitz WJC, et al. The genetics of atypical hemolytic uremic syndrome. Med Genet. 2018;30(4):400–9.
13. Fremeaux-Bacchi V, et al. Genetics and outcome of atypical hemolytic uremic syndrome: a nationwide French series comparing children and adults. Clin J Am Soc Nephrol. 2013;8(4):554–62.
14. Noris M, et al. Relative role of genetic complement abnormalities in sporadic and familial aHUS and their impact on clinical phenotype. Clin J Am Soc Nephrol. 2010;5(10):1844–59.
15. Zuber J, et al. Use of eculizumab for atypical haemolytic uraemic syndrome and C3 glomerulopathies. Nat Rev Nephrol. 2012;8(11):643–57.
16. Loirat C, Fremeaux-Bacchi V. Hemolytic uremic syndrome recurrence after renal transplantation. Pediatr Transplant. 2008;12(6):619–29.
17. Noris M, Ruggenenti P, Remuzzi G. Kidney transplantation in patients with atypical Hemolytic uremic syndrome: a therapeutic dilemma (or not)? Am J Kidney Dis. 2017;70(6):754–7.
18. Zuber J, et al. New insights into postrenal transplant hemolytic uremic syndrome. Nat Rev Nephrol. 2011;7(1):23–35.
19. Loirat C, et al. An international consensus approach to the management of atypical hemolytic uremic syndrome in children. Pediatr Nephrol. 2016;31(1):15–39.
20. Noris M, Remuzzi G. Managing and preventing atypical hemolytic uremic syndrome recurrence after kidney transplantation. Curr Opin Nephrol Hypertens. 2013;22(6):704–12.
21. Renner B, et al. Cyclosporine induces endothelial cell release of complement-activating microparticles. J Am Soc Nephrol. 2013;24(11):1849–62.
22. Duineveld C, et al. Living donor kidney transplantation in atypical Hemolytic uremic syndrome: a case series. Am J Kidney Dis. 2017;70(6):770–7.
23. Artz MA, et al. Renal transplantation in patients with hemolytic uremic syndrome: high rate of recurrence and increased incidence of acute rejections. Transplantation. 2003;76(5):821–6.
24. Verhave JC, Wetzels JF, van de Kar NC. Novel aspects of atypical haemolytic uraemic syndrome and the role of eculizumab. Nephrol Dial Transplant. 2014;29(Suppl 4):iv131–41.
25. Noris M, Remuzzi G. Atypical hemolytic-uremic syndrome. N Engl J Med. 2009;361(17):1676–87.
26. Wijnsma KL, et al. Eculizumab in atypical hemolytic uremic syndrome: strategies toward restrictive use. Pediatr Nephrol. 2019;34(11):2261–77.
27. Benamu E, Montoya JG. Infections associated with the use of eculizumab: recommendations for prevention and prophylaxis. Curr Opin Infect Dis. 2016;29(4):319–29.
28. Nester CM, Smith RJ. Complement inhibition in C3 glomerulopathy. Semin Immunol. 2016;28(3):241–9.
29. Sethi S, et al. C3 glomerulonephritis: clinicopathological findings, complement abnormalities, glomerular proteomic profile, treatment, and follow-up. Kidney Int. 2012;82(4):465–73.
30. Pickering MC, et al. C3 glomerulopathy: consensus report. Kidney Int. 2013;84(6):1079–89.
31. Hou J, et al. Toward a working definition of C3 glomerulopathy by immunofluorescence. Kidney Int. 2014;85(2):450–6.
32. Smith RJ, et al. New approaches to the treatment of dense deposit disease. J Am Soc Nephrol. 2007;18(9):2447–56.
33. Smith RJH, et al. C3 glomerulopathy – understanding a rare complement-driven renal disease. Nat Rev Nephrol. 2019;15(3):129–43.
34. Denton MD, Singh AK. Recurrent and de novo glomerulonephritis in the renal allograft. Semin Nephrol. 2000;20(2):164–75.
35. Floege J. Recurrent glomerulonephritis following renal transplantation: an update. Nephrol Dial Transplant. 2003;18(7):1260–5.
36. Braun MC, et al. Recurrence of membranoproliferative glomerulonephritis type II in renal allografts: the north American Pediatric renal transplant cooperative study experience. J Am Soc Nephrol. 2005;16(7):2225–33.
37. Zand L, et al. Clinical findings, pathology, and outcomes of C3GN after kidney transplantation. J Am Soc Nephrol. 2014;25(5):1110–7.

38. Angelo JR, Bell CS, Braun MC. Allograft failure in kidney transplant recipients with membranoproliferative glomerulonephritis. Am J Kidney Dis. 2011;57(2):291–9.
39. Alasfar S, et al. Membranoproliferative glomerulonephritis recurrence after kidney transplantation: using the new classification. BMC Nephrol. 2016;17:7.
40. Chadban SJ, et al. KDIGO clinical practice guideline on the evaluation and management of candidates for kidney transplantation. Transplantation. 2020;104(4S1 Suppl 1):S11–S103.
41. Lu DF, et al. Clinical features and outcomes of 98 children and adults with dense deposit disease. Pediatr Nephrol. 2012;27(5):773–81.
42. Panzer SE, et al. Glomerular C3 deposition is an independent risk factor for allograft failure in kidney transplant recipients with transplant Glomerulopathy. Kidney Int Rep. 2019;4(4):582–93.
43. Gonzalez Suarez ML, et al. Treatment of C3 glomerulopathy in adult kidney transplant recipients: a systematic review. Med Sci (Basel). 2020;8(4)
44. Gonzalez Suarez ML, et al. Outcomes of kidney transplant patients with atypical hemolytic uremic syndrome treated with eculizumab: a systematic review and meta-analysis. J Clin Med. 2019;8(7)
45. Wong EK, et al. LNP023: a novel oral complement alternative pathway factor b inhibitor safely and effectively reduces proteinuria in C3 glomerulopathy. In: American Society of Nephrology. Virtual; 2020.
46. Donadio JV, Grande JP. IgA nephropathy. N Engl J Med. 2002;347(10):738–48.
47. Gharavi AG, et al. Genome-wide association study identifies susceptibility loci for IgA nephropathy. Nat Genet. 2011;43(4):321–U68.
48. Ronkainen J, et al. Long-term outcome 19 years after childhood IgA nephritis: a retrospective cohort study. Pediatr Nephrol. 2006;21(9):1266–73.
49. Barbour SJ, Reich HN. Risk stratification of patients with IgA nephropathy. Am J Kidney Dis. 2012;59(6):865–73.
50. Moroni G, et al. Immunoglobulin A nephropathy. Recurrence after renal transplantation. Front Immunol. 2019:10.
51. Jiang SH, Kennard AL, Walters GD. Recurrent glomerulonephritis following renal transplantation and impact on graft survival. BMC Nephrol. 2018;19
52. Ortiz F, et al. IgA nephropathy recurs early in the graft when assessed by protocol biopsy. Nephrol Dial Transplant. 2012;27(6):2553–8.
53. Odum J, et al. Recurrent Mesangial Iga nephritis following renal-transplantation. Nephrol Dial Transplant. 1994;9(3):309–12.
54. Habib R, et al. Glomerular-lesions in the transplanted kidney in children. Am J Kidney Dis. 1987;10(3):198–207.
55. Avasare RS, et al. Predicting post-transplant recurrence of IgA nephropathy: the importance of crescents. Am J Nephrol. 2017;45(2):99–106.
56. Andresdottir MB, et al. Exclusive characteristics of graft survival and risk factors in recipients with immunoglobulin a nephropathy: a retrospective analysis of registry data. Transplantation. 2005;80(8):1012–8.
57. Wang AY, et al. Recurrent IgA nephropathy in renal transplant allografts. Am J Kidney Dis. 2001;38(3):588–96.
58. Freese P, et al. Clinical risk factors for recurrence of IgA nephropathy. Clin Transpl. 1999;13(4):313–7.
59. Han SS, et al. Impact of recurrent disease and chronic allograft nephropathy on the long-term allograft outcome in patients with IgA nephropathy. Transpl Int. 2010;23(2):169–75.
60. Kim YS, et al. Live donor renal allograft in end-stage renal failure patients from immunoglobulin a nephropathy. Transplantation. 2001;71(2):233–8.
61. Ponticelli C, et al. Kidney transplantation in patients with IgA mesangial glomerulonephritis. Kidney Int. 2001;60(5):1948–54.
62. McDonald SP, Russ GR. Recurrence of IgA nephropathy among renal allograft recipients from living donors is greater among those with zero HLA mismatches. Transplantation. 2006;82(6):759–62.

63. Kennard AL, Jiang SH, Walters GD. Increased glomerulonephritis recurrence after living related donation. BMC Nephrol. 2017;18(1):25.
64. Kiryluk K, et al. Discovery of new risk loci for IgA nephropathy implicates genes involved in immunity against intestinal pathogens. Nat Genet. 2014;46(11):1187–96.
65. Zhai YL, et al. Rare variants in the complement factor H-related protein 5 gene contribute to genetic susceptibility to IgA nephropathy. J Am Soc Nephrol. 2016;27(9):2894–905.
66. Schena FP, et al. Increased risk of end-stage renal disease in familial IgA nephropathy. J Am Soc Nephrol. 2002;13(2):453–60.
67. Chandrakantan A, et al. Recurrent IgA nephropathy after renal transplantation despite immunosuppressive regimens with mycophenolate mofetil. Nephrol Dial Transplant. 2005;20(6):1214–21.
68. Berthoux F, et al. Antithymocyte globulin (ATG) induction therapy and disease recurrence in renal transplant recipients with primary IgA nephropathy. Transplantation. 2008;85(10):1505–7.
69. Berthoux F, et al. Prognostic value of serum biomarkers of autoimmunity for recurrence of IgA nephropathy after kidney transplantation. J Am Soc Nephrol. 2017;28(6):1943–50.
70. Pascual J, et al. Alemtuzumab induction and recurrence of glomerular disease after kidney transplantation. Transplantation. 2007;83(11):1429–34.
71. Nehus E, Goebel J, Abraham E. Outcomes of steroid-avoidance protocols in pediatric kidney transplant recipients. Am J Transplant. 2012;12(12):3441–8.
72. Zhang H, et al. Steroid avoidance or withdrawal regimens in paediatric kidney transplantation: a meta-analysis of randomised controlled trials. PLoS One. 2016;11(3):e0146523.
73. Leeaphorn N, et al. Recurrence of IgA nephropathy after kidney transplantation in steroid continuation versus early steroid-withdrawal regimens: a retrospective analysis of the UNOS/OPTN database. Transpl Int. 2018;31(2):175–86.
74. Clayton P, McDonald S, Chadban S. Steroids and recurrent IgA nephropathy after kidney transplantation. Am J Transplant. 2011;11(8):1645–9.
75. Nehus EJ, et al. Graft survival of pediatric kidney transplant recipients selected for de novo steroid avoidance-a propensity score-matched study. Nephrol Dial Transplant. 2017;32(8):1424–31.
76. Kasiske BL, et al. KDIGO clinical practice guideline for the care of kidney transplant recipients: a summary. Kidney Int. 2010;77(4):299–311.
77. Messina M, et al. Treatment protocol with pulse and oral steroids for IgA nephropathy after kidney transplantation. J Nephrol. 2016;29(4):575–83.
78. Matsukuma Y, et al. Effect of steroid pulse therapy on post-transplant immunoglobulin a nephropathy. Nephrology (Carlton). 2018;23(Suppl 2):10–6.
79. Chancharoenthana W, et al. Rituximab for recurrent IgA nephropathy in kidney transplantation: a report of three cases and proposed mechanisms. Nephrology (Carlton). 2017;22(1):65–71.
80. Kennoki T, et al. Proteinuria-reducing effects of tonsillectomy alone in IgA nephropathy recurring after kidney transplantation. Transplantation. 2009;88(7):935–41.
81. Hotta K, et al. Tonsillectomy ameliorates histological damage of recurrent immunoglobulin a nephropathy after kidney transplantation. Nephrology (Carlton). 2013;18(12):808–12.
82. Ushigome H, et al. Efficacy of tonsillectomy for patients with recurrence of IgA nephropathy after kidney transplantation. Clin Transpl. 2009;23(Suppl 20):17–22.
83. Fellstrom BC, et al. Targeted-release budesonide versus placebo in patients with IgA nephropathy (NEFIGAN): a double-blind, randomised, placebo-controlled phase 2b trial. Lancet. 2017;389(10084):2117–27.
84. Briganti EM, et al. Recurrent glomerulonephritis and risk of renal allograft loss. N Engl J Med. 2002;347(19):1531–2.
85. Andresdottir MB, et al. Favorable outcome of renal transplantation in patients with IgA nephropathy. Clin Nephrol. 2001;56(4):279–88.
86. Samuel JP, et al. Long-term outcome of renal transplantation patients with Henoch-Schonlein purpura. Clin J Am Soc Nephrol. 2011;6(8):2034–40.

87. Kanaan N, et al. Recurrence and graft loss after kidney transplantation for henoch-schonlein purpura nephritis: a multicenter analysis. Clin J Am Soc Nephrol. 2011;6(7):1768–72.
88. Amaral B, et al. A comparison of the outcome of adolescent and adult-onset systemic lupus erythematosus. Rheumatology (Oxford). 2014;53(6):1130–5.
89. Feng X, et al. Associations of clinical features and prognosis with age at disease onset in patients with systemic lupus erythematosus. Lupus. 2014;23(3):327–34.
90. North American Pediatric Renal Transplant Cooperative Study Annual Report. 2014.
91. Wenderfer SE, Ruth NM, Brunner HI. Advances in the care of children with lupus nephritis. Pediatr Res. 2017;81(3):406–14.
92. Rianthavorn P, Buddhasri A. Long-term renal outcomes of childhood-onset global and segmental diffuse proliferative lupus nephritis. Pediatr Nephrol. 2015;30(11):1969–76.
93. Askenazi D, et al. Outcomes of children with proliferative lupus nephritis: the role of protocol renal biopsy. Pediatr Nephrol. 2007;22(7):981–6.
94. Lee BS, et al. Clinical outcomes of childhood lupus nephritis: a single center's experience. Pediatr Nephrol. 2007;22(2):222–31.
95. Nathanson S, et al. Prognosis of lupus membranous nephropathy in children. Pediatr Nephrol. 2006;21(8):1113–6.
96. Hugle B, et al. Presentation and outcome of paediatric membranous non-proliferative lupus nephritis. Pediatr Nephrol. 2015;30(1):113–21.
97. Marks SD, et al. Clinicopathological correlations of paediatric lupus nephritis. Pediatr Nephrol. 2007;22(1):77–83.
98. Norby GE, et al. Recurrent lupus nephritis after kidney transplantation: a surveillance biopsy study. Ann Rheum Dis. 2010;69(8):1484–7.
99. Ponticelli C, Moroni G, Glassock RJ. Recurrence of secondary glomerular disease after renal transplantation. Clin J Am Soc Nephrol. 2011;6(5):1214–21.
100. Contreras G, et al. Recurrence of lupus nephritis after kidney transplantation. J Am Soc Nephrol. 2010;21(7):1200–7.
101. Moroni G, et al. The long-term prognosis of renal transplantation in patients with lupus nephritis. Am J Kidney Dis. 2005;45(5):903–11.
102. Winchester RJ, Nunez-Roldan A. Some genetic aspects of systemic lupus erythematosus. Arthritis Rheum. 1982;25(7):833–7.
103. Cats S, et al. Increased vulnerability of the donor organ in related kidney transplants for certain diseases. Transplantation. 1984;37(6):575–9.
104. Albuquerque BC, et al. Outcome and prognosis of patients with lupus nephritis submitted to renal transplantation. Sci Rep. 2019;9(1):11611.
105. Ponticelli C, Moroni G. Renal transplantation in lupus nephritis. Lupus. 2005;14(1):95–8.
106. Wagenknecht DR, et al. Risk of early renal allograft failure is increased for patients with antiphospholipid antibodies. Transpl Int. 2000;13(Suppl 1):S78–81.
107. Vaidya S, Gugliuzza K, Daller JA. Efficacy of anticoagulation therapy in end-stage renal disease patients with antiphospholipid antibody syndrome. Transplantation. 2004;77(7):1046–9.
108. McIntyre JA, Wagenknecht DR. Antiphospholipid antibodies and renal transplantation: a risk assessment. Lupus. 2003;12(7):555–9.
109. Pham PT, Pham PC. The impact of mycophenolate mofetil versus azathioprine as adjunctive therapy to cyclosporine on the rates of renal allograft loss due to glomerular disease recurrence. Nephrol Dial Transplant. 2012;27(7):2965–71.
110. Bartosh SM, Fine RN, Sullivan EK. Outcome after transplantation of young patients with systemic lupus erythematosus: a report of the north American pediatric renal transplant cooperative study. Transplantation. 2001;72(5):973–8.
111. Danpure CJ, Jennings PR. Peroxisomal alanine: glyoxylate aminotransferase deficiency in primary hyperoxaluria type I. FEBS Lett. 1986;201(1):20–4.
112. Danpure CJ, Jennings PR, Watts RW. Enzymological diagnosis of primary hyperoxaluria type 1 by measurement of hepatic alanine: glyoxylate aminotransferase activity. Lancet. 1987;1(8528):289–91.

113. Bergstralh EJ, et al. Transplantation outcomes in primary hyperoxaluria. Am J Transplant. 2010;10(11):2493–501.
114. Leumann E, Hoppe B. The primary hyperoxalurias. J Am Soc Nephrol. 2001;12(9):1986–93.
115. Harambat J, et al. Characteristics and outcomes of children with primary oxalosis requiring renal replacement therapy. Clin J Am Soc Nephrol. 2012;7(3):458–65.
116. Lorenzo V, et al. Presentation and role of transplantation in adult patients with type 1 primary hyperoxaluria and the I244T AGXT mutation: single-center experience. Kidney Int. 2006;70(6):1115–9.
117. Malla I, et al. Two-step transplantation for primary hyperoxaluria: cadaveric liver followed by living donor related kidney transplantation. Pediatr Transplant. 2009;13(6):782–4.
118. Ruder H, et al. Excessive urinary oxalate excretion after combined renal and hepatic transplantation for correction of hyperoxaluria type 1. Eur J Pediatr. 1990;150(1):56–8.
119. Cibrik DM, et al. Renal allograft survival in patients with oxalosis. Transplantation. 2002;74(5):707–10.
120. Dabade TS, et al. Recurrent idiopathic membranous nephropathy after kidney transplantation: a surveillance biopsy study. Am J Transplant. 2008;8(6):1318–22.
121. Grupper A, et al. Recurrent membranous nephropathy after kidney transplantation: treatment and long-term implications. Transplantation. 2016;100(12):2710–6.
122. El-Zoghby ZM, et al. Recurrent idiopathic membranous nephropathy: early diagnosis by protocol biopsies and treatment with anti-CD20 monoclonal antibodies. Am J Transplant. 2009;9(12):2800–7.
123. Leon J, et al. Membranous nephropathy Posttransplantation: an update of the pathophysiology and management. Transplantation. 2019;103(10):1990–2002.
124. Kattah A, et al. Anti-phospholipase a(2) receptor antibodies in recurrent membranous nephropathy. Am J Transplant. 2015;15(5):1349–59.
125. Quintana LF, et al. Antiphospholipase A2 receptor antibody levels predict the risk of Posttransplantation recurrence of membranous nephropathy. Transplantation. 2015;99(8):1709–14.
126. Patel K, et al. De novo membranous nephropathy in renal allograft associated with antibody-mediated rejection and review of the literature. Transplant Proc. 2013;45(9):3424–8.
127. Cosyns JP, et al. Recurrence of membranous nephropathy after renal transplantation: probability, outcome and risk factors. Clin Nephrol. 1998;50(3):144–53.
128. Debiec H, et al. Autoantibodies specific for the phospholipase A2 receptor in recurrent and De novo membranous nephropathy. Am J Transplant. 2011;11(10):2144–52.

Nephrotic Syndrome Challenges: An Old Recurring Problem

9

German Lozano Guzman and Joshua J. Zaritsky

This chapter will address several aspects of disease recurrence in the setting of renal transplantation. Much of the focus will be on nephrotic syndrome and the risk factors for its recurrence after transplant. In addition, some attention will be placed on treatment of disease recurrence.

APOL1

The high incidence of chronic kidney disease (CKD) in those with African ancestry is very well documented [5] and is likely the result of a complex interplay of genetic and environmental factors. In 2008, variations in the APOL1 gene, located on chromosome 22, were linked to an increased risk of kidney disease. Specifically, two variants of APOL1 gene (G1/G2) confer increased risk for non-diabetic kidney disease, and it is thought that the high prevalence of these variants in African descendants is secondary to a natural selection advantage against infection by *Trypanosoma brucei rhodesiense* [6].

APOL1 is a unique gene only found in humans and higher order primates that became part of the human genome around 33 million years ago [7]. It encodes the apolipoprotein L1 protein which is found in circulation mainly associated with high-density lipoprotein (HDL). This complex confers protection against infection by *Trypanosoma brucei* [8]. However, strains of trypanosome parasite such as *T.b. rhodesiense*, *T. brucei,* and *T.b. gambiense* can develop resistance to APOL1-mediated lysis. The APOL1 G1/G2 polymorphisms confer counter resistance to this

G. L. Guzman (✉)
Section of Nephrology St Christopher Hospital, Philadelphia, PA, USA
e-mail: German.lozanoguzman@towerhealth.org

J. J. Zaritsky
Division Chief Section of Nephrology St Christopher Hospital, Philadelphia, PA, USA
e-mail: Joshua.Zaritsky@towerhealth.org

K. E. Twombley (ed.), *Challenges in Pediatric Kidney Transplantation*,
https://doi.org/10.1007/978-3-030-74783-1_9

parasite adaptation, and this likely explains their high prevalence in those of African descendant [9 10]. However, these variants also confer a higher risk of kidney disease via an unclear mechanism, and in this section, we will review the current state of knowledge with a focus on possible implications for kidney transplantation.

Mechanism of Renal Injury

In addition to its circulatory form, the APOL1 protein is expressed in podocytes, proximal tubule cells, and the endothelium of extraglomerular arterioles and small arteries [9]. Initially there was thought that abnormal levels of the circulatory form could be a contributing factor toward the development of kidney disease. However, there does not appear to be a correlation between APOL1 genotype, circulatory APOL1 protein levels, and CKD prevalence [11, 12]. Additionally, APOL1 G1/G2 variants do not appear to influence renal allograft survival [13]. Animal models have instead suggested that the G1/G2 variants induce mitochondrial dysfunction and intracellular potassium loss leading to cell apoptosis via stress-activated protein kinase (SAPK) pathways [14, 15].

Second Hit Modifiers

Despite a body of evidence that the G1/G2 variants can lead to intracellular dysfunction, only 20% of African Americans with them will develop kidney disease. This has given rise to the hypothesis that there needs to be a "2nd" hit for kidney disease to manifest in the setting of these variants. One of the better described "second hits" is HIV infection as patients with the G1/G2 variants have a significantly increased incidence of HIV-associated nephropathy (HIVAN) [16]. Interestingly, there is a decreased risk of kidney disease in JC polyomavirus in G1/G2 patients [17]. Currently both The Chronic Kidney Disease in Children Cohort Study (CiKD) and Nephrotic Syndrome Study Network (NEPTUNE) are actively studying how the G1/G2 variants affect the incidence of FSGS in children with a hypothesis that prematurity could represent a second hit [18].

Clinical Implications

In the current CKiD study, African American children make up 23% of the population with CKD and account for 19% and 36% of the non-glomerular and glomerular disease, respectively. Interestingly in CKiD, patients with glomerular disease have a more rapid decrease in renal function [19] with FSGS as the leading cause of End-Stage Kidney Disease (ESKD) in this group. Given that APOL1 risk alleles in adults are associated with a higher rate of CKD and that allograft failure is higher in African Americans compared to other groups [27], the question remains whether it is beneficial to ascertain APOL1 status prior to kidney transplant.

APOL1 status has a potential implication for both deceased and living donor kidney transplant selection. A kidney transplant from a deceased donor with two copies of the G1/G2 variants has a high graft failure rate when compared to those from donors with only one copy of the risk variant [20, 21], and there are reports of rapid decline of residual kidney function in donors with 2 APOL1 risk variants [22]. This has recently raised significant ethical questions on whether individuals with the risk variants should be allowed to donate.

Currently there is no consensus between transplant centers on the need for APOL1 variations screening nor on how it should alter clinical practice. Clearly before considering establishing APOL1 genetic testing as the standard of care in the transplant setting, there are some aspects that need to be taken into consideration. First is who should be tested? While individuals with West African descent have a high incidence of the G1/G2 variants, those of East African descent have a much lower likelihood of carrying the risk alleles [6]. Individuals from the Caribbean (Dominican Republic, Cuba, Haiti) are less likely to identify as African but often have a West African heritage. Thus, screening for APOL1 variants needs to be individualized on a case-to-case basis.

Assuming a population can be targeted for testing, the next hurdle is the clinical consequences of the results. From the donor perspective, the presence of the APOL1 G1/G2 alleles carries a higher risk of non-diabetic CKD, but this risk is not 100% and it remains unclear who will go on to develop disease. This poor genotype-phenotype correlation makes it extremely difficult to advise those with risk alleles on the ability to donate a kidney. Even if the donor decides not to move forward with donation, a G1/G2 genotype could have medical insurance or even family planning implications. Consider the hypothetical scenario that the presence of APOL1 risk alleles is a contraindication to living donor kidney transplantation (LDKT). This would disproportionally affect an ethnic group that already has decreased access to LDKT [23, 24]. However, since there is evidence of kidney function decline in donors with the risk alleles, some transplant programs now consider it a contraindication to LDKT.

From the recipient perspective, the challenges are focused on the potential risk of receiving a graft from a donor with the G1/G2 alleles. There is evidence that an allograft from a deceased donor with the risk variants has decreased longevity [25, 26]. Most likely this risk exists with LDKT as well. The APOL1 Long-term Kidney Transplantation Outcomes Network (APOLLO) study, a National Institutes of Health (NIH) prospective observation study, is evaluating the effects of APOL1 variants on both deceased- and living-donor renal transplantation. It is due to be completed in 2023 and will hopefully shed much needed light on this issue.

Currently allografts from African American donors have a higher Kidney Donor Risk Index (KDRI). APOL1 genotyping could be used to identify lower risk grafts from this population and in turn facilitate organ allocation. Clearly there is much study to be done on the implications of APOL1 genotyping, and there is hope that studies like APOLLO will help to standardize practice and result in improved transplant outcomes.

Pre-transplant Nephrectomy

Due to the lack of consensus, native kidney nephrectomy prior to kidney transplantation remains a controversial topic. Nephrectomy remains an invasive procedure and comes with a host of potential complications and along with implications on clinical management. The rationale for nephrectomy varies tremendously between adults and children since the etiology of ESKD is biased toward congenital abnormalities of the kidney and urinary tract. In general, these patients continue to have urine output despite ESKD, so a nephrectomy can further complicate fluid management in a population that is very dependent on nutrition for proper growth. While the most common reason for nephrectomy is severe proteinuria, there are some other indications, and this section will address some of the clinical considerations and challenges around this topic.

Proteinuria

Nephrectomy is often advocated in patients with severe proteinuria as the low albumin that accompanies it has been associated with several complications including increased infections and impaired healing and growth. In addition, the nephrotic state comes with an increased risk of thrombosis and thromboembolic events, which can affect the future graft [28–30]. One consideration in the setting of proteinuria is whether a unilateral or bilateral nephrectomy should be performed. Unilateral nephrectomy is an appealing option in pediatrics as the tight fluid restriction that accompanies anuria can present nutritional challenges. Ghane et al. examined 22 pediatric patients who underwent nephrectomy due to severe proteinuria. In the patients that had a unilateral nephrectomy, urine protein excretion decreased from 3.7 to 2.4 g/24 h (158 to 102 mg/m2/h). Serum albumin, total protein, and fibrinogen showed modest increases with most returning to the normal range for the majority of these patients. Patients undergoing bilateral nephrectomies showed larger increases in serum albumin, protein, and fibrinogen concentration, but it was noted that they tended to have more proteinuria to start with, hence needed a more radical approach [32]. Similar results were seen in a European cohort of patients with congenital nephrotic syndrome. Following unilateral nephrectomy serum albumin increased significantly with a reduction in albumin infusion requirements by 5 [29–36] g/kg/week. Interestingly, a comparison of this group with patients who did not undergo nephrectomy and patients undergoing bilateral nephrectomies did not show any differences in complications such as sepsis and thrombotic episodes. Growth was comparable between these three groups. At the end of follow-up, median age was 34 months and 80% of children in the nephrectomy group had been transplanted, while in the non-nephrectomy group only 24% had been transplanted with another 53% remaining off dialysis. This led the authors to postulate that that conservative management is an alternative to early single or even bilateral nephrectomy [4]. Clearly additional prospective studies need to be done in order to elucidate the benefit of unilateral versus bilateral nephrectomy on the management of severe proteinuria.

WT1 Mutation

Another reason to consider pre-transplant nephrectomy is the risk of malignancy such as Wilms' tumor (WT) in patients with WT1 mutations. The WT1 gene is an essential regulator of kidney development, critical to the survival and subsequent differentiation of kidney cells and gonadal development [33]. WT is a heterogeneous tumor with several genetic and epigenetic abnormalities involving oncogenes and tumor suppressor genes like WT1. One of the diseases caused by WT1 mutations is Denys-Drash syndrome (DDS) defined as the clinical triad of congenital/infantile nephrotic syndrome, Wilms' tumor, and ambiguous genitalia. Patients with DDS usually progress to ESKD early in life with renal histopathology exhibiting diffuse mesangial sclerosis or focal segmental glomerulosclerosis (FSGS) [34]. Due to the concern of WT, two main approaches have been taken historically, nephrectomy before or after ESKD has occurred. A recent publication of an international survey indicated that the vast majority of nephrologists prefer to follow serial ultrasounds and only perform nephrectomies after ESKD [35]. In this publication, of the four patients that underwent preemptive nephrectomies, only one had WT identified via pathology. Not unexpectedly those patients had a much shorter median time to dialysis initiation (1–35 months) compared to the group undergoing nephrectomy after ESKD (7–78 months). Given the inherent challenges in beginning dialysis earlier [36] and the fact that most centers require a minimum cutoff weight of 10 kg for transplantation, this leads most nephrologists to take a wait and see approach. Indeed, there can be very variable disease courses in DDS patients with some remaining tumor-free with normal renal function for many years [37]. In our experience the conservative approach with regular interval ultrasound every 3 months and ideally nephrectomy at the time of transplant is preferred, but this decision needs to consider the additional technical challenges at the time of transplant.

Disease Recurrence

Since the initial report by Hoyer et al. [38] in 1972, allograft disease recurrence (DR) has remained a challenge and is the second leading cause of graft loss in this population. FSGS is the most common cause of DR with an estimated incidence of 30% for the first transplant and over 50% in subsequent transplants in which the first graft was lost to the disease [39]. Fortunately, there have been recent advances in our knowledge of recurrence risk which will hopefully reduce DR. In this section we address risk factors and novel treatments of DR.

DR is a devastating event, especially in cases of rapid recurrence and resistance to intensive treatment. In addition, it remains difficult to identify which patients will have DR. One specific disease state, which highlight this, is idiopathic childhood nephrotic syndrome (NS). Current classification of NS is based on the International Study of Kidney Disease in Children (ISKDC) 1967 [40] that recommends the initial use of high dose of steroids for 6–8 weeks. Depending on the response, the patient is classified as: (1) steroid responsive nephrotic syndrome, (2) steroid dependent nephrotic syndrome, or (3) steroid resistance nephrotic syndrome. Patients in the steroid responsive nephrotic group that go into remission within 8 weeks of treatment have a high likelihood of minimal change disease and usually have a better prognosis [41]. However, this simplified approach can prove to be much more complex, since patients initially labeled as steroid responsive can develop resistance later in time and up to 30% of patients with FSGS show an initial response to steroids. In fact, patients with secondary steroid resistance have a higher incidence of DR after transplant than those who were initially steroid resistant [42]. In summary, although an empiric steroid trial is broadly used in clinical practice, it does not necessarily predict which patients will go on to have DR.

Genetic Mutations

Next-generation sequencing has ushered in an era of low-cost rapid screening of patients in which there is a concern for a genetic basis of disease. There is mounting evidence that patients with a known monogenic cause of NS have a much lower rate of DR [43]. To date, over 50 genes have been linked to the pathogenesis of nephrotic syndrome and have allowed gene panels to become a routine part of the pre-transplant evaluation of patients who have ESKD due to nephrotic syndrome. However, the genotype-phenotype relationship is not always clear, especially when variants of unknown pathogenic significance are found. So, while genetic testing shows promise in stratifying patients based on DR, the results must be interpreted in a cautious case by case basis.

Living vs Deceased Donation

Based on largely anecdotal experiences, some centers view FSGS as a contraindication to living-related donation (LRD) due to the high DR rate. However, a recent study of the North American Renal Pediatric Trials and Collaborative Studies (NAPRTCS) database has shown that while allograft survival is worse in patients with FSGS, it is not inferior when LRD is compared to deceased donor (DD) [44]. In other words, while the advantage of the graft survival normally seen with LRD is blunted in patients with FSGS, outcomes are comparable to those without a history of FSGS receiving a DD. Additionally, data from the United States Renal Data System (USRDS) has not shown any differences in DR between LRD and DD [78]. Previous studies showing a positive correlation between LD and disease recurrence may have been the result of selection bias.

Below is one approach to taking into consideration whether a LD should be considered in the setting of ESKD due to nephrotic syndrome:

1. If an autosomal dominant genetic mutation is identified, LD is not recommended since it can have variable penetrance and phenotype expression, placing both the donor and recipient at increased risk.
2. In the cases of an autosomal recessive mutation (with the exclusion of APOL1 variants), LD is a viable option.

3. In cases without an identifiable genetic cause, LD remains a viable option but must include sufficient education of the family as to the risks of DR.

Clinical Features Predictive of DR

One clinical feature that has shown an association with higher DR incidence is pre-transplant nephrectomy [45, 46]. Most likely, this is a reflection of the fact that patients with lower serum albumins, significant proteinuria, and rapid progression to dialysis are more likely to undergo bilateral nephrectomy. In other words, the higher rate of DR is due to underlying aggressive disease rather than bilateral nephrectomy. In fact, probably the most consistent risk factors associated with DR in the literature are early age at the time of diagnosis and degree of proteinuria. Finally, even though no other clinical features show a strong correlation with DR, patients who have an initial aggressive course of disease, mesangial proliferation on biopsy, or being less than 15 years old are considered to be at high risk of DR [47].

Circulating Factor and DR

As discussed previously, an initial steroid responsive course is often predictive of a benign disease course. However, those patients with subsequent steroid resistance show a high rate of DR [48]. One possible explanation for this phenomenon is that this group of patients develops an immune mediated circulating factor. Enforcing the possibility of a circulating factor is a multitude of case reports showing severe recurrent proteinuria occurring immediately after transplantation. One particularly unique case was that of a patient who had immediate DR and subsequent poor graft function. The allograft pathology showed podocyte foot process effacement consistent with the early reappearance of FSGS. Remarkably, re-transplant of the same allograft into a separate patient without a history of FSGS resulted in full resolution of proteinuria and glomerular lesions [49]. Similar results in animal models point to a circulating factor as a mediator of DR in FSGS [50].

To date, identification of this circulating factor remains elusive. Although potential factors, such as suPAR, have been identified, they are not consistently present in all patients with DR [51]. Delville et al. recently identified a panel of seven antibodies (CD40, PTPRO, CGB5, FAS, P2RY11, SNRPB2, and APOL2) that predict DR with 92% accuracy [52]. Unfortunately, this set of bio-markers has not yet been re-validated and is not available for clinical use.

Treatment of Disease Recurrence

Management of disease recurrence remains a controversial topic with little consensus as there is a lack of well-designed randomized controlled trials. The following subsections touch on a variety of treatments.

Plasmapheresis

Therapeutic plasma exchange (TPE) is one of the most widely used modalities to treat recurrent disease in patients with primary FSGS. TPE efficacy is thought to be due to removal of the circulating factor which can be achieved by either centrifugal or filtration-based techniques. In centrifugal TPE (cTPE) blood components are separated utilizing centrifugal forces, and plasma is removed and replaced with 5% albumin or fresh frozen plasma (FFP). In contrast, membrane therapeutic plasma exchange (mTPE) utilizes a highly permeable membrane to achieve plasma separation. Plasma removal efficiency, a measure of how efficient the plasma is removed with a single exchange, is usually much higher in cTPE (~70%) versus mTPE (~30–35%). This results in longer treatment times with mTPE. Another consideration is that cTPE can be performed via peripheral veins using regional citrate anticoagulation whereas mTPE usually needs central access and systemic heparin [53].

The America Society for Apheresis guidelines consider TPE for FSGS recurrence as category 1 (i.e., strong) recommendation [54]. Since its initial use in 1985 [55], it has been the subject of several clinical trials with differing outcomes. A review by Ponticelli et al. showed partial or complete remission of proteinuria using TPE in 70% of children and 63% of adult patients with FSGS recurrence. More encouraging results were seen if therapy was instituted earlier [56]. In a pediatric series, Dall'Amico et al. reported remission in 9 of 11 patients who were treated with TPE in combinations with a cyclophosphamide regimen [57].

Currently, there is no unified consensus on a TPE protocol nor duration of therapy. A common prescription consists of 1–1.5x plasma exchange volume, 3–4 times per week for a total of 8–12 treatments [58]. Other more intensive regimens consist of daily exchanges for 3 days followed by two to three exchanges per week for the first 2 weeks and continue with one or two exchanges per week until partial or complete remission is achieved [56].

There is an immunomodulatory effect associated with TPE with a decline of B and natural killer cells and an increase in regulatory T cells [59]. This effect, which presumably increases the susceptibility of cell mediated and humoral immunity to immunosuppressive agents, is the rationale behind the use of TPE and immunosuppressive medication protocols. Canaud et al. used high dose steroids and intravenous (IV) cyclosporine for 14 days, followed by oral cyclosporine to treat DR. This protocol resulted in remission in 9 out of 10 adult patients with a follow-up of 12 months [60].

Prophylactic use of TPE has been tried in patients at high risk of DR, but to date there has been no proven benefit on the incidence of DR [47, 61].

Immunoadsorption

The success of TPE has also prompted the use of immunoadsorption (IA) techniques in the setting of DR. IA relies on the same principle as TPE, but in theory the circulating factor is removed via selective antibody binding using high affinity columns. Lionaki et al. demonstrated an approach in which IA was used prophylactically in all patients with idiopathic FSGS. Patients undergoing LRD received IA as much as 1 week prior to transplant. IA was then individualized according to response with a case-by-case taper. Using this protocol, 66.7% of the patients had sustained remission and prevention of graft loss over a 4-year follow-up [62]. The benefits of IA versus TPE include no need for plasma replacement (FFP or 5% albumin). The use of IA seems to be more available in Asia and Europe and in the USA seems to be restricted only on research settings; the main obstacle for use of IA remains its cost, complexity, and lack of FDA-approved absorption columns.

Rituximab

Rituximab is a human chimera monoclonal antibody against the B-lymphocyte antigen CD20. Since its first reported successful use in a child with lymphoproliferative disorder and FSFG DR [63], there have been several subsequent studies demonstrating mixed results. In a small case series, rituximab was used in TPE-resistant patients and resulted in remission rates of 40% [64]. There have been reports of both success and failure when rituximab is used in combination with TPE [65, 66]. While rituximab's mechanism of action remains unclear, there is evidence that by preventing the downregulation of sphingomyelin phosphodiesterase acid-like 3b (SMPDL-3b) and acid sphingomyelinase (ASMase), it has a protective effect in podocytes. SMPDL-3b and ASMase were depleted on podocyte culture exposed to sera from a patient with recurrent FSGS. In this study, overexpression of SMPDL-3b was able to prevent disruption of podocyte cytoskeleton and podocyte apoptosis [67]. Typical protocols utilizing rituximab consist of 2–4 doses of 375 mg/m2/dose administered every 1 to 2 weeks. Ideally, if TPE is also used, the dosing of rituximab is done at least 24–72 hours prior to or after TPE to prevent its removal via TPE.

Cyclosporine

Cyclosporine is an immunosuppressant agent that inhibits T-cell signaling of nuclear factor in activated T-cells. However, the anti-proteinuric effect is likely multifactorial as it also appears to decrease production of T cell mediated cytokines. Cyclosporine in combination with IV steroids has been used with success in inducing remission of primary FSFG, but its efficacy in post-transplant recurrence remains unclear. It is important to note that case reports describing its use have often utilized high intravenous dosing of cyclosporine [68]. Cyclosporine entry into lymphocytes is via an LDL receptor, so given the high levels of lipoproteins seen in nephrotic syndrome, it is thought that high free levels of the drug are needed to overcome this competition for entry into the cell.

Lipid Apheresis

Lipid apheresis is a novel treatment for dyslipidemia in patients with nephrotic syndrome and is a well-established extracorporeal technique used to treat patients with homozygous familial hypercholesterolemia. A study utilizing lipid apheresis in combination with prednisone in children with treatment-resistant nephrotic syndrome found reductions in both cholesterol and triglyceride levels [69], similar to previous reports using lipid apheresis in adults [70]. However, this treatment in children with nephrotic syndrome is unique in that a significant number of patients went into either complete or partial remission of their nephrotic syndrome 13%—5 of 11 patients (45%) went into complete remission, and 2 of 11 patients (18%) went into partial remission. Remarkably, all of the patients that responded to therapy remained in remission with follow-up as long as 10 years. The mechanism by which lipid apheresis leads to remission remains unclear, but possible explanations include a direct effect of improving the dyslipidemia, removal of pathogenic vascular permeability factors, and/or enhancement of the response to immunosuppressants [71]. One potential but unexplored hypothesis is that lipid apheresis, by lowering the level of free fatty acids, could reduce or prevent podocyte damage and reduce proteinuria [72].

A more recent publication [73] was able to demonstrate successful treatment of post-transplant FSGS recurrence in seven pediatric patients from four different centers. Using a 9-week course of lipid apheresis in combination with pulse solumedrol, all seven patients experienced reductions in their protein to creatinine ratios resulting in partial or complete remission. Significantly, all of these patients had previously undergone extensive alternative treatments including extended courses of plasmapheresis.

The prospective multicenter POLARIS trial in Japan assessed the efficacy of lipid apheresis for treating dyslipidemia and inducing remission in patients with nephrotic syndrome. Initial results demonstrated nearly 50% reductions in both total cholesterol and LDL cholesterol levels during treatment [74]. A follow-up paper [75] demonstrated complete remission in 25% of the 44 patients enrolled in the study, and an additional 23% of patients had partial remission (defined as <1 g of urinary protein per day). Furthermore, a case report demonstrated induction of remission by lipid apheresis in an adult with rituximab-resistant nephrotic syndrome [76].

The high cost and the need in most cases for central venous access may play a part in limiting the potential adoption of lipid apheresis. One system of lipid apheresis, the Liposorber LA-15 (Kaneka), is being utilized in a prospective study for the treatment of focal segmental glomerulosclerosis in children (NCT02235857) and adults (NCT04065438). This study is a post-approval trial mandated by the FDA after the LA-15 system received a humanitarian device exemption for the treatment of patients with drug-resistant focal segmental glomerulosclerosis. Preliminary results from the pediatric study noted two out of seven patients achieving either a partial or complete remission [77].

Questions

1. *According to the evidence cited in this chapter, the incidence of disease recurrence on living donation vs deceased is:*
   A. Higher on the group that received a living donor kidney.
   B. Higher on the group that received a deceased donor kidney.
   C. There was no difference between the two groups.
   Answer: C.
   There is no evidence of benefit between living vs deceased donors in terms of increased incidence of recurrent disease. LD transplants given to FSGS patients have worse graft survival rates compared to patients without FSGS, but deceased donor graft survival rates in FSGS patients were not inferior to patients without FSGS [7]. In other words, the advantage of graft survival from LD is lost on patients with FSGS.
2. *Which of the following is not a risk factor for a disease recurrence of FSGS on the allograft?*
   A. Initial steroids responsive nephrotic syndrome
   B. Identified genetic mutation
   C. Presence of a circulation factor
   Answer: B.
   Patients with monogenic generic mutation have no predisposition to DR post-transplant except for some variant mutations of NPHS2. The incidence of recurrent disease is higher in patients who were initially steroid responsive and then became steroid resistant.
3. *Which of the following is true about APOL1 renal-related variants and non-diabetic renal disease:*
   A. There is a clear correlation between the presence of two copies of APOL1 RRV and phenotypic expression of renal disease.
   B. Presence of APOL1 is considered by some to be a contraindication for donation.
   C. Incidence is higher on East African descendants or those with mixed heritage.
   Answer: B.
   Despite a body of evidence that the G1/G2 variants can lead to intracellular dysfunction, only 20% of African Americans with them will develop kidney disease. APOL1 status has a potential implication for both deceased and living donor kidney transplant selection. Kidney transplant from a deceased donor with two copies of the G1/G2 variants has high graft failure rates when compared to those from donors with only one copy of the risk variant, and some evidence suggest rapid decline on residual kidney function on donors with 2 APOL risk variants after donation. The incidence is higher in West African descendants and lower in East Africans.

Bibliography

1. Chadwick J. The medical works of Hippocrates: A new translation from the original Greek (Vol. 174). Oxford: Blackwell; 1950. (Section 7, No 34).
2. Roelans C. Liber de Aegritudinibus Infantium. München: Verl. der Mu¨nchner Dr; 1484.
3. Arneil GC. The nephrotic syndrome. Pediatr Clin N Am. 1971;18(2):547–59.
4. Report of the International Study of Kidney Disease in Children, Barnett HL, Edelmann CM. Minimal change nephrotic syndrome in chil-dren: deaths during the first 5 to 15 years' observation. Pediatrics. 1984;73(4):497–501.
5. Tarver-Carr ME, Powe NR, Eberhardt MS, et al. Excess risk of chronic kidney disease among African-American versus white subjects in the United States: a population-based study of potential explanatory factors. J Am Soc Nephrol. 2002;13(9):2363–70. https://doi.org/10.1097/01.asn.0000026493.18542.6a.
6. Cooper A, Capewell P, Clucas C, et al. A primate APOL1 variant that kills trypanosoma brucei gambiense. PLoS Negl Trop Dis. 2016;10(8):e0004903. https://doi.org/10.1371/journal.pntd.0004903.
7. Kumar V, Singhal PC. APOL1 and kidney cell function [published online ahead of print, 2019 Jun 26]. Am J Physiol Renal Physiol. 2019;317(2):F463–77. https://doi.org/10.1152/ajprenal.00233.2019.
8. Vanhamme L, Paturiaux-Hanocq F, Poelvoorde P, et al. Apolipoprotein L-I is the trypanosome lytic factor of human serum. Nature. 2003;422(6927):83–7. https://doi.org/10.1038/nature01461.
9. O'Toole JF, Bruggeman LA, Madhavan S, Sedor JR. The cell biology of APOL1. Semin Nephrol. 2017;37(6):538–45. https://doi.org/10.1016/j.semnephrol.2017.07.007.
10. Nadkarni GN, Gignoux CR, Sorokin EP, et al. Worldwide frequencies of APOL1 renal risk variants. N Engl J Med. 2018;379(26):2571–2. https://doi.org/10.1056/NEJMc1800748.
11. Weckerle A, Snipes JA, Cheng D, et al. Characterization of circulating APOL1 protein complexes in African Americans. J Lipid Res. 2016;57(1):120–30. https://doi.org/10.1194/jlr.M063453.
12. Bruggeman LA, O'Toole JF, Ross MD, et al. Plasma apolipoprotein L1 levels do not correlate with CKD. J Am Soc Nephrol. 2014;25(3):634–44. https://doi.org/10.1681/ASN.2013070700.
13. Lee BT, Kumar V, Williams TA, et al. The APOL1 genotype of African American kidney transplant recipients does not impact 5-year allograft survival. Am J Transplant. 2012;12(7):1924–8. https://doi.org/10.1111/j.1600-6143.2012.04033.x.
14. Olabisi OA, Zhang JY, VerPlank L, et al. APOL1 kidney disease risk variants cause cytotoxicity by depleting cellular potassium and inducing stress-activated protein kinases. Proc Natl Acad Sci U S A. 2016;113(4):830–7. https://doi.org/10.1073/pnas.1522913113.
15. Granado D, Müller D, Krausel V, et al. Intracellular APOL1 risk variants cause cytotoxicity accompanied by energy depletion. J Am Soc Nephrol. 2017;28(11):3227–38. https://doi.org/10.1681/ASN.2016111220.
16. Kasembeli AN, Duarte R, Ramsay M, et al. APOL1 risk variants are strongly associated with HIV-associated nephropathy in black south Africans. J Am Soc Nephrol. 2015;26(11):2882–90. https://doi.org/10.1681/ASN.2014050469.
17. Ma L, Divers J, Freedman BI. Mechanisms of injury in APOL1-associated kidney disease. Transplantation. 2019;103(3):487–92. https://doi.org/10.1097/TP.0000000000002509.
18. Ng DK, Robertson CC, Woroniecki RP, et al. APOL1-associated glomerular disease among African-American children: a collaboration of the chronic kidney disease in children (CKiD) and nephrotic syndrome study network (NEPTUNE) cohorts. Nephrol Dial Transplant. 2017;32(6):983–90. https://doi.org/10.1093/ndt/gfw061.
19. Warady BA, Abraham AG, Schwartz GJ, et al. Predictors of rapid progression of glomerular and nonglomerular kidney disease in children and adolescents: the chronic kidney disease in children (CKiD) cohort. Am J Kidney Dis. 2015;65(6):878–88. https://doi.org/10.1053/j.ajkd.2015.01.008.

20. Freedman BI, Locke JE, Reeves-Daniel AM, Julian BA. Apolipoprotein L1 gene effects on kidney transplantation. Semin Nephrol. 2017;37(6):530–7. https://doi.org/10.1016/j.semnephrol.2017.07.006.
21. Reeves-Daniel AM, DePalma JA, Bleyer AJ, et al. The APOL1 gene and allograft survival after kidney transplantation. Am J Transplant. 2011;11(5):1025–30. https://doi.org/10.1111/j.1600-6143.2011.03513.x.
22. Doshi MD, Ortigosa-Goggins M, Garg AX, et al. APOL1 genotype and renal function of black living donors. J Am Soc Nephrol. 2018;29(4):1309–16. https://doi.org/10.1681/ASN.2017060658.
23. Freedman BI, Langefeld CD, Turner J, et al. Association of APOL1 variants with mild kidney disease in the first-degree relatives of African American patients with non-diabetic end-stage renal disease. Kidney Int. 2012;82(7):805–11. https://doi.org/10.1038/ki.2012.217.
24. Harding K, Mersha TB, Pham PT, et al. Health disparities in kidney transplantation for African Americans. Am J Nephrol. 2017;46(2):165–75. https://doi.org/10.1159/000479480.
25. Reeves-Daniel AM, DePalma JA, Bleyer AJ, et al. The APOL1 gene and allograft survival after kidney transplantation. Am J Transplant. 2011;11(5):1025–30. https://doi.org/10.1111/j.1600-6143.2011.03513.x.
26. Freedman BI, Julian BA, Pastan SO, et al. Apolipoprotein L1 gene variants in deceased organ donors are associated with renal allograft failure. Am J Transplant. 2015;15(6):1615–22. https://doi.org/10.1111/ajt.13223.
27. Guan I, Singer P, Frank R, Chorny N, Infante L, Sethna CB. Role of race in kidney transplant outcomes in children with focal segmental glomerulosclerosis. Pediatr Transplant. 2016;20(6):790–7. https://doi.org/10.1111/petr.12766.
28. Lau SO, Tkachuck JY, Hasegawa DK, Edson JR. Plasminogen and antithrombin III deficiencies in the childhood nephrotic syndrome associated with plasminogenuria and antithrombinuria. J Pediatr. 1980;96(3 Pt 1):390–2. https://doi.org/10.1016/s0022-3476(80)80678-0.
29. Singhal R, Brimble KS. Thromboembolic complications in the nephrotic syndrome: pathophysiology and clinical management. Thromb Res. 2006;118(3):397–407. https://doi.org/10.1016/j.thromres.2005.03.030.
30. Suri D, Ahluwalia J, Saxena AK, et al. Thromboembolic complications in childhood nephrotic syndrome: a clinical profile. Clin Exp Nephrol. 2014;18(5):803–13. https://doi.org/10.1007/s10157-013-0917-2.
31. Dufek S, Holtta T, Trautmann A, et al. Management of children with congenital nephrotic syndrome: challenging treatment paradigms. Nephrol Dial Transplant. 2019;34(8):1369–77. https://doi.org/10.1093/ndt/gfy165.
32. Ghane Sharbaf F, Bitzan M, Szymanski KM, et al. Native nephrectomy prior to pediatric kidney transplantation: biological and clinical aspects. Pediatr Nephrol. 2012;27(7):1179–88. https://doi.org/10.1007/s00467-012-2115-y.
33. Dome JS, Huff V. In: Pagon RA, Bird TD, Dolan CB, Stephans K, editors. Wilms Tumor overview. GeneReviews. Seattle: University of Washington; 2011.
34. Denys P, Malvaux P, Van Den Berghe H, Tanghe W, Proesmans W. Association d'un syndrome anatomo-pathologique de pseudohermaphrodisme masculin, d'une tumeur de Wilms, d'une nephropathie parenchymateuse et d'un mosaicisme XX/XY [association of an anatomopathological syndrome of male pseudohermaphroditism, Wilms' tumor, parenchymatous nephropathy and XX/XY mosaicism]. Arch Fr Pediatr. 1967;24(7):729–39.
35. Gariépy-Assal L, Gilbert RD, Žiaugra A, Foster BJ. Management of Denys-Drash syndrome: a case series based on an international survey. Clin Nephrol Case Stud. 2018;6:36–44. https://doi.org/10.5414/CNCS109515. Published 2018 Nov 12.
36. Weaver DJ Jr, Somers MJG, Martz K, Mitsnefes MM. Clinical outcomes and survival in pediatric patients initiating chronic dialysis: a report of the NAPRTCS registry. Pediatr Nephrol. 2017;32(12):2319–30. https://doi.org/10.1007/s00467-017-3759-4.
37. Habib R, Loirat C, Gubler MC, et al. The nephropathy associated with male pseudohermaphroditism and Wilms' tumor (Drash syndrome): a distinctive glomerular lesion--report of 10 cases. Clin Nephrol. 1985;24(6):269–78.

38. Hoyer JR, Raij L, Vernier RL, Simmons RL, Najarian JS, Michael AF. Recurrence of idiopathic nephrotic syndrome after renal transplantation. Lancet. 1972; https://doi.org/10.1016/S0140-6736(72)91734-5.
39. Striegel JE, Sibley RK, Fryd DS, Mauer SM. Recurrence of focal segmental sclerosis in children following renal transplantation. Kidney Int Suppl. 1986;19:S44–50.
40. Gipson DS, Massengill SF, Yao L, et al. Management of childhood onset nephrotic syndrome. Pediatrics. 2009;124(2):747–57. https://doi.org/10.1542/peds.2008-1559.
41. The primary nephrotic syndrome in children: identification of patients with minimal change nephrotic syndrome from initial response to prednisone—a report of the International Study of Kidney Disease in Children. J Pediatr. 1981;98(4):561–4.
42. Ding WY, Koziell A, McCarthy HJ, et al. Initial steroid sensitivity in children with steroid-resistant nephrotic syndrome predicts post-transplant recurrence. J Am Soc Nephrol. 2014;25(6):1342–8. https://doi.org/10.1681/ASN.2013080852.
43. Bertelli R, Ginevri F, Caridi G, et al. Recurrence of focal segmental glomerulosclerosis after renal transplantation in patients with mutations of podocin. Am J Kidney Dis. 2003;41(6):1314–21. https://doi.org/10.1016/s0272-6386(03)00364-0.
44. Baum MA, Stablein DM, Panzarino VM, Tejani A, Harmon WE, Alexander SR. Loss of living donor renal allograft survival advantage in children with focal segmental glomerulosclerosis. Kidney Int. 2001;59(1):328–33. https://doi.org/10.1046/j.1523-1755.2001.00494.x.
45. Odorico JS, Knechtle SJ, Rayhill SC, et al. The influence of native nephrectomy on the incidence of recurrent disease following renal transplantation for primary glomerulonephritis. Transplantation. 1996;61(2):228–34. https://doi.org/10.1097/00007890-199601270-00012.
46. Bierzynska A, McCarthy HJ, Soderquest K, et al. Genomic and clinical profiling of a national nephrotic syndrome cohort advocates a precision medicine approach to disease management. Kidney Int. 2017;91(4):937–47. https://doi.org/10.1016/j.kint.2016.10.013.
47. Gohh RY, Yango AF, Morrissey PE, et al. Preemptive plasmapheresis and recurrence of FSGS in high-risk renal transplant recipients. Am J Transplant. 2005;5(12):2907–12. https://doi.org/10.1111/j.1600-6143.2005.01112.x.
48. Ding WY, Koziell A, McCarthy HJ, et al. Initial steroid sensitivity in children with steroid-resistant nephrotic syndrome predicts post-transplant recurrence. J Am Soc Nephrol. 2014;25(6):1342–8. https://doi.org/10.1681/ASN.2013080852.
49. Gallon L, Leventhal J, Skaro A, Kanwar Y, Alvarado A. Resolution of recurrent focal segmental glomerulosclerosis after retransplantation. N Engl J Med. 2012;366(17):1648–9. https://doi.org/10.1056/NEJMc1202500.
50. Le Berre L, Godfrin Y, Günther E, et al. Extrarenal effects on the pathogenesis and relapse of idiopathic nephrotic syndrome in Buffalo/Mna rats. J Clin Invest. 2002;109(4):491–8. https://doi.org/10.1172/JCI12858.
51. Thunø M, Macho B, Eugen-Olsen J. suPAR: the molecular crystal ball. Dis Markers. 2009;27(3):157–72. https://doi.org/10.3233/DMA-2009-0657.
52. Delville M, Sigdel TK, Wei C, et al. A circulating antibody panel for pretransplant prediction of FSGS recurrence after kidney transplantation. Sci Transl Med. 2014;6(256):256ra136. https://doi.org/10.1126/scitranslmed.3008538.
53. Salvadori M, Tsalouchos A. Therapeutic apheresis in kidney transplantation: an updated review. World J Transplant. 2019;9(6):103–22. https://doi.org/10.5500/wjt.v9.i6.103.
54. Schwartz J, Winters JL, Padmanabhan A, et al. Guidelines on the use of therapeutic apheresis in clinical practice-evidence-based approach from the writing Committee of the American Society for apheresis: the sixth special issue. J Clin Apher. 2013;28(3):145–284. https://doi.org/10.1002/jca.21276.
55. Zimmerman SW. Plasmapheresis and dipyridamole for recurrent focal glomerular sclerosis. Nephron. 1985;40(2):241–5. https://doi.org/10.1159/000183469.
56. Ponticelli C. Recurrence of focal segmental glomerular sclerosis (FSGS) after renal transplantation. Nephrol Dial Transplant. 2010;25(1):25–31. https://doi.org/10.1093/ndt/gfp538.

57. Dall'Amico R, Ghiggeri G, Carraro M, et al. Prediction and treatment of recurrent focal segmental glomerulosclerosis after renal transplantation in children. Am J Kidney Dis. 1999;34(6):1048–55. https://doi.org/10.1016/S0272-6386(99)70010-7.
58. Rudnicki M. FSGS recurrence in adults after renal transplantation. Biomed Res Int. 2016;2016:3295618. https://doi.org/10.1155/2016/3295618.
59. Dau PC, Callahan JP. Immune modulation during treatment of systemic sclerosis with plasmapheresis and immunosuppressive drugs. Clin Immunol Immunopathol. 1994;70(2):159–65. https://doi.org/10.1006/clin.1994.1024.
60. Canaud G, Zuber J, Sberro R, et al. Intensive and prolonged treatment of focal and segmental glomerulosclerosis recurrence in adult kidney transplant recipients: a pilot study. Am J Transplant. 2009;9(5):1081–6. https://doi.org/10.1111/j.1600-6143.2009.02580.x.
61. Gohh RY, Yango AF, Morrissey PE, et al. Preemptive plasmapheresis and recurrence of FSGS in high-risk renal transplant recipients. Am J Transplant. 2005;5(12):2907–12. https://doi.org/10.1111/j.1600-6143.2005.01112.x.
62. Lionaki S, Vlachopanos G, Georgalis A, et al. Individualized scheme of immunoadsorption for the recurrence of idiopathic focal segmental glomerulosclerosis in the graft: a single center experience. Ren Fail. 2015;37(5):777–83. https://doi.org/10.3109/0886022X.2015.1015366.
63. Pescovitz MD, Book BK, Sidner RA. Resolution of recurrent focal segmental glomerulosclerosis proteinuria after rituximab treatment. N Engl J Med. 2006;354(18):1961–3. https://doi.org/10.1056/NEJMc055495.
64. Dello Strologo L, Guzzo I, Laurenzi C, et al. Use of rituximab in focal glomerulosclerosis relapses after renal transplantation. Transplantation. 2009;88(3):417–20. https://doi.org/10.1097/TP.0b013e3181aed9d7.
65. Tsagalis G, Psimenou E, Nakopoulou L, Laggouranis A. Combination treatment with plasmapheresis and rituximab for recurrent focal segmental glomerulosclerosis after renal transplantation. Artif Organs. 2011;35(4):420–5. https://doi.org/10.1111/j.1525-1594.2010.01068.x.
66. Yabu JM, Ho B, Scandling JD, Vincenti F. Rituximab failed to improve nephrotic syndrome in renal transplant patients with recurrent focal segmental glomerulosclerosis. Am J Transplant. 2008;8(1):222–7. https://doi.org/10.1111/j.1600-6143.2007.02021.x.
67. Fornoni A, Sageshima J, Wei C, et al. Rituximab targets podocytes in recurrent focal segmental glomerulosclerosis. Sci Transl Med. 2011;3(85):85ra46. https://doi.org/10.1126/scitranslmed.3002231.
68. Raafat RH, Kalia A, Travis LB, Diven SC. High-dose oral cyclosporin therapy for recurrent focal segmental glomerulosclerosis in children. Am J Kidney Dis. 2004;44(1):50–6. https://doi.org/10.1053/j.ajkd.2004.03.028.
69. Hattori M, et al. A combined low-density lipoprotein apheresis and prednisone therapy for steroid-resistant primary focal segmental glomerulosclerosis in children. Am J Kidney Dis. 2003;42:1121–30.
70. Muso E, et al. Low density lipoprotein apheresis therapy for steroid-resistant nephrotic syndrome. Kansai-FGS-apheresis treatment (K-FLAT) study group. Kidney Int Suppl. 1999;71:S122–5.
71. Muso E. Beneficial effect of LDL-apheresis in refractory nephrotic syndrome. Clin Exp Nephrol. 2014;18:286–90.
72. Chung JJ, et al. Albumin-associated free fatty acids induce macropinocytosis in podocytes. J Clin Invest. 2015;125:2307–16.
73. Shah L, et al. LDL-apheresis-induced remission of focal segmental glomerulosclerosis recurrence in pediatric renal transplant recipients. Pediatric Neph. 2019;34:2343–50.
74. Muso E, et al. Immediate therapeutic efficacy of low-density lipoprotein apheresis for drug-resistant nephrotic syndrome: evidence from the short-term results from the POLARIS study. Clin Exp Nephrol. 2015;19:379–86.
75. Muso E, et al. A prospective observational survey on the long-term effect of LDL apheresis on drug-resistant nephrotic syndrome. Nephron Extra. 2015;5:58–66.

76. Suzuki H, Tsukamoto T, Muso E. Rituximab-resistant nephrotic syndrome with successful induction of remission by low-density lipoprotein apheresis. Ther Apher Dial. 2017;21: 295–6.
77. Raina R, et al. Dextran-sulfate plasma adsorption lipoprotein apheresis in drug resistant primary focal segmental glomerulosclerosis patients: results from a prospective, multicenter, single-arm intervention study. Front Pediatr. 2019;7:454.
78. Abbott KC, Sawyers ES, Oliver JD III, et al. Graft loss due to recurrent focal segmental glomerulosclerosis in renal transplant recipients in the United States. Am J Kidney Dis. 2001;37(2):366–73.

Challenges of Maintaining Adequate Health and Well-Being, Growth, Nutrition, and Development in Pediatric Transplant Recipients

10

Kristen Sgambat, Kaushalendra Amatya, and Asha Moudgil

Vaccinations

Vaccinations to prevent infections by vaccine-preventable diseases are very important for prospective transplant recipients. All efforts should be made to vaccinate these children during early chronic kidney disease (CKD) and prior to transplant as in the late stages of CKD and post-transplant immune response to vaccines may be blunted and live vaccines are contraindicated post-transplant.

Pre-transplant

Patients with CKD and end-stage kidney disease (ESKD) need to be up to date with all recommended childhood vaccines prior to transplantation. Achieving timely and adequate immunization pre-transplantation is critical since children are unable to get live vaccines after transplant. Some of these children may be missing routine vaccination due to frequent illness or hospitalizations. Pre-transplant consultation with infectious disease, when possible, can help to optimize a patient's pre-transplant immunization status.

The Centers for Disease Control (CDC) and Prevention immunization schedule for children and adolescents can be found at:

https://www.cdc.gov/vaccines/schedules/hcp/imz/child-adolescent.html [1]

In some situations, where the transplant is more imminent, an accelerated vaccine schedule can be undertaken especially for live viral vaccines. Measles, mumps, rubella, and varicella can be given as early as 6 months of life. Hepatitis B vaccine

K. Sgambat · K. Amatya · A. Moudgil (✉)
Children's National Hospital Washington DC, Division of Nephrology, Washington, DC, USA
e-mail: Ksgambat@childrensnational.org; Kamatya@childrensnational.org; Amoudgil@childrensnational.org

K. E. Twombley (ed.), *Challenges in Pediatric Kidney Transplantation*,
https://doi.org/10.1007/978-3-030-74783-1_10

series can be started at birth, and human papilloma virus vaccine can be started as early as 9 years of age [2].

It is important to measure titers against hepatitis A, hepatitis B, and live virus vaccines including measles, mumps, rubella, and varicella 1 month after vaccination, and children should be revaccinated if noted to be non-immune. Children over the age of 2 years old should also receive the pneumococcal vaccine polyvalent (Pneumovax®23) in addition to pneumococcal 13-valent conjugate vaccine (Prevnar 13®) for expanded immunity to pneumococcal strains. It is recommended that high-risk children, such as transplant patients, receive 2 doses 5 years apart. General pediatricians do not routinely carry Pneumovax®23 since it is not a routine childhood vaccine. It is not cost-effective for pediatricians to order the vaccine for a child since it is not distributed as a single dose. This vaccine may be available to the pediatricians working in academic institutions or those in family practice. Alternately, nephrologists and transplant physicians should make special arrangements to give this vaccine in their own specialty clinics.

It is important for all household members and caregivers to remain up to date with their scheduled immunizations to prevent spread of infection to transplant recipients. Household members of transplant recipients can receive live virus vaccines safely.

Post-transplant

While every effort should be made to vaccinate prior to transplantation, inactivated vaccines are generally safe after solid organ transplantation. Transplant recipients and their family members should receive yearly influenza vaccination. While it is desirable to wait until 3–6 months after transplant to give the influenza vaccine to transplant recipients, it can be given after about 1 month of transplant if needed. Some centers give a dose at the time of transplant if it is high season and give a booster 1 month later. Both children and household members should get the injectable vaccine. Immunogenicity of the influenza vaccine in kidney transplant recipients varies widely. This variation could be attributed to the vaccine strain, the time after transplantation, the immunosuppressive regimen, as well as the net state of immunosuppression of the recipient [3]. For example, patients on mycophenolate mofetil (MMF) have a lower seroprotective rate.

There have been concerns about the influenza vaccine triggering acute rejections, but these concerns were not substantiated in large-scale studies [4]. In large registry data, influenza vaccine use in transplant recipients was associated with lower rates of allograft loss and death [5]. However, use of adjuvanted Influenza vaccines (typically recommended for patients 65 years of age and older) has been shown to cause a rise in anti-HLA antibodies, but this has not been shown to lead to acute rejection episodes [6]. It is, therefore, advisable not to use adjuvanted influenza vaccines in kidney transplant recipients.

Though live vaccines are contraindicated, occasionally live vaccines have been given when an outbreak has occurred and there is no alternative type of vaccine. However, this should be done only with strict observation and oversight and in conjunction with an infectious disease specialist.

Vaccines and Travel

Need for travel vaccines depends upon the place and season of travel. Vaccines against hepatitis A, typhoid, cholera, and Japanese encephalitis and a repeat dose of meningococcal and injectable polio may be needed, whereas yellow fever vaccine is contraindicated. It is ideal to check the CDC website on the recommendations for specific areas of travel. A consultation with an infectious disease specialist may also be helpful for travel planning.

Nutritional Challenges

The aims of nutritional management of children with CKD, both pre- and post-transplant, are to maintain healthy weight, promote growth and development, ensure adequate intake of macro- and micro-nutrients, avoid and treat metabolic imbalances, and optimize bone and muscle health. Monitoring and early intervention to promote cardiovascular health are also key to reducing the risks of morbidity and mortality, which may become more evident as pediatric patients transition into young adulthood. Children with CKD often struggle to achieve optimal growth and nutrition due to a variety of reasons which include altered taste, restricted diet, increased prevalence of vomiting, metabolic acidosis, gastrointestinal symptoms, recurrent infections, increased catabolism, lack of physical activity, and growth hormone resistance. In addition, factors such as depression, non-adherence, and food insecurity are often additional barriers to achieving optimal nutrition in this population. These challenges are especially marked in those with early onset of CKD and worsen as CKD progresses into ESKD and dialysis. After kidney transplantation, some of these nutritional issues resolve, but new and different nutritional challenges can emerge. Therefore, a multidisciplinary team approach is important to optimize the nutrition of the pediatric patient both pre-transplant and post-transplant and should be at the forefront of CKD management. Nutritional management by a registered dietitian nutritionist (RDN) with expertise in pediatric renal nutrition is recommended for children with CKD and ESKD [7].

Pre-transplant

CKD 2–5 Pre-dialysis

The journey to successful kidney transplantation begins in the early stages of CKD. The CKD milieu is associated with a cascade of disturbances in the regulation of numerous physiologic systems that contribute to impaired appetite, stunted growth, and compromised nutrition. The topic of growth in children with CKD will be reviewed in more detail in the section. Growth Challenges of this chapter. Factors contributing to decreased appetite in CKD include dysregulation of appetite-regulating hormones [8], increased release of inflammatory cytokines [9], altered taste sensation [10, 11], and adverse changes in the gut microbiome. Alteration in gastrointestinal microbiota has also been linked with increased cardiovascular risk in children with CKD [12].

Early nutrition assessment and intervention are the key to optimizing growth and nutritional status and preventing onset of protein-energy wasting (PEW) in children with CKD. Once PEW occurs, it cannot be easily corrected by nutritional supplementation alone due to the presence of additional factors, including persistent inflammation, metabolic acidosis, endocrine disorders, hypermetabolism, poor physical activity, and frailty that lead to breakdown of protein and muscle stores. Diagnosis of PEW in children with CKD is based on five key criteria: (1) decreased appetite, (2) serum biochemistry (low cholesterol, albumin and transferrin, and high C-reactive protein [CRP]), (3) reduced body mass, (4) reduced muscle mass, and (5) short stature or poor growth [13]. Frailty in children with CKD is a similar but distinct condition which is defined by presence of at least three of the following four criteria: (1) suboptimal growth and/or weight gain, (2) low muscle mass, (3) fatigue, and/or (4) inflammation (CRP >3 mg/l). Children with frailty in the setting of CKD have increased risk for infections and hospitalizations [14].

Hemodialysis

Children receiving chronic hemodialysis (HD) typically undergo treatments 3–4 times a week and therefore often require strict restrictions on dietary intake of sodium, potassium, phosphorus, and fluid. Provision of adequate nutrition is particularly challenging in infants and young children who are anuric, as they may require highly concentrated formula to prevent fluid overload between HD treatments. In older children, it may be challenging to meet macro- and micro-nutrient needs due to the elimination of favorite foods that are commonly consumed by children in North America, such as milk, ice cream, pizza, French fries, and macaroni and cheese.

Factors associated with the hemodialysis procedure itself may induce inflammation and catabolism, further predisposing patients to development of PEW [8]. Therefore, protein requirements for pediatric HD patients are estimated to be slightly higher than the daily recommended intake (DRI) for age (by 0.1 g/kg/day) [7]. The normalized catabolic protein rate (nPCR) is an important marker of protein and overall nutritional status in HD patients. In adolescents and adults, an nPCR value below 1 g/kg/day indicates that the patient is at risk for weight loss and malnutrition [15], but this has not yet been validated in infants and young children. In addition to protein, water-soluble vitamins and carnitine are also removed during the HD treatment. All chronic HD patients should receive an oral water-soluble vitamin supplement daily [7], and intravenous levocarnitine supplementation can be considered in those with dialysis-related carnitine deficiency [16].

HD adequacy also impacts nutrition and growth. Evidence suggests that providing enhanced dialytic clearance may promote better nutrition and growth in children receiving chronic HD [17, 18]. More frequent and/or intensified hemodialysis regimens have been shown to promote normal growth in children, without the need for growth hormone therapy [19].

Peritoneal Dialysis

In addition to the hormonal and inflammatory effects that suppress appetite in renal failure, patients receiving chronic peritoneal dialysis (PD) face additional challenges to meeting nutritional needs. Gastrointestinal symptoms, such as early satiety, delayed gastric emptying, vomiting, and gastroesophageal reflux (GER), are very common in PD patients due to the presence of increased intra-abdominal pressure [20]. In addition to decreased appetite and gastrointestinal symptoms, nutrition in PD patients may be further compromised by loss of protein in the PD effluent, which varies by age and has been estimated to range from 0.28 g/kg/day in infants to 0.1 g/kg/day in adolescents [21].

Conversely, caution should be taken in PD patients who are at risk for obesity or diabetes, as absorption of dextrose from the peritoneal dialysate can contribute to excess weight gain or increase in blood sugars [22]. This is especially concerning in patients requiring higher concentrations of dextrose in the dialysate.

Nutritional Management in CKD and Dialysis

Comprehensive pediatric renal nutrition guidelines were published by the National Kidney Foundation Kidney Disease Quality Outcomes Initiative (KDOQI) in 2009 [7]. A series of updated pediatric renal nutrition clinical practice guidelines have since been published by the Pediatric Renal Nutrition Taskforce, an international team of pediatric nephrologists and renal dietitians [23–25]. The most current guidelines for nutritional management of children with CKD stages 2–5 and dialysis are summarized in Table 10.1.

Table 10.1 Nutritional management for CKD stage 2–5 and dialysis

Calories	100% DRI for age, with adjustments to promote weight gain or loss as needed
Protein	Stage 3: Limit to 140% of DRI for age Stage 4–5: Limit to 120% of DRI for age Hemodialysis: DRI for age + 0.1 g/kg/day Peritoneal dialysis: Infant: DRI for age + 0.3 g/kg/day Child (1–3 years): DRI for age + 0.25 g/kg/day Child (4–18 years): DRI for age + 0.15 g/kg/day
Fluid	Restrict fluid in glomerular disease and anuric patients Polyuric patients may require supplemental fluid
Fats	Encourage a heart-healthy diet, limited in saturated and trans fats
Potassium	1–3 mmol/kg/day; adjust as needed to maintain K levels within normal range
Sodium	Typically restrict in setting of glomerular diseases Salt-wasting polyuric infants may require sodium supplementation
Calcium	Goal to meet 100% of DRI for age Limit to no greater than 2 times the DRI from diet and supplemental sources
Phosphorus	Limit intake to 100% of the DRI for age if serum phosphorus levels are normal but PTH level elevated based on target range for stage of CKD Limit intake to 80% of the DRI for age when serum phosphorus level and PTH level are both elevated
Vitamin D	Goal to meet 100% of DRI for age Supplement breastfed infants with 400 IU per day of vitamin D Monitor 25-hydroxyvitamin D level and treat for 25-hydroxyvitamin D deficiency (<30 ng/dL)
Water-soluble vitamins	All dialysis patients should take a daily water-soluble vitamin supplement to replace dialytic losses
Physical activity	Aerobic and resistance exercise to promote aerobic fitness and muscle strength Goal to preserve muscle mass and prevent PEW

Enteral Nutrition Support

Enteral nutrition support via enteral tube feeding has been shown to improve growth and nutrition in infants and young children on dialysis [26–29]. The Pediatric Renal Nutrition Taskforce has published clinical practice guidelines for enteral tube feeding in children with CKD stages 2–5 and on dialysis [24]. The guidelines recommend partial or exclusive enteral tube feeding in infants and children who are unable to meet their nutritional requirements orally. The guidelines advise that intervention with enteral tube feeding should occur promptly in any infant or child noted to have decline in weight percentile [24].

In addition to improved nutrition, enteral feeding tubes can also be used for medication administration. This can improve quality of life for the child, as they can avoid the negative experience of taking medications by mouth, which may help to minimize development of oral aversions. It may also improve quality of life for the parents by reducing the stress associated with medication administration. It should be noted that certain medications, such as the active form of 1,25 dihydroxy vitamin-D, may not be appropriate for administration via the enteral tube, and a pharmacist should be consulted to help determine which medications are safe to put in enteral tubes.

Post-transplant

Appetite and Weight

Following successful kidney transplantation, dietary restrictions can typically be liberalized, and the child may be encouraged to consume a regular healthy balanced diet for age. Increased dietary options in combination with reversal of the uremic state result in improved appetite and taste perception. This typically leads to increased oral intake and rapid post-transplant weight gain. Corticosteroids and other immunosuppressive medications compound the risks associated with obesity and metabolic sequela as they also can stimulate weight. Pediatric transplant recipients have been reported to double their weight in the first-year post-transplant, after which time body mass index (BMI) tends to stabilize [30]. Post-transplant obesity and metabolic syndrome are common and are associated with adverse outcomes, including increased risk of allograft failure, surgical complications, cardiovascular morbidity, and new onset of diabetes after transplant (NODAT) [31, 32].

While obesity and metabolic complications are common post-transplant, it should also be noted that failure to thrive may persist in a smaller subset of children after kidney transplantation. In a single-center study of pediatric kidney transplant recipients, 21.9% and 17.9% of patients had failure to thrive at 1- and 3-year post-transplantation, respectively [33]. Compared to other recipients, patients with failure to thrive were more likely to experience infections and hospitalization in the first 3 years post-transplantation. These patients may benefit from ongoing oral or enteral nutrition supplementation post-transplant under the supervision of an RDN.

Transition from Enteral to Oral Feeding

While many infants and young children with CKD require enteral nutrition support prior to transplant, generally the goal is to transition to 100% oral feeds after successful kidney transplantation. Recent evidence suggests that the majority of children (70%) are able to discontinue enteral tube feeding at a median time of 6 weeks post-transplant [34]. In children who remain feeding tube-dependent after 3 months post-transplant, referral to oral feeding therapy is recommended, if such therapy is not already in place [34].

Medication Effects

Immunosuppressive medications are essential for preventing rejection of the allograft; however, these medications also carry increased risk of numerous nutrition-related side effects. Some of the most common medication-associated adverse effects experienced by pediatric transplant recipients include magnesium wasting, hyperkalemia, gastrointestinal symptoms, and cardiovascular complications such as hypertension and dyslipidemia. Effects associated with specific medications are as follows:

- *Calcineurin inhibitors (CNI)*: increased risk of hyperglycemia, NODAT, hypomagnesemia, hyperkalemia, and hypertension
- *Corticosteroids*: increased risk of hypertension, dyslipidemia, hyperglycemia, NODAT, increased appetite leading to weight gain/obesity, metabolic syndrome, and osteoporosis
- *Mycophenolate mofetil*: increased risk of adverse gastrointestinal symptoms such as nausea, diarrhea, and altered taste acuity

Nutritional Management Post-transplant

Post-transplant diet and nutrition recommendations are summarized in Table 10.2. In order to optimize nutrition while promoting weight management and minimize common complications such as hypertension, dyslipidemia, and NODAT after transplant, a healthy balanced diet limited in sodium, saturated fats, and simple sugars is recommended. Ensuring adequate fluid intake to maintain perfusion of the transplanted kidney is critical. The diet should also aim to provide at least 100% of the DRI for calcium, phosphorus, and vitamin D in order to optimize bone health, particularly in children with post-transplant hypophosphatemia or those receiving corticosteroid therapy [7]. Obtaining phosphorus through the diet is preferred to supplementation, as oral phosphate supplements may be ineffective in correcting post-transplant hypophosphatemia due to stimulation of fibroblast growth factor 23 (FGF-23) secretion, and supplemental phosphate may also induce diarrhea. The recommended daily intake for maintenance (not repletion) of normal vitamin D levels is 400 international units (IU) of vitamin D_3 for infants and 600 IU of vitamin D_3 for individuals 1–30 years of age. Exclusively breast-fed infants as well as infants taking <1000 mL/day of fortified formula should be supplemented with 400 IU of vitamin D_3 daily [35]. Bone health of pediatric transplant recipients is discussed in further detail later in this chapter.

Table 10.2 Nutrition and activity recommendations after kidney transplant

Calories	100% DRI for age, with adjustments to promote weight gain or loss as needed
Protein	100% DRI for age; avoid excessive protein intake long term
Fluid	Adequate fluid intake is critical for perfusion of the transplanted kidney
Sugars	Limit intake of concentrated sweets and refined carbohydrates Choose water, low fat dairy, or sugar-free beverages Choose whole grains with fiber content >3 grams per serving
Fats	Encourage a heart-healthy diet, limited in saturated and trans fats
Potassium	Monitor for CNI-induced hyperkalemia Initiate low K diet restriction if needed
Sodium	Avoid excessive sodium intake to prevent or control hypertension
Magnesium	Encourage intake of high magnesium foods Monitor for hypomagnesemia, a common side effect of CNI therapy Initiate oral magnesium supplementation as needed
Calcium	Goal to meet 100% of DRI for age Avoid intake of colas, which impair calcium absorption
Phosphorus	Goal to meet 100% DRI for age Monitor for hypophosphatemia, which is common in the early post-transplant period Target normal phosphorus levels and correct hypophosphatemia with high phosphorus diet (low-fat dairy, legumes, nuts)
Vitamin D	Goal to meet 100% of DRI for age Supplement breastfed infants with 400 IU per day of vitamin D Monitor 25-hydroxyvitamin D level and supplement if deficient (<30 ng/dL)
DASH diet	Consider DASH diet, which incorporates foods rich in potassium, phosphorus, calcium, magnesium, and fiber (fruits, vegetables, legumes, nuts, whole grains, and low-fat dairy), and limits sodium, saturated fats, and refined carbohydrates by avoiding foods such as red meats, processed foods, and sugar-sweetened beverages
Physical activity	Aerobic and resistance exercise promotes aerobic fitness and muscle strength. Goal to manage weight and decrease the risk of metabolic comorbidities post-transplant
Food safety	Follow the four basic steps to food safety, "Clean, separate, cook, and chill," in order to minimize risk of foodborne illness

"The Dietary Approaches to Stop Hypertension (DASH)" eating plan is known to promote healthy blood pressure and help to maintain a healthy weight post-transplant [36]. The principles of the DASH diet include increased intake of foods rich in potassium, phosphorus, calcium, magnesium, fiber, and protein (fruits, vegetables, legumes, nuts, whole grains, and low-fat dairy), as well as limiting the intake of sodium, saturated fats, and refined carbohydrates by avoiding foods such as red meats, processed foods, and sugar-sweetened beverages. Following the DASH diet after kidney transplant is independently associated with improved allograft function and lower all-cause mortality [37].

As the DASH diet promotes foods that are high in both phosphorus and magnesium, it should be especially encouraged in patients who experience post-transplant hypophosphatemia and hypomagnesemia. In patients who experience persistent hypomagnesemia despite consuming a high magnesium diet, oral magnesium supplementation may be necessary while monitoring for side effects of oral magnesium, such as diarrhea. As the DASH diet is rich in potassium-containing foods, the diet may need to be modified for transplant recipients who experience CNI-related hyperkalemia. In addition to a healthy diet, physical activity, including both aerobic and resistance exercises, is important to building fitness and strength after kidney transplant.

Food Safety

Food safety is an important consideration for prevention of foodborne illness in immunosuppressed pediatric kidney transplant recipients. Immunosuppressed patients are significantly more susceptible to developing foodborne illness after exposure to an opportunistic pathogen compared to healthy peers, and children are at particularly high risk. Effects of chronic immunosuppression can weaken the defenses of gut-associated lymphoid tissue, allowing foodborne pathogens to penetrate the gastrointestinal tract [38]. Transplant patients and families should be educated about the "Four Basic Steps to Food Safety: Clean, Separate, Cook, and Chill." The basic principles involve (1) proper washing of hands, cooking surfaces, and raw produce, (2) avoiding cross-contamination by keeping raw foods separate from ready-to-eat foods, (3) cooking foods to the proper internal temperatures, and (4) refrigerating chilled foods to the proper temperature. Patients and clinicians may refer to the educational booklet published by the Unites States Department of Agriculture (USDA) and food and drug administration (FDA), "Food Safety for Transplant Recipients: A need-to-know guide for bone marrow and solid organ transplant recipients" for detailed guidelines. This booklet is patient-friendly and can be easily accessed online [39].

Growth Challenges

Growth Hormone Physiology

The physiology of growth is regulated by human growth hormone and the growth hormone/insulin like growth factor-1 (GH/IGF-1) axis. In healthy children, hypothalamic growth hormone-releasing hormone (HGHR) stimulates the production and release of GH from the somatotroph cells of the pituitary gland. GH then binds to receptors in the liver to stimulate production and secretion of insulin-like growth factor-1 (IGF-1). Under normal conditions, IGF-1 promotes growth via various pathways, including proliferation of osteoblasts and pre-chondrocytes, bone remodeling, and bone mineralization [40]. IGF-1 is also important for building muscle mass and strength via stimulation of proliferation and differentiation of myoblasts and inhibition of muscle breakdown [40].

Growth and CKD

In children with CKD, multiple disturbances and abnormalities converge to impair growth and development. Most notably, the GH/IGF-1 axis is altered, creating a state of growth hormone resistance which is characterized by decreased growth hormone receptor expression and function and reduced circulating IGF-1 levels and activity related to increased production of inhibitory IGF-1 binding proteins by the liver. As CKD progresses, other factors contributing to impaired growth may include poor nutrition, metabolic acidosis, mineral and bone disorders (MBD), and altered regulation of sex hormones. By the time children present for kidney transplantation, they exhibit significant growth delay, with a height deficit of around −1.72 standard deviation (SD) below the mean, with the greatest height deficits seen in younger children (2–5 years old) and second transplant recipients [41].

Growth After Kidney Transplant

Although successful kidney transplantation typically restores normal function of the GH/IGF-1 axis, suboptimal growth may persist in some children post-transplant. Age at time of transplant is a significant determinant of growth after transplant. Studies have shown that children who are less than 6 years old at the time of transplant exhibit spontaneous catch-up growth post-transplant, while older children may not [42]. The other major determinants of poor growth in children after kidney transplant are related to glucocorticoid therapy and poor or declining function of the allograft. Use of steroid avoidance or minimization protocols may help improve growth in transplant recipients [43, 44]. However, in those who require maintenance steroid immunosuppression or do not exhibit catch-up growth in the first-year post-transplant, recombinant human growth hormone (GH) therapy may be beneficial [45].

Recombinant human GH is an effective therapy, evidenced by numerous randomized control trials (RCTs) which have shown improvement in growth velocity and height standard deviation score (SDS) in children with CKD [46] and after kidney transplant [47–50]. In transplant recipients with steroid-related growth impairment, GH helps to block the action of the glucocorticoids on the GH/IGF-1 axis, thereby restoring more normal post-transplant growth patterns. In those with declining allograft function, a state of CKD-associated growth hormone resistance will re-emerge. This GH insensitivity can be overcome by the administration of supraphysiologic levels of exogenous GH, which will increase production of IGF-1 and promote growth [45].

Outcomes

Treatment of growth failure in children with kidney disease has important implications beyond cosmetic effects. Short stature is associated with poor outcomes in pediatric kidney transplant recipients, including increased hospitalizations, infections, higher risk of cardiac and infection-related mortality, and increased all-cause mortality [51–53]. The Chronic Kidney Disease in Children (CKiD) study showed that short stature is associated with a faster decline in kidney allograft function after transplant, evidenced by 40% shorter time to estimated glomerular filtration rate (eGFR) <45 ml/min/1.73 m^2 among short children [54]. Short stature is also associated with adverse psychosocial outcomes, such as lower health-related quality of life (HRQOL), including poor physical, school, emotional, and social functioning during childhood [55]. This lower HRQOL persists into adulthood, as young adults who were diagnosed with CKD during infancy and have short stature report lower HRQOL scores [56]. Treatment with GH has been associated not only with improved linear growth and greater adult height, but also with improved physical and social functioning [57].

Growth Hormone Utilization

Despite its proven efficacy, GH is still under-utilized, especially post-transplant. A study of North American children with CKD revealed that 51% of those with short stature do not receive GH therapy [58]. Across Europe, just 24% of children with growth impairment on dialysis receive GH therapy [59]. Post-transplant usage of GH is even lower, with only 7.6% of pediatric kidney transplant recipients with short stature receiving GH [59]. Barriers to GH therapy may include 1) family refusal due to fear of injections or side effects; 2) medical contraindications such as secondary hyperparathyroidism, malignancy, or fused epiphyseal growth plates; and 3) difficulties with insurance approval [58, 60].

Indications and Contraindications for Growth Hormone

GH is FDA-approved in the USA for children with short stature for several indications, including chronic kidney disease [61]; however it is not specifically approved for use in pediatric kidney allograft recipients.

Indications: GH therapy is indicated in pediatric kidney transplant recipients who fail to exhibit spontaneous catch-up growth during the first year post-transplant and have growth failure as defined by height less than the third percentile for age and sex, and a height velocity below the 25th percentile [45].

Contraindications: GH is typically not initiated until the patient is around one-year post-transplant to allow for possible spontaneous catch-up growth [45]. Additional contraindications to GH therapy include the following [45]:

- Closed epiphyses
- Secondary hyperparathyroidism (iPTH >500 pg/ml)
- Active malignancy
- Acute critical illness
- Diabetic retinopathy
- Patient or family refusal

Work-Up, Treatment, and Monitoring

Work-Up

The following parameters should be evaluated as part of the work-up process prior to initiation of GH [7, 45]:

- Rate of spontaneous growth should be monitored for the first 12 months after kidney transplantation prior to initiating GH in children with normal renal function.
- Growth potential should be assessed in the context of mid-parental height and bone age.
- Nutritional status should be optimized prior to initiation of GH, as nutrition is the key driver of growth in infants and young children. The following nutritional components should be corrected prior to GH initiation [7]:
  - Protein-energy malnutrition: ensure energy and protein intake >80% of estimated needs and implement enteral nutrition support if indicated.
  - Urine sodium wasting: sodium/fluid supplementation should be provided in children with salt-wasting polyuria.
  - Dialysis adequacy: increased dialytic clearance promotes improved nutrition and growth [62].
- Any additional factors affecting growth should be controlled prior to initiation of GH, including metabolic acidosis, secondary hyperparathyroidism, and mineral and electrolyte balance.
- The following baseline studies should be obtained prior to initiation of GH:
  - Serum creatinine and estimated glomerular filtration rate (eGFR)
  - Bone health indicators: serum calcium, phosphorus, alkaline phosphatase, parathyroid hormone, and 25 OH vitamin D levels
  - Fasting glucose and HbA1c% levels
  - Thyroid studies (TSH and free T3)
  - IGF-1 level
  - Bone age by radiography of left wrist
  - Pubertal status/Tanner stage

Treatment

The recommended dose of GH for children with CKD is 0.045 to 0.05 mg/kg of body weight per day, administered by subcutaneous injection daily. Ideally, the GH injection should be given in the evening, to simulate the body's natural circadian rhythm of endogenous GH secretion [45, 63]. The treatment goal is to achieve a growth velocity greater than 2 cm per year over the baseline growth velocity.

Monitoring

The following parameters should be assessed every 3–6 months while on GH therapy [7, 45]:

- Height-for-age SDS and growth velocity
- Bone age
- Pubertal development
- Biochemical indicators: thyroid studies, serum creatinine, glucose, bicarbonate, calcium, and phosphorus levels
- Parathyroid hormone (PTH): Due to increased risk of slipped capital femoral epiphysis, GH therapy should be held in patients with PTH >500 pg/mL. GH can be resumed when PTH levels return to the desired target range

In transplant recipients, GH therapy should be discontinued in the following circumstances [45]:

- Closed epiphyses or attainment of genetic target height for age SDS
- Slipped capital femoral epiphysis or accelerated bone maturation
- Intracranial hypertension
- Unexplained decrease in eGFR
- Lack of adequate growth on GH therapy, despite optimization of nutrition and metabolic parameters and good adherence to therapy

Safety of Growth Hormone in Transplant Recipients

Studies indicate that GH is generally safe for use in pediatric kidney transplant recipients. GH usage does not appear to increase the risk for malignancy in children with CKD or in pediatric kidney transplant recipients [64, 65]. In addition, transplant recipients treated with GH do not experience more allograft rejection episodes or impairment in eGFR compared with transplant recipients not treated with GH [66]. However, GH can decrease insulin sensitivity, and therefore monitoring of glucose tolerance is recommended, particularly in patients with other risk factors for diabetes mellitus such as obesity or family history [45].

Metabolic Bone Disease

Progression of CKD precipitates a chain of disturbances in bone and mineral metabolism which predispose children to chronic kidney disease-mineral and bone disorder (CKD-MBD). CKD-BMD begins in the early stages of CKD and persists throughout ESKD. After kidney transplantation, new factors emerge which pose continued threats to bone health and growth. Factors impacting bone health post-transplant may include hypophosphatemia, hypomagnesemia, nutritional vitamin D deficiency, effects of immunosuppressive therapies, and alteration of sex hormones.

Pathophysiology of CKD-BMD

In the early stages of CKD, increased dietary phosphorus load stimulates increased secretion of FGF-23 by osteoblasts and osteocytes. FGF-23, a phosphaturic hormone, attempts to maintain phosphorus homeostasis by binding to the FGF receptor and co-receptor Klotho in the renal proximal tubule, promoting downregulation of sodium phosphate cotransporters and inhibition of 1-alpha-hydroxylase production. This prompts increased excretion of urine phosphate, decreased absorption of phosphate from the gastrointestinal tract, and decreased production of 1,25-dihydroxy vitamin D (calcitriol) [67]. As kidney disease progresses, serum phosphorus levels rise, and hyperphosphatemia in combination with decreased 1,25-dihydroxy vitamin D production results in hypocalcemia, which stimulates release of parathyroid hormone. Thus, this series of events culminates in secondary hyperparathyroidism leading to CKD-BMD.

Consequently, most children will already have some degree of pre-existing bone disease when they present for kidney transplant. In addition, late-stage CKD and ESKD patients are likely to have impaired growth as well as disproportionate stunting, characterized by longer trunk length and shorter limb length at the time of transplant [68].

Bone Mineral Monitoring

Regular monitoring of serum calcium, phosphorus, total carbon dioxide (CO_2), alkaline phosphatase, PTH, and 25-hydroxy vitamin D should occur beginning at stage 2 CKD and continuing throughout the cycle of CKD, dialysis, and transplantation. In the immediate post-transplant period, it is recommended to monitor serum calcium and phosphorus levels at least weekly, and thereafter monitor these and other parameters, including magnesium, based on the degree of abnormalities and rate of CKD progression [69]. Measurement of bone mineral density (BMD) in the first 3 months after kidney transplant may be considered in patients who have risk factors for osteoporosis, i.e., those with low BMD or severe CKD-MBD pre-transplant or those receiving maintenance corticosteroids post-transplant [69].

Post-transplant Bone Metabolism

PTH, FGF-23, and Hypophosphatemia

Elevation of FGF-23 and PTH levels at the time of transplant precipitate urinary phosphorus wasting after transplant. Therefore, hypophosphatemia is common in the early post-transplant period due to decreased phosphorus reabsorption in the proximal tubule, but this typically resolves within a few months. However, in 10–60% of transplant recipients, elevation of PTH and associated hypophosphatemia may persist beyond 1-year post-transplant [70, 71]. This phenomenon is typically observed in those who had severe elevation of FGF-23, severe secondary hyperparathyroidism, or tertiary hyperparathyroidism prior to transplant [72]. Persistent renal phosphate wasting contributes to decreased osteoblast activity and progressive bone demineralization over the long term. In children with chronic allograft nephropathy, FGF-23 and PTH levels increase with the degree of chronic allograft failure, reactivating the cycle of CKD-MBD [73]

Hypomagnesemia

Urinary magnesium wasting and use of CNIs predispose pediatric kidney transplant recipients to hypomagnesemia. Magnesium is essential for the physiological function of osteoblasts and osteoclasts and regulation of PTH, and is also an integral component of the hydroxyapatite structure of bone. Magnesium deficiency contributes to osteoporosis by impairing the magnesium-dependent hydrogen-potassium-ATPase pump within the cells of the periosteum, lowering the pH of extracellular bone fluid leading to bone demineralization. Magnesium deficiency has numerous effects on PTH regulation by impairing PTH secretion, inducing PTH resistance, and decreasing production of calcitriol [74].

Vitamin D

Vitamin D deficiency and/or insufficiency occurs commonly across the USA with a rate of about 27% of children being vitamin D deficient (25-hydroxyvitamin D level <20 ng/mL) [75]. In children with chronic kidney disease, including those with a renal transplant, these rates have been shown to be much higher. In a study of 59 pediatric patients on dialysis (mean age: 14.4 ± 5.1 years), 83% (n = 49) had 25-hydroxy vitamin D levels less than 30 ng/ml [76]. Sadlier et al. reported that only 12% of patients at the time of kidney transplant had 25-hydroxy vitamin D concentration >30 ng/mL, and 29% of patients had 25-hydroxy vitamin D levels <10 ng/mL [77]. Ebbert et al. reported a similar prevalence of vitamin D insufficiency and deficiency of 76% in a study of pediatric renal transplant patients [78].

In the pediatric renal transplant population, vitamin D deficiency has been shown to correlate with hyperparathyroidism, short stature, and hypophosphatemia [79]. KDOQI guidelines for the nutritional management of pediatric kidney transplant recipients recommend intake of at least 100% of the DRI for vitamin D from diet and/or supplements to promote optimal bone mineralization [7].

Immunosuppression

Although maintenance immunosuppressive therapies are required to sustain the kidney allograft, these medications have been implicated in causing impairment of bone health in children after transplant. It is well known that corticosteroids inhibit bone formation by decreasing intestinal calcium absorption, reducing osteoblast proliferation, inducing osteoblast apoptosis, and impairing osteoblast function via interference with the GH/IGF-1 axis. These changes result in decreased bone formation, trabecular bone loss, and increased risk for fractures [80, 81].

CNI medications, such as tacrolimus and cyclosporine, also exert negative effects on bone by stimulating osteoclast differentiation and inhibiting synthesis of the vitamin D receptor and osteoprotegerin [82]. CNIs, including tacrolimus and cyclosporine, have been linked to bone loss and increased fracture risk in adult renal transplant recipients [83]. Mammalian target of rapamycin (mTOR) inhibitors such as sirolimus and everolimus may also impair bone formation and growth by interfering with osteoblast proliferation and inhibiting growth plate structure and function [84]. Further studies are needed to elucidate the effect of mTOR inhibitors on bone in the pediatric transplant population.

Role of Sex Hormones

Delayed sexual maturation may negatively impact bone development and mineralization post-transplant. Delayed puberty and sexual maturation are common in this population and may be attributed in part to glucocorticoids, which reduce the production of sex hormones and interfere with bone maturation by impairing differentiation of the growth plate.

Prevention Strategies

Whenever possible, prevention strategies should be implemented to preserve and optimize post-transplant bone health. The following are potentially modifiable risk factors which should be considered.

Steroid Minimization

The introduction of steroid minimization protocols in the early 2000s has resulted in a decrease in the use of post-transplant steroid immunosuppression therapy in certain populations. Kidney disease improving global outcome (KDIGO) guidelines recommend minimizing or avoiding corticosteroid use in children who still have growth potential if possible [85]. Steroid avoidance and withdrawal protocols are associated with improved growth and decreased fracture risk in pediatric kidney transplant recipients, and the continued development of strategies to minimize steroid exposure in the pediatric transplant population is important.

Diet and Physical Activity

Healthy diet and physical activity are key components of promoting bone health after kidney transplant.

- **Adequate dietary intake of key nutrients**. Goal to meet 100% of the DRI for nutrients that affect bone health, including calcium, phosphorus, vitamin D, copper, zinc, and magnesium [7].
- **Limit sodium intake.** High dietary sodium intake increases urinary calcium excretion and losses of calcium from bone and decreases bone formation. The DASH diet is low in sodium and also incorporates the key nutrients that promote bone health; therefore it may be beneficial for kidney transplant recipients [86].

- **Avoid cola beverages:** In animal studies, cola intake was associated with decreased osteogenesis, delayed bone formation, and thinner trabeculae [87]. Intake of cola beverages has been linked with decreased BMD, increased fracture risk in children, and increased risk of osteoporosis in adult women. Possible etiologies may include replacement of more nutrient-rich foods and beverages in the diet by cola, reduction of vitamin D synthesis and calcium absorption by the phosphoric acid in the cola, and/or accelerated bone resorption induced by the acid load of cola.

Weight-bearing exercise: Physical activity plays a key role in maintaining bone mass throughout life and is important for promoting bone health and strength after transplant. Bones strengthen in response to mechanical loading forces but weaken if not subjected to loading and weight bearing. Moderate weight-bearing physical activity of at least 30 minutes per day on most days of the week is recommended to promote increase or preservation of bone mass.

Treatment

Nutritional vitamin D: 25-hydroxy vitamin D insufficiency and deficiency should be treated with oral supplementation, both before and after renal transplantation. There is some evidence to suggest that supplementation with cholecalciferol (D_3) is more effective than ergocalciferol (D_2) for repletion of vitamin D [88]. Treatment guidelines for the pediatric CKD population have been established, as follows. Severe deficiency (25-hydroxy vitamin D levels <5 ng/mL) should be treated with 8000 IU per day for 1 month followed by 4000 IU per day for 2 months. Mild deficiency (5–15 ng/mL) should be treated with 4000 IU per day for 3 months. Insufficiency (16–30 ng/mL) should be treated with 2000 IU per day for 3 months. After vitamin D repletion (≥30 ng/mL), a maintenance dose of 200–1000 IU per day should be provided [7]. There are presently no clinical practice guidelines for treatment of vitamin D deficiency specifically targeted to pediatric transplant recipients. The level of vitamin D sufficiency is not well defined, with the target levels varying from >20 to 30 ng/mL.

Parathyroid hormone: levels should be maintained within the target range based on stage of CKD. As allograft function declines, 1,25-vitamin D_3 should be initiated if nutritional vitamin D is replete and PTH is above the target range for CKD stage [7].

Metabolic acidosis: should be corrected and CO_2 level maintained ≥22 mEq/L to promote resolution of electrolyte abnormalities, decrease the risk of post-transplant osteoporosis, and maximize growth [7].

Magnesium: post-transplant hypomagnesemia should be corrected with either increased dietary intake of high magnesium containing foods or oral magnesium supplementation to achieve and maintain magnesium homeostasis and promote optimization of BMD.

Pharmacologic Therapies

The KDIGO guidelines recommend consideration of using vitamin D, vitamin D analogs, and/or antiresorptive medications to treat bone disease during the first-year post-transplant in adult kidney transplant recipients [69]. Clinicians should use levels of calcium, phosphorus, PTH, alkaline phosphatase, and vitamin D to guide treatment [69]. Very little data is available on the safety and efficacy of pharmacologic treatment of post-transplant bone disease in children. Further research is needed to identify the most appropriate therapies to treat bone disease in children after transplant.

Developmental and Psychosocial Impairments

Deficits in neurocognitive functioning are prominent in children both before and after transplant. Children with severe CKD frequently have low intellectual abilities [89] and difficulties in executive functioning, such as attention, memory, task initiation, and planning/organization [90]. While some improvements in intellectual functioning is observed after transplantation, transplant does not normalize developmental status or intellectual functioning compared to healthy controls [91]. Children and adolescents continue to face challenges after transplant and display an intelligence quotient (IQ) of 11.2 points lower than healthy peers [92]. Among the identified risk factors for lower cognitive abilities are earlier age of dialysis onset, longer dialysis duration, duration of hospitalization, malnutrition, infections, and reduced age-appropriate environmental stimulation [93]. Similarly, academic performance is also found to be lower in the transplant population, likely due to learning disabilities and poorer neurocognitive functioning as well as poor school attendance [94]. Children on hemodialysis prior to transplantation in particular are also at higher risk of poorer adaptive functioning as defined by everyday living skills [95].

Pediatric renal transplant recipients also exhibit poorer emotional/behavioral and social development compared to healthy peers. A significant number of dialysis patients experience mental health difficulties, and while some studies note reductions in psychiatric symptoms post-transplant [96], others have noted no differences in reports of anxiety, depression, or behavioral concerns between dialysis and post-transplant groups [97]. Overall, children after kidney transplant have higher rates of depression and anxiety (17–36.4%), attention deficit/hyperactivity disorder (ADHD, 22.5%), and post-traumatic stress symptoms (PTSS, 65%) in comparison to healthy peers [98, 99]. On measures of social functioning, post-transplant patients' scores are comparable to scores of those with CKD or on dialysis [100] but lower than those of healthy controls [101].

Neurocognitive and emotional/behavioral difficulties have significant implications on youth's health literacy and healthcare engagement. Intellectual delays and executive functioning deficits can impact how well patients understand, retain, and utilize healthcare information. As such, developmental delays can complicate youth's readiness to transition to adult care and impact post-transition success [102]. Furthermore, developmental difficulties may persist into adolescence and young adulthood in ESKD patients, characterized by dependence on parents or other adults as well as decrease in motor performance [103]. Autonomy development (adaptive skills, independent daily functioning), social functioning, and psycho-sexual behaviors are also found to be delayed among adults who were on ESKD in childhood despite renal transplantation [104]. Additionally, young adults on renal replacement therapies are also more likely to be unemployed and live in the family home, and less likely to be married or have a partner compared to healthy peers [105].

It is important to screen for developmental functioning as well as their risk factors to adequately intervene and address these various challenges. Empirically validated age-appropriate batteries and measures of developmental, intellectual, executive, psychological, and social functioning should be used for early detection [106]. The results of such neuropsychological testing are essential in guiding early interventions such as academic accommodations, special education services, and cognitive interventions such as problem-solving skills training and computerized progressive attentional training. An evaluation for Individualized Education Plan both before and after transplantation is critical in addressing developmental delays globally and in school environment where children and adolescent have more opportunities to receive appropriate services. Comprehensive psychological assessment with measures of emotional/behavioral health should be used at pre-transplant evaluation, or better yet at onset of dialysis. Furthermore, developmental evaluation should continue regularly after transplantation to address deficits in readiness to transition to adulthood and guide appropriate clinical practices [107].

Questions

- Question 1. Influenza vaccine increases the risk of acute rejection in renal transplant recipients:

  A. True

  B. False

  B. There have been concerns about the influenza vaccine triggering acute rejections, but these concerns were not substantiated in large-scale studies. In large registry data, influenza vaccine use in transplant recipients was associated with lower rates of allograft loss and death.

  Question 2: A kidney transplant recipient is fully immunized with PCV13 and has received one dose of the PPSV23, what needs to be done after transplant?

  A. Repeat the PPSV23 every 5 years.

  B. Repeat the PPSV23 once after 5 years.

  C. Restart the PCV13 and the PPSV23 vaccination series after 5 years.

  B. It is typically recommended that high-risk patients, such as transplant patients, receive 2 doses of PPSV23 5 years apart.

  Question 3: Growth and metabolic changes after transplant TYPICALLY include the following:

A. Hypomagnesemia, hypophosphatemia, excessive weight gain, hyperkalemia, and metabolic acidosis
B. Hypokalemia, improved growth, new onset diabetes post-transplant, dyslipidemia
C. Hypomagnesemia, hypophosphatemia, failure to thrive and growth retardation
D. A and B

D. Transplant typically leads to growth improvement and not growth retardation. Although successful kidney transplantation typically restores normal function of the GH/IGF-1 axis, suboptimal growth may persist in some children post-transplant, but is not retarded. Age at time of transplant is a significant determinant of growth after transplant. Studies have shown that children who are less than 6 years old at the time of transplant exhibit spontaneous catch-up growth post-transplant, while older children may not.

Question 4. Risk factors for lower cognitive abilities post-transplant include the following:

A. Younger age at dialysis onset
B. Longer dialysis duration
C. Duration of hospitalization
D. Malnutrition and infections
E. All of the above

E. Among the identified risk factors for lower cognitive abilities are earlier age of dialysis onset, longer dialysis duration, duration of hospitalization, malnutrition, infections, and reduced age-appropriate environmental stimulation.

References

1. CDC. [https://www.cdc.gov/vaccines/schedules/hcp/imz/child-adolescent.html].
2. Kelgeri C, Kelly DF, Brant A, Patel M, Gupte GL. Principles of immunisation in children with solid organ transplant. Arch Dis Child. 2020.
3. Kumar D, Blumberg EA, Danziger-Isakov L, Kotton CN, Halasa NB, Ison MG, Avery RK, Green M, Allen UD, Edwards KM, et al. Influenza vaccination in the organ transplant recipient: review and summary recommendations. Am J Transplant. 2011;11(10):2020–30.
4. Nailescu C, Xu X, Zhou H, Hall H, Wilson AC, Leiser JD, Chand DH, Valentini RP, Hebert D, Mahan JD. Influenza vaccine after pediatric kidney transplant: a Midwest pediatric nephrology consortium study. Pediatr Nephrol. 2011;26(3):459–67.
5. Hurst FP, Lee JJ, Jindal RM, Agodoa LY, Abbott KC. Outcomes associated with influenza vaccination in the first year after kidney transplantation. Clin J Am Soc Nephrol. 2011;6(5):1192–7.
6. Katerinis I, Hadaya K, Duquesnoy R, Ferrari-Lacraz S, Meier S, van Delden C, Martin PY, Siegrist CA, Villard J. De novo anti-HLA antibody after pandemic H1N1 and seasonal influenza immunization in kidney transplant recipients. Am J Transplant. 2011;11(8):1727–33.
7. Group KW: KDOQI clinical practice guideline for nutrition in children with CKD: 2008 update. Executive summary. Am J Kidney Dis. 2009;53(3 Suppl 2):S11–104.
8. Iorember FM. Malnutrition in chronic kidney disease. Front Pediatr. 2018;6:161.

9. Cheung WW, Paik KH, Mak RH. Inflammation and cachexia in chronic kidney disease. Pediatr Nephrol. 2010;25(4):711–24.
10. Correa M, Laing DG, Hutchinson I, Jinks AL, Armstrong JE, Kainer G. Reduced taste function and taste papillae density in children with chronic kidney disease. Pediatr Nephrol. 2015;30(11):2003–10.
11. Manley KJ. Taste genetics and gastrointestinal symptoms experienced in chronic kidney disease. Eur J Clin Nutr. 2015;69(7):781–5.
12. Hsu CN, Chang-Chien GP, Lin S, Hou CY, Lu PC, Tain YL. Association of trimethylamine, trimethylamine n-oxide, and dimethylamine with cardiovascular risk in children with chronic kidney disease. J Clin Med. 2020;9(2).
13. Abraham AG, Mak RH, Mitsnefes M, White C, Moxey-Mims M, Warady B, Furth SL. Protein energy wasting in children with chronic kidney disease. Pediatr Nephrol. 2014;29(7):1231–8.
14. Sgambat K, Matheson MB, Hooper SR, Warady B, Furth S, Moudgil A. Prevalence and outcomes of fragility: a frailty-inflammation phenotype in children with chronic kidney disease. Pediatr Nephrol. 2019;34(12):2563–9.
15. Juarez-Congelosi M, Orellana P, Goldstein SL. Normalized protein catabolic rate versus serum albumin as a nutrition status marker in pediatric patients receiving hemodialysis. J Ren Nutr. 2007;17(4):269–74.
16. Eknoyan G, Latos DL, Lindberg J, National Kidney Foundation Carnitine Consensus C. Practice recommendations for the use of L-carnitine in dialysis-related carnitine disorder. National Kidney Foundation Carnitine Consensus Conference. Am J Kidney Dis. 2003;41(4):868–76.
17. Tom A, McCauley L, Bell L, Rodd C, Espinosa P, Yu G, Yu J, Girardin C, Sharma A. Growth during maintenance hemodialysis: impact of enhanced nutrition and clearance. J Pediatr. 1999;134(4):464–71.
18. Fischbach M, Terzic J, Menouer S, Dheu C, Soskin S, Helmstetter A, Burger MC. Intensified and daily hemodialysis in children might improve statural growth. Pediatr Nephrol. 2006;21(11):1746–52.
19. Fischbach M, Fothergill H, Zaloszyc A, Menouer S, Terzic J. Intensified daily dialysis: the best chronic dialysis option for children? Semin Dial. 2011;24(6):640–4.
20. Rees L, Brandt ML. Tube feeding in children with chronic kidney disease: technical and practical issues. Pediatr Nephrol. 2010;25(4):699–704.
21. Quan A, Baum M. Protein losses in children on continuous cycler peritoneal dialysis. Pediatr Nephrol. 1996;10(6):728–31.
22. Bodnar DM, Busch S, Fuchs J, Piedmonte M, Schreiber M. Estimating glucose absorption in peritoneal dialysis using peritoneal equilibration tests. Adv Perit Dial. 1993;9:114–8.
23. Shaw V, Polderman N, Renken-Terhaerdt J, Paglialonga F, Oosterveld M, Tuokkola J, Anderson C, Desloovere A, Greenbaum L, Haffner D, et al. Energy and protein requirements for children with CKD stages 2-5 and on dialysis-clinical practice recommendations from the pediatric renal nutrition taskforce. Pediatr Nephrol. 2020;35(3):519–31.
24. Rees L, Shaw V, Qizalbash L, Anderson C, Desloovere A, Greenbaum L, Haffner D, Nelms C, Oosterveld M, Paglialonga F, et al. Delivery of a nutritional prescription by enteral tube feeding in children with chronic kidney disease stages 2-5 and on dialysis-clinical practice recommendations from the pediatric renal nutrition taskforce. Pediatr Nephrol. 2020.
25. McAlister L, Pugh P, Greenbaum L, Haffner D, Rees L, Anderson C, Desloovere A, Nelms C, Oosterveld M, Paglialonga F, et al. The dietary management of calcium and phosphate in children with CKD stages 2-5 and on dialysis-clinical practice recommendation from the pediatric renal nutrition taskforce. Pediatr Nephrol. 2020;35(3):501–18.
26. Rees L, Azocar M, Borzych D, Watson AR, Buscher A, Edefonti A, Bilge I, Askenazi D, Leozappa G, Gonzales C, et al. Growth in very young children undergoing chronic peritoneal dialysis. J Am Soc Nephrol. 2011;22(12):2303–12.
27. Ledermann SE, Scanes ME, Fernando ON, Duffy PG, Madden SJ, Trompeter RS. Long-term outcome of peritoneal dialysis in infants. J Pediatr. 2000;136(1):24–9.

28. Parekh RS, Flynn JT, Smoyer WE, Milne JL, Kershaw DB, Bunchman TE, Sedman AB. Improved growth in young children with severe chronic renal insufficiency who use specified nutritional therapy. J Am Soc Nephrol. 2001;12(11):2418–26.
29. Norman LJ, Macdonald IA, Watson AR. Optimising nutrition in chronic renal insufficiency--growth. Pediatr Nephrol. 2004;19(11):1245–52.
30. Wilson AC, Mitsnefes MM. Cardiovascular disease in CKD in children: update on risk factors, risk assessment, and management. Am J Kidney Dis. 2009;54(2):345–60.
31. Sgambat K, Clauss S, Moudgil A. Cardiovascular effects of metabolic syndrome after transplantation: convergence of obesity and transplant-related factors. Clin Kidney J. 2018;11(1):136–46.
32. Ladhani M, Lade S, Alexander SI, Baur LA, Clayton PA, McDonald S, Craig JC, Wong G. Obesity in pediatric kidney transplant recipients and the risks of acute rejection, graft loss and death. Pediatr Nephrol. 2017;32(8):1443–50.
33. Sgambat K, Cheng YI, Charnaya O, Moudgil A. The prevalence and outcome of children with failure to thrive after pediatric kidney transplantation. Pediatr Transplant. 2019;23(1):e13321.
34. Khweir S, Mcalister L, Marks SD. Feeding patterns and outcomes of enterally tube fed paediatric kidney transplant recipients. Pediatr Nephrol. 2020.
35. Misra M, Pacaud D, Petryk A, Collett-Solberg PF, Kappy M, Drug, Therapeutics Committee of the Lawson Wilkins Pediatric Endocrine S. Vitamin D deficiency in children and its management: review of current knowledge and recommendations. Pediatrics. 2008;122(2):398–417.
36. Sacks FM, Appel LJ, Moore TJ, Obarzanek E, Vollmer WM, Svetkey LP, Bray GA, Vogt TM, Cutler JA, Windhauser MM, et al. A dietary approach to prevent hypertension: a review of the dietary approaches to stop hypertension (DASH) study. Clin Cardiol. 1999;22(7 Suppl):III6–10.
37. Oste MCJ, Gomes-Neto AW, Corpeleijn E, Gans ROB, de Borst MH, van den Berg E, Soedamah-Muthu SS, Kromhout D, Navis GJ, Bakker SJL. Dietary approach to stop hypertension (DASH) diet and risk of renal function decline and all-cause mortality in renal transplant recipients. Am J Transplant. 2018;18(10):2523–33.
38. Obayashi PA. Food safety for the solid organ transplant patient: preventing foodborne illness while on chronic immunosuppressive drugs. Nutr Clin Pract. 2012;27(6):758–66.
39. U.S. department of agriculture and the food and drug administration. food safety for transplant recipents. [https://Www.fsis.usda.gov/shared/PDF/Food_Safety_for_Transplant_Recipients.pdf].
40. Bikle DD, Tahimic C, Chang W, Wang Y, Philippou A, Barton ER. Role of IGF-I signaling in muscle bone interactions. Bone. 2015;80:79–88.
41. Chua A, Cramer C, Moudgil A, Martz K, Smith J, Blydt-Hansen T, Neu A, Dharnidharka VR, Investigators N. Kidney transplant practice patterns and outcome benchmarks over 30 years: the 2018 report of the NAPRTCS. Pediatr Transplant. 2019;23(8):e13597.
42. Tejani A, Fine R, Alexander S, Harmon W, Stablein D. Factors predictive of sustained growth in children after renal transplantation. The north American pediatric renal transplant cooperative study. J Pediatr. 1993;122(3):397–402.
43. Sarwal MM, Ettenger RB, Dharnidharka V, Benfield M, Mathias R, Portale A, McDonald R, Harmon W, Kershaw D, Vehaskari VM, et al. Complete steroid avoidance is effective and safe in children with renal transplants: a multicenter randomized trial with three-year follow-up. Am J Transplant. 2012;12(10):2719–29.
44. Grenda R, Watson A, Trompeter R, Tonshoff B, Jaray J, Fitzpatrick M, Murer L, Vondrak K, Maxwell H, van Damme-Lombaerts R, et al. A randomized trial to assess the impact of early steroid withdrawal on growth in pediatric renal transplantation: the TWIST study. Am J Transplant. 2010;10(4):828–36.
45. Drube J, Wan M, Bonthuis M, Wuhl E, Bacchetta J, Santos F, Grenda R, Edefonti A, Harambat J, Shroff R, et al. Clinical practice recommendations for growth hormone treatment in children with chronic kidney disease. Nat Rev Nephrol. 2019;15(9):577–89.
46. Fine RN, Kohaut EC, Brown D, Perlman AJ. Growth after recombinant human growth hormone treatment in children with chronic renal failure: report of a multicenter randomized

double-blind placebo-controlled study. Genentech Cooperative Study Group. J Pediatr. 1994;124(3):374–82.
47. Fine RN, Stablein D, Cohen AH, Tejani A, Kohaut E. Recombinant human growth hormone post-renal transplantation in children: a randomized controlled study of the NAPRTCS. Kidney Int. 2002;62(2):688–96.
48. Guest G, Berard E, Crosnier H, Chevallier T, Rappaport R, Broyer M. Effects of growth hormone in short children after renal transplantation. French Society of Pediatric Nephrology. Pediatr Nephrol. 1998;12(6):437–46.
49. Hokken-Koelega AC, Stijnen T, de Jong RC, Donckerwolcke RA, Groothoff JW, Wolff ED, Blum WF, de Muinck Keizer-Schrama SM, Drop SL. A placebo-controlled, double-blind trial of growth hormone treatment in prepubertal children after renal transplant. Kidney Int Suppl. 1996;53:S128–34.
50. Ahmad S, Robertson HT, Golper TA, Wolfson M, Kurtin P, Katz LA, Hirschberg R, Nicora R, Ashbrook DW, Kopple JD. Multicenter trial of L-carnitine in maintenance hemodialysis patients. II. Clinical and biochemical effects. Kidney Int. 1990;38(5):912–8.
51. Wong CS, Gipson DS, Gillen DL, Emerson S, Koepsell T, Sherrard DJ, Watkins SL, Stehman-Breen C. Anthropometric measures and risk of death in children with end-stage renal disease. Am J Kidney Dis. 2000;36(4):811–9.
52. Furth SL, Hwang W, Yang C, Neu AM, Fivush BA, Powe NR. Growth failure, risk of hospitalization and death for children with end-stage renal disease. Pediatr Nephrol. 2002;17(6):450–5.
53. Ku E, Fine RN, Hsu CY, McCulloch C, Glidden DV, Grimes B, Johansen KL. Height at first RRT and mortality in children. Clin J Am Soc Nephrol. 2016;11(5):832–9.
54. Li Y, Greenbaum LA, Warady BA, Furth SL, Ng DK. Short stature in advanced pediatric CKD is associated with faster time to reduced kidney function after transplant. Pediatr Nephrol. 2019;34(5):897–905.
55. Gerson AC, Wentz A, Abraham AG, Mendley SR, Hooper SR, Butler RW, Gipson DS, Lande MB, Shinnar S, Moxey-Mims MM, et al. Health-related quality of life of children with mild to moderate chronic kidney disease. Pediatrics. 2010;125(2):e349–57.
56. Mekahli D, Ledermann S, Gullett A, Rees L. Evaluation of quality of life by young adult survivors of severe chronic kidney disease in infancy. Pediatr Nephrol. 2014;29(8):1387–93.
57. Al-Uzri A, Matheson M, Gipson DS, Mendley SR, Hooper SR, Yadin O, Rozansky DJ, Moxey Mims M, Furth SL, Warady BA, et al. The impact of short stature on health-related quality of life in children with chronic kidney disease. J Pediatr. 2013;163(3):736–41. e731
58. Greenbaum LA, Hidalgo G, Chand D, Chiang M, Dell K, Kump T, Peschansky L, Smith HK, Boyle M, Kopf M, et al. Obstacles to the prescribing of growth hormone in children with chronic kidney disease. Pediatr Nephrol. 2008;23(9):1531–5.
59. van Huis M, Bonthuis M, Sahpazova E, Mencarelli F, Spasojevic B, Reusz G, Caldas-Afonso A, Bjerre A, Baiko S, Vondrak K, et al. Considerable variations in growth hormone policy and prescription in paediatric end-stage renal disease across European countries-a report from the ESPN/ERA-EDTA registry. Nephrol Dial Transplant. 2016;31(4):609–19.
60. Akchurin OM, Kogon AJ, Kumar J, Sethna CB, Hammad HT, Christos PJ, Mahan JD, Greenbaum LA, Woroniecki R. Approach to growth hormone therapy in children with chronic kidney disease varies across North America: the Midwest pediatric nephrology consortium report. BMC Nephrol. 2017;18(1):181.
61. [https://www.fda.gov/drugs/postmarket-drug-safety-information-patients-and-providers/somatropin-information].
62. Warady BA, Fischbach M, Geary D, Goldstein SL. Frequent hemodialysis in children. Adv Chronic Kidney Dis. 2007;14(3):297–303.
63. Hodson EM, Willis NS, Craig JC. Growth hormone for children with chronic kidney disease. Cochrane Database Syst Rev. 2012;2:CD003264.
64. Dharnidharka VR, Talley LI, Martz KL, Stablein DM, Fine RN. Recombinant growth hormone use pretransplant and risk for post-transplant lymphoproliferative disease--a report of the NAPRTCS. Pediatr Transplant. 2008;12(6):689–95.

65. Longmore DK, Conwell LS, Burke JR, McDonald SP, McTaggart SJ. Post-transplant lymphoproliferative disorder: no relationship to recombinant human growth hormone use in Australian and New Zealand pediatric kidney transplant recipients. Pediatr Transplant. 2013;17(8):731–6.
66. Wu Y, Cheng W, Yang XD, Xiang B. Growth hormone improves growth in pediatric renal transplant recipients--a systemic review and meta-analysis of randomized controlled trials. Pediatr Nephrol. 2013;28(1):129–33.
67. Musgrove J, Wolf M. Regulation and effects of FGF23 in chronic kidney disease. Annu Rev Physiol. 2020;82:365–90.
68. Franke D, Thomas L, Steffens R, Pavicic L, Gellermann J, Froede K, Querfeld U, Haffner D, Zivicnjak M. Patterns of growth after kidney transplantation among children with ESRD. Clin J Am Soc Nephrol. 2015;10(1):127–34.
69. Ketteler M, Block GA, Evenepoel P, Fukagawa M, Herzog CA, McCann L, Moe SM, Shroff R, Tonelli MA, Toussaint ND, et al. Executive summary of the 2017 KDIGO chronic kidney disease-mineral and bone disorder (CKD-MBD) guideline update: what's changed and why it matters. Kidney Int. 2017;92(1):26–36.
70. Sirilak S, Chatsrisak K, Ingsathit A, Kantachuvesiri S, Sumethkul V, Stitchantrakul W, Radinahamed P, Disthabanchong S. Renal phosphate loss in long-term kidney transplantation. Clin J Am Soc Nephrol. 2012;7(2):323–31.
71. Van de Cauter J, Sennesael J, Haentjens P. Long-term evolution of the mineral metabolism after renal transplantation: a prospective, single-center cohort study. Transplant Proc. 2011;43(9):3470–5.
72. Haffner D, Leifheit-Nestler M. CKD-MBD post kidney transplantation. Pediatr Nephrol. 2019.
73. van Husen M, Lehnhardt A, Fischer AK, Brinkert F, Loos S, Oh J, Kemper MJ. Fibroblast growth factor 23 and calcium phosphate homeostasis after pediatric renal transplantation. Pediatr Transplant. 2012;16(5):443–50.
74. Castiglioni S, Cazzaniga A, Albisetti W, Maier JA. Magnesium and osteoporosis: current state of knowledge and future research directions. Nutrients. 2013;5(8):3022–33.
75. Moore CE, Liu Y. Low serum 25-hydroxyvitamin D concentrations are associated with total adiposity of children in the United States: National Health and examination survey 2005 to 2006. Nutr Res. 2016;36(1):72–9.
76. Cho HY, Hyun HS, Kang HG, Ha IS, Cheong HI. Prevalence of 25(OH) vitamin D insufficiency and deficiency in pediatric patients on chronic dialysis. Peritoneal Dialysis International: Journal of the International Society for Peritoneal Dialysis. 2013;33(4):398–404.
77. Sadlier DM, Magee CC. Prevalence of 25(OH) vitamin D (calcidiol) deficiency at time of renal transplantation: a prospective study. Clin Transpl. 2007;21(6):683–8.
78. Ebbert K, Chow J, Krempien J, Matsuda-Abedini M, Dionne J. Vitamin D insufficiency and deficiency in pediatric renal transplant recipients. Pediatr Transplant. 2015;19(5):492–8.
79. Shroff R, Knott C, Gullett A, Wells D, Marks SD, Rees L. Vitamin D deficiency is associated with short stature and may influence blood pressure control in paediatric renal transplant recipients. Pediatr Nephrol. 2011;26(12):2227–33.
80. Terpstra AM, Kalkwarf HJ, Shults J, Zemel BS, Wetzsteon RJ, Foster BJ, Strife CF, Foerster DL, Leonard MB. Bone density and cortical structure after pediatric renal transplantation. J Am Soc Nephrol. 2012;23(4):715–26.
81. Nikkel LE, Mohan S, Zhang A, McMahon DJ, Boutroy S, Dube G, Tanriover B, Cohen D, Ratner L, Hollenbeak CS, et al. Reduced fracture risk with early corticosteroid withdrawal after kidney transplant. Am J Transplant. 2012;12(3):649–59.
82. Hofbauer LC, Shui C, Riggs BL, Dunstan CR, Spelsberg TC, O'Brien T, Khosla S. Effects of immunosuppressants on receptor activator of NF-kappaB ligand and osteoprotegerin production by human osteoblastic and coronary artery smooth muscle cells. Biochem Biophys Res Commun. 2001;280(1):334–9.
83. Panday K, Gona A, Humphrey MB. Medication-induced osteoporosis: screening and treatment strategies. Ther Adv Musculoskelet Dis. 2014;6(5):185–202.

84. Alvarez-Garcia O, Carbajo-Perez E, Garcia E, Gil H, Molinos I, Rodriguez J, Ordonez FA, Santos F. Rapamycin retards growth and causes marked alterations in the growth plate of young rats. Pediatr Nephrol. 2007;22(7):954–61.
85. Kasiske BL, Zeier MG, Chapman JR, Craig JC, Ekberg H, Garvey CA, Green MD, Jha V, Josephson MA, Kiberd BA, et al. KDIGO clinical practice guideline for the care of kidney transplant recipients: a summary. Kidney Int. 2010;77(4):299–311.
86. Doyle L, Cashman KD. The DASH diet may have beneficial effects on bone health. Nutr Rev. 2004;62(5):215–20.
87. Teofilo JM, Leonel DV, Lamano T. Cola beverage consumption delays alveolar bone healing: a histometric study in rats. Braz Oral Res. 2010;24(2):177–81.
88. Armas LA, Hollis BW, Heaney RP. Vitamin D2 is much less effective than vitamin D3 in humans. J Clin Endocrinol Metab. 2004;89(11):5387–91.
89. Ferris M, Cohen S, Haberman C, Javalkar K, Massengill S, Mahan JD, Kim S, Bickford K, Cantu G, Medeiros M, et al. Self-management and transition readiness assessment: development, reliability, and factor structure of the STARx questionnaire. J Pediatr Nurs. 2015;30(5):691–9.
90. Hooper SR, Laney N, Radcliffe J, Moodalbail D, Hartung EA, Ruebner RL, Jawad AF, Furth SL. Executive functioning in children, adolescents, and young adults with chronic kidney disease. J Dev Behav Pediatr. 2015;36(9):734–42.
91. Icard P, Hooper SR, Gipson DS, Ferris ME. Cognitive improvement in children with CKD after transplant. Pediatr Transplant. 2010;14(7):887–90.
92. Harshman LA, Johnson RJ, Matheson MB, Kogon AJ, Shinnar S, Gerson AC, Warady BA, Furth SL, Hooper SR. Academic achievement in children with chronic kidney disease: a report from the CKiD cohort. Pediatr Nephrol. 2019;34(4):689–96.
93. Szabo R, Lantsman T, Peters DE, Bugge TH. Delineation of proteolytic and non-proteolytic functions of the membrane-anchored serine protease prostasin. Development. 2016;143(15):2818–28.
94. Gulleroglu K, Baskin E, Bayrakci US, Aydogan M, Alehan F, Kantar A, Karakayali F, Moray G, Haberal M. Neurocognitive functions in pediatric renal transplant patients. Transplant Proc. 2013;45(10):3511–3.
95. Popel J, Joffe R, Acton BV, Bond GY, Joffe AR, Midgley J, Robertson CMT, Sauve RS, Morgan CJ. Neurocognitive and functional outcomes at 5 years of age after renal transplant in early childhood. Pediatr Nephrol. 2019;34(5):889–95.
96. Roscoe JM, Smith LF, Williams EA, Stein M, Morton AR, Balfe JW, Arbus GS. Medical and social outcome in adolescents with end-stage renal failure. Kidney Int. 1991;40(5):948–53.
97. Fielding D, Brownbridge G. Factors related to psychosocial adjustment in children with end-stage renal failure. Pediatr Nephrol. 1999;13(9):766–70.
98. McCormick King ML, Mee LL, Gutierrez-Colina AM, Eaton CK, Lee JL, Blount RL. Emotional functioning, barriers, and medication adherence in pediatric transplant recipients. J Pediatr Psychol. 2014;39(3):283–93.
99. Dobbels F, Decorte A, Roskams A, Van Damme-Lombaerts R. Health-related quality of life, treatment adherence, symptom experience and depression in adolescent renal transplant patients. Pediatr Transplant. 2010;14(2):216–23.
100. McKenna AM, Keating LE, Vigneux A, Stevens S, Williams A, Geary DF. Quality of life in children with chronic kidney disease-patient and caregiver assessments. Nephrol Dial Transplant. 2006;21(7):1899–905.
101. Anthony SJ, Hebert D, Todd L, Korus M, Langlois V, Pool R, Robinson LA, Williams A, Pollock-BarZiv SM. Child and parental perspectives of multidimensional quality of life outcomes after kidney transplantation. Pediatr Transplant. 2010;14(2):249–56.
102. Aylor DL, Valdar W, Foulds-Mathes W, Buus RJ, Verdugo RA, Baric RS, Ferris MT, Frelinger JA, Heise M, Frieman MB, et al. Genetic analysis of complex traits in the emerging collaborative cross. Genome Res. 2011;21(8):1213–22.

103. Eijsermans RM, Creemers DG, Helders PJ, Schroder CH. Motor performance, exercise tolerance, and health-related quality of life in children on dialysis. Pediatr Nephrol. 2004;19(11):1262–6.
104. Grootenhuis MA, Stam H, Last BF, Groothoff JW. The impact of delayed development on the quality of life of adults with end-stage renal disease since childhood. Pediatr Nephrol. 2006;21(4):538–44.
105. Hamilton AJ, Clissold RL, Inward CD, Caskey FJ, Ben-Shlomo Y. Sociodemographic, psychologic health, and lifestyle outcomes in young adults on renal replacement therapy. Clin J Am Soc Nephrol. 2017;12(12):1951–61.
106. Gerson AC, Butler R, Moxey-Mims M, Wentz A, Shinnar S, Lande MB, Mendley SR, Warady BA, Furth SL, Hooper SR. Neurocognitive outcomes in children with chronic kidney disease: current findings and contemporary endeavors. Ment Retard Dev Disabil Res Rev. 2006;12(3):208–15.
107. Watson AR, Harden PN, Ferris ME, Kerr PG, Mahan JD, Ramzy MF, International Society of N, International Pediatric Nephrology A. Transition from pediatric to adult renal services: a consensus statement by the International Society of Nephrology (ISN) and the international pediatric nephrology association (IPNA). Kidney Int. 2011;80(7):704–7.

Part IV
Medication Challenges

11 Challenges Surrounding Induction Protocols in Children

Raphael H. Parrado and Satish N. Nadig

The birth of pediatric transplantation followed the first successful adult kidney transplantation in 1954 in the United States by Dr. Joseph Murray. The first successful pediatric kidney transplant was performed in 1966 [1]. This was followed by the first pediatric liver transplantation in 1967 and the first pediatric heart and lung transplantation in 1984 and 1987, respectively. Since then, the field of transplantation has evolved and continues to progress rapidly with the development and optimization of techniques, protocols, and better donor and organ selection. Approximately two thirds of pediatric transplantation consists of liver and/or kidney allografts with around 800 pediatric kidney transplants performed in the United States annually [2].

The cornerstone of the development of transplantation is the growth of transplant immunology. This is exemplified by the discovery of the immune response to alloantigen and the development of molecular targets for modern immunosuppression regimens. The purpose of the immunosuppressive therapy is to achieve low rates of acute rejection and to improve long-term survival of the graft while minimizing short- and long-term effect of the immunosuppression itself (such as infections or malignancies). Traditionally the immunosuppressive therapies are divided into induction, maintenance, and treatment of rejection. In this chapter, we will focus in the scientific basis and the clinical use of induction immunosuppression in pediatric patients as well as complications arising from it.

R. H. Parrado
Department of General Surgery, Medical University of South Carolina, Charleston, SC, USA
e-mail: parrado@musc.edu

S. N. Nadig (✉)
Division of Transplant Surgery, Department of Surgery, Medical University of South Carolina, Charleston, SC, USA
e-mail: nadigsn@musc.edu

K. E. Twombley (ed.), *Challenges in Pediatric Kidney Transplantation*,
https://doi.org/10.1007/978-3-030-74783-1_11

Immunologic Basis of Current Induction Protocols

As with any foreign peptide, there is an interaction between the host's immune system and the transplanted organ which becomes vital in the process of developing methods to prevent an immune reaction that will lead to rejection. The objective is to achieve operational tolerance which refers to the immunologic acceptance of a transplanted allograft while maintaining global immune function. To achieve this objective, T- and B-cell activation and regulatory pathways have been targeted. The continued development of immunotherapy has permitted therapies to become more specific resulting in a decrease in systemic toxicity and other short- and long-term effects.

T-Cell Activation and the Immune Response

T lymphocytes are the cornerstone in the control and development of an immune response as they regulate cell-mediated injury and regulate the antigen response by activating/inactivating other immune cells. T-cell development starts from hematopoietic stem cells that migrate into the bone marrow and become nascent thymocytes that contain T-cell receptors (TCRs) that are rearranged in a random manner in the thymus. Then a process of antigen presentation takes place in these TCR-containing thymocytes in a process of "positive" or "negative" selection. "Self" antigens are presented to these TCR-containing thymocytes, and if they elicit a response, they undergo programmed cell death (positive selection); if they don't elicit any response, they do not receive a "survival" signal and ultimately undergo apoptosis (negative selection). If these thymocytes express intermediate affinity, they differentiate into double positive thymocytes (CD4+/CD8+) and migrate into the thymic cortex. After migration into the thymic cortex, they interact with the major histocompatibility complex molecules (MHC1–MHC2) and differentiate into CD4+ or CD8+ lymphocytes that will interact with antigen-presenting cells (APCs) such as dendritic cells or macrophages. The objective of this thymic selection process is to ensure that autoimmunity does not occur [3].

With mature T cells that can mount an immune response, the basis of the immune response revolves around antigen presentation by APCs (macrophages, B cells, and dendritic cells) allowing for adaptive (or acquired) immunity to be specific and respond to both intracellular and extracellular pathogens.

In one of the most common scenarios, the immune response starts when dendritic cells present their MHC class I or II molecules to the CD8+ or CD4+ T cells. If the peptide presented is a "self" antigen, the bond is very weak, and the T cell removes itself from the complex and recirculates. However, in settings such as infection or transplantation where a "non-self" molecule is presented, the cascade of T-cell activation and clonal expansion results in an immune response. Interestingly and uniquely, in the setting of transplantation, the entire MHC along with the peptide can be presented as well and elicit T-cell activation [4].

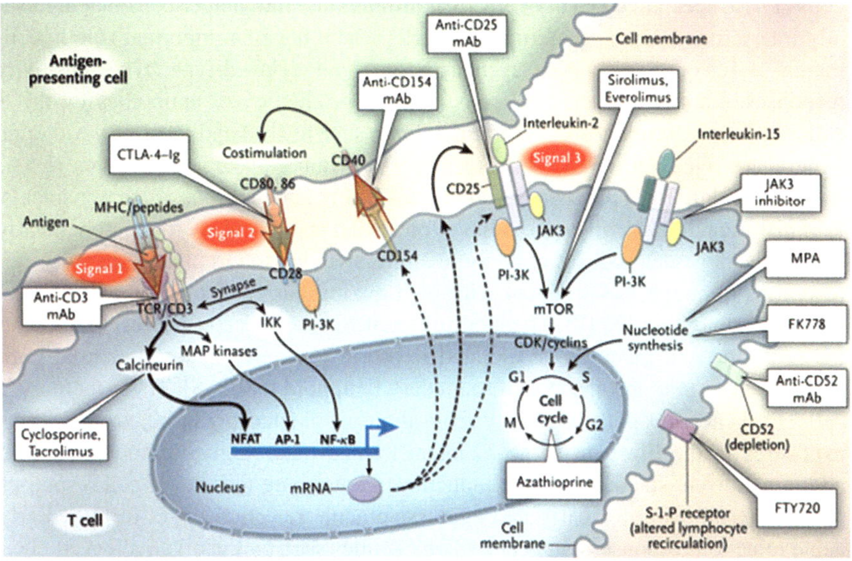

Fig. 11.1 Action of the multiple immunosuppressive medications used nowadays in the field of transplant medicine. MPA denotes mycophenolic acid. (Reproduced with permission from Halloran [5])

T-cell activation is a complex process that involves three signals that occur sequentially (Fig. 11.1) [5]:

- *Signal 1*: First interaction that occurs between the T-cell receptor (TCR) on a CD4+ cell and the MHC complex attached to the antigen presented by an APC (macrophage, B cells, and dendritic cells).
- *Signal 2*: Occurs after the TCR MHC interaction and involves the activation of multiple costimulatory molecules that are located on the periphery of both the APCs and the T cells resulting in a cascade of signaling pathways. Some of the pathways include the activation of the nuclear factor kappa-light-chain-enhancer of activated B cells (NFκB) and the translocation of the nuclear factor of activation and transcription (NFAT) to the nucleus of the T cell that promotes the production of T-cell-activating factors such as interleukin-2 (IL-2).
- *Signal 3*: IL-2 engages with the CD25 on the T cell resulting in the activation of a complex known as the mammalian target of rapamycin (mTOR). Activation of mTOR starts the cell cycle machinery resulting in T-cell activation and proliferation.

Following transplantation and reperfusion of the organ allograft, many inflammatory markers are upregulated. These inflammatory markers act as signals for the effector T cells and subsequently allow a more optimal uptake of antigens by APCs. Dendritic cells derived from the organ (also called passenger leukocytes) are then released to the host's secondary lymphoid tissue to present antigen to naïve host T cells. These specialized CD4+ cells then differentiate into helper cells that are usually interferon-γ (IFNγ)-secreting TH1 cells which have an important role in cell-mediated rejection responses such as acute- and delayed-type hypersensitivity responses. Another subset, TH2 cells, support production of antibodies by the B cells and secrete immunosuppressive cytokines such as IL-4 and IL-10 [6]. Although hyperacute rejection, resulting from preformed donor-specific antibodies (DSA) most commonly from pregnancy, blood transfusion, and previous organ transplants, is of historical interest given the reliance on virtual and physical crossmatches, early acute rejection seen today can be more aggressive due to circulating memory cell responses although less frequent with high-quality current induction and maintenance immunotherapies [7]. The vital subset of memory T cells can react rapidly to the graft and can incite an accelerated rejection response causing potential graft destruction even in the absence of secondary lymphoid tissue [8]. These memory T cells are generated not necessarily from the transplanted organ but from various exposures in the lifespan of the recipient termed heterologous immunity [9]. In addition, current standard-of-care induction agents spare memory T-cell responses potentially allowing for early and aggressive acute rejection to set in [10]. Early acute rejection responses can occur when peptides seen by the organ allograft elicit a circulating memory T-cell response with antigenic mimicry, for example [11]. It is the role of induction therapies to dampen the early response and create a "window" for the newly transplanted organ to heal and accommodate to its new environment.

Overview of Induction Therapy in Pediatric Renal Transplantation

During the induction therapy, powerful immunosuppressive agents are administered at the time of the transplantation with the aim of preventing acute rejection early. Biologically the most important factors that contribute to the need for an induction therapy are the presence of donor-specific T-cell precursor cells that directly affect the effector response and the association of transplantation with tissue injury that, by itself, can promote complement activation, ischemia, and reperfusion that can exacerbate the immune response [12]. The major benefit in terms of decreasing rejection in kidney transplantation is within the first 6 months and slowly fades for which maintenance therapy becomes an important mainstay [12, 13].

Historically, the induction protocols were based on complete immune cell depletion at the time of the transplant with the use of total lymphocyte irradiation (TLI) or splenectomy; however, currently there are more targeted and safer agents. All the agents can be divided by their own mechanism but more broadly into biologic agents (antibodies) and chemical agents (such as steroids) [14].

Typically, all agents are administered intravenously at the time of transplant with subsequent doses given in the immediate post-transplant period. The choice of induction agent depends on how highly sensitized a recipient is, planned maintenance regimen, diagnosis of renal failure, risk of post-transplant infection, and the recipient's comorbidities. Thus, the overall advantage of induction therapy is to decrease the risk of acute rejection, whereas the main disadvantage is the risk for adverse effects associated with each of the agents used for induction such as malignancies, especially post-transplant lymphoproliferative disease (PTLD) or infections [15].

PTLD is defined as an heterogenous group of abnormal lymphoid proliferations (usually from B cells) that occur in the setting of ineffective T-cell production because of pharmacologic immunosuppression after organ transplantation. It has been linked with the Epstein-Barr virus (EBV) infection as it will infect and immortalize B cells that in the absence of a T-cell regulation response will continue to grow in number. The spectrum of conditions can range from infectious mononucleosis-like illnesses, polyclonal lymphoid hyperplasia, and monoclonal malignancies such as B-cell lymphoma that can be fulminant. The mainstay of therapy is reduction of immunosuppression. Other options include antiviral therapy, anti-B-cell antibodies, chemotherapy, or most recently immunotherapy [16].

Anti-inflammatory Steroids

Corticosteroids are popularly used as immunosuppressants for many diseases as they reduce the synthesis of prostaglandins and cytokines which are vital in the immune response. The most commonly used corticosteroid in pediatric transplantation induction is methylprednisolone which is administered immediately pre- and post-transplantation followed by an oral/intravenous tapering regimen. Due to the high prevalence of adverse effects and the development of new medications, many programs have tried to minimize use of steroids in children. Reported side effects include growth impairment, diabetes mellitus, bone metabolism disruption, peptic ulcers, delayed wound healing, emotional fluctuation, and Cushing syndrome among others [15, 17]. The practice has shifted into developing induction and maintenance regimens that limit the use of steroids after 1–2 weeks or with rapid "steroid withdrawal" tapering off after weeks 1–2 [18–21]. Further, transplant programs have seen a shift to a limited steroid pathway in general [21].

A meta-analysis performed by Zhang et al. concluded that steroid avoidance regimens have no difference in acute rejection rates when compared to steroid withdrawal regimens in low-risk Caucasian patients. Also, there was a reported decreased risk of diabetes and hypertension requiring medication in the steroid withdrawal group [22]. Another reason to avoid steroids is based on the increased risk of PTLD in steroid regimens which was shown in a randomized controlled trial by Benfield et al. [23].

In terms of the induction agent alternative, many studies have reported "steroid-free" protocols based off IL-2 receptor blockers such as basiliximab and daclizumab. Sarwal et al. compared 57 pediatric renal transplant recipients undergoing induction with daclizumab with tacrolimus and mycophenolate mofetil maintenance with 50 historical-matched children with corticosteroid-dependent regimens [24]. At 1 year, the "steroid-free" group had improvements in acute rejection, graft function, hypertension, and growth without increase in infectious complications.

On a follow-up study by the same author with 77 children vs 300 children matched from the North American Pediatric Renal Trials and Collaborative Studies (*NAPRTCS*) database, the authors showed the same results with 90% of children free from hypertension and hyperlipidemia drug therapy in the "steroid-free" cohort vs 40% in the comparison group. Finally, a follow-up clinical trial comparing matched patients with panel reactive antigen (PRA) <20% to the same regimens previously described showed no differences in acute rejection 3 years after transplantation (16.7 vs 17%, $p = 0$, $p = 0.94$), no differences in patient survival (100% in both), and no differences in graft survival (95% in "steroid-free" vs 93% in steroid based). Importantly, children on the "steroid-free" group had lower systolic blood pressure and lower cholesterol levels ($p < 0.05$) [14, 24].

IL-2 Cell Surface Receptor Blockade

These induction agents target signal 3 of the T-cell activation pathway resulting in a dampened clonal proliferation of effector T cells. Medications in this class include monoclonal antibodies as well as recombinant fusion proteins [5, 15].

Basiliximab and Daclizumab

Basiliximab (Simulect®; Novartis Pharmaceuticals Corp, East Hanover, NJ, USA) is a chimeric monoclonal antibody (75% human, 25% murine) that targets the alpha chain of the CD25 (IL-2) receptor. Daclizumab (Zenapax®; Roche Laboratories, Nutley, NJ, USA) is a more humanized form (90% human and 10% murine) with the same pharmacological target. When compared to basiliximab, daclizumab has a longer half-life (13–20 days vs 9 days) and a longer duration of effect (90 vs 45 days in infants) [25]. However, daclizumab was found to have severe adverse events and fatal immune reactions affecting multiple organs such as autoimmune hepatitis with liver failure, central nervous system vasculitis, encephalitis, and meningoencephalitis [26]. Both are produced by hybridoma technology resulting from murine myeloma cells fused with immunized murine B cells [14]. Chemically they bind to the IL-2 receptor preventing T-cell activation and proliferation of the T cells. Due to the lower rate of hypersensitivity reactions with basiliximab, pre-medication is not often used.

Basiliximab is the only FDA-approved antibody for pediatric solid organ transplantation. It has been shown to reduce acute rejection rates in renal and pancreas transplant recipients. In clinical trials, it has shown to decrease the rate of acute rejection without an increase in postoperative infections when compared to patients with no treatment [27]. The dose of basiliximab is 10 mg for patients <35 kg and 20 mg for patients >20 kg administered on day 0 and day 4 after transplant. The dose of daclizumab is 1 mg/kg/dose on day 0 and every 2 weeks for a total of 5 doses [28]. There are multiple studies using these agents with concomitant cyclosporine or tacrolimus and MMF or azathioprine and corticosteroids achieving a 1-year graft survival of 86–98% with acute rejection between 6% and 17% [29–31].

Regarding safety, data pooled from the North American Pediatric Renal Trials and Collaborative Studies (*NAPRTCS*) database on 284 patients treated with daclizumab, 166 with basiliximab, and 711 with no induction showed an increased graft survival (95–97% vs 93%) and a lower rate of acute rejection (23% vs 34%) [32] in patient treated with IL-2 receptor blockers compared to no induction, respectively. Most studies converge on the fact that these agents reduce the rate of acute rejection with no increase in the rate of adverse effects. When compared to other agents such as Thymoglobulin®, there have been some promising results. A study performed by Clark et al. compared 42 pediatric transplant recipients receiving Thymoglobulin® vs 42 receiving basiliximab with a lower acute rejection rate in the basiliximab group (45% vs 62%, $p < 0.05$) [33]. However, in patients with focal segmental glomerulosclerosis (FSGS), Il-2 receptor blockers when used in conjunction with cyclosporine or tacrolimus with MMF and corticosteroids showed an increased rate of recurrence when compared to Thymoglobulin® (83% vs 38%, $p < 0.05$) [33]. Of note, it is reported that that IL-2 receptor antagonists might increase cyclosporine serum levels and consequently a possible reduction in the dose could be required [34].

Abatacept and Belatacept

As previously described, a part of the second signal involves the costimulation of the T cell by the ligation of CD80/CD86 to CD28 for activation of CTLA4 (CD152) for inhibition of the immune response [35]. In this pathway, only the agonism of CTLA4 has shown promising results. Abatacept or CTLA4-Ig is an immunoglobulin fusion protein of CTLA4 that has been shown to inhibit graft rejection [15]. The early benefits of abatacept prompted the development of variants of this CTLA4-Ig such as LEA29Y (belatacept) which has twice the ligation affinity to both CD80 and CD86. As a result, there is a tenfold greater suppression on the clonal expansion of the cell [15]. In early Phase II studies, belatacept showed improved renal function, reduction in chronic allograft nephropathy, decreased calcineurin-related toxicity, and no thromboembolic susceptibility [36]. In adults, the Phase III trials (BENEFIT and BENEFIT-Ext) have shown improvements in the glomerular filtration rate but showed an increase in the incidence of post-transplant lymphoproliferative disease and acute rejection when compared to calcineurin inhibitor therapy [36–38].

Leukocyte Depletion Agents

Antithymocyte Globulin

The depletion of effector T cells which mediate early rejection responses is imperative in the early perioperative period as early insults to the graft lead to long-term failure. Complete depletion of the effector T cells not only provides a "window" so that the allograft can "settle in" without being at risk of rejection but also mitigates the early B-cell response given the dependency B-cell proliferation has on T-cell activation [12, 39].

Antithymocyte globulin (rATG or Thymoglobulin) is a polyclonal antibody produced by sensitizing either rabbit or equine cells with human lymphoid cells.

Thymoglobulin is formulated using human thymus cells and induces T-cell apoptosis and complement-dependent lysis. The depletion of helper CD4+ T cells not only abrogates T-cell-mediated rejection responses but removes the assistance given to the activation of alloreactive B cells. In addition, the lysis induced by complement is agnostic of lymphocyte domain and surface markers (i.e., MHC I/II, CD95, CD28, CD45) leading to B-cell depletion as well [40]. The pharmacological effect of rATG is the depletion and modulation of the activity of effector circulating T cells by binding to multiple T-cell (CD3, CD4, CD8, CD28, CD2, CD5, CD45, CD154), B-cell (CD20), and NK cell (CD16, CD56) antigens [15].

The rabbit antithymocyte globulin (rATG, Thymoglobulin®, Genzyme, Cambridge, MA, USA) is ten times more potent than the equine antithymocyte globulin (eATG, ATGAM®, Pfizer, New York, NY, USA) and as a result is more commonly used [14, 41]. Studies have shown that Thymoglobulin® has superior outcomes when compared to ATGAM® in terms of decreased mortality, decreased acute rejection, and decreased graft loss [42]. The half-life of Thymoglobulin® is 2–3 days; however, it has been described that its T-cell depletion effects can last more than 9–12 months [15]. These prolonged immunosuppressive effects result in a decrease on the incidence and recurrence of rejection. However, this number is variable; historically, the dose of Thymoglobulin® was adjusted with the CD3+ counts with <25 cells/ul as a goal. This provided same lymphocyte depletion efficacy with less opportunistic infection and malignancies [43]. The usual dose of Thymoglobulin® is 1.5 mg/kg/d in an infusion over 4–6 hours for 5–10 days.

Thymoglobulin® is the mainstay for both induction in high-risk recipients and treatment of acute rejection in pediatric renal transplantation. The infusion is started prior to starting the graft anastomosis as postoperative administration has been associated with ischemia-reperfusion injury and delayed graft function [15, 44]. Doses and frequency of Thymoglobulin® administration are often adjusted by CD3 count, white blood cell count, and/or platelet count. In addition, in the pediatric population, doses and frequency of induction depend heavily on the etiology of disease and risk of recurrence (in the case of FSGS, e.g.) as well as level of sensitization and steroid burden [15, 44]. It can be administered by a central or peripheral route, but the time must be lengthened with peripheral administration. The deleterious ramifications of Thymoglobulin® can happen in early phases post-administration or in a delayed response. Given the depleting nature of Thymoglobulin®, effector T cells chalk-full of inflammatory mediators and cytokines can be released once the induction therapy is given leading to a cytokine release syndrome. This is typically characterized by fevers, rigors, hypo- or hypertension, nausea/vomiting, or anaphylaxis. The treatment of the early-phase responses is often thwarted by the routine uses of steroids and diphenhydramine and/or Tylenol prior to administration or epinephrine after administration in severe circumstances [15, 44, 45]. In later phases, the use of Thymoglobulin® has also shown to increase the risks of chronic leukopenia and thrombocytopenia, infection, and malignancy.

There has been extensive research in the adult transplantation field with few studies in the pediatric population and mostly in high-risk renal transplant recipients. A retrospective, single-institution study included 17 recipients with 11 receiving deceased organ allografts and 7 living related allografts. In all of them, Thymoglobulin® was utilized with tacrolimus (62%) or cyclosporine (38%), mycophenolate mofetil, and prednisone. At 1 year, the patient survival was 100% and the graft survival was 93%. The authors did not report acute rejection, infections, or malignancies [46].

Another study included a larger retrospective cohort of 198 patients comparing Thymoglobulin® ($n = 127$) and ATGAM® ($n = 81$) with maintenance with cyclosporine, azathioprine, or mycophenolate mofetil and prednisone. This study showed a lower rate of acute rejection in the Thymoglobulin® group (33% vs 50%; $p = 0.02$) but with higher rates of EBV infection (8% vs 3%; $p = 0.002$). There were no differences in graft survival, chronic rejection, or malignancy [47].

Induction Therapies Targeted at B Cells

Another important aspect of selecting the appropriate induction agent is the level of sensitization. As therapies improve and increased patient survival is achieved, re-transplants occur more often. Furthermore, organ shortage (especially in pediatric patients) has pushed the pediatric transplant community of practice to aggressively pursue the listing and transplantation of high PRA individuals and in some cases ABO-incompatible transplants [14]. In our own center, living donation is highly sought after for these individuals with the use of internal matching software. In the case of altruistic donors, attempts are also made to identify children to "end a chain." Strategies for these high-risk groups include rituximab, plasmapheresis, intravenous immunoglobulin (IVIG), and splenectomy always in conjunction with a lymphocyte depletion agent (such as alemtuzumab) due to the high risk of acute rejection.

Plasmapheresis will partially remove any pre-existing antibodies, whereas IVIG will downregulate production of antibodies and neutralize pre-existing ones [48]. Therapeutic apheresis has been used to desensitize both adult and pediatric patients undergoing both deceased and living donor renal transplantation showing decrease in waitlist times [49]. Likewise, treatment with IVIG has shown good success rates with decreasing HLA antibody titers as well as lower transplant waitlist times [50]. In the pediatric population, there have been reports of highly sensitized children (PRA > 80%) that with IVIG they were able to be desensitized and transplanted successfully with follow-ups between 11 and 17 months [50–52].

Rituximab is a chimeric/murine human antibody directed against the CD20 antigen in B cells. As a result, it depletes B cells through cellular apoptosis. It is used in a dose of 100–375 mg/m^2 in adults with 1–4 doses. Rituximab was first used for treating antibody-mediated rejection and PTLD [53]. A clinical trial in adults using rituximab induction vs placebo in 280 adult patients undergoing renal transplant showed that immunological high-risk patients (PRA > 6) had a lower incidence of acute rejection (38% vs 18%, $P < 0.05$). In this same study at 24 months, there was no difference in the incidence of infection or malignancy [54]. Additionally, there have been multiple reports of the use of rituximab in ABO-incompatible renal transplant children with graft and patient survival over 90% in 1 year with ages from 12 months to 6 years [55].

Selecting the Most Appropriate Induction Agent

When selecting the most appropriate induction agent, there are multiple factors that should be considered such as race, immunological risk, underlying disease, and planned maintenance therapy [56]. Currently, over 90% of pediatric transplant recipients receive induction with either a lymphocyte-depleting agent (antithymocyte globulin, alemtuzumab) or a non-depleting agent (basiliximab/corticosteroids) [57]. It is important to have in mind that there is no standardized consensus and induction protocols are mostly center dependent. Some studies have failed to show a clear benefit of depleting agents for induction on low-risk patients, and the most benefit we have seen is in high-risk groups such as African Americans, recipients of kidneys with prolonged cold ischemia time, and sensitized individuals.

For patients without a high risk or sensitization, IL-2 receptor antagonists have been increasingly used based on its safety profile and lower incidence of adverse effects. Patients with a higher risk for rejection or centers using steroid avoidance will often need stronger induction protocols such as the use of leukocyte depletion agents. Multiple authors have recommended the use of potent leukocyte depletion agents such as Thymoglobulin® or alemtuzumab for high-risk pediatric renal transplant patients such as re-transplant candidates, highly sensitized recipients, or those with a high risk of recurrent FSGS [14, 58]. The Kidney Disease: Improving Global Outcomes (KDIGO) guidelines recommend antithymocyte globulin (ATG) for kidney recipients with high risk of acute rejection after transplantation [59]. Another option for patients with high risk and sensitization, and now being increasingly used, is alemtuzumab with adjuvant therapies such as plasmapheresis, rituximab, or IVIG. Still, more studies are needed, and protocols vary per institution.

Alemtuzumab is the most powerful lymphocyte-depleting agent that acts as an antibody against the CD52 protein in T and B cells as well as monocytes and natural killer cells [60]. One of the larger studies evaluated alemtuzumab with tacrolimus in 42 pediatric living donor transplant recipients showing graft survival of 85% and acute cellular rejection of 5% at 4 years [61]. Another report on 101 pediatric living donor recipients with alemtuzumab induction and maintenance with CNI and MMF showed a graft survival of 93% in 3 years [60]. In highly sensitized pediatric patients (PRA >30%), a combination of IVIG, rituximab, and alemtuzumab in 15 patients showed 100% patient and graft survival in 1 year with no difference when compared to IL-2 receptor blockers [62].

There has been increased interest in tailoring the induction and maintenance immunosuppressive therapy based on the underlying disease. As an example, retrospective analyses showed a significant risk reduction of IgA nephropathy recurrence in 116 kidney transplant recipients when comparing Thymoglobulin® with no induction or IL-2 receptor antagonist [63]. Furthermore, and as previously discussed, patients with FSGS have a high risk of recurrence when IL-2 receptor antagonists are used for which leukocyte depletion agents such as Thymoglobulin® are recommended [64].

The overall concept of induction therapy can be summarized as follows [58]:

- Identification and stratification of ESRD etiology (this should inform the induction agent used).
- Patient with low immunological risk + steroids: Use of IL-2r blockade.
- Patient with low immunological risk, steroid-free, or early withdrawal: consider leukocyte depletion.
- Patient with high immunological risk: leukocyte depletion with Thymoglobulin® or alemtuzumab.

Conclusions and Future Challenges

The field of transplantation has gone through a variety of evolutionary changes over the past six decades. Through it all, the development and understanding of transplant immunology has served as the backbone of transplant medicine. From the early days of total lymphocyte irradiation in combination with corticosteroids and splenectomy to the development of calcineurin inhibitors, the field of pediatric transplantation has grown exponentially. Along the way, Thymoglobulin® became increasingly used as an induction agent to allow for the improved efficacy of maintenance regimens. Years later, alemtuzumab and the IL-2 receptors antagonist appeared with a better safety profile. With the concurrent development of other maintenance agents such as tacrolimus and mycophenolate mofetil, newer protocols are now avoiding the use of steroids and leukocyte depletion agents which were vital in the past.

The next era of transplantation is undoubtedly dedicated to the pursuits of tolerance and personalized immunosuppressive strategies along with possible pretreatment strategies to minimize the harmful side effects incurred by current systemic immunotherapies [65].

Questions

1. Which of the signals involved in the activation of T cells involves stimulating the mTOR complex?
   (a) Signal 1
   (b) Signal 2
   (c) Signal 3
   (d) Signal 4

   (c). The first signal involves the interaction of the T-cell receptor (TCR) and an antigen bounded to the MHC complex. The second signal involves the activation of costimulatory molecules reacting to signal 1 that coalesce around the immunologic synapse. These interactions include the activations of nuclear factor kappa-light-chain-enhancer of activated B cells (NFκB) and the translocation of the nuclear factor of activation and transcription (NFAT) producing activating factors such as IL-2. Finally, the third signal involves the engaging of IL-2 with CD25 (IL-2 receptor) stimulating the mTOR complex and resulting in T-cell activation and proliferation. There is no fourth signal.

2. Which of the below best describes induction therapy?
   (a) Administration of immunosuppressive agents at the time of transplantation to prevent accelerated acute rejection
   (b) Administration of immunosuppressive agents after the time of transplant to prevent chronic antibody-mediated rejection
   (c) Administration of immunosuppressive agents intravenously monthly to prevent acute cellular rejection
   (d) Administration of immunosuppressive agents orally to prevent transplant glomerulopathy

   (a). Administration of immunosuppressive agents at the time of transplantation to prevent accelerated acute rejection.
3. Which of the following is a polyclonal antibody produced by sensitizing either rabbit or equine cells with human lymphoid cells and works by inducing T-cell apoptosis and complement-dependent lysis causing as a result depletion of T cells and modulation of the effector response?
   (a) Belatacept
   (b) Antithymocyte globulin
   (c) Tacrolimus
   (d) Simulect

   (b). Antithymocyte globulin is a polyclonal antibody produced by sensitizing either rabbit or equine cells with human lymphoid cells and works by inducing T-cell apoptosis and complement-dependent lysis causing as a result depletion of T cells and modulation of the effector response.

References

1. Verghese PS. Pediatric kidney transplantation: a historical review. Pediatr Res. 2017;81(1–2):259–64.
2. Van Arendonk KJ, Boyarsky BJ, Orandi BJ, et al. National trends over 25 years in pediatric kidney transplant outcomes. Pediatrics. 2014;133(4):594–601.
3. Kumar BV, Connors TJ, Farber DL. Human T cell development, localization, and function throughout life. Immunity. 2018;48(2):202–13.
4. Kumbala D, Zhang R. Essential concept of transplant immunology for clinical practice. World J Transplant. 2013;3(4):113–8.
5. Halloran PF. Immunosuppressive drugs for kidney transplantation. N Engl J Med. 2004;351(26):2715–29.
6. Santana MA, Esquivel-Guadarrama F. Cell biology of T cell activation and differentiation. Int Rev Cytol. 2006;250:217–74.
7. Rohan VS, Pilch N, Moussa O, et al. Virtual crossmatching in kidney transplantation: the wait is over. J Am Coll Surg. 2020;230(4):373–9.

8. Lakkis FG, Chalasani G, Hariharan S. Antibody-mediated rejection of solid-organ allografts. N Engl J Med. 2018;379(26):2580.
9. Adams AB, Pearson TC, Larsen CP. Heterologous immunity: an overlooked barrier to tolerance. Immunol Rev. 2003;196:147–60.
10. Trzonkowski P, Zilvetti M, Chapman S, et al. Homeostatic repopulation by CD28-CD8+ T cells in alemtuzumab-depleted kidney transplant recipients treated with reduced immunosuppression. Am J Transplant. 2008;8(2):338–47.
11. Chen W, Ghobrial RM, Li XC. The evolving roles of memory immune cells in transplantation. Transplantation. 2015;99(10):2029–37.
12. Kirk AD. Induction immunosuppression. Transplantation. 2006;82(5):593–602.
13. Szczech LA, Berlin JA, Feldman HI. The effect of antilymphocyte induction therapy on renal allograft survival. A meta-analysis of individual patient-level data. Anti-Lymphocyte Antibody Induction Therapy Study Group. Ann Intern Med. 1998;128(10):817–26.
14. Moudgil A, Puliyanda D. Induction therapy in pediatric renal transplant recipients: an overview. Paediatr Drugs. 2007;9(5):323–41.
15. Crowther B. Immunosuppression in pediatric SOT. In: Newland D, Soliman M, Zorn Y. ed. PedSAP. 2019;2.
16. Loren AW, Porter DL, Stadtmauer EA, Tsai DE. Post-transplant lymphoproliferative disorder: a review. Bone Marrow Transplant. 2003;31(3):145–55.
17. Buchman AL. Side effects of corticosteroid therapy. J Clin Gastroenterol. 2001;33(4):289–94.
18. Naesens M, Berger S, Biancone L, et al. Lymphocyte-depleting induction and steroid minimization after kidney transplantation: a review. Nefrologia. 2016;36(5):469–80.
19. Pascual J, Galeano C, Royuela A, Zamora J. A systematic review on steroid withdrawal between 3 and 6 months after kidney transplantation. Transplantation. 2010;90(4):343–9.
20. Pascual J, Royuela A, Galeano C, Crespo M, Zamora J. Very early steroid withdrawal or complete avoidance for kidney transplant recipients: a systematic review. Nephrol Dial Transplant. 2012;27(2):825–32.
21. Pascual J, Zamora J, Galeano C, Royuela A, Quereda C. Steroid avoidance or withdrawal for kidney transplant recipients. Cochrane Database Syst Rev. 2009;(1):CD005632.
22. Zhang H, Zheng Y, Liu L, et al. Steroid avoidance or withdrawal regimens in paediatric kidney transplantation: a meta-analysis of randomised controlled trials. PLoS One. 2016;11(3):e0146523.
23. Benfield MR, Bartosh S, Ikle D, et al. A randomized double-blind, placebo controlled trial of steroid withdrawal after pediatric renal transplantation. Am J Transplant. 2010;10(1):81–8.
24. Sarwal MM, Vidhun JR, Alexander SR, Satterwhite T, Millan M, Salvatierra O Jr. Continued superior outcomes with modification and lengthened follow-up of a steroid-avoidance pilot with extended daclizumab induction in pediatric renal transplantation. Transplantation. 2003;76(9):1331–9.
25. Di Filippo S. Anti-IL-2 receptor antibody vs. polyclonal anti-lymphocyte antibody as induction therapy in pediatric transplantation. Pediatr Transplant. 2005;9(3):373–80.
26. Avasarala J. DRESS syndrome and daclizumab failure-were potentially dangerous signs missed in clinical trials? Drug Target Insights. 2018;12:1177392818785136.
27. Mincham CM, Wong G, Teixeira-Pinto A, et al. Induction therapy, rejection, and graft outcomes in pediatric and adolescent kidney transplant recipients. Transplantation. 2017;101(9):2146–51.
28. Swiatecka-Urban A. Anti-interleukin-2 receptor antibodies for the prevention of rejection in pediatric renal transplant patients: current status. Paediatr Drugs. 2003;5(10):699–716.
29. Ciancio G, Burke GW, Suzart K, et al. Effect of daclizumab, tacrolimus, and mycophenolate mofetil in pediatric first renal transplant recipients. Transplant Proc. 2002;34(5):1944–5.
30. Garcia CD, Barros VR, Schneider L, Alves MD, Silveira CG, Garcia VD. IL-2 antibody induction and the outcome of pediatric renal transplants. Transplant Proc. 2002;34(7):2914–5.
31. Garcia Meseguer C, Vila Lopez A, Luque de Pablos A, Vallo Boado A, Simon JM, Pediatric ESG. Immunoprophylaxis with Simulect (basiliximab) in pediatric kidney transplant recipients: results from routine clinical practice at 5 kidney transplant units. Transplant Proc. 2003;35(5):1697–8.

32. Benfield MR, Ping-Leung H. Comparative study of the safety, efficacy, and practice patterns of monoclonal antibodies in pediatric renal transplantation [abstract]. Am J Transplant. 2002;2(Suppl. 3):S192.
33. Clark G, Walsh G, Deshpande P, Koffman G. Improved efficacy of basiliximab over antilymphocyte globulin induction therapy in paediatric renal transplantation. Nephrol Dial Transplant. 2002;17(7):1304–9.
34. Strehlau J, Pape L, Offner G, Nashan B, Ehrich JH. Interleukin-2 receptor antibody-induced alterations of cyclosporine dose requirements in paediatric transplant recipients. Lancet. 2000;356(9238):1327–8.
35. Larsen CP, Elwood ET, Alexander DZ, et al. Long-term acceptance of skin and cardiac allografts after blocking CD40 and CD28 pathways. Nature. 1996;381(6581):434–8.
36. Vincenti F, Blancho G, Durrbach A, et al. Ten-year outcomes in a randomized phase II study of kidney transplant recipients administered belatacept 4-weekly or 8-weekly. Am J Transplant. 2017;17(12):3219–27.
37. Vincenti F, Rostaing L, Grinyo J, et al. Belatacept and long-term outcomes in kidney transplantation. N Engl J Med. 2016;374(4):333–43.
38. Durrbach A, Pestana JM, Pearson T, et al. A phase III study of belatacept versus cyclosporine in kidney transplants from extended criteria donors (BENEFIT-EXT study). Am J Transplant. 2010;10(3):547–57.
39. Penninga L, Wettergren A, Wilson CH, Chan AW, Steinbruchel DA, Gluud C. Antibody induction versus placebo, no induction, or another type of antibody induction for liver transplant recipients. Cochrane Database Syst Rev. 2014;(6):CD010253.
40. Zand MS, Vo T, Huggins J, et al. Polyclonal rabbit antithymocyte globulin triggers B-cell and plasma cell apoptosis by multiple pathways. Transplantation. 2005;79(11):1507–15.
41. Brophy PD, Thomas SE, McBryde KD, Bunchman TE. Comparison of polyclonal induction agents in pediatric renal transplantation. Pediatr Transplant. 2001;5(3):174–8.
42. Hardinger KL, Rhee S, Buchanan P, et al. A prospective, randomized, double-blinded comparison of thymoglobulin versus Atgam for induction immunosuppressive therapy: 10-year results. Transplantation. 2008;86(7):947–52.
43. Uber WE, Uber LA, VanBakel AB, et al. CD3 monitoring and thymoglobulin therapy in cardiac transplantation: clinical outcomes and pharmacoeconomic implications. Transplant Proc. 2004;36(10):3245–9.
44. Shapiro R, Sarwal MM. Pediatric kidney transplantation. Pediatr Clin North Am. 2010;57(2):393–400, table of contents.
45. Thiyagarajan UM, Ponnuswamy A, Bagul A. Thymoglobulin and its use in renal transplantation: a review. Am J Nephrol. 2013;37(6):586–601.
46. Ault BH, Honaker MR, Osama Gaber A, et al. Short-term outcomes of Thymoglobulin induction in pediatric renal transplant recipients. Pediatr Nephrol. 2002;17(10):815–8.
47. Khositseth S, Matas A, Cook ME, Gillingham KJ, Chavers BM. Thymoglobulin versus ATGAM induction therapy in pediatric kidney transplant recipients: a single-center report. Transplantation. 2005;79(8):958–63.
48. Jordan SC, Tyan D, Czer L, Toyoda M. Immunomodulatory actions of intravenous immunoglobulin (IVIG): potential applications in solid organ transplant recipients. Pediatr Transplant. 1998;2(2):92–105.
49. Salvadori M, Tsalouchos A. Therapeutic apheresis in kidney transplantation: an updated review. World J Transplant. 2019;9(6):103–22.
50. Valentini RP, Nehlsen-Cannarella SL, Gruber SA, et al. Intravenous immunoglobulin, HLA allele typing and HLAMatchmaker facilitate successful transplantation in highly sensitized pediatric renal allograft recipients. Pediatr Transplant. 2007;11(1):77–81.
51. Al-Uzri AY, Seltz B, Yorgin PD, Spier CM, Andreoni K. Successful renal transplant outcome after intravenous gamma-globulin treatment of a highly sensitized pediatric recipient. Pediatr Transplant. 2002;6(2):161–5.

52. Tyan DB, Li VA, Czer L, Trento A, Jordan SC. Intravenous immunoglobulin suppression of HLA alloantibody in highly sensitized transplant candidates and transplantation with a histo-incompatible organ. Transplantation. 1994;57(4):553–62.
53. O'Dwyer ME, Launder T, Rabkin JM, Nichols CR. Successful treatment of aggressive post transplant lymphoproliferative disorder using rituximab. Leuk Lymphoma. 2000;39(3–4):411–9.
54. van den Hoogen MW, Kamburova EG, Baas MC, et al. Rituximab as induction therapy after renal transplantation: a randomized, double-blind, placebo-controlled study of efficacy and safety. Am J Transplant. 2015;15(2):407–16.
55. Chauhan K, Mehta AA. Rituximab in kidney disease and transplant. Animal Model Exp Med. 2019;2(2):76–82.
56. Gabardi S, Martin ST, Roberts KL, Grafals M. Induction immunosuppressive therapies in renal transplantation. Am J Health Syst Pharm. 2011;68(3):211–8.
57. Hart A, Smith JM, Skeans MA, et al. OPTN/SRTR 2017 annual data report: kidney. Am J Transplant. 2019;19 Suppl 2:19–123.
58. Pape L. State-of-the-art immunosuppression protocols for pediatric renal transplant recipients. Pediatr Nephrol. 2019;34(2):187–94.
59. Khwaja A. KDIGO guidelines for care of the kidney transplant recipient. Nephron Clin Pract. 2010;116(1):c27–8.
60. Kaabak MM, Babenko NN, Samsonov DV, Sandrikov VA, Maschan AA, Zokoev AK. Alemtuzumab induction in pediatric kidney transplantation. Pediatr Transplant. 2013;17(2):168–78.
61. Tan HP, Donaldson J, Ellis D, et al. Pediatric living donor kidney transplantation under alemtuzumab pretreatment and tacrolimus monotherapy: 4-year experience. Transplantation. 2008;86(12):1725–31.
62. Kim IK, Choi J, Vo AA, et al. Safety and efficacy of alemtuzumab induction in highly sensitized pediatric renal transplant recipients. Transplantation. 2017;101(4):883–9.
63. Berthoux F, El Deeb S, Mariat C, Diconne E, Laurent B, Thibaudin L. Antithymocyte globulin (ATG) induction therapy and disease recurrence in renal transplant recipients with primary IgA nephropathy. Transplantation. 2008;85(10):1505–7.
64. Infante B, Rossini M, Leo S, et al. Recurrent glomerulonephritis after renal transplantation: the clinical problem. Int J Mol Sci. 2020;21(17):5954.
65. Zhu P, Atkinson C, Dixit S, et al. Organ preservation with targeted rapamycin nanoparticles: a pre-treatment strategy preventing chronic rejection in vivo. RSC Adv. 2018;8(46):25909–19.

Post-transplant Medication Challenges

12

Nida Siddiqi and Alesa Campbell

Introduction

Transplantation remains the treatment of choice for renal replacement therapy in eligible pediatric patients with end-stage renal disease. As is the case while managing other chronic disease states, prolonging a young patient's life expectancy and enhancing quality of life with kidney transplantation are of the utmost priority. In addition to advancements in donor and recipient selection, surgical techniques, and post-transplant care strategies, the development of potent immunosuppressive agents over time has significantly improved patient and allograft outcomes (Fig. 12.1).

Immunosuppression plays a vital role in increasing allograft survival by inhibiting the alloimmune response and preventing acute and chronic rejection. With dramatic improvements seen in short-term survival over the last few decades, the focus remains on selecting an ideal immunosuppressive regimen that optimizes long-term survival in pediatric kidney transplant recipients. Children and adolescents are more prone to therapy-related challenges following transplantation than adults, including serious chronic adverse effects, pharmacokinetic variability, administration barriers, as well as medication nonadherence. The focus of this chapter is to highlight the nature of these challenges and discuss strategies for managing them post-transplant in pediatric kidney transplant recipients.

N. Siddiqi (✉)
Department of Pharmacy, Sidra Medicine, Doha, Qatar
e-mail: nsiddiqi@sidra.org

A. Campbell
Department of Pharmacy, Montefiore Medical Center, Bronx, NY, USA

K. E. Twombley (ed.), *Challenges in Pediatric Kidney Transplantation*,
https://doi.org/10.1007/978-3-030-74783-1_12

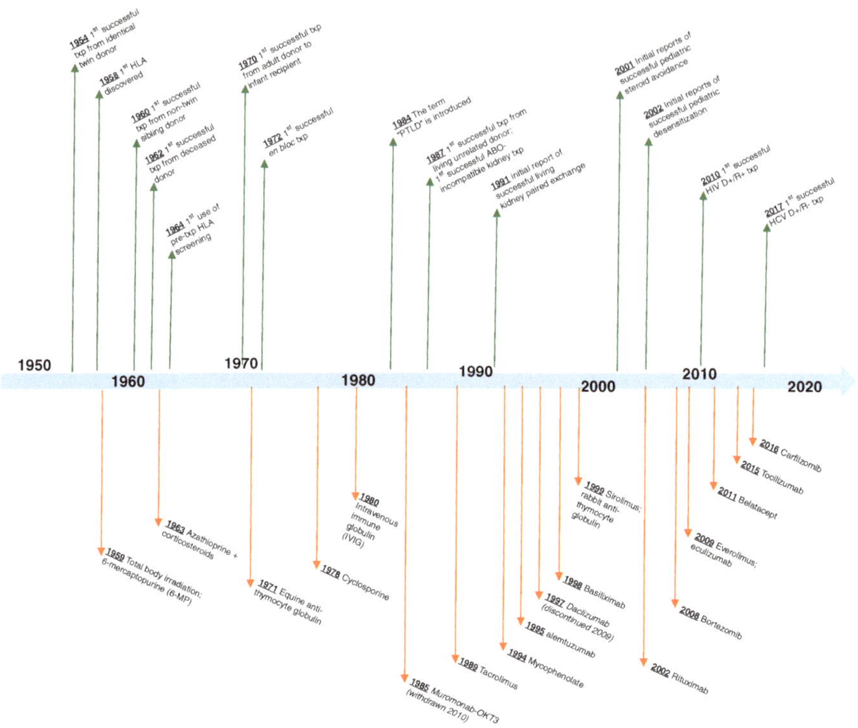

Fig. 12.1 Timeline of transplant milestones and immunosuppression approval in kidney transplantation [299–321]. *ABO* blood goup system; *D* donor; *HCV* hepatitis C virus; *HIV* human immunodeficiency virus; *HLA* human leukocyte antigen; *PTLD* post-transplant lymphoproliferative disorder; *R* recipient; *Txp* transplant

Section I: Post-transplant Immunosuppression Strategies

Maintenance Immunosuppression

Antiproliferative Agents

The use of chemotherapeutic agents for the prevention of organ rejection was first attempted with 6-mercaptopurine, methotrexate, and cyclophosphamide. In 1963, successful use of azathioprine with corticosteroids to prolong patient survival and treat allograft rejection was established. Since then, two antiproliferative agents, azathioprine and subsequently mycophenolate, have become an integral part of post-transplant immunosuppression. With varying specificity, both azathioprine and mycophenolate exert their actions by inhibiting *de novo* and/or salvage pathways of purine synthesis, a mechanism different from other immunosuppressive agents. Although selection of one agent over the other is often patient-driven, mycophenolate is considered the antiproliferative of choice in modern-day protocols.

Azathioprine

Azathioprine (AZA) was one of the first immunosuppressants to be routinely utilized for prevention of rejection in solid organ transplant (SOT) recipients, receiving U.S. Food and Drug Administration (FDA) approval for use in kidney transplantation (KTx) in 1968 [1–3]. A prodrug of 6-mercaptopurine (6-MP), AZA exerts its immunosuppressive effects via metabolites that incorporate into DNA to halt replication and inhibit both *de novo* and salvage pathways of nucleotide synthesis. This leads to cell cycle arrest and inhibition of lymphocyte activation and differentiation. Upon administration, AZA undergoes non-enzymatic conversion to 6-MP. This is followed by enzymatic metabolism to its active metabolite 6-thioguanine nucleotide (6-TGN) via hypoxanthine-guanine phosphoribosyltransferase (HGPRT) and to its inactive metabolites as follows: 6-methylmercaptopurine via thiopurine s-methyltransferase (TPMT), active 6-TGN to 6-TG monophosphates via nucleotide diphosphate (NUDT15), and 6-thiouric acid via xanthine oxidase [4]. Of note, these metabolic pathways play a vital role in determining AZA's immunosuppressive and toxic effects, particularly the thioguanine-associated nucleotides.

In order to overcome the slow circulation and prolonged elimination half-life of the AZA metabolites responsible for its immunosuppressive effects, a single loading dose of 3–5 mg/kg is recommended at the time of transplant, followed by a maintenance dose of 1–3 mg/kg/day administered once daily. Empiric dose reductions, however, may be necessary in patients experiencing AZA-related adverse effects, particularly myelotoxicity. Oral AZA is commercially available in the form of tablets that can be split or crushed, and a suspension can be extemporaneously prepared to allow for more accurate administration in children [5]. As previously mentioned, the use of AZA in modern immunosuppression regimens has been widely replaced by mycophenolic acid derivatives [6, 7].

Mycophenolic Acid Derivatives

Mycophenolate mofetil (MMF) received FDA approval for its use in KTx in 1995 and quickly replaced AZA as the preferred antiproliferative immunosuppressant agent in both adults and pediatrics. MMF is a prodrug that undergoes pre-systemic hydrolysis in the intestinal tract to form mycophenolic acid (MPA) [8]. The biologically active MPA exerts its immunosuppressive effects by nonselective inhibition of inosine 5′-monophosphate dehydrogenase (IMPDH), an enzyme vital for purine synthesis via the *de novo* pathway. The result is inhibition of several key pro-inflammatory processes of allograft rejection: T- and B-lymphocyte proliferation, B-lymphocyte-mediated antibody production, and recruitment of cytotoxic leukocytes to areas of tissue inflammation [8]. Unlike AZA, which causes non-specific cell cycle arrest, MPA exerts a more targeted inhibition of T- and B-cell proliferation [8].

Mycophenolic acid derivatives are available as mycophenolate mofetil (MMF) and enteric-coated mycophenolate sodium (MPS). As opposed to the fixed dosing recommended in adults, dosing for children is 600 mg/m^2/dose twice daily for MMF or 400 mg/m^2/dose twice daily for MPS. Of note, the two products are not interchangeable. Oral MMF is commercially available in tablet, capsule, and suspension form, allowing for ease of administration in pediatric patients. If the commercial suspension product is not available, data also supports extemporaneous preparation of an oral suspension utilizing the oral capsules [9, 10]. On the other hand, as MPS cannot be broken or crushed due to its enteric coating, its use is limited in patients who are unable to swallow whole tablets. Furthermore, doses must be rounded to the nearest 180 mg or 360 mg tablet of MPS, which may be too high in children with low body surface areas.

Following oral administration, mycophenolate undergoes swift conversion to MPA, which is either rapidly absorbed in the proximal duodenum if MMF is administered, or more slowly in the distal duodenum if MPS is administered. Uridine diphosphate glucuronosyltransferase (UGT) enzymes are primarily responsible for the metabolism of MPA to its three by-products: (1) the major, pharmacologically inactive metabolite 7-O-glucuronide (MPAG) via UGT1A9, (2) the minor, pharmacologically active metabolite acyl-glucuronide (AcMPAG) via UGT2B7, and (3) the minor, inactive MPA-phenyl-glucoside (glucoside-MPA). De-glucuronidation of MPAG via the multidrug resistance-associated protein 2 (MRP2) leads to enterohepatic recycling and elicits a second, smaller MPA peak that accounts for 10–60% of the total MPA exposure [11]. Approximately 97% of MPA and 82% of MPAG are albumin bound; thus patients with hepatic impairment may experience more drug toxicity in the setting of hyperbilirubinemia- and hypoalbuminemia-driven MPA displacement from albumin [12, 13]. Furthermore, over 90% of the administered MPA dose is renally excreted as glucuronide metabolites. Hence, patients with renal impairment may have higher exposure and are at risk for drug toxicity secondary to accumulation of unbound MPA available to undergo enterohepatic recirculation [13].

Due to its complex pharmacokinetic profile, wide interpatient variability in drug exposure, drug-disease interactions, and ontogeny of drug pharmacodynamics, MPA therapeutic drug monitoring is an area of great interest and challenge in pediatric patients [11, 13]. The recommended target MPA area under the concentration curve (AUC) in the initial post-transplant period is 30–70 mg·hr/L depending on laboratory assay technique used [11]. Although plasma MPA AUC monitoring provides the most accurate estimate of overall drug exposure, the process is cumbersome and requires ten blood samples to assess concentrations at 0, 0.5, 1, 1.5, 2, 3, 4, 6, 8, and 12 hours after MMF dose administration ($C_{0.5-12}$). Alternatively, abbreviated AUC formulas have been found to provide an acceptable correlation to the full AUC measurement with only four blood samples (C_0, C_1, C_2, and C_4) [14]. A more practical approach shared in the pediatric SOT literature advocates for monitoing MPA trough levels with targets in the 1–3 mcg/mL range, highlighting the concern that younger children may be at a higher risk of MPA under-dosing when compared to adolescents and adults [15, 16]. Of note, target MPA troughs and abbreviated AUC extrapolation algorithms cannot be utilized in patients receiving MPS due to its prolonged gastrointestinal release and inconsistent pharmacokinetic behavior [17].

Efficacy

In addition to a less toxic adverse effect profile, clinical trials demonstrated lower rates of acute and chronic rejection and prolonged allograft survival at 3, 4, and 5 years post-KTx with MMF when compared to AZA [18–21]. Moreover,

MMF-based immunosuppression regimens have been found to reduce the incidence of chronic allograft nephropathy within the first post-transplant year, as well as improve renal function in pediatric kidney transplant (pKTx) recipients with chronic rejection [22, 23]. The survival benefit of MMF over AZA thus explains the dramatic decrease in AZA use from 50% in 1996 to 5% in 2013 [24]. Utilizing MMF-based regimens also allows for lower calcineurin inhibitor (CNI) trough goals, which may subsequently lower the risk of serious CNI-related adverse effects such as hypertension, hyperlipidemia, post-transplant diabetes mellitus, neurotoxicity, and nephrotoxicity [25].

Although no longer first-line, AZA maintains its utility in certain patient-specific scenarios like pregnancy, need for once-daily dosing to improve compliance, or presence of severe gastrointestinal (GI) adverse effects such as diarrhea, esophagitis, or colitis with mycophenolate-based products [8, 9]. In addition, while the post-transplant immunosuppression regimen of choice should not be driven solely by medication cost, AZA may provide a less expensive option for patients who lack insurance coverage or in countries where mycophenolate may not be available. Although drug pricing varies around the world, one study found that mycophenolate-based regimens could cost up to 15 times more than AZA [26].

Steroids

Between the two classes of systemically-administered corticosteroids (glucocorticoids and mineralocorticoids), glucocorticoids are primarily utilized in KTx regimens. The mechanism of action of glucocorticoids is complex, and both anti-inflammatory and immunosuppressive effects contribute to their role in post-transplant immunosuppression. Specifically, glucocorticoids regulate gene transcription and induction, destabilize cytokines such as interleukin-1 and interleukin-6, inhibit T-cell proliferation, and block production of interleukin-2 [27, 28]. They also decrease inflammation by suppressing migration of monocytes to the site of inflammation and decrease capillary permeability [29]. Lastly, glucocorticoids elicit a wide array of effects on fluid homeostasis and musculoskeletal, endocrine, and neurologic physiology [30]. The glucocorticoids used in post-transplantation protocols are oral prednisone and prednisolone, with methylprednisolone succinate available as an intravenous option particularly when higher doses are indicated. Steroids are hepatically metabolized, where prednisone is converted to its active metabolite, prednisolone [31]. The exclusive utilization of prednisone is seen more commonly in North America, with prednisolone used prevalently in other parts of the world including Europe. Although there is no data suggesting a clinical advantage of one over the other, prednisolone may be warranted in patients with moderate to severe liver dysfunction to bypass the need for hepatic activation [32, 33]. Furthermore, prednisolone oral solution may also be preferred due to availability as a more concentrated oral solution allowing for smaller administration volumes. It is also reported to have better palatability and faster resolution of aftertaste when compared to prednisone [34]. Both prednisone and prednisolone reach peak plasma concentrations within 1–2 hours and have a short half-life of 2–3 hours [31, 35]. Of note, this half-life may become prolonged in children as well as in the setting of liver disease, and theoretically shortened in the presence of drugs that induce hepatic enzyme activity. The duration of effect lasts 12–36 hours, allowing for once- to twice-daily dosing regimens.

There are no FDA-labeled dosing recommendations for methylprednisolone, prednisone, or prednisolone for use in adult or pediatric renal transplant recipients. Rather, this data has been accumulated through clinical use and practice. A common dosing range in children for intravenous methylprednisolone as part of an induction or rejection protocol typically ranges from 5 to 20 mg/kg per dose, while initial maintenance dose with oral prednisone or prednisolone is 1–5 mg/kg per day. Some centers utilize body surface area instead of body weight for dosing steroids, which is also considered an acceptable strategy. It is important to note that the ideal dose and duration of steroids to optimize patient and allograft survival in pKTx recipients has not been established [7, 36]. On the other hand, adverse effects may be linked to the intensity of steroid exposure. For example, a clinically significant improvement in physical growth with respect to height has been reported with alternate day dosing when compared to daily dosing of steroids [37, 38]. Consequently, post-transplant steroid dosing strategies, including tapering or discontinuation, are ultimately driven by institution-specific protocols.

Efficacy

Given the adverse effects associated with steroid therapy, there has been a significant evolution in dosing strategies in the last 20 years leading to the emergence of steroid minimization protocols. Certain transplant centers implement late steroid withdrawal (LSW), with discontinuation months to years post-transplant, while others may utilize steroid continuation (SC), remain completely steroid-free (SF), or practice early steroid withdrawal (ESW) strategies in which steroids are discontinued within 7–10 days post-transplant. Use of non-depleting antibody (e.g., basiliximab, daclizumab) versus lymphocyte-depleting antibody (e.g., antithymocyte globulin, alemtuzumab) induction agents, the combination of other maintenance immunosuppressive agents such as CNI, MMF, or sirolimus (SIR), as well as patient population risk factors often influence which steroid dosing strategy is used.

One of the first pediatric studies to retrospectively compare LSW versus SC in low immunologic risk pKTx recipients ≥1 year post-transplant maintained on MMF and cyclosporine reported similar biopsy-proven acute rejection (BPAR) rates and allograft survival, but improved growth and body mass index (BMI) and decreased hypertension ($p < 0.05$) in the LSW group [39]. To counteract withdrawal of steroids, an intensified immunosuppression approach using basiliximab induction and CNI-SIR-steroid maintenance followed by randomization to LSW versus SC ≥ 6 months post-transplant was evaluated [40]. The study was terminated prior to reaching target enrollment, however, due to high rates of post-transplant lymphoproliferative disorder attributed to over-immunosuppression. Perhaps this may have been related to the aggressive targeting of both CNI and mTOR troughs titrated to achieve levels comparable to those targeted when either agent is used separately. Interestingly, although the rejection rates in the cohorts were similar, the LSW group was noted to have higher 3-year allograft survival ($p = 0.002$) [40].

With promising outcomes of LSW trials and more frequent utilization of induction agents, SF and ESW protocols also emerged. Overall, acceptable BPAR and similar patient and allograft survival rates were reported, with significantly improved height Z-scores and reductions in BMI in SF and ESW groups [41–46]. Of note, the development of anti-human leukocyte antigen (anti-HLA) antibodies in up to 25% of pKTx recipients noted within the first 2 years post-transplantation was not linked to steroid withdrawal; SF protocols did not demonstrate higher development of *de novo* anti-HLA donor-specific antibodies (DSA) and subsequent antibody-mediated rejection when compared to steroid-based regimens at 2 years post-transplant [47–49]. Studies with longer follow-up, however, may still be warranted. In addition, it is also worth mentioning that most steroid minimization studies have excluded immunologically high-risk patients and used induction agents such as daclizumab and alemtuzumab which are not as commonly utilized in modern-day protocols, making it difficult to extrapolate their results to today's patient population. Furthermore, although minimization in steroid exposure has been associated with lower incidences of hyperglycemia, hypercholesteremia, hyperlipidemia, and need for antihypertensives, these findings have not been consistently established [44, 45, 50]. One possible explanation for this might be attributed to the co-administration of CNIs, which are associated with a similar adverse effect profile.

Undoubtedly, there is a clinical need for well-designed trials in pKTx recipients that are inclusive of immunologically high-risk and racially diverse populations and incorporate modern regimens of basiliximab or antithymocyte globulin induction with TAC, MMF, or SIR maintenance at recommended levels. It is perhaps due to the lack of such data that many centers still opt to continue steroids, either as part of an LSW strategy or indefinitely. Despite the absence of a widely accepted dosing consensus, it is prudent for transplant practitioners to assess the risks and the benefits of available steroid minimization data in their patient population given the high prevalence of negative adverse effects associated with steroids. Lastly, some transplant recipients may warrant continued steroid use to treat underlying disease states such as focal segmental glomerulosclerosis or lupus nephritis, requiring a detailed evaluation of their chronic immunosuppression regimen [51].

Calcineurin Inhibitors

Since the discovery of cyclosporine (CsA) in the 1970s and tacrolimus (TAC) in the 1990s, calcineurin inhibitors (CNIs) have revolutionized the field of renal transplantation. Despite being structurally different, both CNIs exhibit a similar mechanism of action, with TAC demonstrating greater potency than CsA [52]. Both CsA and TAC suppress the activation of T-cells by inhibiting the phosphatase activity of calcineurin [53]. CsA binds to cyclophilin, while TAC binds to FK-binding protein 12, inhibiting the signaling of transcription factors into the nucleus and halting the production of vital cytokines involved in the alloimmune response [54]. Ultimately, this results in inhibition of T-cell proliferation. Some studies suggest additional mechanisms exerted by TAC such as blockade of cytokine receptor expression and downregulation of cytokine effects on other target cells [55]. Given their nearly identical mechanism, CsA and TAC are never administered in combination, but rather are alternatives to one other as the backbone of immunosuppressive regimens.

Cyclosporine

Cyclosporine is commercially available as a modified microemulsion and a conventional non-modified formulation, with the microemulsion providing better solubility of the drug in an aqueous environment [56]. Due to its improved bioavailability and oral absorption leading to more reliable drug exposure, modified CsA has mostly replaced conventional CsA in clinical practice. These two products are not bioequivalent and thus cannot be used interchangeably. If a switch between the non-modified and modified version is needed, a 1:1 conversion is suggested with close therapeutic drug monitoring and an anticipated dose reduction of the modified formulation relative to the conventional formulation [56]. Both CsA formulations are commercially available in oral capsule and oral liquid dosage forms. Although transplant centers commonly establish institutional-based protocols to define therapeutic goals, the most commonly recommended starting dose in pKTx recipients for modified CsA is 9 ± 3 mg/kg per day divided every 12 hours, with goal trough levels ranging between 100 and 400 ng/mL. The average dose requirement often decreases toward the end of the first posttransplant year, ranging from 4.36 to 8.4 mg/kg per day [57]. Within this dosing range, a correlation between long-term CsA maintenance dose and risk of late rejection and chronic allograft failure has been reported [58]. Published data also suggests that every 1 mg/kg increase in CsA maintenance dose directly correlates to a 5–6% reduction in the risk of chronic allograft failure [59].

Tacrolimus

Oral absorption of TAC in children is incomplete and highly variable, with a reported bioavailability of immediate release formulations ranging from 5% to 70% [60]. Tacrolimus is best administered on an empty stomach as the absorption decreases in the presence of food, particularly high-fat meals. Because more than 90% of TAC present in the plasma is protein-bound, whole blood concentrations are utilized in clinical practice to measure trough concentrations [61]. The elimination half-life of TAC is approximately 12 hours, and it relies heavily on hepatic and intestinal cytochrome-P450 3A4 (CYP3A4) and cytochrome-P450 3A5 (CYP3A5) enzymes, as well as the p-glycoprotein (PgP)/ABCB1 efflux transporter for metabolism and elimination [62]. Thus, one can expect to see an impact on drug levels in the setting of hepatic impairment. On the contrary, because TAC is not renally cleared, no major change in levels is expected with renal dysfunction.

An understanding of marked differences in TAC pharmacokinetics between children and adults is crucial for appropriate dosing and monitoring in this specialized patient population. Studies demonstrate that younger children require significantly higher mg per kg TAC doses compared to adolescents and adults [63]. Although this phenomenon is not clearly understood, possible explanations may include altered PgP activity, immature CYP3A4/5 enzymatic pathways, differences in hepatic blood flow, and liver-size-to-body-weight ratio in younger children [63, 64]. There is also a steady decline in the relative dosing requirements of TAC noted in children greater than 5 years old and as they approach puberty [65]. Thus, based on available data, the suggested initial dose for immediate-release TAC in pKTx recipients as supported by the Kidney Disease: Improving Global Outcomes (KDIGO) guidelines is 0.2–0.3 mg/kg per day divided every12 hours; this is in contrast to the recommended initial dosing of 0.1 mg/kg per day suggested in adults [66]. Trough levels are guided by institution-specific protocols with a general recommended range of 5–15 ng/mL post-transplant and subsequent reductions over time [66]. When examined in older children and adults, minimal to no benefit of thrice-daily TAC in increasing therapeutic exposure and reducing adverse effects has been found; however, data focused on children less than 5 years old remains sparse [67–69]. Thus, due to the lack of available literature and difficulty of appropriately timing administration of doses and trough level measurements, thrice-daily dosing cannot be recommended as a routine strategy in pKTx recipients at this time.

Since TAC became available on the market, several oral dosage forms have emerged. With an end in patent of innovator immediate-release TAC (IR-TAC, Prograf®, Astellas), the FDA approved bioequivalent generic IR-TAC formulations in 2009. When assessing the efficacy and safety of switching from brand to generic, studies report a 1:1 conversion is clinically acceptable but recommend additional therapeutic drug monitoring as patients may require dose adjustments [70–72]. Additionally, it is prudent to maintain patients on formulations from one consistent generic manufacturer to minimize intra-patient trough variability. Although an immediate-release granule formulation is available on the market, due to high cost and lack of dosing flexibility, oral suspensions are commonly compounded with the immediate-release capsules for administration in children. Of note, a standard suspension concentration of 1 mg/mL has been suggested from a medication safety standpoint; however, 0.5 mg/mL is also utilized by many centers [73].

In addition to immediate-release formulations, the FDA also approved extended-release tacrolimus (ER-TAC, Advagraf XL®/Astagraf XL®, Astellas) in 2013 and subsequently once-daily tacrolimus (LCPT, Envarsus XR®, Veloxis Pharmaceuticals) in 2015. Early data demonstrated that although ER-TAC had similar patient and allograft outcomes to IR-TAC [74], a substantial increase in total daily milligram (mg) dose was required upon conversion from IR-TAC to ER-TAC [75]. In the ASTCOFF study, Tremblay and colleagues conducted a pharmacokinetic study comparing all three formulations of TAC [76]. The authors found higher exposure on a per milligram basis, lower intraday fluctuation, prolonged time to peak concentration, and lower dose requirements with LCPT compared to IR-TAC and ER-TAC [76]. In relation to adverse effects, the STRATO study reported that LCPT was associated with fewer neurologic adverse effects in adult KTx recipients, regardless of race or time after transplant [77]. Unfortunately, data for use of LCPT in pediatrics, albeit promising, is still limited to case reports [78]. Of note, the extended-release capsules and tablets cannot be split or crushed, further limiting its utility in younger patients. However, once-daily TAC formulations may have a potential role in improving adherence in adolescents.

Efficacy

The most recent North American Pediatric Renal Transplant Cooperative Study (NAPRTCS) registry data indicates that the majority of pKTx recipients are maintained on TAC post-transplant. A randomized controlled trial comparing TAC versus CsA in 196 pediatric patients reported significantly lower rates of acute rejection and steroid-resistant rejection with TAC [79]. In addition, although patient survival was similar between the two groups, allograft survival at 4-year follow-up and reported glomerular filtration rate (GFR) were significantly higher in the TAC group compared to CsA [79]. A larger retrospective study of 986 pKTx recipients in the NAPRTCS database found a higher mean GFR and lower requirement for antihypertensives with TAC compared to CsA [57]. There was no difference noted in the risk of allograft failure, time to first rejection, and allograft survival between CsA and TAC at 1 and 2 years post-transplant, raising the question of whether one CNI is truly advantageous over the other [57]. Other studies have also corroborated similar findings, but with fewer cosmetic complications in patients receiving TAC, a significant aspect to consider in adolescent patients [80]. One should note that most data comparing CsA and TAC was published over 15 years ago and likely requires re-evaluation with modern-day induction and maintenance strategies in an ever-evolving patient population.

Target of Rapamycin Inhibitors

Approved nearly a decade after TAC for use in SOT, target of rapamycin inhibitors (TOR-Is), namely, sirolimus (SIR) and everolimus (EVR), have steadily gained acceptance in pKTx. The primary advantage of TOR-Is over CNIs is a decrease in nephrotoxicity; however, other benefits have also emerged. Activation of the TOR pathway occurs further downstream in the alloimmune activation cascade in response to cytokine proliferation [81]. Both SIR and EVR bind to the immunophilin FKBP-12 to form a complex that inhibits the function of TOR [82]. This inhibits mRNA synthesis, arresting the cell cycle and inhibiting T-cell proliferation [81, 82].

In addition to immunosuppressive effects, TOR-Is are shown to have antineoplastic, antiviral, and anti-atherogenic effects not seen with other agents, providing a theoretical advantage in both preventing and managing BK polyomavirus, chronic allograft nephropathy and transplant allograft vasculopathy [83, 84]. Reductions in angiogenesis have also been reported due to the agents' inhibition of vascular endothelial growth factor [83, 84]. It is important to note that the actions of TOR-Is extend beyond T-cell inhibition, as TOR is required for B-cell proliferation as well [85]. Thus, inhibition of TOR prevents B-cell receptor signaling and increases apoptosis of B-lymphocytes [86]. These mechanistic differences make TOR-Is an appealing option to consider either for CNI avoidance or in the presence of other risk factors, such as pos-ttransplant lymphoproliferative disorder (PTLD) or post-transplant malignancy, which will be discussed later in this chapter.

Sirolimus

SIR exhibits a predictable and rapid absorption in the small intestines, reaching peak concentrations within approximately one hour. It is commercially available as both an oral solution and oral tablet, with a reported bioavailability of 15–30% [87,

88]. These two products are not bioequivalent and therefore are not interchangeable. It is also worth mentioning that as per manufacturer recommendations, SIR tablets should not be crushed or split, limiting younger children to the oral solution. Similar to TAC, SIR is highly protein-bound, metabolized extensively via CYP3A4, and excreted via PgP transporters. Children exhibit a significantly faster metabolism and thus shorter half-life of SIR when compared to adults; the mean reported half-life in adults is 62 hours, compared to only 13.7 hours in children [87, 88]. This significant pharmacokinetic difference explains the twice-daily dosing recommendations in infants and children and once-daily dosing in adolescents and adults, with the highest SIR clearance in children younger than 5 years of age [89]. In children weighing less than 40 kg, the manufacturer recommends an initial loading dose of 3 mg/m^2 followed by 1 mg/m^2 per day either divided twice daily or administered once daily, with goal trough levels ranging between 5 and 15 ng/mL based on institutional protocols. Initial dosing and goal trough levels may differ when used in combination with a CNI.

Everolimus

Although the mechanism of action of EVR is identical to that of SIR, there are some important pharmacokinetic differences to note. The hydrophilic character of EVR increases its GI absorption and systemic clearance, while speeding up its elimination half-life [90]. Everolimus is commercially available in 0.25 mg, 0.5 mg, 0.75 mg, and 1 mg tablets and also should not be split or crushed, thus limiting administration in children. Although not FDA approved for use in pKTx recipients, studies suggest initial EVR dosing of 1.6 mg/m^2/day in combination with CsA or 2 mg/m^2/day in combination with TAC, divided twice daily, with goal trough targets of 3–8 ng/mL [91–93]. The lower dosing requirement in combination with cyclosporine is likely attributed to CsA-mediated inhibition of CYP3A4 and PgP that is not seen with TAC [93].

Efficacy

As longevity of the allograft is of utmost priority in pKTx recipients, the "nephro-sparing" effects of TOR-Is compared to CNIs are the primary reason for their addition to or switching from CNI-based regimens. When utilized at baseline as part of a maintenance regimen, high patient and allograft survival, acceptable rejection rates, and a tolerable adverse effect profile have been reported [94, 95]. A study of 274 pKTx recipients, however, found that combining SIR, CNIs, and steroids after basiliximab induction resulted in a high incidence of infections and PTLD, suggestive of significant over-immunosuppression [96]. Converting patients from a CNI-based to SIR-based regimen in the presence of CNI-induced nephrotoxicity or chronic allograft vasculopathy may improve GFR while decreasing the prevalence of CNI-related adverse effects [97–99]. It is imperative, however, to optimize the timing of this conversion, as reversal of severe allograft injury is unlikely and late withdrawal of CNI may not provide any clinical benefit [100]. Further clinical trials to evaluate long-term efficacy and safety outcomes of TOR-Is, particularly without CNIs in pKTx recipients, may be warranted.

While clinical data for EVR use in pKTx recipients is limited, it has generally shown to be safe and effective in preventing rejection. *De novo* immunosuppression in pediatrics with corticosteroids and reduced goal troughs of CsA and EVR demonstrated comparable EVR pharmacokinetics to those found in adults, no allograft loss, tolerable side effects, with an acceptable incidence of reversible, mild to moderate acute rejection during a 6-month follow-up period [92]. Similar studies examining the efficacy of an EVR and CsA combination with or without steroids reported high patient and allograft survival, stable allograft function, low incidence of BPAR and chronic rejection at 1–3 years posttransplant, with tolerable adverse effects and infection rates [101–103]. In the setting of modern-day immunosuppression regimens and push for steroid withdrawal, the results of the recent CRADLE study are worth noting [92]. Pediatric patients were randomized to undergo conversion to low-dose EVR and TAC with steroid withdrawal at 6 months or standard TAC, MMF, and steroid maintenance regimen. Allograft function, incidence of biopsy-proven acute rejection, allograft loss, and changes in height and weight were similar in both groups. Interestingly, while growth was significantly less affected in prepubertal patients maintained on EVR therapy, rejection was the leading cause of drug discontinuation in this group, suggesting that TOR-I-containing regimens may be associated with suboptimal immunosuppression in the setting of steroid withdrawal [92]. Of note, no head-to-head comparative trials examining SIR versus EVR in pKTx recipients have been completed at this time.

Costimulatory Blockade

Belatacept

The first-in-class costimulation blocker, belatacept, received FDA approval in 2011 for use in adult KTx recipients. Belatacept is a human fusion protein that binds to the CD80/CD86 ligands on antigen-presenting cells, blocks their interaction with the CD28 receptors on T-lymphocytes, and selectively inhibits T-lymphocyte activation via the costimulatory signal [104]. The fusion protein also activates an inhibitory signal that terminates the T-cell response, inhibits acute and chronic rejection pathways, and may play a significant role in promoting donor-specific tolerance [104]. The primary role of belatacept is CNI avoidance; thus, it is typically used in combination with basiliximab induction, MMF, and steroid maintenance.

Belatacept is commercially available as an intravenous solution approved for two distinct indications with different dosing: *de novo* induction and CNI conversion. For *de novo* induction, belatacept 10 mg/kg is infused over 30 minutes on the day of transplant prior to allograft implantation (day 1), then again on day 5, and at the end of post-operative weeks 2, 4, 8, and 12. By the end of week 16, belatacept is reduced to a maintenance dose of 5 mg/kg and infused every 4 weeks thereafter [105, 106]. For CNI conversion, belatacept 5 mg/kg is administered every 2 weeks for 4 doses and then every 4 weeks thereafter, in addition to a gradual CNI dose withdrawal (Table 12.1). A significant benefit of belatacept is its lack of drug-drug interactions, as well as the absence of the effect of renal or hepatic dysfunction on drug metabolism and clearance.

Table 12.1 Summary of immunosuppression utilization and monitoring in pediatric kidney transplant recipients

Drug	Dosage forms	Initial dosing	Adverse effects	Monitoring parameters	Drug interactions	Comments
Antiproliferative agents						
Azathioprine (AZA; *Imuran®*)	*PO*: 50, 75, 100 mg tablets *IV*: 5 mg/mL vials	*LD*: 3–5 mg/kg ×1 dose *MD*: 1–3 mg/kg once daily	*Frequent*: nausea, fever, fatigue, pancytopenia *Serious*: hepatotoxicity, hypersensitivity, pancreatitis, macrocytic anemia	BMP, CBC, LFT; TPMT activity prior to initiation or if refractory myelosuppression; Pancreatic enzymes if suspected pancreatitis; Routine dermatologic screening	Allopurinol, febuxostat: reduce AZA dose by 75% if cannot avoid combination	Food may alleviate GI irritation following dose administration
Mycophenolate mofetil (MMF; *CellCept®*)	*PO*: 250 mg capsules; 500 mg tablets; 200 mg/mL suspension *IV*: 25 mg/mL vials	*General*: 1200 mg/m²/day divided every 12 hours; max 1500 mg/dose *With CsA*: 1200–1800 mg/m²/day *With TAC*: 600 mg/m²/day	*Frequent*: nausea, diarrhea, vomiting, abdominal pain, pancytopenia *Serious*: esophagitis, gastritis, colitis, PML, pulmonary fibrosis, pure red cell aplasia, autoimmune hemolytic anemia, teratogenicity with fetal exposure	BMP, CBC, LFT; MPA TDM may be considered; Pregnancy in female TXP recipients of childbearing potential; Routine dermatologic screening; Renal/hepatic dysfunction may lead to increased toxicity	Antacids (PPI, H2RA): may lower drug absorption; Aluminum-/magnesium-containing antacids: may chelate MPA, lowering drug exposure; Bile acid resins: may bind MPA, lowering drug exposure; CsA: inhibits enterohepatic re-circulation of MPA, lowering drug exposure; Antibiotics: inhibit normal gut flora, lowering drug exposure; MPS may be less affected by gastric acid-lowering agents	MMF and MPS are not bioequivalent nor interchangeable Food decreases AUC but may alleviate GI irritation following dose administration Conversion from MPS to MMF may be required in patients who cannot swallow whole tablets; 1000 mg MMF is approximately equivalent to 720 mg MPS The use of mycophenolate derivatives is contraindicated during pregnancy due to significant teratogenicity
Mycophenolate sodium (MPS; *Myfortic®*)	*PO*: 180, 360 mg delayed-release tablets	*General*: 800 mg/m²/day divided every 12 hours; max 1080 mg/dose *Doses must be rounded to the nearest 180 mg; tablets should not be cut or crushed*				

(continued)

Table 12.1 (continued)

Drug	Dosage forms	Initial dosing	Adverse effects	Monitoring parameters	Drug interactions	Comments
Corticosteroids						
Methylprednisolone (*Solu-Medrol*®) **Prednisone** (*Deltasone*®) **Prednisolone** (*Orapred*®)	*IV*: multiple vial sizes/ concentrations *Prednisone PO*: 1, 2.5, 5, 10, 20, 50 mg tablets; 1 mg/mL solution *Prednisolone PO*: 5 mg tablets; 10, 15, 30 mg ODT; multiple syrup/solution formulations	*PO (general)*: 1–5 mg/kg/day *IV (general)*: 5–20 mg/kg/dose	*Frequent*: HTN, HLD, hyperglycemia, edema, polyphagia, weight gain, leukocytosis, psychosis/mood changes *Serious*: DM, cardiovascular disease, impaired wound healing, adrenal suppression, Cushingoid changes, impaired growth, cataracts, osteoporosis	BMP, CBC, LFT; Serum lipids, blood glucose/HbA1c, blood pressure, weight; Routine bone mineral density screening; Routine eye exam	Weak CYP3A4, PgP, and MRP2 inhibition may impact concomitantly administered immunosuppression; Psychiatric therapy: steroids may decrease the efficacy of concomitantly administered antipsychotics and antidepressants	Prednisolone is preferred in patients with hepatic dysfunction Steroid dosing should be slowly tapered in patients maintained on ≥20 mg of prednisone dose equivalent for ≥2 weeks

Drug	Dosage forms	Initial dosing	Adverse effects	Monitoring parameters	Drug interactions	Comments
Calcineurin inhibitors						
Cyclosporine (CsA) Non-modified (*SandIMMUNE®*) Modified (*Neoral®*, *Gengraf®*)	*Non-modified PO*: 25, 100 mg capsules; 100 mg/mL solution *Non-modified IV*: 50 mg/mL vials *Modified PO*: 25, 50, 100 mg capsules	*PO (general)*: 6–12 mg/kg/day divided every 12 hours *IV (general)*: ~1/4 of total daily PO dose *Maintenance dosing adjusted to target troughs*	*Frequent*: afferent arteriolar vasospasm, diarrhea, hyperkalemia, hypomagnesemia, hyperuricemia, tremors, headaches, hyperglycemia, HTN, HLD (CsA > TAC) *Serious*: PTDM (TAC > CsA), QTc prolongation, IF/TA, glomerulosclerosis, proteinuria, RTA, seizures (TAC > CsA), behavioral changes, gingival hyperplasia (CsA > TAC), hirsutism (CsA > TAC), alopecia (TAC > CsA), thrombotic microangiopathy	BMP, LFT; Serum lipids, blood glucose/HbA1c, blood pressure, weight; Routine trough TDM	CYP3A4 inducers (list not inclusive) phenobarbital, phenytoin, primidone, carbamazepine, rifampin, rifabutin, St. John's wort, griseofulvin: increase CNI metabolism, lowering drug exposure and increasing risk of rejection; CYP3A4 inhibitors (list not inclusive) triazole antifungals, macrolide antibiotics, protease inhibitors, non-DHP CCB, amiodarone, ranolazine, fluoxetine, fluvoxamine, cimetidine: decrease CNI metabolism, increasing drug exposure and risk of toxicity; Potassium binders, phosphate binders, bile acid resins: bind CNI in the GI tract, lower drug exposure; SMX/TMP, potassium-sparing diuretics, ACEI, ARB: potentiate CNI-induced hyperkalemia; QT-prolonging agents: potentiate CNI-induced QT prolongation	Acute elevations in CNI troughs may occur with liver dysfunction, diarrhea, or drug interactions IR-TAC capsules may be opened and administered sublingually at a 50% dose reduction in patients who have small bowel obstruction or impaired GI absorption with persistently subtherapeutic TAC troughs
Tacrolimus (TAC) Immediate-release (IR-TAC; *Prograf®*) Extended-release (ER-TAC; *Astagraf®*, *Advagraf®*) LCP-tacrolimus (LCPT; *Envarsus®*)	*IR-TAC PO*: 0.5, 1, 5 mg capsules; 0.5 mg, 1 mg granule packets *IR-TAC IV*: 5 mg/mL vials *ER-TAC PO*: 0.5, 1, 5 mg capsules *LCPT PO*: 0.75, 1, 4 mg tablets	*PO (general)*: 0.2–0.3 mg/kg/day divided every 12 hours *IV (general)*: ~¼ of total daily PO dose *Maintenance dosing adjusted to target troughs*				

(continued)

Table 12.1 (continued)

Drug	Dosage forms	Initial dosing	Adverse effects	Monitoring parameters	Drug interactions	Comments
Target of rapamycin inhibitors						
Sirolimus (SIR; *Rapamune*®)	*PO*: 0.5, 1, 2 mg tablets; 1 mg/mL solution	*LD*: 3 mg/m^2 ×1 dose (<40 kg), 6 mg/m^2 ×1 dose (≥40 kg) *MD*: 1 mg/m^2/day, administered either once daily or divided every 12 hours *Maintenance dosing adjusted to target troughs*	*Frequent*: thrombocytopenia, hyperlipidemia, proteinuria, delayed AKI recovery, peripheral edema *Serious*: impaired wound healing, impaired growth, hepatic artery thrombosis (SIR), renal arterial and venous thrombosis (EVR), aphthous ulceration, lymphocele, angioedema, interstitial pneumonitis	BMP, CBC, LFT; Serum lipids, weight; Urine protein; Routine trough TDM	CYP3A4 inducers (list not inclusive) phenobarbital, phenytoin, primidone, carbamazepine, rifampin, rifabutin, St. John's wort, griseofulvin: increase TOR-I metabolism, lowering drug exposure and increasing risk of rejection; CYP3A4 inhibitors (list not inclusive) triazole antifungals, macrolide antibiotics, protease inhibitors, non-DHP CCB, amiodarone, ranolazine, fluoxetine, fluvoxamine, cimetidine, cyclosporine: decrease TOR-I metabolism, increasing drug exposure and risk of toxicity; Potassium binders, phosphate binders, bile acid resins: bind TOR-I in the GI tract, lower drug exposure	Acute elevations in TOR-I troughs may occur with liver dysfunction, diarrhea, or drug interactions
Everolimus (EVR; *Zortress*®)	*PO*: 0.25, 0.5, 0.75, 1 mg tablets	*With CsA*: 1.6 mg/m^2/day divided every 12 hours *With TAC*: 2 mg/m^2/day divided every 12 hours *Maintenance dosing adjusted to target troughs*				

Drug	Dosage forms	Initial dosing	Adverse effects	Monitoring parameters	Drug interactions	Comments
Costimulation blocker						
Belatacept (*Nulojix®*)	*IV*: 250 mg vials	*De novo*: 10 mg/kg intraoperatively and on day 5, end of weeks 2, 4, 8, and 12 post-transplant; followed by 5 mg/kg every 4 weeks (±3 days) thereafter *CNI conversion*: 5 mg/kg on days 1, 15, 29, 43, and 57; followed by 5 mg/kg every 4 weeks (±3 days) thereafter; combined with gradual CNI withdrawal *Doses must be rounded to the nearest 12.5 mg for accurate reconstitution*	Mild infusion-related reactions have been reported, which resolved without necessitating drug discontinuation	EBV serostatus prior to therapy initiation; New or worsening neurological/cognitive decline	No significant drug interactions have been reported; MMF/MPS dose reduction may be required in patients transitioned from CsA to belatacept due to the elimination of CsA's effects on MPA metabolism	The use of belatacept is contraindicated in patients who are EBV-seronegative due to the increased risk of PTLD

Abbreviations
ACEI angiotensin-converting enzyme inhibitors, *ARB* angiotensin receptor blockers, *AUC* area under the curve, *AZA* azathioprine, *BMP* basic metabolic panel, *CBC* complete blood count, *CNI* calcineurin inhibitor, *CsA* cyclosporine, *CYP3A4* cytochrome P450-3A4, *DM* diabetes mellitus, *EBV* Epstein-Barr virus, *ER-TAC* extended-release tacrolimus, *EVR* everolimus, *GI* gastrointestinal, *H2RA* histamine-2 receptor antagonist, *HbA1c* hemoglobin A1c, *HLD* hyperlipidemia, *HTN* hypertension, *IF/TA* interstitial fibrosis/tubular atrophy, *IR-TAC* immediate-release tacrolimus, *IV* intravenous, *LCPT* LCP-tacrolimus, *LD* loading dose, *LFT* liver function tests, *MD* maintenance dose, *MMF* mycophenolate mofetil, *MPA* mycophenolic acid, *MPS* mycophenolate sodium, *non-DHP CCB* non-dihydropyridine calcium channel blockers, *ODT* orally disintegrating tablets, *PML* progressive multifocal leukoencephalopathy, *PO* oral, *PPI* proton pump inhibitor, *PTLD* posttransplant lymphoproliferative disorder, *RTA* renal tubular acidosis, *SIR* sirolimus, *SMX/TMP* sulfamethoxazole/trimethoprim, *TAC* tacrolimus, *TDM* therapeutic drug monitoring, *TOR-I* target of rapamycin inhibitor, *TXP* transplant

Efficacy

Clinical studies evaluating the benefits and drawbacks of belatacept in adults have yielded consistent results. Overall, initial phase II trials demonstrated non-inferiority to CsA-based regimens with respect to acute rejection, patient and allograft survival, infection, and cardiovascular (CV) or metabolic effects [105, 106]. The major benefits of belatacept were found to lie in its preservation of GFR and lower incidence of chronic allograft nephropathy (CAN) at 6 and 12 months post-transplant [105, 106]. However, belatacept patients experienced a higher incidence and grade of acute rejection and significantly higher rates of PTLD, with cases occurring months after belatacept therapy was discontinued. Of note, despite the higher incidence and severity of rejection, no difference in patient or allograft survival was seen at 12 months post-transplant [106].

Data on belatacept for use in pKTx recipients is limited to anecdotal case reports and retrospective, non-randomized conversion studies. A phase I study of a single dose of belatacept in adolescent KTx recipients resulted in therapeutic pharmacokinetic and pharmacodynamic measurements comparable to adults [107]. In another small group of adolescent KTx recipients who required long-term CNI avoidance, conversion to belatacept at a median time of 27 months post-transplant resulted in either stabilization or improvement of allograft function while avoiding rejection [108]. This benefit was only corroborated in patients converted well before significant deterioration of allograft function had occurred, suggesting that there may be a small window of opportunity in which belatacept conversion is most beneficial [109].

Belatacept's significant advantage in CNI avoidance, improved long-term renal allograft outcomes, and benign side effect profile make it an attractive option warranting further investigation for approval in the pediatric population. Of note, due to high rates of reported PTLD, belatacept remains contraindicated in Epstein-Barr virus (EBV)-naïve patients. As younger children are often EBV-negative at the time of transplant, this creates a limitation for use in pediatrics. Moreover, while monthly infusions may improve medication adherence, other limitations include significant treatment cost, strict administration schedules, and more frequent healthcare exposures that may increase nosocomial infectious risks.

Section II: Post-transplant Immunosuppression Challenges

Adverse Effects

Beyond efficacy, other primary drivers for drug selection are related to an agent's adverse effects and toxicities. It is imperative for both patients/caregivers and providers to be familiar with each individual immunosuppressant's unique adverse effect profile (Table 12.1). Overall, all immunosuppressants carry an inherent risk of infection and malignancy; these risks should be monitored frequently and treated swiftly. Several factors predispose patients to infections post-transplant, including high-dose antiproliferative therapy and cumulative myelosuppressive effects of induction and maintenance immunosuppression [110]. Immunosuppressant doses are frequently reduced in the setting of acute and life-threatening infections, as well as opportunistic fungal or viral infections [111], depending on each agent's immune target and the target's role in each particular infection [110]. Given that transplantation commits a pKTx recipient to lifelong immunosuppression, appropriately recognizing and coping with adverse effects is key to improving adherence and minimizing the long-term impact on patient and allograft outcomes.

Antiproliferative Agents

The adverse effects of AZA most frequently encountered post-transplant include fatigue, myelosuppression, hepatotoxicity, and hypersensitivity reactions. AZA-induced myelosuppression commonly manifests as leukopenia and thrombocytopenia, which are also dose-dependent and may be exacerbated by thiopurine methyltransferase (TPMT) and NUDT15 genetic polymorphisms (*see Pharmacogenetics section*). Hepatotoxicity may appear early in the treatment course with transient hepatic enzyme elevations and resolve with medication discontinuation, or after years of therapy in the form of nodular regenerative hyperplasia [112]. Hypersensitivity reactions may also occur, and present with fever, chills, arthralgias, or rash, which also resolve with cessation of therapy [112, 113]. Rarely encountered adverse effects of AZA include diarrhea, pancreatitis, megaloblastic anemia, and malignancy. It is recommended to test for TPMT enzyme activity prior to initiation of AZA and to monitor complete blood count and liver function tests weekly for the first 1–2 months of therapy, followed by every 3 months thereafter. Lastly, serum amylase and lipase should be checked in patients with severe abdominal pain, nausea, or vomiting to rule out pancreatitis [112, 113].

The most common adverse effects encountered with mycophenolate are related to its GI toxicity and myelotoxicity. The incidence and severity are comparable between the adult and pediatric population. Patients younger than 6 years of age, however, may be most susceptible to MMF-induced adverse effects [114, 115]. Of note, the reported incidence of MMF dose reductions or therapy interruption secondary to its adverse effect profile ranges from 13% to 16% [11], which may potentially increase the risk of allograft rejection in new pKTx recipients or those maintained on steroid-sparing immunosuppressive regimens [116].

Mycophenolate-induced GI toxicity presents as nausea, vomiting, diarrhea, and abdominal pain and tends to be dose-related; these symptoms are most likely to occur at the initiation of therapy and often improve over time [117]. Patients with persistent GI discomfort, however, may require the total daily MMF dose to be divided more frequently throughout the day. Although small case series in pKTx recipients suggest reduction in GI adverse effects and increased MPA absorption with MPS versus MMF [118, 119], larger studies fail to report a difference between MPS and MMF therapy [120–124]. Lastly, hematologic toxicities with MMF present as leukopenia, thrombocytopenia, or anemia, and may be further amplified by the co-administration of myelotoxic therapies such as lymphocyte-depleting antibodies for induction, valganciclovir for cytomegalovirus (CMV) prophylaxis, and sulfamethoxazole/trimethoprim or dapsone for *Pneumocystis* prophylaxis.

Supportive therapy with granulocyte colony-stimulating factor (G-CSF) may be considered when an MMF dose reduction is not feasible, such as in recipients who are highly sensitized, recently transplanted, or undergoing treatment of allograft rejection.

Steroids

Despite being a cornerstone of initial immunosuppressive regimens, the physical, psychological, and economic burden of steroid therapy related to both short- and long-term adverse effects have in part contributed to a 20% decreased incidence of steroid use as initial or maintenance immunosuppression in the last 20 years [125]. The adverse effect profile of glucocorticoids is partially attributed to their mechanism of action and often linked to higher doses and prolonged use [126]. Secondary to the inhibition of leukocyte migration to injury sites, poor wound healing is of concern in patients receiving higher steroid doses immediately post-transplant [29]. Steroid-induced leukocytosis is also observed; this effect is primarily due to demargination of neutrophils from the endovascular lining and delayed migration of polymorphonuclear leukocytes into tissues [127, 128]. Other less contributory mechanisms include release of immature neutrophils from the bone marrow into the circulation [129]. Given the risk of infections in transplant patients, it is important for clinicians to consider monitoring white blood cell counts with differential to rule out leukocytosis related to an acute infection, which typically presents with a "left shift" [130]. Additional short-term adverse effects include hyperglycemia and hypertension, particularly in patients with pre-existing metabolic risk factors.

Long-term adverse effects noted with steroid therapy include obesity, osteoporosis, growth impairment, peptic ulcer disease, vision changes, behavioral changes, and Cushing syndrome. Additionally, adrenal suppression is expected with prolonged steroid exposure, warranting administration of "stress dose" steroids to meet physiological needs in the setting of trauma, infection, surgery, or other clinical stressors. In the era of combination therapy with CNIs, chronic hypertension, hypercholesterolemia, hyperlipidemia, and hyperglycemia may also be potentiated, as similar adverse effects are associated with this drug class.

Over 10 years of data from the NAPRTCS registry highlights the contributing negative impact of steroids on both post-transplant growth and weight. With the goal of reaching normal adult height in pKTx recipients, the primary factors shown to influence post-transplant growth include age at transplantation, allograft function, and steroid dosage and duration of exposure [131]. Overall, registry data reported that children less than 5 years old exhibited a more negative Z-score at the time of KTx and significant catch-up growth in the 1–2 years after KTx, followed by a subsequent plateau or decline in Z-score in the years thereafter [125]. When assessing growth with regard to steroids specifically, daily use contributed to a significant decrease in height Z-score, with some improvement in growth deficits seen with alternate-day regimens. The highest but still only modest catch-up growth was noted in patients receiving no steroids after the immediate post-transplant period [125]. At 3 years post-transplant, a significantly greater improvement in growth rate was observed in pKTx less than 5 years old and on steroid-free regimens, with no significant difference noted in other age groups [132]. Thus, although crucial to carefully evaluate steroid use, this reiterates that other factors may also have an impact on growth following transplantation.

National registry data has also shown that at the time of transplant, 15.5% of pKTx recipients were overweight and 15.8% were obese; these proportions increased to 22.9% and 33.8%, respectively, at 6 months post-transplant and remained elevated at 21.3% and 33.6%, respectively, at 2 years post-transplant. Furthermore, the absence of corticosteroid therapy at 6 and 48 months post-transplant was associated with smaller increases in BMI% at 12- and 48-month follow-up; of those patients still on corticosteroids, there was no difference seen between daily and alternate-day dosing [133]. When combined with the worldwide rise in childhood obesity, it is noteworthy for transplant teams to evaluate the potential impact of prolonged steroid maintenance regimens on cardiovascular mortality risk in pediatric transplant recipients [134].

Calcineurin Inhibitors

There are several key adverse effects attributed to calcineurin inhibitors as a class. These include hyperkalemia, hypomagnesemia, hyperuricemia, diarrhea, alopecia, nausea, nephrotoxicity, hepatotoxicity, and neurotoxicity. In addition, metabolic adverse effects reported with CNIs include hypertension, hyperlipidemia, worsening hyperglycemia, and posttransplant diabetes mellitus (PTDM) [135]. Of note, the driver of PTDM is thought to be related to CNI-induced pancreatic β-cell toxicity, rather than insulin resistance as seen with corticosteroids [136, 137]. While hyperlipidemia is more commonly observed with CsA, hyperglycemia and PTDM are more frequently reported with TAC [63]. These complications often require pharmacotherapeutic intervention and are likely potentiated with concurrent corticosteroid therapy. Thus, weighing the role of immunosuppressive therapy in the development of metabolic disorders is crucial as their correlation to cardiovascular disease in the pediatric population is alarming [138, 139]. In fact, 10-year and beyond post-transplant follow-up data shows that following infections, cardiovascular events remain the second leading cause of death in pKTx recipients with a functioning allograft, with a reported mortality rate of 15–30% [140, 141].

Secondary to vasoconstriction at the afferent renal arteriole, both CsA and TAC may cause acute kidney injury marked by oliguria, anuria, and a rapid decline in GFR [142]. This is typically linked to supratherapeutic drug levels as well as concomitant therapy with other medications that also target the renal vasculature. The injury is often reversible by withdrawing the CNI or decreasing the dose. Over time, however, CsA and TAC can also lead to chronic nephrotoxicity, presenting as glomerulosclerosis, interstitial fibrosis, tubular atrophy, proteinuria, and a steady decline in GFR [137]. These structural changes can be progressive and are independent of CNI dose. Some data suggests that CsA is more nephrotoxic than TAC, while others found no difference between the two [138, 139]. Nephrotoxicity may also be greater in protocols that maintain higher CNI trough levels to compensate for steroid withdrawal. Ultimately, to preserve remaining function in deteriorating allografts, patients may require a switch to an alternate class of immunosuppressive agents.

Cyclosporine may cause hirsutism, gingival hyperplasia, and facial dysmorphism, which may have negative and lasting psychosocial impacts in children and adolescents and contribute to medication non-adherence. These adverse effects have not been observed with TAC, particularly adding to its appeal for use in adolescents. Although neurotoxicity is reported with both agents, this is far more prevalent with TAC and can present in the form of headaches, tremors, and seizures [63, 135]. Other rare but serious adverse effects to consider include QT prolongation, myocardial hypertrophy, posterior reversible encephalopathy syndrome (PRES), and thrombotic microangiopathy (TMA) [63]. Although reported with both TAC and CsA, switching from one CNI agent to the other has resulted in resolution of TMA, as has complete CNI withdrawal and conversion to TOR-I [143–146]. It is worth noting, however, that TMA has also been reported with SIR and EVR [145]. More evidence is emerging for successful transition to belatacept in patients with CNI-induced TMA, but this data is still limited to adult renal transplant recipients [142, 147, 148].

Target of Rapamycin Inhibitors

Although one of the reported advantages of TOR-Is is their minimal nephrotoxicity, both SIR and EVR are associated with other adverse effects worth noting. Poor wound healing seen with TOR-Is has the potential to delay surgical recovery, discouraging practitioners from its use in the immediate post-transplant period [149]. SIR and EVR may also cause aphthous ulcers, myelosuppression, peripheral edema, skin rash, and proteinuria [93, 150]. These adverse effects are often reversible by dose reduction. Elevations in total cholesterol, triglyceride, and low- and high-density lipoprotein concentrations have also been reported with both SIR and EVR therapy in a dose-dependent fashion, although more frequently associated with SIR [151].

Rare but serious adverse effects that will usually require discontinuation of TOR-Is include TMA and pulmonary toxicity in the form of interstitial pneumonitis. Should these occur, TOR-I discontinuation is likely warranted to maximize the chance of reversibility and recovery [152, 153]. In addition, TOR-Is may also be associated with delayed recovery from acute tubular necrosis and delayed graft function due to their impact on normal cell growth [154]. Angioedema has also been reported with TOR-Is, particularly at higher levels or in combination with angiotensin-converting enzyme inhibitors. Furthermore, both SIR and EVR carry black box warnings for their pro-thrombotic complications leading to an increased risk of hepatic artery thrombosis with SIR and kidney arterial and venous thrombosis in the first 30 days post-transplant with EVR.

Despite a few small reports of suggesting growth impairment in pKTx recipients maintained on SIR versus CsA [155, 156], a substantial amount of evidence exists supporting the use of reduced-dose EVR in combination with CNIs due to its lack of effect on growth and development [102, 152, 157, 158]. In addition, abnormalities in production of testosterone and luteinizing hormone have been reported in pKTx recipients on SIR [159, 160]. These findings, however, were not seen in more recent studies of reduced EVR dosing regimens, raising the question of whether these are class effects [102, 157].

Costimulatory Blockade (Belatacept)

Belatacept's adverse effect profile is considered relatively benign compared to other maintenance immunosuppressive agents. The increased incidence of PTLD in patients receiving belatacept maintenance is an important adverse effect that limits its use, especially in EBV-seronegative pediatric transplant recipients of EBV-seropositive donor allografts. Atypical EBV infections involving the central nervous system have also been reported [161]. Due to its intravenous route of administration, mild infusion-related reactions have been reported in 5% of patients receiving belatacept, which were similar to placebo and did not require pre-medications or lead to drug discontinuation [162, 163]. Furthermore, chronic venipuncture from monthly belatacept infusions may compromise future vascular dialysis access due to the increased risk of venous sclerosis and thrombosis [164].

Drug Interactions

Another significant challenge present in transplant recipients is the management of drug interactions, which must be addressed with extra caution in order to avoid subtherapeutic or supratherapeutic drug exposure. If managed inappropriately, these interactions may affect immunosuppressive efficacy and ultimately long-term allograft function and survival. In addition, unrecognized interactions may also potentiate serious and harmful adverse effects and contribute to increased healthcare visits, cost of care, and medication nonadherence. This section reviews the most common drug interactions encountered in the post-transplant setting.

Antiproliferative Agents

As previously mentioned, xanthine oxidase is required for the metabolism of 6-MP to its non-myelotoxic by-products. Thus, co-administration of AZA with xanthine oxidase inhibitors, such as allopurinol and febuxostat, should be avoided. In patients where co-administration cannot be avoided, a 75% AZA dose reduction is warranted [165]. As mycophenolate requires a lower gastric pH for hydrolysis in the stomach, acid-suppressing therapies such as proton pump inhibitors may decrease MPA exposure, thereby leading to increased risk of allograft rejection [166, 167]. Of note, this drug interaction appears to affect MMF products more so than MPS and is somewhat disputed in the literature [168–170]. Additionally, aluminum- and magnesium-containing antacids decrease the absorption of MMF and should be separated in administration by at least 2 hours in order to minimize chelation and formation of insoluble complexes in the GI lumen. Lastly, it is best to avoid bile resin sequestrants in combination with MMF due to their binding to MPA and prohibition of its enterohepatic recycling [171]. One small study of seven healthy individuals found a 91% reduction in MPA AUC with concomitant MMF and ferrous sulfate administration [172]. However, this finding has not been duplicated by follow-up studies. In fact, multiple studies have demonstrated a lack of significant effect of oral iron supplements on mycophenolate absorption and MPA exposure [173–175].

Calcineurin Inhibitors and Target of Rapamycin Inhibitors

Both CNIs and TOR-Is are major substrates of CYP3A4/3A5 enzymes and PgP efflux transporters, which are primarily expressed in the liver and small intestine. Due to their metabolism and elimination via these pathways, inducers and inhibitors of either system will impact pharmacokinetics of CsA, TAC, SIR, and EVR. Clinically significant interactions have been reported with CYP3A4-inducing antiepileptics such as phenytoin, phenobarbital, carbamazepine, and oxcarbazepine, as well as the anti-mycobacterials rifampin and rifabutin, leading to decreases in CNI and TOR-I therapeutic levels and requiring dose agumentation [176–178]. Conversely, CYP3A4/3A5 inhibitors, particularly triazole antifungals, non-dihydropyridine calcium channel blockers, macrolide antibiotics, and protease inhibitors can significantly increase CNI/TOR-I levels and may require preemptive dose reductions by approximately 30–50% or greater [179–181]. By the same mechanism, grapefruit juice increases CNI and mTOR-I levels and is considered contraindicated in transplant recipients. With judicious use, these drug interactions can also be applied advantageously. Several reports indicate use of CYP3A4 inhibitors such as diltiazem or clotrimazole to decrease overall CNI dosing requirement and boost levels in patients with difficulty achieving therapeutic trough goals [182–184]; others have successfully administered CYP3A4 inducers such as phenytoin to increase metabolism in the management of tacrolimus toxicity [185, 186].

Moderate- to high-intensity antihyperlipidemic agents such as atorvastatin which utilize CYP3A4 and OATP1B1/SLCO1B1 metabolic pathways are contraindicated in patients on CsA. Because of its inhibitory effects on CYP3A4 and OATP1B1/SLCO1B1, CsA dramatically raises statin concentrations leading to severe myopathy and increased risk of rhabdomyolysis [181]. Although this interaction is not well-observed with TAC or TOR-Is, other statins that forego these metabolic pathways, such as pravastatin, are considered safer options for use in transplant recipients.

Combination therapy of CNI with medications known to induce QT prolongation should be monitored closely, particularly in patients with cardiovascular disease. A few examples of agents that are notorious for prolonging the QT interval and are likely to be administered to a transplant recipient include macrolide or fluoroquinolone antibiotics, triazole antifungals, and amiodarone. Lastly, onset of diarrhea, irrespective of cause, may also increase the possibility of supratherapeutic CNI and TOR-I blood concentrations due to diarrhea-induced sloughing of PgP efflux pumps lining the GI tract [187].

Interactions Between Immunosuppressants

It is crucial to understand how immunosuppressants interact with one another as well to determine the optimal dose when used in combination. Unlike TAC, in addition to inhibition of CYP3A4 and OATP1B1/SLCO1B1, CsA also inhibits CYP2C9, multidrug-resistant protein (MRP)-2, and PgP/ABCB1. One of the resulting significant interactions is seen with mycophenolate, which utilizes MRP-2 to transport 7-O-MPHA glucuronide into the bile for conversion to the active MPA moiety that is reabsorbed via enterohepatic recirculation [11]. Inhibition of MRP-2 by CsA leads to a lower total MPA AUC, leading to higher MMF dose requirements compared to patients on TAC to achieve therapeutic exposure [188]. Thus, in order to overcome this drug interaction, higher MMF starting doses of 1200–1800 mg/m^2/day have been suggested when combined with CsA, compared to 600 mg/m^2/day when combined with tacrolimus [11, 189]. Moreover, if patients are converted from CsA to TAC or belatacept, MMF may require dose reductions to minimize the risk of MMF-associated adverse effects. Although no specific dose reduction recommendations are documented in the literature, practitioners may opt to dose-reduce either empirically or based on institution-specific protocols in the setting of acute infection, myelosuppression, and GI toxicities [163].

Simultaneous administration of CsA and SIR results in 67–85% higher SIR trough levels attributed to CYP450 and PgP substrate competition. Although initial recommendations suggested separating CsA and SIR administration by 4 hours, most practitioners will administer the 2 agents concomitantly for improved adherence but start with a lower SIR dose. Similarly, CsA has also been noted to increase the AUC of EVR, thus explaining the need for lower starting dose requirements when used in combination [93]. Interestingly, a decrease in TAC AUC and trough levels is expected when used in combination with SIR. The mechanism of this interaction is also attributed to competition for the same metabolic pathways and significant protein binding by both TAC and SIR [190]. When used in combination, close therapeutic drug monitoring to adjust levels is warranted.

Lastly, corticosteroids are both substrates and weak inhibitors of CYP3A4, as well as substrates of PgP transporters [30]. Although the likelihood of interaction seems higher with CsA, data demonstrating clinical relevance among other immunosuppressants remains conflicting [191–194]. Corticosteroids may also have inducing properties for both MRP-2 and UGT, with possible effect on mycophenolate exposure [30]. Therapeutic drug monitoring of concomitant immunosuppressants, particularly while receiving high-dose steroids, may be prudent. The lack of major drug-drug interactions and nonenzymatic metabolism of belatacept allows for ease in use as maintenance immunosuppression.

Perhaps one of the biggest challenges in minimizing the incidence and impact of drug interactions in transplant recipients is attributed to non-transplant healthcare interactions, such as those with general practice pediatricians and emergency departments. Oftentimes, medications are prescribed in these settings without knowledge of the clinical interactions with transplant immunosuppression, leading to adverse effects and poor patient outcomes. Thus, a general awareness regarding the nuances of transplant pharmacotherapy among healthcare providers and educating patients and caregivers regarding the importance of communication prior to initiation of any new therapies is essential [195]. Additionally, consulting with pharmacists and other trained practitioners for therapeutic alternatives to avoid the drug interaction altogether may increase the impact and safety of the intervention. Close therapeutic drug monitoring and dose adjustments paired with a comprehensive understanding of these dynamics is key to ensuring both safety and efficacy of immunosuppressive therapy in transplant patients.

Role of Pharmacogenetics

There is significant inter- and intra-patient variability in both the pharmacokinetics and pharmacodynamics of immunosuppression. Although the relationship between pharmacogenetics and pharmacokinetics is now better understood than it was previously, the link between pharmacogenetics and pharmacodynamics remains unclear. For example, we can now anticipate a patient's TAC dosing requirements based on the presence or absence of certain genetic alleles, but we struggle to answer questions such as why one patient develops allograft rejection at therapeutic TAC levels but another patient with subtherapeutic TAC levels does not. Nonetheless, pharmacogenetic testing has become a major area of interest over the last decade, with the goal of personalizing immunosuppressive regimens in transplant recipients and optimizing patient and allograft outcomes. The vast majority of pharmacogenetic research in maintenance immunosuppression targets CNIs and antiproliferative agents, which will be the focus of this section.

Both CNIs and TOR-Is are metabolized via CYP3A enzymatic pathways and eliminated via the PgP efflux transport system. Cyclosporine and TOR-Is' metabolism is mainly dependent upon CYP3A4, while TAC relies heavily on CYP3A5 pathways [196, 197]. Although certain CYP3A4 polymorphisms which affect drug metabolism have been identified, a strong clinical association has not been consistently reported [198]. On the contrary, particular single nucleotide polymorphisms (SNPs) of CYP3A5 alleles play a prominent role in determining its function, thereby contributing to alterations in TAC pharmacokinetics. Because of this, neither CsA nor TOR-Is exhibit as significant inter-patient variability as is seen with TAC.

Of the known genetic variants, the CYP3A5*1 SNP has demonstrated the strongest correlation with changes in TAC dosing requirement [199]. The wild-type allele, CYP3A5*1, is associated with the greatest metabolic function, while the CYP3A5*3 allele is associated with loss of metabolic function. Homozygous (*1/*1) expressors require higher TAC dosing due to more rapid metabolism, while *1/*3 and *3/*3 expressors require lower TAC dosing due to slower metabolism. In fact, expressors (*1/*1 and *1/*3) may require up to 50% higher doses than non-expressors (*3/*3), highlighting the challenges of applying a "one-size-fits-all" dosing model to all patients [200]. This finding is consistent among adult and pKTx recipients [201–203]. Furthermore, there is also a clear role of ethnicity in defining polymorphism frequency that cannot be dismissed; CYP3A5*1 SNPs have been noted to occur in 5–10% of Caucasian, 30% of Asian, and 70% of African patients. This is confirmed with clinical findings of African Americans requiring significantly higher TAC doses to maintain similar trough levels compared to the rest of the transplant patient population [204, 205].

After multiple reports of retrospective findings, the first prospective, randomized, controlled clinical trial to assess genotype-driven TAC dosing was conducted in 2010 by Thervet and colleagues in 280 adult KTx recipients [206]. A greater number of patients in the genotype-driven dosing group achieved target TAC levels by post-transplant day 3 compared to the standard dosing group (43.2% vs. 29.1%, respectively, $p = 0.03$) and required fewer dose modifications [206]. One should note, however, that aside from reaching the therapeutic goal faster, no consistent link between CYP3A5 allele polymorphism and incidence of rejection, delayed graft function, TAC toxicity, or patient and allograft survival has been established [207, 208]. One explanation for this lack of pharmacodynamic correlation in studies may be the inclusion of immunologically low-risk patients and use of lymphocyte-depleting induction therapy [208]. Thus, further prospective trials to examine the relationship with clinical outcomes are warranted before routine genetic testing can be recommended for all transplant patients.

As previously mentioned, PgP and ABCB-1 efflux transporters play a major role in TAC absorption and subsequent distribution. Working collectively with CYP3A enzymes, PgP transporters continuously pump drug out of intestinal enterocytes, decreasing absorption of CNI in the small intestine [209, 210]. Furthermore, presence of PgP transporters at the blood-brain barrier, kidneys, and liver may also affect CNI distribution at these various sites [209, 210]. Of the 50 ABCB-1 SNPs identified, the ABCB1 3435 C > T has received the most attention as it is thought to alter overall transporter expression [211, 212]. Although the expected finding would suggest altered bioavailability, studies have not been able to replicate a clinically relevant impact on TAC pharmacokinetics. It is also postulated that given its role in CNI distribution, ABCB-1 SNPs may instead play a wider role in explaining the adverse effects of TAC [213, 214]. The significance of these polymorphisms, however, remains unclear, and further studies are needed.

Severe adverse effects of AZA may be attributable to loss-of-function genetic polymorphisms in TPMT, the enzyme responsible for inactivating thioguanine nucleotides (TGN). Non-functionality in the TPMT alleles decreases TGN inactivation, causing mild to life-threatening myelotoxicity upon AZA exposure in heterozygous and homozygous carriers, respectively [215]. One in 300 patients may be predisposed to low or nonexistent TPMT function [4], with Afro-Caribbean and female patients being at higher risk than Caucasians, South-Asians, and males [216]. More recently, NUDT15 loss of function genetic polymorphisms have also been implicated as significant contributors to AZA intolerance. The function of NUDT15 is to inactivate AZA's metabolites and neutralize their cytotoxicity. Thus, patients with enzymatic deficiency are at a greater risk of AZA-induced myelotoxicity, especially in the presence of concomitant TPMT deficiency [217]. Finally, genetic variations in enzymes UGT1A9, UGT2B7, and MRP2 have been identified as predictors of interpatient variability of both MPA exposure and MPA-associated leukopenia [218]. Although testing of TPMT status for patients taking AZA is now fairly common, no routine genetic testing has been recommended for patients on mycophenolate derivatives.

Infections

A leading cause of mortality in pKTx recipients, infectious complications account for the greatest proportion of hospital readmissions within the first 2 years posttransplant [219, 220]. The primary driver of infectious risk is long-term immunosuppression, blunting the host's ability to mount an appropriate immune response. In addition, younger children often lack the exposure to opportunistic pathogens such as EBV, CMV, and tuberculosis (TB) to establish lifelong latency prior to transplant, and may develop disseminated infections far more easily than an immunocompetent host [221]. Fortunately, donors are now routinely screened for infections such as CMV, EBV, human immunodeficiency virus (HIV), hepatitis B virus (HBV), and hepatitis C virus (HCV) to minimize inadvertent transmission to the recipient or to allow for risk assessment and initiation of prophylactic therapy where appropriate [222]. In addition to opportunistic infections, the pediatric KTx recipient also remains susceptible to other common childhood infections, including acute otitis media, bronchiolitis, and gastroenteritis.

Viral infections in the setting of chronic immunosuppression complicate treatment and may have long-term effects on allograft function. The incidence of chronic rejection is higher in the setting of CMV infection due to the temporary reduction in immunosuppression during treatment, as well as an increase in the presence of pro-inflammatory mediators in the allograft during the acute infectious process [223]. Post-transplant lymphoproliferative disorder is also more prevalent in EBV-negative pediatric recipients of EBV-positive organs [224]. Moreover, the cumulative hematologic dyscrasias caused by the viral infections themselves may be exacerbated by concomitant immunosuppression with antiproliferative agents and TOR-Is. Although impractical to only accept CMV- and EBV-negative donor allografts due to a significant worldwide organ shortage, exposure prevention and early detection is vital. For example, the use of CMV-seronegative blood product transfusions may reduce the risk of transfusion-transmitted exposure [225].

Another challenge to consider in pKTx recipients is maintaining an up-to-date vaccination schedule both pre-and post-transplantation. If transplanted at a young age, the recipient may not have yet completed their recommended immunization series. In addition, chronic kidney disease (CKD) patients and those on dialysis are often unable to mount a sufficient response to vaccines due to poor immunocompetence and may require repeated doses [226, 227]. Although small studies in pediatric liver transplant recipients have suggested the safety of using live vaccines such as measles, mumps, rubella, and varicella, the consensus remains to avoid live vaccines post-transplant due to the potential risk of disseminated disease [228–230].

Malignancy

Malignancies are well-known complications post-KTx and occur at a higher rate compared to the general population. The types of malignancies initially seen in pKTx recipients differ significantly from that of the adult transplant population. Furthermore, when compared to the general pediatric population, the occurrence of malignancies is reportedly 5–20 times higher in SOT recipients [231]. The most recent NAPRTCS data reports that approximately 11–23% of all deaths after pKTx are secondary to cancer, with PTLD and skin cancers being the first and second most common, respectively [134, 232].

The incidence of PTLD reported in pKTx recipients is 1–2.5% albeit substantially lower when compared to other organ transplants [233]. Often seen within the first post-transplant year, the median time from transplant to PTLD diagnosis is 12.7 months [134]. The most common risk factors associated with development of PTLD are younger age at time of transplant, EBV viremia, and overall level of induction and maintenance immunosuppression. The association with age is likely attributed to the fact that infants and children are typically EBV-seronegative; thus, *de novo* exposure leading to viremia while immunosuppressed creates an opportune environment for development of PTLD.

Interestingly, although the impact of overall immunosuppression is certainly well acknowledged, it is unclear if specific immunosuppressive agents increase this risk or provide a protective advantage. Although some have suggested that induction with lymphocyte-depleting agents correlates with development of PTLD, this finding is not consistently reported [234–237]. Older studies suggest greater PTLD risk with TAC over CsA, but this is likely more related to previously higher TAC trough goals leading to over-immunosuppression rather than individual drug effect [238, 239]. The incidence of PTLD is also significantly higher in belatacept- versus CNI-treated patients, particularly in the setting of EBV donor/recipient serology mismatch [240]. Lastly, MMF demonstrates a low correlation to PTLD, and TOR-Is' effects on the cell cycle make them a preferred option for maintenance immunosuppression after treatment of malignancies, including PTLD [235, 236]. Treatment options for PTLD include minimization of the maintenance immunosuppression regimen, antivirals like ganciclovir, low-dose chemotherapy, and rituximab. Two year patient survival following PTLD diagnosis in pediatrics ranges from 70% to 85% [241–243].

When considering non-lymphoproliferative malignancies, skin cancers in the form of melanoma or squamous cell carcinoma are the most frequent tumor types found in SOT recipients [244]. Malignancies related to chronic viral infections, such as human herpesvirus 8 (HHV8) associated Kaposi sarcoma and human papillomavirus (HPV)-associated genital cancers, also occur. Additionally, cancers of the liver, kidney, soft tissue, ovary, testis, bladder, and thyroid have all been reported [231]. Non-lymphoproliferative malignancies are observed at a much lower rate and seen later on after transplantion compared to PTLD [134]. Pharmacotherapeutic treatment options in addition to chemotherapy also entail overall reduction in immunosuppression and use of a TOR-I [245]. It is essential to note that as patient and allograft survival outcomes continuously improve, pKTx recipients living into adulthood acquire additional age-related cancer risks as well. Ultimately, identifying risk factors and minimizing immunosuppression without jeopardizing allograft function may be beneficial in preventing malignancies in pKTx recipients.

Pregnancy and Fertility

Kidney transplantation allows for rapid resolution of abnormalities in the hypothalamus-pituitary-ovarian axis that can be seen in females with CKD. This restoration can occur within weeks to months post-transplant and thus provides an opportunity for women to regain fertility and conceive. Pregnancies in KTx recipients carry high maternal and fetal risk and are complicated by the presence of proteinuria, hypertension, time elapsed since transplant, immunologic factors, and immunosuppressive agents [246]. Additionally, adolescent and teen pregnancies may further add to these risk factors [247]. Unfortunately, outcomes data on pregnancies in adolescent and adult KTx recipients is limited to registries such as the Transplant Pregnancy Registry International and retrospective reports, further minimizing insight. With expected survial to adulthood, fertility and pregnancy must be addressed as the pKTx recipient matures. It is therefore crucial for healthcare providers to educate adolescents and young adults on the need for highly effective contraception to avoid unwanted pregnancies. In addition, an emphasis should be placed on the importance of planned pregnancy to ideally minimize risk factors for both the mother and fetus prior to conception.

The immunosuppressive agents that are commonly used post-transplant cross the placenta and are detectable to varying degrees in the fetal circulation [248]. CNIs are FDA Pregnancy Category C (human risk not ruled out) and are considered safe in pregnancy and breastfeeding. The extent of exposure detected in blood levels of the fetus is estimated to be half of that seen by the mother [248]. Notably, there is an approximate 25% dose increase required for CNIs during pregnancy to maintain adequate trough levels; this is attributed to an increase in volume of distribution and overactive CYP3A metabolic function [249]. When taken during pregnancy, CsA may increase the risk of pre-eclampsia, cause development of immature T-cells, and decrease production of B-cells [250]. Theoretically, this can predispose the fetus to autoimmune diseases; the long-term impact, however, is still unknown. Such findings are not yet reported with TAC but also cannot be ruled out. Lastly, the incidence of congenital malformations in women maintained on CNIs throughout pregnancy is consistent with the general population, ranging from 3% to 5%, and is similar between TAC and CsA [251].

Although both antiproliferative agents are categorized as FDA Pregnancy Category D (evidence of human risk), AZA is the preferred agent over MPA [66, 252]. This is primarily because the fetal liver lacks the enzyme inosinate pyrophosphorylase, protecting the fetus from the toxic adverse effects of AZA [253]. It is also worth noting that teratogenicity with AZA has been primarily reported at higher doses of ≥6 mg/kg, well above the recommended doses of ≤3 mg/kg/day in KTx recipients [253]. Following administration of AZA, 6-MP reaches its peak at 4 hours and is also present in breastmilk [254]. Although the reported risk is low, pumping and discarding any breastmilk within the 4 hours after each AZA dose may be a strategy to decrease the infant's 6-MP exposure [254]. This is in stark contrast to MPA, which is linked to spontaneous abortions and numerous birth defects [250]. Compared to women who discontinue MPA prior to conception, there is a significantly higher rate of miscarriages around 45–49% in women still taking MPA during the first trimester [251, 255]. In addition, fetal exposure to MPA causes congenital malformations in 20–27% of births. The most commonly observed birth defects include cleft lip and palate, microphthalmos, finger malformations, and congenital heart defects [256, 257]. In light of these findings, MPA derivatives are contraindicated in pregnancy. Consequently, it is strongly recommended to discontinue MMF at least 6 weeks prior to conception [258, 259]. Despite these findings and FDA's black box warning regarding the same, both MMF and MPS remain Pregnancy Category D. Given the high risk, it is required for prescribers to complete a risk evaluation and mitigation strategy (REMS) with all female patients of childbearing potential prior to initiation of MMF. In addition, women should be counseled on pregnancy prevention, use of reliable and effective contraception methods when sexually active, and importance of planned pregnancies. In the young adult population, however, avoiding unplanned pregnancies poses a significant challenge, particularly in adolescents that may engage in "high-risk" sexual behavior [250]. Lastly, it is important to note that the risk of congenital malformations has not been reported in pregnancies fathered by patients receiving MMF or AZA [260, 261].

Limited data is available regarding clinical outcomes of TOR-I exposure in pregnancy. Both SIR and EVR have shown to cause infertility and are FDA Pregnancy Category C. In males, TOR-Is can cause azoospermia and oligospermia, while menstrual irregularities and amenorrhea have been observed in females [262]. Although teratogenicity in women has not been reported [263, 264], animal studies suggest increased fetal mortality, decreased fetal weight, and delayed ossification of skeletal structures [265, 266]. Thus, EVR and SIR should be discontinued at least 8 weeks and 12 weeks, respectively, prior to conception in females and at least 4 weeks in male KTx recipients fathering a pregnancy. Finally, prednisone, prednisolone, and methylprednisolone are considered safe in pregnancy and breastfeeding, with both categorized as FDA Pregnancy Category B and Category C, respectively. This safety is likely due to low fetal exposure as 90% of corticosteroid maternal dose is metabolized in the placenta before reaching the fetus [267]. Orofacial clefts and congenital malformations in newborns exposed to glucocorticoids are reported, but the prevalence is very low [268]. In actuality, adverse effects related to steroid use such as hypertension and preeclampsia are far greater of a concern in the pregnant female and must be closely monitored.

In summary, CNI treatment ideally with TAC and close therapeutic drug monitoring, a switch of mycophenolate to AZA, and utilization of low-dose prednisone is the recommended regimen in pregnant KTx recipients [252]. The risk of rejection is potentiated significantly in the presence of proteinuria and hypertension. Thus, signs of high blood pressure should be monitored and promptly treated; hydralazine, beta-blockers, or calcium channel blockers are considered safe and effective options in pregnancy. More robust registries and studies, however, are needed in this unique patient population.

Medication Nonadherence

Medication nonadherence (MNA) is the age-old challenge that carries a tremendous impact on short- and long-term outcomes following SOT. Nonadherence refers to a deviation from the medication regimen prescribed by the healthcare provider that is sufficient enough to adversely impact the regimen's intended effect [269, 270]. Adherence to complex, lifelong immunosuppressive regimens after transplantation is often burdensome, particularly among adolescents, with rates of MNA in pKTx recipients ranging from 30% to 70% [271]. Expectedly, nonadherence is associated with clinically worse outcomes such as development of *de novo* donor-specific antibodies leading to immunological sensitization and allograft rejection, increased hospitalizations, healthcare costs, treatment-related adverse effects, allograft loss, and death [272, 273].

Rather than an isolated clinical issue, MNA is a modifiable behavior, and interventions to improve adherence must focus on addressing barriers to behavioral change. The World Health Organization has identified five broad categories of factors that are most commonly associated with and contribute to MNA, which include socioeconomic, condition-related, psychosocial, health system-related, and treatment-related factors [274]. Medication nonadherence is rarely triggered by a single risk factor, but rather a combination of multiple barriers with various etiologies that occur simultaneously and ultimately lead to nonadherence [275]. Given its multifactorial etiology, MNA remains one of the biggest long-term challenges for transplant recipients and providers alike.

Socioeconomic factors such as financial instability, lack of a cohesive family structure, as well as adolescent age are perhaps the most common barriers known to affect adherence in the pediatric population [275, 276]. Adolescents have the highest reported incidence of acute rejection within the first post-transplant year and the lowest 5-year allograft survival compared to all other age groups below 65 years [277]. As the adolescent begins transitioning to the ownership of being responsible for self-care, the presence of parental supervision and family support in this crucial developmental stage fosters adherence [278]. Furthermore, socioeconomic status, often associated with racial and ethnic disparities in the United States, is also a major factor linked to significantly higher rates of MNA in pKTx recipients of African-American background [279, 280]. Lastly, post-transplant medication regimens and monitoring are costly; lack of means to secure sufficient medical and prescription insurance coverage puts patients at risk for incurring catastrophic medical costs, driving them to avoid the healthcare system [272]. It is still debatable where the ethical burden of support rests to alleviate such socioeconomic drivers of poor allograft outcomes as a way to maximize the life of the allograft in an era where there is already a shortage of available organs for transplantation [280].

The cause and duration of CKD prior to KTx, time spent on dialysis, and time since transplantation are all condition-related factors that may contribute to MNA [274]. Patients who slowly progress to end-stage renal disease typically have more familiarity with complex medication regimens and have better adherence compared to those with acute renal failure requiring urgent transplantation [275]. Additionally, the more time that has passed after transplant, the less attention and urgency patients allot to their day-to-day routine [281, 282]. From a psychosocial standpoint, low health literacy and incomprehension of one's disease state and a false overestimation of one's own immortality are additional factors that further increase the risk of

MNA, especially in adolescent transplant recipients [274]. It is therefore crucial for providers to discuss the challenging aspects of life after transplantation with patients and families, such as lifelong immunosuppression, monitoring requirements, potential adverse effects, and complications. Clinical pharmacists and transplant coordinators play a significant role in educating transplant candidates and caregivers about post-transplant medication regimens and setting realistic expectations, while social workers are key for identifying psychosocial risk factors that may contribute to MNA. Lastly, other patient-related factors such as depression, low self-esteem, anger, denial, behavioral disturbances, and cognitive impairment must be appropriately identified to allow for necessary intervention by the transplant team.

Treatment-related factors such as high pill burden, cumbersome dosing schedules, and medication side effects are some of the most obvious and common barriers to adherence [271, 274]. Given that the overall pill burden is at its highest immediately following transplantation, it is essential for the medical team to avoid adding medications that are not imperative to immediate post-transplant clinical needs. For example, individual antihypertensive doses should be maximized before adding additional agents, and medications dosed once-daily are usually preferred over those that require multiple-daily dosing [275]. Since younger children are not able to swallow tablets or capsules and rely on oral liquid formulations, medication palatability is another challenge. Pharmacies may offer medication-flavoring services to improve the taste of oral liquids. It is also important for the provider to keep in mind the patient's age and offer the parent or caregiver the option of switching from oral liquids to pills as soon as the child is able to swallow them. Extended-release TAC and LCPT formulations may also be considered in patients who are able to swallow tablets and have a tendency to miss doses of immediate-release TAC.

In line with these challenges, healthcare system-related factors such transitions of care (TOC) from pediatrics to adult and patient-provider relationship present significant barriers as well. The limited time allotted for the provider to spend with the patient, lack of explanation around treatment provided and about adherence, mistrust in the healthcare system, and patient perception that they are burdening the provider all contribute to MNA [283]. Additionally, although studies have not consistently demonstrated a direct link between TOC and MNA in particular, patients who transition from pediatric to adult care under the age of 21 years are more likely to experience allograft loss than those who transition at an older age [284]. Furthermore, the incidence of allograft loss appears to be highest during the "adaptation period" from 6 months before to 2.5 years after TOC, indicating that this high-risk period requires heightened attention and additional resources [285]. Implementation of pediatric-to-adult transition protocols and use of published guidelines and educational resources may significantly decrease the incidence of acute rejection while empowering providers, patients, and caregivers with the tools they need to improve long-term outcomes [286–290].

Currently, there is no gold standard for measuring MNA for ensuring reliability and accuracy in assessment or in predicting allograft outcomes [291]. As no single strategy has shown high sensitivity or specificity, heterogeneous methods such as electronic pill dispensers, pharmacy refill data, therapeutic drug monitoring, and parent or patient self-reporting have all been utilized [292]. Furthermore, instruments and scales, such as the Parent and Adolescent Medication Barriers Scales (PMBS and AMBS, respectively) and Multidimensional Adherence Classification System (MACS), have been developed and validated to measure adherence and assess perceived barriers, while assisting providers in identifying MNA and improving outcomes [273, 293].

Once barriers are identified, addressing behavioral factors that impact adherence likely requires intervention both pre- and post-transplantation. Establishing a strong patient-provider relationship and the use of a multidisciplinary team approach combining the expertise of physicians, surgeons, pharmacists, nurses, dieticians, and social workers may also positively impact post-transplant care and increase adherence [272]. In addition, implementation of strategies such as the Pediatric Psychosocial Preventative Health Model (PPPHM) has been found particularly useful during the pre-transplant patient evaluation process in identifying psychosocial barriers and implementing solutions that minimize the risk of MNA [294]. The impact of post-transplant intervention was demonstrated by the TAKE-IT trial, in which teenage pKTx recipients who received adherence support via electronic dose reminders, routine clinic visits, and feedback on overcoming patient-identified adherence barriers demonstrated significantly better medication adherence compared to the non-intervention group [295]. Other strategies to reduce MNA and improve patient and allograft outcomes include minimization of polypharmacy, decreasing frequency of medication administrations per day, and utilization of adherence contracts. In addition, pillboxes and mobile health reminder applications have demonstrated to significantly reduce the number of missed doses and increase overall adherence in pediatric and adult transplant recipients [270, 291, 296–298].

Nonadherence in the pKTx recipient is a health behavior that may be modified through a collaborative relationship between the transplant team, the patient, and the caretakers. Fostering positive medication adherence habits requires an understanding of the patient-specific barriers and implementation of individualized strategies to ultimately promote positive behavioral changes. Because MNA can occur at any time following transplantation and requires continuous monitoring for long-term patient and allograft survival, it remains an ongoing challenge in the transplant population.

Conclusion

While patient and allograft outcomes have drastically improved over the last few decades, complications of lifelong immunosuppression remain a challenge in pediatric kidney transplant recipients. Concerning long-term adverse effects include short stature, obesity, post-transplant diabetes, hypertension, nephrotoxicity, infections, and malignancy. Adherence to complicated medication regimens poses yet another challenge for both the patient and the caretaker. Furthermore, pharmacokinetic and pharmacogenetic factors such as drug clearance and altered enzymatic metabolism play an evolving role in children. Lastly, despite numerous publications in the adult population, clinical trials in the pediatric transplant population remain limited. An ideal regimen would maintain high allograft survival rates while minimizing adverse effects and providing a simple dosing strategy. As newer immunosuppressive agents come to market, robust clinical trials involving children and adolescents are needed to guide our strategies. Ultimately, however, shifting toward a personalized approach to immunosuppression selection through evaluation of patient-specific factors may yield the most promising outcomes.

Self-Assessment Questions

1. Which of the following classes of immunosuppression is most commonly associated with nephrotoxicity (such as oliguria, rise in serum creatinine, hyperkalemia) and neurotoxicity (such as tremors and headaches)?
   (a) Antiproliferative agents (azathioprine, mycophenolate)
      (i) Antiproliferatives are most commonly associated with gastrointestinal toxicities (such as nausea, vomiting, diarrhea, and gastritis) and hematologic toxicities (such as leukopenia and thrombocytopenia).
   (b) ***Calcineurin inhibitors (cyclosporine, tacrolimus)***
      (i) ***The most common adverse effects of CNIs include nephrotoxicity and neurotoxicity.***
   (c) Corticosteroids (prednisone, prednisolone)
      (i) Steroids are most commonly associated with metabolic adverse effects, such as hypertension, hyperglycemia, edema, and polyphagia.
   (d) Target of rapamycin inhibitors (sirolimus, everolimus)
      (i) TOR-Is are most commonly associated with poor wound healing, proteinuria, aphthous ulceration, and hyperlipidemia.
2. Which of the following approaches would be most appropriate in a pediatric kidney transplant recipient with persistently worsening pancytopenia after being converted to azathioprine due to mycophenolate-induced gastrointestinal toxicity?
   (a) Measure mycophenolic acid (MPA) trough.
      (i) No need to monitor MPA as patient is no longer on mycophenolate.
   (b) Measure an abbreviated MPA area under the curve (AUC).
      (i) No need to monitor MPA AUC as patient is no longer on mycophenolate.
   (c) ***Measure thiopurine methyltransferase (TPMT) function.***
      (i) ***TPMT enzymatic deficiency predisposes patients to mild to life-threatening myelotoxicity due to accumulation of thioguanine nucleotides (TGN) and should be monitored prior to azathioprine initiation or in cases of refractory myelosuppression after therapy initiation.***
   (d) Measure uridine diphosphate glucuronosyltransferase (UGT) function.
      (i) No need to monitor UGT, which is an enzyme responsible for metabolizing mycophenolic acid to mycophenolic acid glucuronide.
3. Which of the following is an absolute contraindication to belatacept administration?

(a) ***Epstein-Barr virus (EBV) seronegativity***
   (i) ***Belatacept carries a black box warning against its use in patients who are EBV-seronegative due to the significant risk of posttransplant lymphoproliferative disorder (PTLD).***
(b) History of previous transplantation
   (i) Patients who undergo re-transplantation may be candidates for belatacept therapy as long as they are EBV-seropositive.
(c) Pregnancy
   (i) Although the data for belatacept use throughout pregnancy is limited, it is classified as Pregnancy Category C.
(d) Presence of proteinuria
   (i) Belatacept has not been associated with inducing or worsening proteinuria; on the contrary, it has shown to improve renal function in kidney transplant recipients with calcineurin inhibitor-induced kidney injury.

4. A kidney transplant recipient is admitted with fever and is found to have leukocytosis, elevated galactomannan, and ground-glass opacities with halo sign on computerized tomography (CT) scan suggestive of invasive fungal pneumonia. The infectious disease team recommends initiating voriconazole until more definitive testing can be performed. Which of the following modifications to the patient's immunosuppression regimen is most appropriate?
   (a) Increase the tacrolimus dose by 50% in order to overcome the CYP3A4-inducing effects of voriconazole.
      (i) Voriconazole is a CYP3A4 inhibitor, not inducer.
   (b) ***Decrease the tacrolimus dose by 50% in order to overcome the CYP3A4-inhibiting effects of voriconazole.***
   (c) Add grapefruit juice to the patient's daily diet in order to increase the absorption of voriconazole.
      (i) Grapefruit juice should be avoided in patients maintained on calcineurin inhibitors, such as tacrolimus, due to its inhibitory effects on CYP3A4 and increased risk of calcineurin inhibitor toxicity.
   (d) Add atorvastatin to the patient's regimen in order to treat voriconazole-induced hyperlipidemia.
      (i) Voriconazole is not associated with significant changes in serum lipids.
5. Which of the following pharmacogenetic characteristics is expected to exert the most significant effect on drug metabolism?
   (a) G6PD deficiency and azathioprine toxicity
      (i) Glucose-6-phosphate dehydrogenase is primarily involved in protecting red blood cells from premature destruction; it is not involved in azathioprine metabolism.
   (b) CYP3A4 polymorphism and decreased sirolimus metabolism
      (i) CYP3A4 polymorphisms are uncommon; additionally, TOR inhibitors do not exhibit significant interpatient variability in metabolic function.
   (c) ***CYP3A5*1 polymorphism and increased tacrolimus metabolism***
      (i) ***CYP3A5 single nucleotide polymorphisms have shown the strongest correlation with determination of tacrolimus interpatient variability;***

CYP3A5*1 wild-type alleles are associated with increased tacrolimus metabolism, leading to an increase in the risk of rejection due to subtherapeutic drug exposure

(d) NUDT15 polymorphism and belatacept toxicity

  (i) NUDT15 polymorphisms are associated with azathioprine toxicity; belatacept is not known to be subject to any genetic polymorphism effects.

References

1. Halloran PF. Immunosuppressive drugs for kidney transplantation. N Engl J Med. 2004;351(26):2715–29.
2. Allison AC. Immunosuppressive drugs: the first 50 years and a glance forward. Immunopharmacology. 2000;47(2–3):63–83.
3. Klintmalm GB, Kaplan B, Kirk AD. FDA jeopardizes the lives of lung transplant recipients and in the process severely increases the cost to develop new immunosuppression. Am J Transplant. 2019;19(4):971–2.
4. Anstey A, Lear JT. Azathioprine: clinical pharmacology and current indications in autoimmune disorders. BioDrugs. 1998;9(1):33–47.
5. Allen LV, Erickson MA. Stability of acetazolamide, allopurinol, azathioprine, clonazepam, and flucytosine in extemporaneously compounded oral liquids. Am J Health Syst Pharm. 1996;53(16):1944–9.
6. Saeed B. Pediatric renal transplantation. Int J Organ Transplant Med. 2012;3(2):62–73.
7. Pape L. State-of-the-art immunosuppression protocols for pediatric renal transplant recipients. Pediatr Nephrol. 2019;34(2):187–94.
8. Staatz CE, Tett SE. Clinical pharmacokinetics and pharmacodynamics of mycophenolate in solid organ transplant recipients. Clin Pharmacokinet. 2007;46(1):13–58.
9. Anaizi NH, Swenson CF, Dentinger PJ. Stability of mycophenolate mofetil in an extemporaneously compounded oral liquid. Am J Health Syst Pharm. 1998;55(9):926–9.
10. Fahimi F, Baniasadi S, Mortazavi SA, Dehghan H, Zarghi A. Physical and chemical stability of mycophenolate mofetil (MMF) suspension prepared at the hospital. Iran J Pharm Res. 2012;11(1):171–5.
11. Tönshoff B, David-Neto E, Ettenger R, Filler G, van Gelder T, Goebel J, et al. Pediatric aspects of therapeutic drug monitoring of mycophenolic acid in renal transplantation. Transplant Rev (Orlando). 2011;25(2):78–89.
12. Kuypers DR, Le Meur Y, Cantarovich M, Tredger MJ, Tett SE, Cattaneo D, et al. Consensus report on therapeutic drug monitoring of mycophenolic acid in solid organ transplantation. Clin J Am Soc Nephrol. 2010;5(2):341–58.
13. Filler G, Alvarez-Elías AC, McIntyre C, Medeiros M. The compelling case for therapeutic drug monitoring of mycophenolate mofetil therapy. Pediatr Nephrol. 2017;32(1):21–9.
14. Filler G. Abbreviated mycophenolic acid AUC from C0, C1, C2, and C4 is preferable in children after renal transplantation on mycophenolate mofetil and tacrolimus therapy. Transpl Int. 2004;17(3):120–5.
15. Yoo EC, Alvarez-Elías AC, Todorova EK, Filler G. Developmental changes of MPA exposure in children. Pediatr Nephrol. 2016;31(6):975–82.
16. Siddiqi N, Lamour JM, Hsu DT. The effect of MMF dose and trough levels on adverse effects in pediatric heart transplant recipients. Pediatr Transplant. 2015;19(6):618–22.
17. Tett SE, Saint-Marcoux F, Staatz CE, Brunet M, Vinks AA, Miura M, et al. Mycophenolate, clinical pharmacokinetics, formulations, and methods for assessing drug exposure. Transplant Rev (Orlando). 2011;25(2):47–57.

18. Halloran P, Mathew T, Tomlanovich S, Groth C, Hooftman L, Barker C. Mycophenolate mofetil in renal allograft recipients: a pooled efficacy analysis of three randomized, double-blind, clinical studies in prevention of rejection. The International Mycophenolate Mofetil Renal Transplant Study Groups. Transplantation. 1997;63(1):39–47.
19. Jungraithmayr T, Staskewitz A, Kirste G, Böswald M, Bulla M, Burghard R, et al. Pediatric renal transplantation with mycophenolate mofetil-based immunosuppression without induction: results after three years. Transplantation. 2003;75(4):454–61.
20. Jungraithmayr TC, Wiesmayr S, Staskewitz A, Kirste G, Bulla M, Fehrenbach H, et al. Five-year outcome in pediatric patients with mycophenolate mofetil-based renal transplantation. Transplantation. 2007;83(7):900–5.
21. van Gelder T, Hesselink DA. Mycophenolate revisited. Transpl Int. 2015;28(5):508–15.
22. Merville P, Bergé F, Deminière C, Morel D, Chong G, Durand D, et al. Lower incidence of chronic allograft nephropathy at 1 year post-transplantation in patients treated with mycophenolate mofetil. Am J Transplant. 2004;4(11):1769–75.
23. Ferraris JR, Tambutti ML, Redal MA, Bustos D, Ramirez JA, Prigoshin N. Conversion from azathioprine [correction of azathioprina] to mycophenolate mofetil in pediatric renal transplant recipients with chronic rejection. Transplantation. 2000;70(2):297–301.
24. NAPRT, Studies C. North American Pediatric Renal Trials and Collaborative Studies (NAPRTCS) 2014 annual transplant report; 2014.
25. Zimmerhackl LB, Wiesmayr S, Kirste G, Jungraithmayr T. Mycophenolate mofetil (Cellcept) in pediatric renal transplantation. Transplant Proc. 2006;38(7):2038–40.
26. Remuzzi G, Lesti M, Gotti E, Ganeva M, Dimitrov BD, Ene-Iordache B, et al. Mycophenolate mofetil versus azathioprine for prevention of acute rejection in renal transplantation (MYSS): a randomised trial. Lancet. 2004;364(9433):503–12.
27. Amano Y, Lee SW, Allison AC. Inhibition by glucocorticoids of the formation of interleukin-1 alpha, interleukin-1 beta, and interleukin-6: mediation by decreased mRNA stability. Mol Pharmacol. 1993;43(2):176–82.
28. Northrop JP, Crabtree GR, Mattila PS. Negative regulation of interleukin 2 transcription by the glucocorticoid receptor. J Exp Med. 1992;175(5):1235–45.
29. Fauci AS. Mechanisms of the immunosuppressive and anti-inflammatory effects of glucocorticosteroids. J Immunopharmacol. 1978;1(1):1–25.
30. Bergmann TK, Barraclough KA, Lee KJ, Staatz CE. Clinical pharmacokinetics and pharmacodynamics of prednisolone and prednisone in solid organ transplantation. Clin Pharmacokinet. 2012;51(11):711–41.
31. Pickup ME. Clinical pharmacokinetics of prednisone and prednisolone. Clin Pharmacokinet. 1979;4(2):111–28.
32. Burleson RL, Marbarger PD, Jermanovich N, Brennan AM, Scruggs BF. A prospective study of methylprednisolone and prednisone as immunosuppressive agents in clinical renal transplantation. Transplant Proc. 1981;13(1 Pt 1):339–43.
33. Gambertoglio JG, Frey FJ, Holford NH, Birnbaum JL, Lizak PS, Vincenti F, et al. Prednisone and prednisolone bioavailability in renal transplant patients. Kidney Int. 1982;21(4):621–6.
34. Mitchell JC, Counselman FL. A taste comparison of three different liquid steroid preparations: prednisone, prednisolone, and dexamethasone. Acad Emerg Med. 2003;10(4):400–3.
35. Czock D, Keller F, Rasche FM, Häussler U. Pharmacokinetics and pharmacodynamics of systemically administered glucocorticoids. Clin Pharmacokinet. 2005;44(1):61–98.
36. Steiner RW, Awdishu L. Steroids in kidney transplant patients. Semin Immunopathol. 2011;33(2):157–67.
37. Broyer M, Guest G, Gagnadoux MF. Growth rate in children receiving alternate-day corticosteroid treatment after kidney transplantation. J Pediatr. 1992;120(5):721–5.
38. Jabs K, Sullivan EK, Avner ED, Harmon WE. Alternate-day steroid dosing improves growth without adversely affecting graft survival or long-term graft function. A report of the North American Pediatric Renal Transplant Cooperative Study. Transplantation. 1996;61(1):31–6.

39. Höcker B, Weber LT, Feneberg R, Drube J, John U, Fehrenbach H, et al. Prospective, randomized trial on late steroid withdrawal in pediatric renal transplant recipients under cyclosporine microemulsion and mycophenolate mofetil. Transplantation. 2009;87(6):934–41.
40. Benfield MR, Bartosh S, Ikle D, Warshaw B, Bridges N, Morrison Y, et al. A randomized double-blind, placebo controlled trial of steroid withdrawal after pediatric renal transplantation. Am J Transplant. 2010;10(1):81–8.
41. Birkeland SA, Larsen KE, Rohr N. Pediatric renal transplantation without steroids. Pediatr Nephrol. 1998;12(2):87–92.
42. Sarwal MM, Vidhun JR, Alexander SR, Satterwhite T, Millan M, Salvatierra O. Continued superior outcomes with modification and lengthened follow-up of a steroid-avoidance pilot with extended daclizumab induction in pediatric renal transplantation. Transplantation. 2003;76(9):1331–9.
43. Silverstein DM, Aviles DH, LeBlanc PM, Jung FF, Vehaskari VM. Results of one-year follow-up of steroid-free immunosuppression in pediatric renal transplant patients. Pediatr Transplant. 2005;9(5):589–97.
44. Delucchi A, Valenzuela M, Ferrario M, Lillo AM, Guerrero JL, Rodriguez E, et al. Early steroid withdrawal in pediatric renal transplant on newer immunosuppressive drugs. Pediatr Transplant. 2007;11(7):743–8.
45. Grenda R, Watson A, Trompeter R, Tönshoff B, Jaray J, Fitzpatrick M, et al. A randomized trial to assess the impact of early steroid withdrawal on growth in pediatric renal transplantation: the TWIST study. Am J Transplant. 2010;10(4):828–36.
46. Li L, Chang A, Naesens M, Kambham N, Waskerwitz J, Martin J, et al. Steroid-free immunosuppression since 1999: 129 pediatric renal transplants with sustained graft and patient benefits. Am J Transplant. 2009;9(6):1362–72.
47. Chaudhuri A, Ozawa M, Everly MJ, Ettenger R, Dharnidharka V, Benfield M, et al. The clinical impact of humoral immunity in pediatric renal transplantation. J Am Soc Nephrol. 2013;24(4):655–64.
48. Sarwal MM, Yorgin PD, Alexander S, Millan MT, Belson A, Belanger N, et al. Promising early outcomes with a novel, complete steroid avoidance immunosuppression protocol in pediatric renal transplantation. Transplantation. 2001;72(1):13–21.
49. Naesens M, Salvatierra O, Benfield M, Ettenger RB, Dharnidharka V, Harmon W, et al. Subclinical inflammation and chronic renal allograft injury in a randomized trial on steroid avoidance in pediatric kidney transplantation. Am J Transplant. 2012;12(10):2730–43.
50. Mericq V, Salas P, Pinto V, Cano F, Reyes L, Brown K, et al. Steroid withdrawal in pediatric kidney transplant allows better growth, lipids and body composition: a randomized controlled trial. Horm Res Paediatr. 2013;79(2):88–96.
51. Barletta GM, Kirk E, Gardner JJ, Rodriguez JF, Bursach SM, Bunchman TE. Rapid discontinuation of corticosteroids in pediatric renal transplantation. Pediatr Transplant. 2009;13(5):571–8.
52. Maes BD, Vanrenterghem YF. Cyclosporine: advantages versus disadvantages vis-à-vis tacrolimus. Transplant Proc. 2004;36(2 Suppl):40S–9S.
53. Bram RJ, Hung DT, Martin PK, Schreiber SL, Crabtree GR. Identification of the immunophilins capable of mediating inhibition of signal transduction by cyclosporin A and FK506: roles of calcineurin binding and cellular location. Mol Cell Biol. 1993;13(8):4760–9.
54. Miroux C, Morales O, Ghazal K, Othman SB, de Launoit Y, Pancré V, et al. In vitro effects of cyclosporine A and tacrolimus on regulatory T-cell proliferation and function. Transplantation. 2012;94(2):123–31.
55. Salerno A, Bonanno CT, Caccamo N, Cigna D, Dominici R, Ferro C, et al. The effect of cyclosporin A, FK506 and rapamycin on the murine contact sensitivity reaction. Clin Exp Immunol. 1998;112(1):112–9.
56. Colombo D, Egan CG. Bioavailability of Sandimmun® versus Sandimmun Neoral®: a meta-analysis of published studies. Int J Immunopathol Pharmacol. 2010;23(4):1177–83.

57. Neu AM, Ho PL, Fine RN, Furth SL, Fivush BA. Tacrolimus vs. cyclosporine A as primary immunosuppression in pediatric renal transplantation: a NAPRTCS study. Pediatr Transplant. 2003;7(3):217–22.
58. Harmon WE, Sullivan EK. Cyclosporine dosing and its relationship to outcome in pediatric renal transplantation. Kidney Int Suppl. 1993;43:S50–5.
59. Tejani A, Sullivan EK. Higher maintenance cyclosporine dose decreases the risk of graft failure in North American children: a report of the North American Pediatric Renal Transplant Cooperative Study. J Am Soc Nephrol. 1996;7(4):550–5.
60. Scott LJ, McKeage K, Keam SJ, Plosker GL. Tacrolimus: a further update of its use in the management of organ transplantation. Drugs. 2003;63(12):1247–97.
61. Venkataramanan R, Swaminathan A, Prasad T, Jain A, Zuckerman S, Warty V, et al. Clinical pharmacokinetics of tacrolimus. Clin Pharmacokinet. 1995;29(6):404–30.
62. Plosker GL, Foster RH. Tacrolimus: a further update of its pharmacology and therapeutic use in the management of organ transplantation. Drugs. 2000;59(2):323–89.
63. Prytuła A, van Gelder T. Clinical aspects of tacrolimus use in paediatric renal transplant recipients. Pediatr Nephrol. 2019;34(1):31–43.
64. Björkman S. Prediction of cytochrome p450-mediated hepatic drug clearance in neonates, infants and children: how accurate are available scaling methods? Clin Pharmacokinet. 2006;45(1):1–11.
65. Naesens M, Salvatierra O, Li L, Kambham N, Concepcion W, Sarwal M. Maturation of dose-corrected tacrolimus predose trough levels in pediatric kidney allograft recipients. Transplantation. 2008;85(8):1139–45.
66. Group KDIGOKTW. KDIGO clinical practice guideline for the care of kidney transplant recipients. Am J Transplant. 2009;9 Suppl 3:S1–155.
67. Alabdulkarim Z, Al-Jedai A, Alkortas D, Alhasan K, Devol E. Efficacy and safety of three times daily dosing of tacrolimus in pediatric kidney transplantation patients: a single-center comparative study. Pediatr Transplant. 2020;24(6):e13733.
68. Ichikawa Y, Hanafusa T, Kyo M, Fukunishi T, Nagano S. Three-times-daily monotherapy with tacrolimus (FK 506) in kidney transplantation. Int J Urol. 1996;3(3):180–3.
69. Khalaf H, Al-Asseri A, Bhuiyan J, Nafea O, Al-Sebayel M. Tacrolimus (FK 506) given three times daily after liver transplantation for minimizing nephrotoxicity and neurotoxicity. Transplant Proc. 2003;35(7):2787–8.
70. Spence MM, Nguyen LM, Hui RL, Chan J. Evaluation of clinical and safety outcomes associated with conversion from brand-name to generic tacrolimus in transplant recipients enrolled in an integrated health care system. Pharmacotherapy. 2012;32(11):981–7.
71. Abdulnour HA, Araya CE, Dharnidharka VR. Comparison of generic tacrolimus and Prograf drug levels in a pediatric kidney transplant program: brief communication. Pediatr Transplant. 2010;14(8):1007–11.
72. Naicker D, Reed PW, Ronaldson J, Kara T, Wong W, Prestidge C. Nationwide conversion to generic tacrolimus in pediatric kidney transplant recipients. Pediatr Nephrol. 2017;32(11):2125–31.
73. Pharmacists ASoHS. American Society of Health System Pharmacists (ASHP) compounded oral liquids 2017 [Version 1.01]. Available from: https://www.ashp.org/-/media/assets/pharmacy-practice/s4s/docs/s4s-ashp-oral-compound-liquids.ashx.
74. Alloway R, Steinberg S, Khalil K, Gourishankar S, Miller J, Norman D, et al. Two years postconversion from a prograf-based regimen to a once-daily tacrolimus extended-release formulation in stable kidney transplant recipients. Transplantation. 2007;83(12):1648–51.
75. Crespo M, Mir M, Marin M, Hurtado S, Estadella C, Gurí X, et al. De novo kidney transplant recipients need higher doses of Advagraf compared with Prograf to get therapeutic levels. Transplant Proc. 2009;41(6):2115–7.
76. Tremblay S, Nigro V, Weinberg J, Woodle ES, Alloway RR. A steady-state head-to-head pharmacokinetic comparison of all FK-506 (Tacrolimus) formulations (ASTCOFF): an open-label, prospective, randomized, two-arm, three-period crossover study. Am J Transplant. 2017;17(2):432–42.

77. Langone A, Steinberg SM, Gedaly R, Chan LK, Shah T, Sethi KD, et al. Switching STudy of Kidney TRansplant PAtients with Tremor to LCP-TacrO (STRATO): an open-label, multicenter, prospective phase 3b study. Clin Transpl. 2015;29(9):796–805.
78. Szempruch KR, Westreich KD, Toledo AH. Early use of tacrolimus extended-release in a pediatric kidney transplant recipient. Exp Clin Transplant. 2017. https://doi.org/10.6002/ect.2017.0195. Available at: http://ectrx.org/forms/ectrxcontentshow.php?doi_id=10.6002/ect.2017.0195.
79. Filler G, Webb NJ, Milford DV, Watson AR, Gellermann J, Tyden G, et al. Four-year data after pediatric renal transplantation: a randomized trial of tacrolimus vs. cyclosporin microemulsion. Pediatr Transplant. 2005;9(4):498–503.
80. Trompeter R, Filler G, Webb NJ, Watson AR, Milford DV, Tyden G, et al. Randomized trial of tacrolimus versus cyclosporin microemulsion in renal transplantation. Pediatr Nephrol. 2002;17(3):141–9.
81. Gupta P, Kaufman S, Fishbein TM. Sirolimus for solid organ transplantation in children. Pediatr Transplant. 2005;9(3):269–76.
82. Augustine JJ, Bodziak KA, Hricik DE. Use of sirolimus in solid organ transplantation. Drugs. 2007;67(3):369–91.
83. Cao W, Mohacsi P, Shorthouse R, Pratt R, Morris RE. Effects of rapamycin on growth factor-stimulated vascular smooth muscle cell DNA synthesis. Inhibition of basic fibroblast growth factor and platelet-derived growth factor action and antagonism of rapamycin by FK506. Transplantation. 1995;59(3):390–5.
84. Marx SO, Jayaraman T, Go LO, Marks AR. Rapamycin-FKBP inhibits cell cycle regulators of proliferation in vascular smooth muscle cells. Circ Res. 1995;76(3):412–7.
85. Aagaard-Tillery KM, Jelinek DF. Inhibition of human B lymphocyte cell cycle progression and differentiation by rapamycin. Cell Immunol. 1994;156(2):493–507.
86. Ferrer IR, Araki K, Ford ML. Paradoxical aspects of rapamycin immunobiology in transplantation. Am J Transplant. 2011;11(4):654–9.
87. Tejani A, Alexander S, Ettenger R, Lerner G, Zimmerman J, Kohaut E, et al. Safety and pharmacokinetics of ascending single doses of sirolimus (Rapamune, rapamycin) in pediatric patients with stable chronic renal failure undergoing dialysis. Pediatr Transplant. 2004;8(2):151–60.
88. Zimmerman JJ, Kahan BD. Pharmacokinetics of sirolimus in stable renal transplant patients after multiple oral dose administration. J Clin Pharmacol. 1997;37(5):405–15.
89. Schachter AD, Meyers KE, Spaneas LD, Palmer JA, Salmanullah M, Baluarte J, et al. Short sirolimus half-life in pediatric renal transplant recipients on a calcineurin inhibitor-free protocol. Pediatr Transplant. 2004;8(2):171–7.
90. Klawitter J, Nashan B, Christians U. Everolimus and sirolimus in transplantation-related but different. Expert Opin Drug Saf. 2015;14(7):1055–70.
91. Hoyer PF, Ettenger R, Kovarik JM, Webb NJ, Lemire J, Mentser M, et al. Everolimus in pediatric de nova renal transplant patients. Transplantation. 2003;75(12):2082–5.
92. Tönshoff B, Tedesco-Silva H, Ettenger R, Christian M, Bjerre A, Dello Strologo L, et al. Three-year outcomes from the CRADLE study in de novo pediatric kidney transplant recipients receiving everolimus with reduced tacrolimus and early steroid withdrawal. Am J Transplant. 2021;21:123–37.
93. Pape L, Ahlenstiel T. mTOR inhibitors in pediatric kidney transplantation. Pediatr Nephrol. 2014;29(7):1119–29.
94. El-Sabrout R, Weiss R, Butt F, Delaney V, Qadir M, Hanson P, et al. Rejection-free protocol using sirolimus-tacrolimus combination for pediatric renal transplant recipients. Transplant Proc. 2002;34(5):1942–3.
95. Hymes LC, Warshaw BL. Sirolimus in pediatric patients: results in the first 6 months post-renal transplant. Pediatr Transplant. 2005;9(4):520–2.
96. McDonald RA, Smith JM, Ho M, Lindblad R, Ikle D, Grimm P, et al. Incidence of PTLD in pediatric renal transplant recipients receiving basiliximab, calcineurin inhibitor, sirolimus and steroids. Am J Transplant. 2008;8(5):984–9.

97. Ibáñez JP, Monteverde ML, Goldberg J, Diaz MA, Turconi A. Sirolimus in pediatric renal transplantation. Transplant Proc. 2005;37(2):682–4.
98. Ibáñez JP, Monteverde ML, Diaz MA, Goldberg J, Turconi AF. Sirolimus in chronic allograft nephropathy in pediatric recipients. Pediatr Transplant. 2007;11(7):777–80.
99. Höcker B, Tönshoff B. Treatment strategies to minimize or prevent chronic allograft dysfunction in pediatric renal transplant recipients: an overview. Paediatr Drugs. 2009;11(6):381–96.
100. Weintraub L, Li L, Kambham N, Alexander S, Concepcion W, Miller K, et al. Patient selection critical for calcineurin inhibitor withdrawal in pediatric kidney transplantation. Pediatr Transplant. 2008;12(5):541–9.
101. Ettenger R, Hoyer PF, Grimm P, Webb N, Loirat C, Mahan JD, et al. Multicenter trial of everolimus in pediatric renal transplant recipients: results at three year. Pediatr Transplant. 2008;12(4):456–63.
102. Pape L, Lehner F, Blume C, Ahlenstiel T. Pediatric kidney transplantation followed by de novo therapy with everolimus, low-dose cyclosporine A, and steroid elimination: 3-year data. Transplantation. 2011;92(6):658–62.
103. Grushkin C, Mahan JD, Mange KC, Hexham JM, Ettenger R. De novo therapy with everolimus and reduced-exposure cyclosporine following pediatric kidney transplantation: a prospective, multicenter, 12-month study. Pediatr Transplant. 2013;17(3):237–43.
104. Nguyen C, Shapiro R. New immunosuppressive agents in pediatric transplantation. Clinics (Sao Paulo). 2014;69 Suppl 1:8–16.
105. Vincenti F, Larsen C, Durrbach A, Wekerle T, Nashan B, Blancho G, et al. Costimulation blockade with belatacept in renal transplantation. N Engl J Med. 2005;353(8):770–81.
106. Vincenti F, Charpentier B, Vanrenterghem Y, Rostaing L, Bresnahan B, Darji P, et al. A phase III study of belatacept-based immunosuppression regimens versus cyclosporine in renal transplant recipients (BENEFIT study). Am J Transplant. 2010;10(3):535–46.
107. Moudgil A, Dharnidharka VR, Feig DI, Warshaw BL, Perera V, Murthy B, et al. Phase I study of single-dose pharmacokinetics and pharmacodynamics of belatacept in adolescent kidney transplant recipients. Am J Transplant. 2019;19(4):1218–23.
108. Garro R, Winterberg P, Liverman R, Serluco A, Warshaw B, George R. Outcomes and experience with belatacept in pediatric kidney transplantation [abstract]. Am J Transplant. 2020;20(suppl 3). https://atcmeetingabstracts.com/abstract/outcomes-and-experience-with-belatacept-in-pediatrickidney-transplantation/. Accessed May 11, 2021.
109. Lerch C, Kanzelmeyer NK, Ahlenstiel-Grunow T, Froede K, Kreuzer M, Drube J, et al. Belatacept after kidney transplantation in adolescents: a retrospective study. Transpl Int. 2017;30(5):494–501.
110. Fishman JA. Infection in organ transplantation. Am J Transplant. 2017;17(4):856–79.
111. Roberts MB, Fishman JA. Immunosuppressive agents and infectious risk in transplantation: managing the "Net State of Immunosuppression". Clin Infect Dis. 2020. ciaa1189. https://doi.org/10.1093/cid/ciaa1189. Available at: https://watermark.silverchair.com/ciaa1189.pdf?token=AQECAHi208BE49Ooan9kkhW_Ercy7Dm3ZL_9Cf3qfKAc485-ysgAAAsowggLGBgkqhkiG9w0BBwagggK3MIICswIBADCCAqwGCSqGSIb3DQEHATAeBglghkgBZQMEAS4wEQQM-T_6EKQcCCUV4cgkAgEQgIICfSI8yqzd-i05b-Eke6EuJA8idDf27h35BCFVqIgwR9fpaCZ4xYHsJADe4R9-ZxAiDTomq9Chwv0immOPRMN5FSXogF5qbD9REzTXDutS66zwTEyHFyvnuG_877xpGErssqoks62OCpQKajHSyMIgbZ3i2C19_7Rk3bzIUwXL3p9Hw1Yy-LxaZtjHbE4FgaOihZhfamyDZrCr6a-n2iy5akT6xsH7Hn0H4RSC8y8uskBlCYvV5BHxdEgEqCmcc6FBFM07Es0ng3GTFm-Wg362ZcOwyP7EjEfbGjQUZoEmZo5Vne8EqAWLqkOXsNp8rK9atyPwb6jRAi-kNG7r6DoLdb11CJbUnKCW4EsdNwOrFGkHKaPz2EWeYRZg7NwJ0UINUqQ1K-Dh0e-uJPca5DhFCZgj8-UXbG2558ONwvlUERzmwBCLYN6ppXYHiIeUv5u71DL4wS-nQ2wJBGGSKqnxSMO6NYBfqPohr2XGam7I6tXt26TnQE_UkgfiIvzgEROWUiqx-JJjbkqocY5tlwOUfvUfSh8sun-9qgJWDelFrKX3mZaJTfJedkHKjZLR3HKlPvfPX3Su-UIYnSTFwuQWnYqh9_fPt0P1bIyXwkUwrIqtvOzXatW_Ex7MRQITnrt_WcU-wdJj10MS8vtsZ_ApsN_POGodY0EL1vAE098LyaNEHlii9fmiGhMrq_CJmfk7G-fvg97Vhu7z5hgVzK8G7uPSD6khyELtTcD12vRKU8Z79QZlh6A4-x5N_etA1XzVN-

y7o3fnf6nF5-ZYJkHpLG0WTULLzrBfq7rSKLpsWglBSjFccb-K7NqNo3U_LKfc-m4vow3BJIEDSM8LqgvnaAdKIc.
112. Mohammadi O, Kassim TA. Azathioprine. [Updated 2020 Feb 7]. In: StatPearls [Internet]. Treasure Island (FL): StatPearls Publishing; 2020. Available at: https://www.ncbi.nlm.nih.gov/books/NBK542190/.
113. Meggitt SJ, Anstey AV, Mohd Mustapa MF, Reynolds NJ, Wakelin S. British Association of Dermatologists' guidelines for the safe and effective prescribing of azathioprine 2011. Br J Dermatol. 2011;165(4):711–34.
114. Downing HJ, Pirmohamed M, Beresford MW, Smyth RL. Paediatric use of mycophenolate mofetil. Br J Clin Pharmacol. 2013;75(1):45–59.
115. Höcker B, van Gelder T, Martin-Govantes J, Machado P, Tedesco H, Rubik J, et al. Comparison of MMF efficacy and safety in paediatric vs. adult renal transplantation: subgroup analysis of the randomised, multicentre FDCC trial. Nephrol Dial Transplant. 2011;26(3):1073–9.
116. TE Johnson J, Ettenger R. Increase incidence of acute cellular rejection in pediatric renal transplant patients receiving steroid free immune suppression [abstract]. Transplantation. 2008;86:626.
117. Staatz CE, Tett SE. Pharmacology and toxicology of mycophenolate in organ transplant recipients: an update. Arch Toxicol. 2014;88(7):1351–89.
118. Vilalta Casas R, Vila López A, Nieto Rey JL, Lara Moctezuma LE, Madrid Aris A, Quintana Montero M, et al. Mycophenolic acid reaches therapeutic levels whereas mycophenolate mofetil does not. Transplant Proc. 2006;38(8):2400–1.
119. Pape L, Ahlenstiel T, Kreuzer M, Ehrich JH. Improved gastrointestinal symptom burden after conversion from mycophenolate mofetil to enteric-coated mycophenolate sodium in kidney transplanted children. Pediatr Transplant. 2008;12(6):640–2.
120. Granger DK, Group EBRTS, Group EBRTS. Enteric-coated mycophenolate sodium: results of two pivotal global multicenter trials. Transplant Proc. 2001;33(7–8):3241–4.
121. Salvadori M, Holzer H, de Mattos A, Sollinger H, Arns W, Oppenheimer F, et al. Enteric-coated mycophenolate sodium is therapeutically equivalent to mycophenolate mofetil in de novo renal transplant patients. Am J Transplant. 2004;4(2):231–6.
122. Budde K, Curtis J, Knoll G, Chan L, Neumayer HH, Seifu Y, et al. Enteric-coated mycophenolate sodium can be safely administered in maintenance renal transplant patients: results of a 1-year study. Am J Transplant. 2004;4(2):237–43
123. Cooper M, Salvadori M, Budde K, Oppenheimer F, Sollinger H, Zeier M. Enteric-coated mycophenolate sodium immunosuppression in renal transplant patients: efficacy and dosing. Transplant Rev (Orlando). 2012;26(4):233–40.
124. Gardiner KM, Tett SE, Staatz CE. Is conversion from mycophenolate mofetil to enteric-coated mycophenolate sodium justifiable for gastrointestinal quality of life? Drugs R D. 2018;18(4):271–82.
125. Fine RN, Martz K, Stablein D. What have 20 years of data from the North American Pediatric Renal Transplant Cooperative Study taught us about growth following renal transplantation in infants, children, and adolescents with end-stage renal disease? Pediatr Nephrol. 2010;25(4):739–46.
126. Fryer JP, Benedetti E, Gillingham K, Najarian JS, Matas AJ. Steroid-related complications in pediatric kidney transplant recipients in the cyclosporine era. Transplant Proc. 1994;26(1):91–2.
127. Shoenfeld Y, Gurewich Y, Gallant LA, Pinkhas J. Prednisone-induced leukocytosis. Influence of dosage, method and duration of administration on the degree of leukocytosis. Am J Med. 1981;71(5):773–8.
128. Liles WC, Dale DC, Klebanoff SJ. Glucocorticoids inhibit apoptosis of human neutrophils. Blood. 1995;86(8):3181–8.
129. Nakagawa M, Terashima T, D'yachkova Y, Bondy GP, Hogg JC, van Eeden SF. Glucocorticoid-induced granulocytosis: contribution of marrow release and demargination of intravascular granulocytes. Circulation. 1998;98(21):2307–13.

130. Abramson N, Melton B. Leukocytosis: basics of clinical assessment. Am Fam Physician. 2000;62(9):2053–60.
131. Laster ML, Fine RN. Growth following solid organ transplantation in childhood. Pediatr Transplant. 2014;18(2):134–41.
132. Sarwal MM, Ettenger RB, Dharnidharka V, Benfield M, Mathias R, Portale A, et al. Complete steroid avoidance is effective and safe in children with renal transplants: a multicenter randomized trial with three-year follow-up. Am J Transplant. 2012;12(10):2719–29.
133. Foster BJ, Martz K, Gowrishankar M, Stablein D, Al-Uzri A. Weight and height changes and factors associated with greater weight and height gains after pediatric renal transplantation: a NAPRTCS study. Transplantation. 2010;89(9):1103–12.
134. Smith JM, Martz K, Blydt-Hansen TD. Pediatric kidney transplant practice patterns and outcome benchmarks, 1987–2010: a report of the North American Pediatric Renal Trials and Collaborative Studies. Pediatr Transplant. 2013;17(2):149–57.
135. Staatz CE, Tett SE. Clinical pharmacokinetics and pharmacodynamics of tacrolimus in solid organ transplantation. Clin Pharmacokinet. 2004;43(10):623–53.
136. Nam JH, Mun JI, Kim SI, Kang SW, Choi KH, Park K, et al. beta-Cell dysfunction rather than insulin resistance is the main contributing factor for the development of postrenal transplantation diabetes mellitus. Transplantation. 2001;71(10):1417–23.
137. Hagen M, Hjelmesaeth J, Jenssen T, Morkrid L, Hartmann A. A 6-year prospective study on new onset diabetes mellitus, insulin release and insulin sensitivity in renal transplant recipients. Nephrol Dial Transplant. 2003;18(10):2154–9.
138. Ligtenberg G, Hené RJ, Blankestijn PJ, Koomans HA. Cardiovascular risk factors in renal transplant patients: cyclosporin A versus tacrolimus. J Am Soc Nephrol. 2001;12(2):368–73.
139. Artz MA, Boots JM, Ligtenberg G, Roodnat JI, Christiaans MH, Vos PF, et al. Improved cardiovascular risk profile and renal function in renal transplant patients after randomized conversion from cyclosporine to tacrolimus. J Am Soc Nephrol. 2003;14(7):1880–8.
140. McDonald SP, Craig JC, Association AaNZPN. Long-term survival of children with end-stage renal disease. N Engl J Med. 2004;350(26):2654–62.
141. Serrano OK, Bangdiwala AS, Vock DM, Chinnakotla S, Dunn TB, Finger EB, et al. Incidence and magnitude of post-transplant cardiovascular disease after pediatric kidney transplantation: risk factor analysis of 1058 pediatric kidney transplants at the University of Minnesota. Pediatr Transplant. 2018;22(7):e13283.
142. Naesens M, Kuypers DR, Sarwal M. Calcineurin inhibitor nephrotoxicity. Clin J Am Soc Nephrol. 2009;4(2):481–508.
143. Franz M, Regele H, Schmaldienst S, Stummvoll HK, Hörl WH, Pohanka E. Posttransplant hemolytic uremic syndrome in adult retransplanted kidney graft recipients: advantage of FK506 therapy? Transplantation. 1998;66(9):1258–62.
144. Franco A, Hernandez D, Capdevilla L, Errasti P, Gonzalez M, Ruiz JC, et al. De novo hemolytic-uremic syndrome/thrombotic microangiopathy in renal transplant patients receiving calcineurin inhibitors: role of sirolimus. Transplant Proc. 2003;35(5):1764–6.
145. Ponticelli C. De novo thrombotic microangiopathy. An underrated complication of renal transplantation. Clin Nephrol. 2007;67(6):335–40.
146. Abbas F, El Kossi M, Kim JJ, Sharma A, Halawa A. Thrombotic microangiopathy after renal transplantation: current insights in *de novo* and recurrent disease. World J Transplant. 2018;8(5):122–41.
147. Ashman N, Chapagain A, Dobbie H, Raftery MJ, Sheaff MT, Yaqoob MM. Belatacept as maintenance immunosuppression for postrenal transplant de novo drug-induced thrombotic microangiopathy. Am J Transplant. 2009;9(2):424–7.
148. Koppula S, Yost SE, Sussman A, Bracamonte ER, Kaplan B. Successful conversion to belatacept after thrombotic microangiopathy in kidney transplant patients. Clin Transpl. 2013;27(4):591–7.
149. Daly KP. Managing risk of surgical procedures in pediatric transplant recipients taking mTOR inhibitors: what is the optimal strategy? Pediatr Transplant. 2018;22(1):1–2.

150. Ganschow R, Pape L, Sturm E, Bauer J, Melter M, Gerner P, et al. Growing experience with mTOR inhibitors in pediatric solid organ transplantation. Pediatr Transplant. 2013;17(7):694–706.
151. Sindhi R, Seward J, Mazariegos G, Soltys K, Seward L, Smith A, et al. Replacing calcineurin inhibitors with mTOR inhibitors in children. Pediatr Transplant. 2005;9(3):391–7.
152. Zaza G, Tomei P, Ria P, Granata S, Boschiero L, Lupo A. Systemic and nonrenal adverse effects occurring in renal transplant patients treated with mTOR inhibitors. Clin Dev Immunol. 2013;2013:403280.
153. Kranz B, Wingen AM, Vester U, König J, Hoyer PF. Long-term side effects of treatment with mTOR inhibitors in children after renal transplantation. Pediatr Nephrol. 2013;28(8):1293–8.
154. Campistol JM, Sacks SH. Mechanisms of nephrotoxicity. Transplantation. 2000;69(12 Suppl):SS5–10.
155. Huyghe E, Zairi A, Nohra J, Kamar N, Plante P, Rostaing L. Gonadal impact of target of rapamycin inhibitors (sirolimus and everolimus) in male patients: an overview. Transpl Int. 2007;20(4):305–11.
156. González D, García CD, Azócar M, Waller S, Alonso A, Ariceta G, et al. Growth of kidney-transplanted pediatric patients treated with sirolimus. Pediatr Nephrol. 2011;26(6):961–6.
157. Pape L, Offner G, Kreuzer M, Froede K, Drube J, Kanzelmeyer N, et al. De novo therapy with everolimus, low-dose ciclosporine A, basiliximab and steroid elimination in pediatric kidney transplantation. Am J Transplant. 2010;10(10):2349–54.
158. Billing H, Burmeister G, Plotnicki L, Ahlenstiel T, Fichtner A, Sander A, et al. Longitudinal growth on an everolimus- versus an MMF-based steroid-free immunosuppressive regimen in paediatric renal transplant recipients. Transpl Int. 2013;26(9):903–9.
159. Cavanaugh TM, Schoenemen H, Goebel J. The impact of sirolimus on sex hormones in male adolescent kidney recipients. Pediatr Transplant. 2012;16(3):280–5.
160. Lee S, Coco M, Greenstein SM, Schechner RS, Tellis VA, Glicklich DG. The effect of sirolimus on sex hormone levels of male renal transplant recipients. Clin Transpl. 2005;19(2):162–7.
161. Schroder PM, Fitch ZW, Schmitz R, Choi AY, Kwun J, Knechtle SJ. The past, present, and future of costimulation blockade in organ transplantation. Curr Opin Organ Transplant. 2019;24(4):391–401.
162. Perez CP, Patel N, Mardis CR, Meadows HB, Taber DJ, Pilch NA. Belatacept in solid organ transplant: review of current literature across transplant types. Transplantation. 2018;102(9).1440–52.
163. Nulojix® [package insert]. Princeton N, Company B-MS; 2014.
164. Buowari OY. Complications of venepuncture. Adv Biosci Biotechnol. 2013;4:126–8.
165. Gearry RB, Day AS, Barclay ML, Leong RW, Sparrow MP. Azathioprine and allopurinol: a two-edged interaction. J Gastroenterol Hepatol. 2010;25(4):653–5.
166. Schaier M, Scholl C, Scharpf D, Hug F, Bönisch-Schmidt S, Dikow R, et al. Proton pump inhibitors interfere with the immunosuppressive potency of mycophenolate mofetil. Rheumatology (Oxford). 2010;49(11):2061–7.
167. Kofler S, Deutsch MA, Bigdeli AK, Shvets N, Vogeser M, Mueller TH, et al. Proton pump inhibitor co-medication reduces mycophenolate acid drug exposure in heart transplant recipients. J Heart Lung Transplant. 2009;28(6):605–11.
168. Rupprecht K, Schmidt C, Raspé A, Schweda F, Shipkova M, Fischer W, et al. Bioavailability of mycophenolate mofetil and enteric-coated mycophenolate sodium is differentially affected by pantoprazole in healthy volunteers. J Clin Pharmacol. 2009;49(10):1196–201.
169. Kees MG, Steinke T, Moritz S, Rupprecht K, Paulus EM, Kees F, et al. Omeprazole impairs the absorption of mycophenolate mofetil but not of enteric-coated mycophenolate sodium in healthy volunteers. J Clin Pharmacol. 2012;52(8):1265–72.
170. Kiberd BA, Wrobel M, Dandavino R, Keown P, Gourishankar S. The role of proton pump inhibitors on early mycophenolic acid exposure in kidney transplantation: evidence from the CLEAR study. Ther Drug Monit. 2011;33(1):120–3.
171. Bullingham RE, Nicholls AJ, Kamm BR. Clinical pharmacokinetics of mycophenolate mofetil. Clin Pharmacokinet. 1998;34(6):429–55.

172. Morii M, Ueno K, Ogawa A, Kato R, Yoshimura H, Wada K, et al. Impairment of mycophenolate mofetil absorption by iron ion. Clin Pharmacol Ther. 2000;68(6):613–6.
173. Lidgate D, Brandl M, Holper M, Abubakari A, Wu X. Influence of ferrous sulfate on the solubility, partition coefficient, and stability of mycophenolic acid and the ester mycophenolate mofetil. Drug Dev Ind Pharm. 2002;28(10):1275–83.
174. Mudge DW, Atcheson B, Taylor PJ, Sturtevant JM, Hawley CM, Campbell SB, et al. The effect of oral iron administration on mycophenolate mofetil absorption in renal transplant recipients: a randomized, controlled trial. Transplantation. 2004;77(2):206–9.
175. Lorenz M, Wolzt M, Weigel G, Puttinger H, Hörl WH, Födinger M, et al. Ferrous sulfate does not affect mycophenolic acid pharmacokinetics in kidney transplant patients. Am J Kidney Dis. 2004;43(6):1098–103.
176. Siddiqi N, Marfo K. Clinically significant drug-drug interaction between tacrolimus and phenobarbital: the price we pay. J Pharm Pract. 2010;23(6):585–9.
177. Asconapé JJ. Pharmacokinetic considerations with the use of antiepileptic drugs in patients with HIV and organ transplants. Curr Neurol Neurosci Rep. 2018;18(12):89.
178. Wada K, Takada M, Sakai M, Ochi H, Kotake T, Okada H, et al. Drug interaction between tacrolimus and carbamazepine in a Japanese heart transplant recipient: a case report. J Heart Lung Transplant. 2009;28(4):409–11.
179. Marfo K, Greenstein S. Antiretroviral and immunosuppressive drug-drug interactions in human immunodeficiency virus-infected liver and kidney transplant recipients. Transplant Proc. 2009;41(9):3796–9.
180. Billaud EM, Antoine C, Berge M, Abboud I, Lefeuvre S, Benammar M, et al. Management of metabolic cytochrome P450 3A4 drug-drug interaction between everolimus and azole antifungals in a renal transplant patient. Clin Drug Investig. 2009;29(7):481–6.
181. Campana C, Regazzi MB, Buggia I, Molinaro M. Clinically significant drug interactions with cyclosporin. An update. Clin Pharmacokinet. 1996;30(2):141–79.
182. Vasquez E, Pollak R, Benedetti E. Clotrimazole increases tacrolimus blood levels: a drug interaction in kidney transplant patients. Clin Transpl. 2001;15(2):95–9.
183. Choong CL, Wong HS, Lee FY, Lee CK, Kho JV, Lai YX, et al. Dose-response relationship between diltiazem and tacrolimus and its safety in renal transplant recipients. Transplant Proc. 2018;50(8):2515–20.
184. Tsapepas D, Saal S, Benkert S, Levine D, Delfin M, Cremers S, et al. Sublingual tacrolimus: a pharmacokinetic evaluation pilot study. Pharmacotherapy. 2013;33(1):31–7.
185. Bax K, Tijssen J, Rieder MJ, Filler G. Rapid resolution of tacrolimus intoxication-induced AKI with a corticosteroid and phenytoin. Ann Pharmacother. 2014;48(11):1525–8.
186. Lange NW, Salerno DM, Berger K, Tsapepas DS. Using known drug interactions to manage supratherapeutic calcineurin inhibitor concentrations. Clin Transplant. 2017;31(11):1–6.
187. Asano T, Nishimoto K, Hayakawa M. Increased tacrolimus trough levels in association with severe diarrhea, a case report. Transplant Proc. 2004;36(7):2096–7.
188. Braun F, Schöcklmann H, Ziegler E, Kunzendorf U, Armstrong VW, Renders L. Increased mycophenolic acid exposure in stable kidney transplant recipients on tacrolimus as compared with those on sirolimus: implications for pharmacokinetics. Clin Pharmacol Ther. 2009;86(4):411–5.
189. Filler G, Zimmering M, Mai I. Pharmacokinetics of mycophenolate mofetil are influenced by concomitant immunosuppression. Pediatr Nephrol. 2000;14(2):100–4.
190. Prescribing Pt, information. Deerfield IAPU, Inc.; 2012.
191. Griffin PJ, Da Costa CA, Salaman JR. A controlled trial of steroids in cyclosporine-treated renal transplant recipients. Transplantation. 1987;43(4):505–8.
192. Hricik DE, Moritz C, Mayes JT, Schulak JA. Association of the absence of steroid therapy with increased cyclosporine blood levels in renal transplant recipients. Transplantation. 1990;49(1):221–3.
193. van Duijnhoven EM, Boots JM, Christiaans MH, Stolk LM, Undre NA, van Hooff JP. Increase in tacrolimus trough levels after steroid withdrawal. Transpl Int. 2003;16(10):721–5.

194. Kim JS, Aviles DH, Silverstein DM, Leblanc PL, Matti VV. Effect of age, ethnicity, and glucocorticoid use on tacrolimus pharmacokinetics in pediatric renal transplant patients. Pediatr Transplant. 2005;9(2):162–9.
195. Dagenais R, Leung M, Poinen K, Landsberg D. Common questions and misconceptions in the management of renal transplant patients: a guide for health care providers in the post-transplant setting. Ann Pharmacother. 2019;53(4):419–29.
196. Dai Y, Iwanaga K, Lin YS, Hebert MF, Davis CL, Huang W, et al. In vitro metabolism of cyclosporine A by human kidney CYP3A5. Biochem Pharmacol. 2004;68(9):1889–902.
197. Dai Y, Hebert MF, Isoherranen N, Davis CL, Marsh C, Shen DD, et al. Effect of CYP3A5 polymorphism on tacrolimus metabolic clearance in vitro. Drug Metab Dispos. 2006;34(5):836–47.
198. Hesselink DA, Bouamar R, Elens L, van Schaik RH, van Gelder T. The role of pharmacogenetics in the disposition of and response to tacrolimus in solid organ transplantation. Clin Pharmacokinet. 2014;53(2):123–39.
199. Birdwell KA, Grady B, Choi L, Xu H, Bian A, Denny JC, et al. The use of a DNA biobank linked to electronic medical records to characterize pharmacogenomic predictors of tacrolimus dose requirement in kidney transplant recipients. Pharmacogenet Genomics. 2012;22(1):32–42.
200. Allegri L, Baldan F, Vallone C, Tulissi P, Gropuzzo M, Canelles MF, et al. Tacrolimus therapeutic drug monitoring in stable kidney transplantation and individuation of CYP3A5 genotype. Transplant Proc. 2019;51(9):2917–20.
201. Glowacki F, Lionet A, Buob D, Labalette M, Allorge D, Provôt F, et al. CYP3A5 and ABCB1 polymorphisms in donor and recipient: impact on Tacrolimus dose requirements and clinical outcome after renal transplantation. Nephrol Dial Transplant. 2011;26(9):3046–50.
202. Ferraresso M, Tirelli A, Ghio L, Grillo P, Martina V, Torresani E, et al. Influence of the CYP3A5 genotype on tacrolimus pharmacokinetics and pharmacodynamics in young kidney transplant recipients. Pediatr Transplant. 2007;11(3):296–300.
203. Zhao W, Elie V, Roussey G, Brochard K, Niaudet P, Leroy V, et al. Population pharmacokinetics and pharmacogenetics of tacrolimus in de novo pediatric kidney transplant recipients. Clin Pharmacol Ther. 2009;86(6):609–18.
204. Oetting WS, Schladt DP, Guan W, Miller MB, Remmel RP, Dorr C, et al. Genomewide Association Study of tacrolimus concentrations in African American kidney transplant recipients identifies multiple CYP3A5 alleles. Am J Transplant. 2016;16(2):574–82.
205. Hustert E, Haberl M, Burk O, Wolbold R, He YQ, Klein K, et al. The genetic determinants of the CYP3A5 polymorphism. Pharmacogenetics. 2001;11(9):773–9.
206. Thervet E, Loriot MA, Barbier S, Buchler M, Ficheux M, Choukroun G, et al. Optimization of initial tacrolimus dose using pharmacogenetic testing. Clin Pharmacol Ther. 2010;87(6):721–6.
207. MacPhee IA, Fredericks S, Tai T, Syrris P, Carter ND, Johnston A, et al. The influence of pharmacogenetics on the time to achieve target tacrolimus concentrations after kidney transplantation. Am J Transplant. 2004;4(6):914–9.
208. van Gelder T, Hesselink DA. Dosing tacrolimus based on CYP3A5 genotype: will it improve clinical outcome? Clin Pharmacol Ther. 2010;87(6):640–1.
209. Christians U, Strom T, Zhang YL, Steudel W, Schmitz V, Trump S, et al. Active drug transport of immunosuppressants: new insights for pharmacokinetics and pharmacodynamics. Ther Drug Monit. 2006;28(1):39–44.
210. Fromm MF. Importance of P-glycoprotein for drug disposition in humans. Eur J Clin Investig. 2003;33 Suppl 2:6–9.
211. Kimchi-Sarfaty C, Oh JM, Kim IW, Sauna ZE, Calcagno AM, Ambudkar SV, et al. A "silent" polymorphism in the MDR1 gene changes substrate specificity. Science. 2007;315(5811):525–8.
212. Fredericks S, Moreton M, Reboux S, Carter ND, Goldberg L, Holt DW, et al. Multidrug resistance gene-1 (MDR-1) haplotypes have a minor influence on tacrolimus dose requirements. Transplantation. 2006;82(5):705–8.

213. Yamauchi A, Ieiri I, Kataoka Y, Tanabe M, Nishizaki T, Oishi R, et al. Neurotoxicity induced by tacrolimus after liver transplantation: relation to genetic polymorphisms of the ABCB1 (MDR1) gene. Transplantation. 2002;74(4):571–2.
214. Bochud M, Bovet P, Burnier M, Eap CB. CYP3A5 and ABCB1 genes and hypertension. Pharmacogenomics. 2009;10(3):477–87.
215. Rieder MJ, Carleton B. Pharmacogenomics and adverse drug reactions in children. Front Genet. 2014;5:78.
216. Cooper SC, Ford LT, Berg JD, Lewis MJ. Ethnic variation of thiopurine S-methyltransferase activity: a large, prospective population study. Pharmacogenomics. 2008;9(3):303–9.
217. Moriyama T, Nishii R, Perez-Andreu V, Yang W, Klussmann FA, Zhao X, et al. NUDT15 polymorphisms alter thiopurine metabolism and hematopoietic toxicity. Nat Genet. 2016;48(4):367–73.
218. Fukuda T, Goebel J, Cox S, Maseck D, Zhang K, Sherbotie JR, et al. UGT1A9, UGT2B7, and MRP2 genotypes can predict mycophenolic acid pharmacokinetic variability in pediatric kidney transplant recipients. Ther Drug Monit. 2012;34(6):671–9.
219. Renoult E, Buteau C, Lamarre V, Turgeon N, Tapiero B. Infectious risk in pediatric organ transplant recipients: is it increased with the new immunosuppressive agents? Pediatr Transplant. 2005;9(4):470–9.
220. Dharnidharka VR, Stablein DM, Harmon WE. Post-transplant infections now exceed acute rejection as cause for hospitalization: a report of the NAPRTCS. Am J Transplant. 2004;4(3):384–9.
221. Knackstedt ED, Danziger-Isakov L. Infections in pediatric solid-organ transplant recipients. Semin Pediatr Surg. 2017;26(4):199–205.
222. Green M, Michaels MG. Infections in pediatric solid organ transplant recipients. J Pediatric Infect Dis Soc. 2012;1(2):144–51.
223. Humar A, Gillingham KJ, Payne WD, Dunn DL, Sutherland DE, Matas AJ. Association between cytomegalovirus disease and chronic rejection in kidney transplant recipients. Transplantation. 1999;68(12):1879–83.
224. Mynarek M, Hussein K, Kreipe HH, Maecker-Kolhoff B. Malignancies after pediatric kidney transplantation: more than PTLD? Pediatr Nephrol. 2014;29(9):1517–28.
225. Ziemann M, Thiele T. Transfusion-transmitted CMV infection - current knowledge and future perspectives. Transfus Med. 2017;27(4):238–48.
226. Schulman SL, Deforest A, Kaiser BA, Polinsky MS, Baluarte HJ. Response to measles-mumps-rubella vaccine in children on dialysis. Pediatr Nephrol. 1992;6(2):187–9.
227. Mathew R, Mason D, Kennedy JS. Vaccination issues in patients with chronic kidney disease. Expert Rev Vaccines. 2014;13(2):285–98.
228. Pittet LF, Verolet CM, McLin VA, Wildhaber BE, Rodriguez M, Cherpillod P, et al. Multimodal safety assessment of measles-mumps-rubella vaccination after pediatric liver transplantation. Am J Transplant. 2019;19(3):844–54.
229. Posfay-Barbe KM, Pittet LF, Sottas C, Grillet S, Wildhaber BE, Rodriguez M, et al. Varicella-zoster immunization in pediatric liver transplant recipients: safe and immunogenic. Am J Transplant. 2012;12(11):2974–85.
230. Danziger-Isakov L, Kumar D, Practice AICo. Vaccination of solid organ transplant candidates and recipients: guidelines from the American society of transplantation infectious diseases community of practice. Clin Transpl. 2019;33(9):e13563.
231. Yanik EL, Smith JM, Shiels MS, Clarke CA, Lynch CF, Kahn AR, et al. Cancer risk after pediatric solid organ transplantation. Pediatrics. 2017;139(5):e20163893.
232. Foster BJ, Dahhou M, Zhang X, Platt RW, Hanley JA. Change in mortality risk over time in young kidney transplant recipients. Am J Transplant. 2011;11(11):2432–42.
233. Absalon MJ, Khoury RA, Phillips CL. Post-transplant lymphoproliferative disorder after solid-organ transplant in children. Semin Pediatr Surg. 2017;26(4):257–66.
234. Cleper R, Ben Shalom E, Landau D, Weissman I, Krause I, Konen O, et al. Post-transplantation lymphoproliferative disorder in pediatric kidney-transplant recipients - a national study. Pediatr Transplant. 2012;16(6):619–26.

235. Cherikh WS, Kauffman HM, McBride MA, Maghirang J, Swinnen LJ, Hanto DW. Association of the type of induction immunosuppression with posttransplant lymphoproliferative disorder, graft survival, and patient survival after primary kidney transplantation. Transplantation. 2003;76(9):1289–93.
236. Caillard S, Dharnidharka V, Agodoa L, Bohen E, Abbott K. Posttransplant lymphoproliferative disorders after renal transplantation in the United States in era of modern immunosuppression. Transplantation. 2005;80(9):1233–43.
237. Dharnidharka VR, Stevens G. Risk for post-transplant lymphoproliferative disorder after polyclonal antibody induction in kidney transplantation. Pediatr Transplant. 2005;9(5):622–6.
238. Dharnidharka VR, Ho PL, Stablein DM, Harmon WE, Tejani AH. Mycophenolate, tacrolimus and post-transplant lymphoproliferative disorder: a report of the North American Pediatric Renal Transplant Cooperative Study. Pediatr Transplant. 2002;6(5):396–9.
239. Dharnidharka VR, Tejani AH, Ho PL, Harmon WE. Post-transplant lymphoproliferative disorder in the United States: young Caucasian males are at highest risk. Am J Transplant. 2002;2(10):993–8.
240. Martin ST, Tichy EM, Gabardi S. Belatacept: a novel biologic for maintenance immunosuppression after renal transplantation. Pharmacotherapy. 2011;31(4):394–407.
241. Gross TG, Orjuela MA, Perkins SL, Park JR, Lynch JC, Cairo MS, et al. Low-dose chemotherapy and rituximab for posttransplant lymphoproliferative disease (PTLD): a Children's Oncology Group report. Am J Transplant. 2012;12(11):3069–75.
242. Maecker B, Jack T, Zimmermann M, Abdul-Khaliq H, Burdelski M, Fuchs A, et al. CNS or bone marrow involvement as risk factors for poor survival in post-transplantation lymphoproliferative disorders in children after solid organ transplantation. J Clin Oncol. 2007;25(31):4902–8.
243. Webber SA, Naftel DC, Fricker FJ, Olesnevich P, Blume ED, Addonizio L, et al. Lymphoproliferative disorders after paediatric heart transplantation: a multi-institutional study. Lancet. 2006;367(9506):233–9.
244. Morath C, Mueller M, Goldschmidt H, Schwenger V, Opelz G, Zeier M. Malignancy in renal transplantation. J Am Soc Nephrol. 2004;15(6):1582–8.
245. Euvrard S, Morelon E, Rostaing L, Goffin E, Brocard A, Tromme I, et al. Sirolimus and secondary skin-cancer prevention in kidney transplantation. N Engl J Med. 2012;367(4):329–39.
246. Josephson MA, McKay DB. Women and transplantation: fertility, sexuality, pregnancy, contraception. Adv Chronic Kidney Dis. 2013;20(5):433–40.
247. Dalby J, Hayon R, Carlson J. Adolescent pregnancy and contraception. Prim Care. 2014;41(3):607–29.
248. Coscia LA, Constantinescu S, Davison JM, Moritz MJ, Armenti VT. Immunosuppressive drugs and fetal outcome. Best Pract Res Clin Obstet Gynaecol. 2014;28(8):1174–87.
249. Kim H, Jeong JC, Yang J, Yang WS, Ahn C, Han DJ, et al. The optimal therapy of calcineurin inhibitors for pregnancy in kidney transplantation. Clin Transpl. 2015;29(2):142–8.
250. Shah S, Verma P. Overview of pregnancy in renal transplant patients. Int J Nephrol. 2016;2016:4539342.
251. Coscia LA, Constantinescu S, Moritz MJ, Frank AM, Ramirez CB, Maley WR, et al. Report from the National Transplantation Pregnancy Registry (NTPR): outcomes of pregnancy after transplantation. Clin Transpl. 2010:65–85.
252. López LF, Martínez CJ, Castañeda DA, Hernández AC, Pérez HC, Lozano E. Pregnancy and kidney transplantation, triple hazard? Current concepts and algorithm for approach of preconception and perinatal care of the patient with kidney transplantation. Transplant Proc. 2014;46(9):3027–31.
253. Makol A, Wright K, Amin S. Rheumatoid arthritis and pregnancy: safety considerations in pharmacological management. Drugs. 2011;71(15):1973–87.
254. Christensen LA, Dahlerup JF, Nielsen MJ, Fallingborg JF, Schmiegelow K. Azathioprine treatment during lactation. Aliment Pharmacol Ther. 2008;28(10):1209–13.

255. Constantinescu S, Coscia LA, Armenti D, Moritz MJ. Mycophenolic acid product discontinuation prior to conception: analysis of pregnancies in kidney transplant recipients. Am J Transplant. 2016;16:66.
256. Perez-Aytes A, Marin-Reina P, Boso V, Ledo A, Carey JC, Vento M. Mycophenolate mofetil embryopathy: a newly recognized teratogenic syndrome. Eur J Med Genet. 2017;60(1):16–21.
257. Hoeltzenbein M, Elefant E, Vial T, Finkel-Pekarsky V, Stephens S, Clementi M, et al. Teratogenicity of mycophenolate confirmed in a prospective study of the European Network of Teratology Information Services. Am J Med Genet A. 2012;158A(3):588–96.
258. Kasiske BL, Zeier MG, Chapman JR, Craig JC, Ekberg H, Garvey CA, et al. KDIGO clinical practice guideline for the care of kidney transplant recipients: a summary. Kidney Int. 2010;77(4):299–311.
259. Transplantation EEGoR. European best practice guidelines for renal transplantation. Section IV: long-term management of the transplant recipient. Nephrol Dial Transplant. 2002;17 Suppl 4:1–67.
260. Jones A, Clary MJ, McDermott E, Coscia LA, Constantinescu S, Moritz MJ, et al. Outcomes of pregnancies fathered by solid-organ transplant recipients exposed to mycophenolic acid products. Prog Transplant. 2013;23(2):153–7.
261. Teruel C, López-San Román A, Bermejo F, Taxonera C, Pérez-Calle JL, Gisbert JP, et al. Outcomes of pregnancies fathered by inflammatory bowel disease patients exposed to thiopurines. Am J Gastroenterol. 2010;105(9):2003–8.
262. Zuber J, Anglicheau D, Elie C, Bererhi L, Timsit MO, Mamzer-Bruneel MF, et al. Sirolimus may reduce fertility in male renal transplant recipients. Am J Transplant. 2008;8(7):1471–9.
263. Framarino dei Malatesta M, Corona LE, De Luca L, Rocca B, Manzia TM, Orlando G, et al. Successful pregnancy in a living-related kidney transplant recipient who received sirolimus throughout the whole gestation. Transplantation. 2011;91(9):e69–71.
264. Carta P, Caroti L, Zanazzi M. Pregnancy in a kidney transplant patient treated with everolimus. Am J Kidney Dis. 2012;60(2):329.
265. Armenti VT, Moritz MJ, Cardonick EH, Davison JM. Immunosuppression in pregnancy: choices for infant and maternal health. Drugs. 2002;62(16):2361–75.
266. Sifontis NM, Coscia LA, Constantinescu S, Lavelanet AF, Moritz MJ, Armenti VT. Pregnancy outcomes in solid organ transplant recipients with exposure to mycophenolate mofetil or sirolimus. Transplantation. 2006;82(12):1698–702.
267. Beitins IZ, Bayard F, Ances IG, Kowarski A, Migeon CJ. The transplacental passage of prednisone and prednisolone in pregnancy near term. J Pediatr. 1972;81(5):936–45.
268. Bay Bjørn AM, Ehrenstein V, Hundborg HH, Nohr EA, Sørensen HT, Nørgaard M. Use of corticosteroids in early pregnancy is not associated with risk of oral clefts and other congenital malformations in offspring. Am J Ther. 2014;21(2):73–80.
269. Fine RN, Becker Y, De Geest S, Eisen H, Ettenger R, Evans R, et al. Nonadherence consensus conference summary report. Am J Transplant. 2009;9(1):35–41.
270. Chisholm-Burns MA, Spivey CA, Graff Zivin J, Lee JK, Sredzinski E, Tolley EA. Improving outcomes of renal transplant recipients with behavioral adherence contracts: a randomized controlled trial. Am J Transplant. 2013;13(9):2364–73.
271. Dobbels F, Ruppar T, De Geest S, Decorte A, Van Damme-Lombaerts R, Fine RN. Adherence to the immunosuppressive regimen in pediatric kidney transplant recipients: a systematic review. Pediatr Transplant. 2010;14(5):603–13.
272. Steinberg EA, Moss M, Buchanan CL, Goebel J. Adherence in pediatric kidney transplant recipients: solutions for the system. Pediatr Nephrol. 2018;33(3):361–72.
273. Simons LE, Blount RL. Identifying barriers to medication adherence in adolescent transplant recipients. J Pediatr Psychol. 2007;32(7):831–44.
274. Burkhart PV, Sabaté E. Adherence to long-term therapies: evidence for action. J Nurs Scholarsh. 2003;35(3):207.
275. Bunchman TE. Compliance in pediatric transplant. Pediatr Transplant. 2000;4(3):165–9.
276. Rodig NM, Vakili K, Harmon WE. Pediatric renal transplantation. Pediatric nephrology. Berlin, Heidelberg: Springer; 2016. p. 2501–2552.

277. Hart A, Smith JM, Skeans MA, Gustafson SK, Wilk AR, Castro S, et al. OPTN/SRTR 2018 annual data report: kidney. Am J Transplant. 2020;20 Suppl s1:20–130.
278. Guilfoyle SM, Goebel JW, Pai AL. Efficacy and flexibility impact perceived adherence barriers in pediatric kidney post-transplantation. Fam Syst Health. 2011;29(1):44–54.
279. Tucker CM, Fennell RS, Pedersen T, Higley BP, Wallack CE, Peterson S. Associations with medication adherence among ethnically different pediatric patients with renal transplants. Pediatr Nephrol. 2002;17(4):251–6.
280. Moseley KL, Kershaw DB. African American and white disparities in pediatric kidney transplantation in the United States -- unfortunate or unjust? Camb Q Healthc Ethics. 2012;21(3):353–65.
281. Blowey DL, Hébert D, Arbus GS, Pool R, Korus M, Koren G. Compliance with cyclosporine in adolescent renal transplant recipients. Pediatr Nephrol. 1997;11(5):547–51.
282. Raiz LR, Kilty KM, Henry ML, Ferguson RM. Medication compliance following renal transplantation. Transplantation. 1999;68(1):51–5.
283. Wolff G, Strecker K, Vester U, Latta K, Ehrich JH. Non-compliance following renal transplantation in children and adolescents. Pediatr Nephrol. 1998;12(9):703–8.
284. Fernandez HE, Amaral S, Shaw PA, Doyle AM, Bloom RD, Palmer JA, et al. The effect of transfer to adult transplant care on kidney function and immunosuppressant drug level variability in pediatric kidney transplant recipients. Pediatr Transplant. 2019;23(6):e13527.
285. Samuel SM, Nettel-Aguirre A, Hemmelgarn BR, Tonelli MA, Soo A, Clark C, et al. Graft failure and adaptation period to adult healthcare centers in pediatric renal transplant patients. Transplantation. 2011;91(12):1380–5.
286. Remorino R, Taylor J. Smoothing things over: the transition from pediatric to adult care for kidney transplant recipients. Prog Transplant. 2006;16(4):303–8.
287. Raina R, Wang J, Krishnappa V, Ferris M. Pediatric renal transplantation: focus on current transition care and proposal of the "RISE to Transition" protocol. Ann Transplant. 2018;23:45–60.
288. Haddad M, Winnicki E. Transition of care for adolescent kidney transplant recipients. Ann Pediatr Child Health. 2014;2(1):1008.
289. (OPTN) OPaTN. Pediatric transition and transfer guidance document 2018. Available from: https://optn.transplant.hrsa.gov/media/2759/pediatric_guidance_201812.pdf.
290. Transplantation ASo. Pediatric transition portal 2020. Available from: https://www.myast.org/education/specialty-resources/peds-transition.
291. Shellmer DA, Dew MA, Mazariegos G, DeVito Dabbs A. Development and field testing of Teen Pocket PATH(®), a mobile health application to improve medication adherence in adolescent solid organ recipients. Pediatr Transplant. 2016;20(1):130–40.
292. Schäfer-Keller P, Steiger J, Bock A, Denhaerynck K, De Geest S. Diagnostic accuracy of measurement methods to assess non-adherence to immunosuppressive drugs in kidney transplant recipients. Am J Transplant. 2008;8(3):616–26.
293. Simons LE, Gilleland J, Blount RL, Amaral S, Berg A, Mee LL. Multidimensional adherence classification system: initial development with adolescent transplant recipients. Pediatr Transplant. 2009;13(5):590–8.
294. Amatya K, Monnin K, Steinberg CE. Psychological functioning and psychosocial issues in pediatric kidney transplant recipients. Pediatr Transplant. 2021;25:e13842.
295. Foster BJ, Pai ALH, Zelikovsky N, Amaral S, Bell L, Dharnidharka VR, et al. A randomized trial of a multicomponent intervention to promote medication adherence: the Teen Adherence in Kidney Transplant Effectiveness of Intervention Trial (TAKE-IT). Am J Kidney Dis. 2018;72(1):30–41.
296. Zelikovsky N, Schast AP, Palmer J, Meyers KE. Perceived barriers to adherence among adolescent renal transplant candidates. Pediatr Transplant. 2008;12(3):300–8.
297. Levine D, Torabi J, Choinski K, Rocca JP, Graham JA. Transplant surgery enters a new era: increasing immunosuppressive medication adherence through mobile apps and smart watches. Am J Surg. 2019;218(1):18–20.

298. Browning RB, McGillicuddy JW, Treiber FA, Taber DJ. Kidney transplant recipients' attitudes about using mobile health technology for managing and monitoring medication therapy. J Am Pharm Assoc (2003). 2016;56(4):450–4.e1.
299. Verghese PS. Pediatric kidney transplantation: a historical review. Pediatr Res. 2017;81(1):259–64.
300. Murray JE, Tilney NL, Wilson RE. Renal transplantation: a twenty-five year experience. Ann Surg. 1976;184(5):565–73.
301. Meakins JL, Smith EJ, Alexander JW. En bloc transplantation of both kidneys from pediatric donors into adult patients. Surgery. 1972;71:72–5.
302. McCauley J. History of kidney transplantation, A. In: Ramirez C, McCauley J, editors. Contemporary kidney transplantation. Organ and tissue transplantation. Cham: Springer; 2018. https://doi.org/10.1007/978-3-319-14779-6_1-1.
303. Miller LC, Lum CT, Bock GH, et al. Transplantation of the adult kidney into the very small child: technical considerations. Am J Surg. 1983;145:243–7.
304. Starzl TE, Porter KA, Iwatsuki S, et al. Reversibility of lymphomas and lymphoproliferative lesions developing under cyclosporin-steroid therapy. Lancet. 1984;1(8377):583–7.
305. Muramatsu M, Gonzalez HD, Cacciola R, et al. ABO incompatible renal transplants: good or bad? World J Transplant. 2014;4(1):18–29.
306. Gjertson DW, Cecka JM. Living unrelated donor kidney transplantation. Kidney Int. 2000;58:491–9.
307. Kwak JY, Kwon OJ, Lee KS, et al. Exchange-donor program in renal transplantation: a single-center experience. Transplant Proc. 1999;31:344–5.
308. Sarwal MM, Yorgin PD, Alexander S, et al. Promising early outcomes with a novel, complete steroid avoidance immunosuppression protocol in pediatric renal transplantation. Transplantation. 2001;72(1):13–21.
309. Al-Uzri AY, Seltz B, Yorgin PD, et al. Successful renal transplant outcome after intravenous gamma-globulin treatment of a highly sensitized pediatric recipient. Pediatr Transplant. 2002;6:161–5.
310. Werbel WA, Durand CM. Solid organ transplantation in HIV-infected recipients: history, progress, and frontiers. Curr HIV/AIDS Rep. 2019;16(3):191–203.
311. Goldberg DS, Abt PL, Blumberg EA, et al. Trial of transplantation of HCV-infected kidneys into uninfected recipients. New Engl J Med. 2017;376(24):2394–5.
312. Groth CG, Brent LB, Calne RY, et al. Historic landmarks in clinical transplantation: conclusions from the consensus conference at the University of California, Los Angeles. World J Surg. 2000;24(7):834–43.
313. Thiyagarajan UM, Ponnuswamy A, Bagul A. Thymoglobulin and its use in renal transplantation: a review. Am J Nephrol. 2013;37:586–601.
314. Barnett AN, Hadkianastassiou VG, Mamode N. Rituximab in renal transplantation. Transpl Int. 2013;26:563–75.
315. Raghavan R, Jeroudi A, Achkar K, et al. Bortezomib in kidney transplantation. J Transplant. 2010; article ID 698594, 2010:1–6.
316. Friend PJ. Alemtuzumab induction therapy in solid organ transplantation. Transplant Res. 2013;2(S1):S5.
317. Jordan SC, Toyoda M, Kahwaji J, et al. Clinical aspects of intravenous immunoglobulin use in solid organ transplant recipients. Am J Transplant. 2011;11:196–202.
318. Barnett ANR, Asgari E, Chowdhury P, et al. The use of eculizumab in renal transplantation. Clin Transpl. 2013;27:E216–29.
319. Vo AA, Choi J, Kim I, et al. A phase I/II trial of the interleukin-6 receptor specific humanized monoclonal (tocilizumab) + intravenous immunoglobulin in difficult to desensitize patients. Transplantation. 2015;99:2356–63.
320. Sethi S, Choi J, Toyoda M, et al. Desensitization: overcoming the immunologic barriers to transplantation. J Immunol Res. 2017; article ID 6804678, 2017:1–11.
321. Starzl TE, Barker C. The origin of clinical organ transplantation revisited. JAMA. 2009;301(19):2041–3.

Part V

Surgical Challenges

Challenges in Surgical Approach and Complications in Pediatric Renal Transplant

13

Aleah L. Brubaker and Beau Kelly

Introduction

Surgical complications are the dreaded outcomes of the imperfect science of surgery that can limit the quantity and quality of life following a pediatric renal transplant. Thus, transplantation of the neonatal and pediatric patient requires that surgeons are specifically trained in and prepared for the myriad of challenges and opportunities posed by this precious patient population in order to minimize postoperative medical and surgical complications. While similar surgical techniques are utilized for adult and pediatric renal transplant recipients, differences in donor-recipient size, indications for native nephrectomy, vascular anatomic anomalies, and complex urologic conditions make pediatric renal transplantation a unique subspecialty. Patient and graft survival outcomes in children continue to improve for both living and brain-deceased donor transplants, particularly for the youngest age groups, equaling or exceeding outcomes in all adult age categories [1]. Although poor outcomes related to poor surgical technique cannot be salvaged by good medical management, poor medical management can compromise the best of surgical techniques. Thus, it should be emphasized that transplant team communication and collaborative patient-centric management are essential to high-quality outcomes. Herein, we describe the postoperative complications in the context of surgical preoperative evaluation of the recipient and donor, with emphasis on the intraoperative techniques and decision-making that help identify and mitigate postsurgical complications in pediatric renal transplant recipients.

A. L. Brubaker
Division Abdominal Transplantation, Department of Surgery, Stanford University, Stanford, CA, USA
e-mail: Abrubake@stanford.edu

B. Kelly (✉)
DCI Donor Services, West Sacramento, CA, USA

K. E. Twombley (ed.), *Challenges in Pediatric Kidney Transplantation*,
https://doi.org/10.1007/978-3-030-74783-1_13

Recipient Preoperative Evaluation

The most common causes of end-stage renal disease (ESRD) unique to children (>50% of cases) are congenital anomalies of the kidney and urinary tract (CAKUT), focal segmental glomerulosclerosis (FSGS), hemolytic uremic syndrome (HUS), and metabolic disorders (including oxalosis, cystinosis, etc.). Confounding unique challenges to the evaluation and management of pediatric transplant recipients include small size (<7 kg) at disease presentation, late clinical presentation with renal failure, and congenital anatomic anomalies. Of the approximately 24,000 pediatric renal transplants performed since 1987, only 0.5% (n = 116) have been neonates (<1 year old) despite the trend toward earlier diagnosis of renal diseases [2]. This practice tendency has placed an even greater emphasis on medical management strategies for the neonate. In considering the ideal recipient size and level of cognitive development for optimal outcomes following renal transplant, experience varies across transplant centers. The clinical decision to place a patient on the renal waitlist and subsequently perform the transplant entails balancing the risks of renal insufficiency and renal replacement therapy, acquiring a size-appropriate kidney, the projected rate of renal decompensation, the demonstrated benefits to cognitive and physical development that accompany renal transplantation, and the potential lifelong effects of protracted immunosuppression. At this time, >25% of pediatric renal transplants are intentionally performed preemptively, prior to initiation of renal replacement therapy. Of these pre-emptive transplants, >50% come from living donors which further impacts the timing of decision-making and clinical management [3]. Optimizing nutrition and fluid intake prior to and during peritoneal dialysis allows for weight gain to an ideal minimum of 10 kilograms (kg) prior to transplantation. The minimum weight threshold is center-specific with some programs waitlisting patients at weights as low as 7 kg and reserving transplant until a minimum of 8–10 kg if successful dialysis is not possible [4, 5]. This effectively decreases the number of neonates receiving a transplant as most children do not reach an 8–10 kg size until 12–24 months of age. It also increases the probability that the child can tolerate an adult-sized kidney, thus expanding the options for both living and brain-deceased donor kidney access. In summary, when children are of adequate weight, preemptive transplant should be performed when feasible, to minimize the potential growth failure, morbidity, and mortality associated with dialysis [6].

The initial surgical evaluation of prospective pediatric recipients includes a thorough medical/surgical history, appropriate immunizations, physical and psychosocial examination, and proper informed consent for transplant. A dedicated vascular exam including abdominal imaging with either ultrasound or magnetic resonance imaging (MRI) should be performed to evaluate for any vascular anomalies that may alter the operative plan or compromise the transplant outcome. This is particularly valuable in smaller children or for those with known congenital diseases associated with anatomic variations where a more proximal anastomosis to the aorta or vena cava may be necessary. Urologic assessment of the bladder as an adequate functional urinary reservoir begins with simple ultrasound in the renal insufficient child that makes urine to assess the bladder volume. Urodynamic study consisting of a voiding cystourethrogram and/or cystoscopy should be completed in children of age who can cooperate with the study. To avoid the morbidity of chronic pyelonephritis and the associated risk of graft loss, it is imperative to understand the urine flow dynamics for waitlisted patients who produce urine, have a history of vesicoureteral reflux, and demonstrated obstruction secondary to benign stricture or urethral stones or recurrent infections due to neurogenic voiding dysfunction [7]. Renal transplantation in the setting of a dysfunctional bladder is associated with significant urological complications precipitating ~5% lower 1-year graft survival, particularly for anatomic abnormalities like posterior urethral valves [8]. Pretransplant evaluation for preemptive bladder augmentation or an ileo-conduit should also be considered to avoid postoperative renal urodynamics that mimic distal ureteral obstruction or reflux. Cutaneous ureterostomy may be a desirable approach in pediatric recipients with inadequate bladder capacity and function [9].

The most impactful complications contributing to chronic renal dysfunction and possible re-transplantation are disease recurrence, medication nonadherence, acute/chronic rejection, and general lack of transition follow-up care. A multidisciplinary team approach pretransplant and constant engagement posttransplant are necessary strategies for improved long-term graft survival.

Donor Selection

Donor selection for pediatric renal transplant aims to minimize the risk of delayed graft function (DGF) as DGF has been associated with worse long-term outcomes in pediatric transplant recipients [10]. Living donor allografts minimize the risk of DGF in pediatrics; however, selected deceased donor allografts are widely used with similar good outcomes to living donor transplants [11, 12]. While individual transplant centers define specific criteria for organ utility, identifying deceased donors with minimal medical comorbidities, limited low perfusion duration, preserved renal function without significant acute kidney injury or signs of multi-organ dysfunction, and shorter cold ischemia times help reduce the risk of DGF in these patients [2, 12]. Most allografts for children come from brain-deceased adult donors, as younger donors particularly those <5 kg are associated with an increased risk of DGF, vascular thrombosis, and urethral complications secondary to the small size of donor vessels and renal parenchyma [13, 14]. For this reason, renal transplant from donation after cardiac death (DCD) patients is infrequently performed in children. En bloc kidney transplant of small donors has been used with success to mitigate the risk of graft thrombosis [14]. Although pulsatile perfusion of deceased donor kidneys has a role in mitigating DGF in DCD and extended criteria kidneys for adult recipients, there has not been an established role for pulsatile perfusion in pediatric renal transplant.

Surgical Operation Overview

In pediatric kidney transplants, either an intraperitoneal or extraperitoneal approach can be performed. The extraperitoneal approach is feasible in small recipients while minimizing the risk of bowel complications and preserving the peritoneum for future peritoneal dialysis. Several studies support the extraperitoneal approach in pediatric recipients less than <15 kg with good graft outcomes [4, 5]. Studies utilizing the intraperitoneal approach favor this technique for ease of access if a native nephrectomy is necessary and mitigating concerns for adequate space for an adult-sized kidney, especially in younger, smaller children [6, 15]. Complications commonly associated with both an intraperitoneal and extraperitoneal approach include urinomas, lymphoceles, seromas, and vascular complications. Gastrointestinal complications are more common with an intraperitoneal approach and include bowel obstruction, incisional hernia, ileus, and volvulus [15].

For larger recipients with standard anatomy, the vascular anastomosis can be made to the external iliac artery and vein as in adult kidney transplants. However, recipient vessel size or anatomy may make a more proximal anastomosis to either the common iliac vessels or aorta and inferior vena cava (IVC) necessary for sufficient size and inflow [9, 16]. Vascular anastomosis to the aorta and IVC can be made via both the intraperitoneal and extraperitoneal approaches. Congenital abnormalities may result in atypical anatomical locations of the IVC, an atretic IVC, or cava thrombosis, requiring changes to kidney location approach choice (intraperitoneal vs. extraperitoneal), graft laterality (right vs. left when utilizing the extraperitoneal approach), necessity of interposition grafts, and anastomoses to less common venous structures, including the portal vein [17].

As the majority of allografts for pediatric recipients are adult kidneys, a native nephrectomy may be performed in smaller children to create adequate space of the new renal allograft. A native nephrectomy should be considered in cases of recurrent infection, significant proteinuria, extremely large native kidney size, unusually high native urine output, and refractory hypertension, as discussed in previous chapters [18].

For urinary drainage, pediatric recipients with a functional bladder and no outlet obstruction typically undergo ureteroneocystostomy as performed in adults. The use of stents in pediatrics is common, but some studies have reported an increased risk of BK nephritis in pediatric recipients with stent placement [19], especially when left in for long periods of time (>7 days). If the bladder is not suitable for urinary drainage, other surgical options include bladder augmentation, creation of an ileal conduit [20–22], or a cutaneous ureterostomy [9, 19, 20–22]. The experience with living donor kidney recipients has shown that in uncomplicated transplants where postoperative fluid management does not require hourly adjustments based on urine output, the Foley catheter can be safely removed by postoperative day 3 to avoid the 3–7% daily incremental increased risk of UTI. This early Foley removal has not been associated with increased risk of urinary leak [23]. Renal ultrasound to document vascular patency, absence of hydronephrosis, or concerning undrained fluid can be obtained pre- and post-Foley removal.

Postsurgical Complications

Wound Infections

Wound infections after pediatric renal transplant range from peri-incisional cellulitis to subcutaneous tissue abscess in 10–15% of recipients within the first 5–10 postoperative days. Patients who are most at risk for wound complications include children with diabetes mellitus, morbid obesity (BMI > 30), previous ileal conduit, sirolimus-based immunosuppression regimens, pyelonephritis, and recent plasmapheresis. The principles of meticulous tissue handling and sterile technique are critical to minimizing postoperative wound infections after pediatric renal transplant. Most prophylactic antibiotic perioperative administration protocols utilize first- or second-generation cephalosporins for 24 hours postoperatively. For those who are allergic to cephalosporins, a single dose of vancomycin can be administered 1 hour prior to incision. Patients with newly constructed ileal conduits should receive a total of 48 hours of prophylactic antibiotics.

Cellulitis can be managed by local wound treatment consisting of minimal staple removal and wound packing until secondary healing has occurred. For deeper infections requiring debridement or fascial opening, care should be taken to reapproximate the fascia over the kidney in a tension-free fashion to avoid a renal compartment syndrome. Polypropylene, polytetrafluoroethylene (PTFE), or porcine mesh can be used to approximate the fascia over the kidney [24].

Vascular Thrombosis

While occurring in only 1.9–6.5% of pediatric transplants, vascular thrombosis and stenosis are the most ominous surgical complications to affect early graft loss [5, 13, 15, 25, 26]. Vascular thrombosis and/or stenosis are associated with younger recipients and donors, owing to smaller vessel size [13]. A retrospective review of 221 transplants in pediatric recipients also found an increased risk of vascular complications in recipients age 6 years or less, en bloc grafts, and prior nephrectomy [25]. Other studies have reported that use of en bloc grafts may prevent vascular complications [14]. Additional risk factors include intraoperative hypotension, pretransplant peritoneal dialysis, hypercoagulable states, multiple arteries, or prior nephrectomy [13]. Given an overall smaller vessel and anastomotic diameter, antiplatelet therapy with aspirin in the early postoperative period can reduce thrombotic complications.

Early concern for vascular thrombosis in either the renal artery or vein should be surgically explored with thrombectomy and attempted revascularization. Detection of vascular compromise can be made by increased pain over the allograft and an abrupt decrease or cessation in urine output. Suspicion for vascular compromise must be high in these clinical scenarios to prompt quick evaluation and treatment. In addition to the aforementioned risk factors, acute arterial thrombosis can be secondary to a vessel kink, intimal flap, or complete occlusion of the vessel from a technical failure. Ultrasonographic evaluation of the kidney will demonstrate a hypoechoic kidney with no appreciable arterial flow [27]. Renal vein thrombosis can also occur secondary to a technical failure or distortion of the vein. Hypovolemia, hypotension, and compression can also be contributing factors. On ultrasound, the renal vein may have low or no flow with reversal of flow seen in the renal artery [27]. Early emergent surgical exploration to restore flow in both situations is critical to salvage the allograft. Clot that has propagated very distal into the renal allograft may render the graft unsalvageable, and transplant nephrectomy may be required. The surgeon should be prepared to perform intraoperative ultrasound following revascularization and a transplant nephrectomy if vascularization is unsuccessful. Even with successful thrombectomy and revascularization, damage to the allograft may be significant, resulting in DGF or, in worst-case scenarios, primary non-function and graft loss.

Vascular Stenosis

While data in pediatrics is limited, transplant renal artery stenosis (TRAS) can occur in 2–9% of pediatric kidney transplant recipients [26, 28, 29]. Based on adult literature, TRAS typically occurs 3–24 months after renal transplant and can be detected by worsening blood pressure control and a deterioration in renal function [28, 30, 31]. Similar to adult patients, TRAS can be reliably detected in most patients with Doppler ultrasonography. Initial management of TRAS is with antihypertensive agents. However refractory hypertension or decline in renal function warrants further intervention. Percutaneous transluminal angioplasty (PTA) and stenting has become the mainstay of interventional treatment in adults, with a recent study demonstrating PTA as a safe, effective treatment for TRAS in pediatric recipients [28]. For patients that fail PTA or who have severe stenosis not amenable to PTA, surgical correction of TRAS may be indicated.

Urologic Complications

The external ureteroneocystostomy (Lich-Gregoir technique) can be accomplished in pediatric renal transplantation using a continuous suture of the spatulated ureter to the bladder mucosa. An anti-reflux tunnel is then created by closing the bladder myotomy over the hood of the ureter. Urologic complications range from 3.6% to 13.1% following pediatric transplant [25, 26, 32, 33]. Complications include urine leak (2.9–7.6%), ureteral stenosis (3.8%), vesicoureteral reflux (VUR, 3.6%), and stone development (2.7%) [15, 26, 33]. Use of double-J ureteral stents has been found to decrease anastomotic urological complications; however, to avoid the potential infectious complications of UTI and BK virus, the stent should be removed by postoperative day 5 [34].

Urine leak is the most common urological complication occurring after ~5% of transplants. Leaks can be diagnosed by sampling a perirenal fluid collection for fluid creatinine; elevated levels greater than that of serum are diagnostic. Typically, urine leaks are an early complication (most occurring in the first 48 hours post-transplant) that can be managed with bladder decompression for 7 days and percutaneous fluid drainage in most patients. Persistent leaks may indicate significant disruption of the ureteroneocystostomy; in these cases, a percutaneous nephrostomy tube and ureteral stenting may be necessary to control the leak. Although surgical intervention is rarely required, surgical options include a ureteroureterostomy or a new ureteroneocystostomy with closure of the prior cystotomy. The decision for ureteral construction depends on evaluation of the transplant ureter and bladder tissue, taking into consideration if the ureter is under tension or appears devascularized and ensuring to avoid inflammation associated with the original anastomotic failure. The addition of a pyeloureterostomy is indicated for leaks associated with a stricture. There are no distinct differences in complication rates following these surgical options [35]. In all cases, proximal drainage of the transplanted kidney with a nephrostomy tube is recommended to allow decompression of the new anastomosis.

Ureteral stenosis typically presents with impaired graft function and is often secondary to distal ureteral ischemia. Ultrasonographic imaging will typically demonstrate hydroureter and upstream dilation of the renal pelvis. A nephrogram can help determine stricture length. Percutaneous dilation of short segment stricture can be considered; however, most patients will require ureteral reimplantation. Similar to a urine leak, a new ureteroneocystostomy, ureteroureterostomy, or pyeloureterostomy can be considered depending on the length of the stricture, remainder of viable ureter, and health of the patient's native collecting system.

Persistent, symptomatic VUR following transplant can be managed with suppressive antibiotics targeted a causative uropathogens, transurethral polymer injections, or ureteral reimplantation in more severe cases [26]. Risk of posttransplant VUR is associated with underlying urological conditions [33].

Perinephric Lymphoceles, Hematomas, and Abscesses

Perinephric fluid collections can be identified in the wake of presenting symptoms or found incidentally. Diagnosis includes ultrasound and fluid aspiration to distinguish lymphoceles from urinomas, hematomas, and abscesses.

Lymphoceles occur in ~5–6% of post-renal transplant patients and are caused by disruption of lymphatic channels traversing the length of the iliac vessels and the lower IVC and/or aorta during vascular isolation dissection [36, 37]. Fluid aspirate from a lymphocele demonstrates an electrolyte composition consistent with the serum, low protein level, and predominant lymphocytes on the cell count differential. Although most lymphoceles are sterile, some can become secondarily infected. Depending on the intra- or extraperitoneal position of the kidney, patients can present with a spectrum of symptoms including decreased urine output, abdominal "fullness," early satiety, pain, ileus, scrotal edema, wound leakage, or wound infection [38]. In a series of 241 pediatric renal transplants, re-transplant, age >11 years old, male gender, and BMI for age >95% were found to be risk factors for the development of lymphoceles [39].

Asymptomatic lymphoceles are incidentally identified fluid collections which typically resolve spontaneously. Large symptomatic lymphoceles may compress the ureter causing hydronephrosis and should be managed expectantly by percutaneous drainage. Due to the 20% failure rate of percutaneous drains and the 59% recurrence rate with aspiration alone, persistent and large lymphoceles may be surgically treated by laparoscopic peritoneal fenestration, open surgical lymphatic ligation, or sclerotherapy with povidone-iodine or doxycycline preparations. Surgical treatment carries an 84% (open surgical approach) to 92% (laparoscopic fenestration) rate of recurrence-free recovery [37, 40, 41].

Despite improvements in management, lymphoceles can contribute to a lower 1-year graft survival, and thus meticulous surgical technique during the transplant, early diagnosis, and treatment of the complication are essential to good outcomes [36, 38, 40].

Hematomas can occur around the transplanted kidney as a complication of anticoagulation, plasmapheresis, platelet dysfunction, vascular anastomotic bleeding, a biopsy site, liver dysfunction, or thymoglobulin induction [38, 41]. Hematomas are diagnosed by decreases in hemoglobin and hematocrit in combination with imaging studies (ultrasound or IV contrast CT) consistent with heterogenic patterns and septations. Most hematomas are asymptomatic and self-limited and will spontaneously resolve. However, large hematomas may compress the kidney parenchyma activating renin-angiotensin-aldosterone system-related hypertension (Page kidney) [38]. Large compressive hematomas require correction of anticoagulation abnormality and percutaneous drainage or surgical washout.

Fluid around the renal allograft in the setting of pain and fever should raise suspicion for a perirenal abscess. Air-fluid levels demonstrated by CT scan may further assist in the diagnosis. Gram stain and culture results should guide antibiotic therapy in conjunction with percutaneous drainage. Purulent wound drainage in combination with a perirenal abscess should prompt surgical drainage and appropriate wound management.

Surgical Approach and Complications in Pediatric Renal Transplant

(Questions)

1. A 1-year-old 6.5 kg child with renal insufficiency secondary to focal segmental glomerular sclerosis presents as a referral for renal transplant evaluation. Evaluation and early management strategy should consist of:
   A. Dialysis evaluation
   B. Nutritional and fluid optimization
   C. Living donor evaluation options
   D. Child development evaluation

E. All of the above

2. On POD# 6 following an uneventful renal transplant from a brain-deceased donor into a 7-year-old recipient, the patient complains of increased pain at the incision site and decreased urine output. The temperature is 100.9 F and the WBC is 11K. Ultrasound demonstrates patent renal vasculature and a large perinephric fluid collection. Subsequent CT scan demonstrates a large perinephric fluid collection with compression of the distal ureter, hydronephrosis, rim enhancement, and air bubbles in the nondependent aspects of the fluid collection.
   Initial treatment strategy should be:
   A. Broad-spectrum antibiotics
   B. IR-guided percutaneous fluid drainage with gram stain and culture of fluid collection
   C. Reinsertion of Foley catheter
   D. All of the above
3. A 13-year-old 40 kg child is POD#2 s/p living donor renal transplant. No ureteral stent was placed during the transplant operation. The measured Foley urine output decreased to less than 0.5 cc/kg/hr, while the drainage from the intraoperatively placed drain increased to 300 cc/day. The drain fluid was sampled, demonstrating a creatinine of 25 mg/dL. Management strategy should include:
   A. NPO for imminent exploratory operation
   B. Initiation of broad-spectrum antibiotics
   C. Continued Foley bladder decompression
   D. Ultrasound to evaluate presence of undrained fluid collection or hydronephrosis
   E. C and D

Surgical Approach and Complications in Pediatric Renal Transplant

(Answers)

1. *Option E.* Placing a child on the renal waitlist and subsequently performing transplantation entails balancing the risks of renal replacement therapy and the lifelong effects of immunosuppression, against waiting for the child to reach adequate cognitive and physical development to benefit from transplantation. Greater than 25% of pediatric renal transplants are performed preemptively, prior to initiation of renal replacement therapy. Of these preemptive transplants, >50% come from living donors which further impacts the timing of decision-making and clinical management [3]. Optimizing nutrition and fluid intake prior to and during peritoneal dialysis allows for reserving transplant until a minimum of 8–10 kg if successful dialysis is not possible [4, 5].
2. *Option D.* Fluid around the renal allograft in the setting of pain and fever should raise suspicion for a perirenal abscess. Air-fluid levels demonstrated by CT scan may further assist in the diagnosis. Gram stain and culture results should guide

antibiotic therapy in conjunction with percutaneous drainage. In the setting of hydronephrosis and oliguria, bladder decompression with a Foley catheter should be performed. Purulent wound drainage in combination with a perirenal abscess should prompt surgical drainage and appropriate wound management.

3. *Option E.* Urine leak is the most common urological complication (~5%) following pediatric renal transplant. Leaks are diagnosed from a perirenal fluid collection where the fluid creatinine level is greater than serum values. Typically, urine leaks are an early complication (most occurring in the first 48 hours posttransplant) that can be managed with bladder decompression for 7 days and percutaneous fluid drainage. Persistent leaks may indicate significant disruption of the ureteroneocystostomy; in these cases, a percutaneous nephrostomy tube and ureteral stenting may be necessary to control the leak. Although surgical intervention is rarely required, surgical options include a ureteroureterostomy or a new ureteroneocystostomy with closure of the prior cystotomy.

References

1. SRTR data report, www.srtr.org; 2020.
2. UNOS data registry, www.UNOS.org; 2020.
3. Kim JK, Lorenzo AJ, Farhat WA, Chua ME, Ming JM, Dos Santos J, Koyle MA. A comparison of post-transplant renal function in pre-emptive and post-dialysis pediatric kidney transplant recipients. Pediatr Transplant. 2019;23(3):e13377. https://doi.org/10.1111/petr.13377.Epub.
4. Vitola SP, Gnatta D, Garcia VD, Garcia CD, Bittencourt VB, Keitel E, et al. Kidney transplantation in children weighing less than 15 kg: extraperitoneal surgical access-experience with 62 cases. Pediatr Transplant. 2013;17(5):445–53.
5. Raza S, Alahmadi I, Broering D, Alherbish A, Ali T. Kidney transplantation in low weight pediatric recipients from adult donors: the short- And the long-term outcomes. Pediatr Transplant. 2021;25:e13860. https://doi.org/10.1111/petr.13860.
6. Chavers B, Najarian JS, Humar A. Kidney transplantation in infants and small children. Pediatr Transplant. 2007;11(7):702–8.
7. Suhail SM. Bladder augmentation surgery in prospective renal transplant recipients - a nephrologist perspective. Clin Surg. 2017;2:1847.
8. Adams J, Mehls O, Wiesel M. Pediatric renal transplantation and the dysfunctional bladder. Transpl Int. 2004;17(10):596–602. https://doi.org/10.1007/s00147-004-0784-6. Epub 2004 Oct 29.
9. Brubaker AL, Wu HY, Lee A, Vuong P, Stoltz DJ, Chaudhuri A, et al. Ureterostomy as an alternative to ileal conduits in pediatric kidney transplantation. Clin Transplant. 2020;34(2):e13777.
10. Chaudhuri A, Gallo A, Grimm P. Pediatric deceased donor renal transplantation: an approach to decision making II. Acceptability of a deceased donor kidney for a child, a snap decision at 3 AM. Pediatr Transplant. 2015;19(7):785–91.
11. Grenda R. Delayed graft function and its management in children. Pediatr Nephrol. 2017;32(7):1157–67. https://doi.org/10.1007/s00467-016-3528-9. Epub 2016 Oct 24.PMID: 27778091 Review.
12. Solomon S, Hayde N. Utilization of donor kidneys with acute kidney injury in pediatric kidney transplant recipients. Transplantation. 2020;104(3):597–602. https://doi.org/10.1097/TP.0000000000002827. PMID: 32238780.

13. Harmon WE, Stablein D, Alexander SR, Tejani A. Graft thrombosis in pediatric renal transplant recipients. A report of the North American Pediatric Renal Transplant Cooperative Study. Transplantation. 1991;51(2):406–12.
14. Su X, Shang W, Liu L, Li J, Fu Q, Feng Y, Zhang H, Deng R, Wu C, Wang Z, Pang X, Nashan B, Feng G, Wang C. Transplantation of a single kidney from pediatric donors less than 10 kg to children with poor access to transplantation: a two-year outcome analysis. BMC Nephrol. 2020;21(1):250. https://doi.org/10.1186/s12882-020-01895-6.
15. Taher A, Zhu B, Ma S, Shun A, Durkan AM. Intra-abdominal complications after pediatric kidney transplantation: incidence and risk factors. Transplantation. 2019;103(6):1234–9.
16. Donati-Bourne J, Roberts HW, Coleman RA. Donor-recipient size mismatch in paediatric renal transplantation. J Transp Secur. 2014;2014:1–5.
17. Cauley RP, Potanos K, Fullington N, Lillehei C, Vakili K, Kim HB. Reno-portal anastomosis as an approach to pediatric kidney transplantation in the setting of inferior vena cava thrombosis. Pediatr Transplant. 2013;17(3):E88–92.
18. Brubaker AL, Stoltz DJ, Chaudhuri A, Maestretti L, Grimm PC, Concepcion W, et al. Superior hypertension management in pediatric kidney transplant patients after native nephrectomy. Transplantation. 2018;102(7):1172–8.
19. Maliakkal JG, Brennan DC, Goss C, Horwedel TA, Chen H, Fong DK, et al. Ureteral stent placement and immediate graft function are associated with increased risk of BK viremia in the first year after kidney transplantation. Transpl Int. 2017;30(2):153–61.
20. Broniszczak D, Ismail H, Nachulewicz P, Szymczak M, Drewniak T, Markiewicz-Kijewska M, et al. Kidney transplantation in children with bladder augmentation or ileal conduit diversion. Eur J Pediatr Surg Off J Austrian Assoc Pediatr Surg/Zeitschrift fur Kinderchirurgie. 2010;20(1):5–10.
21. Mcloughlin LC, Davis NF, Dowling CM, Power RE, Mohan P, Hickey DP, et al. Outcome of deceased donor renal transplantation in patients with an ileal conduit. Clin Transpl. 2014;28(3):307–13.
22. Surange RS, Johnson RWG, Tavakoli A, Parrott NR, Riad HN, Campbell BA, et al. Kidney transplantation into an ileal conduit: a single center experience of 59 cases. J Urol. 2003;170(5):1727–30.
23. Siskind E, Sameyah E, Goncharuk E, Molmenti E, et al. Removal of Foley catheters in live donor kidney transplant recipients on postoperative day 1 does not increase the incidence of urine leaks. Int J Angiol. 2013;22(1):45–8.
24. Halawa A. Abdominal wall closure of renal transplant recipients: an undermined challenge. Int J Organ Transplant Med. 2010;1(2):73–6.
25. Beetz O, Weigle CA, Nogly R, Klempnauer J, Pape L, Richter N, et al. Surgical complications in pediatric kidney transplantation—incidence, risk factors, and effects on graft survival: a retrospective single-center study. Pediatr Transplant. 2021;25(2):e13871. https://doi.org/10.1111/petr.13871. Epub 2020 Oct 14. PMID: 33053269.
26. Torricelli FCM, Watanabe A, Piovesan AC, Antonopoulos IM, David-Neto E, Nahas WC. Urological complications, vesicoureteral reflux, and long-term graft survival rate after pediatric kidney transplantation. Pediatr Transplant. 2015;19(8):844–8.
27. Kolofousi C, Stefanidis K, Cokkinos DD, Karakitsos D, Antypa E, Piperopoulos P. Ultrasonographic features of kidney transplants and their complications: an imaging review. ISRN Radiol. 2013;2013:1–12.
28. Ghirardo G, De Franceschi M, Vidal E, Vidoni A, Ramondo G, Benetti E, et al. Transplant renal artery stenosis in children: risk factors and outcome after endovascular treatment. Pediatr Nephrol. 2014;29(3):461–7.
29. Seeman T. Hypertension after renal transplantation. Pediatr Nephrol. 2009;24(5):959–72.
30. Granata A, Clementi S, Londrino F, Romano G, Veroux M, Fiorini F, et al. Renal transplant vascular complications: the role of Doppler ultrasound. J Ultrasound [Internet]. 2015;18(2):101–7. Available from: https://doi.org/10.1007/s40477-014-0085-6.

31. Hedegard W, Saad WEA, Davies MG. Management of vascular and nonvascular complications after renal transplantation. Tech Vasc Interv Radiol [Internet] 2009;12(4):240–62. Available from: https://doi.org/10.1053/j.tvir.2009.09.006.
32. Tanabe K, Takahashi K, Kawaguchi H, Ito K, Yamazaki Y, Toma H. Surgical complications of pediatric kidney transplantation: a single center experience with the extraperitoneal technique. J Urol. 1998;160(3 II):1212–5.
33. Routh JC, Yu RN, Kozinn SI, Nguyen HT, Borer JG. Urological complications and vesicoureteral reflux following pediatric kidney transplantation. J Urol. 2013;189(3):1071–6.
34. Patel P, Rebollo-Mesa I, Banga N, et al. TrUST (transplant ureteric stent trial): early versus standard removal. A randomized controlled trial. Transplantation. 2014;98:638.
35. Nie ZL, Zhang KQ, Li QS, Jin FS, Zhu FQ, Huo WQ. Urological complications in 1223 kidney transplantations. Urol Int. 2009;83(3):337–41. https://doi.org/10.1159/000241679. Epub 2009 Oct 13.
36. Giuliani S, Gamba P, Kiblawi R, Midrio P, Ghirardo G, Zanon GF. Lymphocele after pediatric kidney transplantation: incidence and risk factors. Pediatr Transplant. 2014;18(7):720–5. https://doi.org/10.1111/petr/12341. Epub 2014 Aug 27.
37. Lucewicz A, Wong G, Lam VW, Hawthorne WJ, Allen R, Craig JC, Pleass HC. Management of primary symptomatic lymphocele after kidney transplantation: a systemic review. Transplantation. 2011;92(6):663–73. https://doi.org/10.1097/TP.0b013e31822a40ef.
38. Alshamsi I, Alshamsi H, Al Falahi S, Sharma A, Halawa A. Perinephric transplant fluid collection approach and management. Saudi J Kidney Dis Transpl. 2019;30:564–70.
39. Englesbe MJ, Dubay DA, Gillespie BW, Moyer AS, Pelletier SJ, Sung RS, Magee JC, Punch JD, Campbell DA, Merion RM. Risk factors for urinary complications after renal transplantation. Am J Transplant. 2007;7(6):1536–41. https://doi.org/10.1111/j.1600-6143.2007.01790.x.Epub. 2007 Apr 8.
40. Gander R, Arsenio M, Royo GF, Molino JA, Vilalta R, Coma A, Perez M, Ariceta G. Treatment of post-transplant lymphocele in children. Urology. 2017;103:218–23. https://doi.org/10.1016/j.urology.2016.12.039. Epub 2017 Jan 26.
41. Inci MF, Ozkan F, See TC, Tatli S. Renal transplant complications: diagnostic and therapeutic role of radiology. Can Assoc Radiol J. 2014;65:242–52.

Multiorgan Transplantation Challenges 14

Rachel M. Engen and Priya Verghese

Pediatric nephrologists are familiar with the many ways in which renal-associated diseases can cross the boundaries of traditional medical subspecialties, involving the eyes, ears, heart, liver, pancreas, and intestines. In these cases, the kidney may be part of the primary syndrome or a victim of another organ disorder via hypoperfusion or toxic substances. Despite this, multiorgan transplants are uncommon in pediatrics, with 1677 reported cases in the United States since OPTN began collecting data in 1988. Incidence of pediatric multiorgan transplants rose throughout the 1990s and 2000s, peaking at 116 procedures in 2007 before declining to the current average of 55 per year [1] (Fig. 14.1).

Multiorgan transplantation can pose special challenges in pediatrics, especially when one of those organs is a kidney. Pediatric renal transplantation in the United States typically involves an adult- or near-adult-sized donor kidney to minimize the risk of graft thrombosis; however, heart and liver transplants involve matching the size of donor and recipient. Standard postoperative management of renal transplants involves high rates of fluid administration to maintain renal blood flow and urine output; standard management of lung and heart transplants involves limiting fluid intake to avoid pulmonary edema and heart failure. Furthermore, small abdomens may not have adequate domain to fit multiple allografts, especially if the native organs are not being removed.

Related to the relative rarity of multiorgan transplantation in children, there is a paucity of data on postoperative management and, in some cases, indications and outcomes. Here we have collected and summarized the published literature on the allocation, incidence, indications, perioperative management, and outcomes of pediatric multiorgan transplants.

R. M. Engen (✉) · P. Verghese
Department of Pediatrics, Northwestern University Feinberg School of Medicine, Chicago, IL, USA
e-mail: rengen@luriechildrens.org; pverghese@luriechildrens.org

K. E. Twombley (ed.), *Challenges in Pediatric Kidney Transplantation*,
https://doi.org/10.1007/978-3-030-74783-1_14

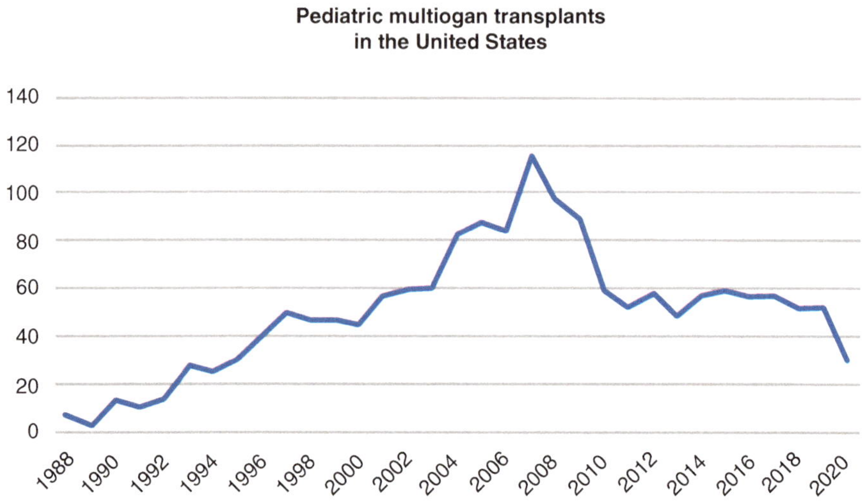

Fig. 14.1 Number of pediatric multiorgan transplants performed in the United States, by year. (Source: OPTN data [1])

Multiorgan Allocation

While the number of pediatric multiorgan transplants has stabilized over the last decade, the number among adults, excluding kidney-pancreas transplants, has more than doubled from 560 transplants in 2010 to 1074 transplants in 2019; 67% of these were combined liver-kidney transplants (CLKT) [1]. With this increase has come rising interest in the impact of multiorgan transplants on access and outcomes for single-organ recipients. The US kidney allocation system prioritizes multiorgan recipients over kidney-alone recipients, and multiorgan transplant outcomes are not included in center-specific reporting [2]. This has led to concerns about the objectivity, variability, and equitability of multiorgan allocation across the country, especially the potential impact on access to transplant for pediatric patients [2, 3]. Multiorgan transplant recipients can be listed for transplant with estimated glomerular filtration rates that would not meet the criteria for receipt of a kidney alone [4]. At the same time, kidneys allocated as part of a multiorgan transplant are not available to candidates for a kidney alone, and in 2016, 6.6% of kidney allografts were allocated with a liver or heart [2]. In the United States, the "Final Rule" governing the development of organ allocation policies requires the creation of policies "specific for each organ type or combination of organ types" [5]; however prior to 2014, there were no policies governing multiorgan transplants.

Organ allocation policies "seek to achieve the best use of donated organs" [5], requiring a balance between equity and organ utility. A multiorgan transplant may be lifesaving for one transplant candidate, but multiple single-organ transplants can save multiple lives. For example, recipients of combined heart-kidney transplant

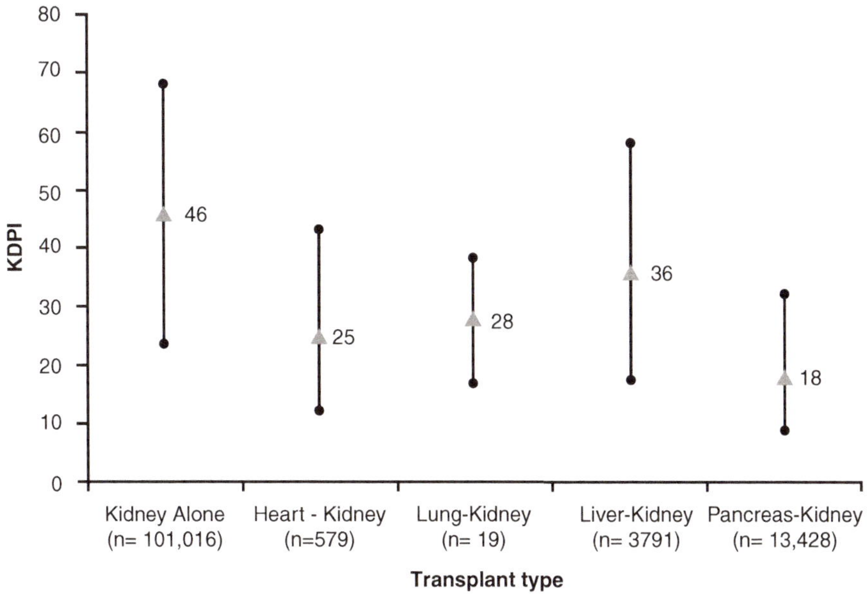

Fig. 14.2 Distribution of kidney donor profile index (KDPI) scores among kidney-alone and multi-organ transplant recipients. (Reprinted with permission from *American Journal of Transplantation* [4])

have significantly lower mortality than heart transplant recipients who remain on dialysis, but have high incidence of primary nonfunction and post-transplant dialysis [2], despite generally receiving higher quality (low kidney donor profile index) kidneys than kidney-alone recipients [3] (Fig. 14.2). Similarly, individual recipients of pediatric liver-kidney transplants have similar graft survival and lower rejection incidence compared to recipients of liver-alone transplants but worse outcomes than kidney-alone transplants, despite 49% of kidneys allocated with a liver-kidney transplant having a KDPI <35% (i.e., better quality organ) [6]. These situations result in improved outcomes for the multiorgan recipients but decrease the availability of kidney allografts [7].

To address these concerns in the United States, the United Network for Organ Sharing (UNOS) has begun developing policies to address multiorgan transplant allocation. Kidney-pancreas allocation policies were added in 2014, establishing listing criteria that included the requirement that patients meet criteria for kidney-alone listing and specific pancreas-specific parameters including insulin use, C-peptide level, and/or body mass index threshold [8]; however, pediatric candidates are exempt from these requirements [9]. Kidney-pancreas candidates accumulate priority based on their kidney waiting time, but receive priority over kidney-alone recipients for all available local kidney-pancreas organs [10]. A 6-month evaluation of the new policy showed no change in pancreas utilization and increased regional sharing [11]. Between 2015 and 2019 there were an average of 802 kidney-pancreas transplants [1] with significant geographic variation in practice [12].

In 2017, UNOS implemented a simultaneous liver-kidney policy that established kidney eligibility criteria (either chronic kidney disease, prolonged acute kidney injury, or metabolic disease) and created a safety net giving priority for kidneys with a KDPI >20% to individuals who have continued dialysis dependency or an eGFR ≤20 ml/min/1.73m^2 2–12 months after liver transplant [2]. Over the following year, the number of CLKT decreased from 740 to 676, while the number of kidney-after-liver transplants increased from 44 to 87 [2], a net decrease of 21 kidney transplants, although there may have been an initial "bolus" effect causing a transient increase in kidney-after-liver transplants immediately after policy implementation [6].

In the United States, there are currently no established national criteria for simultaneous heart-kidney or multivisceral transplant allocation, although proposals similar to the liver-kidney policy have been put forward [2].

Pediatric Heart-Kidney Transplantation

Pediatric simultaneous heart-kidney transplantation (sHKTx) is a rare procedure. The International Thoracic Organ Transplant Registry of the International Society for Heart and Lung Transplantation (ISHLT), which collects data on approximately 80% of thoracic transplants worldwide, recorded only 50 pediatric heart-kidney transplants between January 1990 and June 2017 [13]. The majority of those transplants are in North America; 38 pediatric sHKTxs were performed between 1988 and April 30, 2017, in the United States [14]. The number of sHKTx overall, pediatric and adult, has risen significantly in the past ten years, likely for two main reasons. In part, heart transplant candidates are waiting longer for a transplant, developing more kidney disease related to their heart failure. Additionally, heart transplant recipients are surviving longer; 32.7% of pediatric multiorgan-heart recipients in the International Thoracic Organ Transplant Registry were re-transplants [13].

Individuals considered for heart-kidney transplantation typically have a primary cardiac disease that leads to renal failure due to multiple factors, including low cardiac output, nephrotoxic medications, and concomitant renal anomalies such as agenesis or dysplasia [14, 15]. In the ISHLT registry, 36% were repeat heart transplants with the majority of the remaining having congenital heart disease or dilated cardiomyopathy [13]. However, there is no consensus on the degree of renal dysfunction that indicates a need for renal transplantation in heart transplant candidates; 61.8% of sHKTx recipients in the ISHLT registry received dialysis prior to their transplant [13]. In a study linking Scientific Registry of Transplant Recipients (SRTR) data to the US Renal Data System, pediatric heart transplant recipients who required acute dialysis were significantly more likely to develop ESRD (14% versus 6.6%, HR 7.46 $p = 0.0002$) over the 25-year follow-up time, while an estimated glomerular filtration rate <60 ml/min/1.73m^2 was less strongly associated with ESRD (HR 2.58, $p < 0.001$). The average eGFRs at transplant of patients who did and did not develop end-stage renal disease over the 25 years of the cohort were similar [16]. Complicating matters, renal dysfunction due to hypoperfusion may resolve with improved hemodynamics. In infants with renal failure at the time of cardiac surgery, mortality was high but none of the survivors required dialysis at the time of discharge [15]. Multiple studies in adult liver-kidney transplant recipients have shown that renal function, as measured by radionucleotide scans, demonstrates some level of native kidney function recovery in up to 50% of recipients [2]. These studies only included one heart-kidney recipient, whose results showed that the native kidneys were contributing 26% of the renal function while the transplant was contributing 74% [17].

Much of the discussion about pediatric sHKTx focuses on whether or not to perform the procedure. Simultaneous heart-kidney transplantation offers certain advantages to the recipient. Recipients of a sHKTx were less likely to have an episode of rejection within the first year post-transplant (10%) compared with recipients of a heart alone (25%) [13]. Animal models have shown that recipients of multiorgan transplants seem to develop tolerance to the donor, perhaps in part due to the increased total mass of allograft relative to body size [18]. Similarly, infant recipients of adult-sized kidneys have longer allograft survival than older children receiving similar-sized grafts [19]. Observational studies of adults have also shown decreased mortality among sHKTx recipients compared to heart transplant alone, although there is concern that these studies are subject to bias in that healthier patients were more likely to be listed for sHKTx [2]. A similar improvement in survival has not been reported in pediatric sHKTx recipients (Fig. 14.3). ISHLT data showed no difference in survival or freedom from cardiac allograft vasculopathy among recipients of a pediatric heart-kidney or heart-liver transplant [13] (Fig. 14.4).

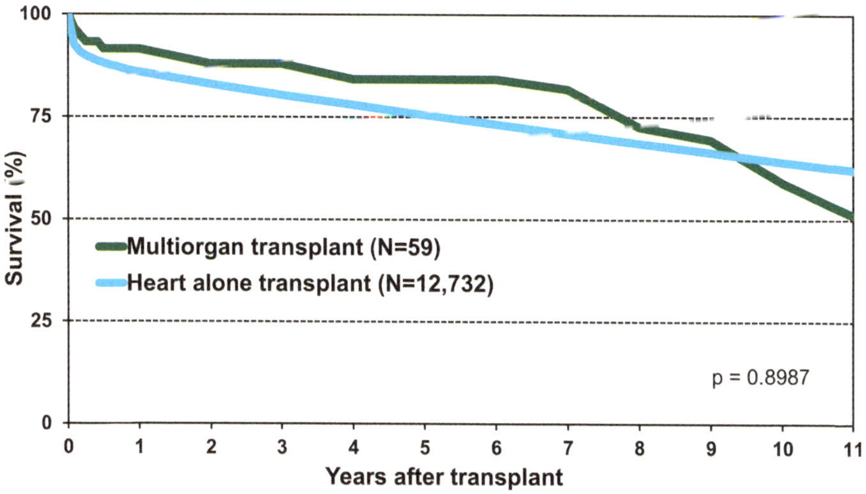

Fig. 14.3 Kaplan-Meier curve comparing survival for pediatric heart-alone transplants to that of pediatric multiorgan transplants that involved a heart, January 1990 to June 2016, 80% of which are heart-kidney transplants. (With permission from *The Journal of Heart and Lung Transplantation* [13])

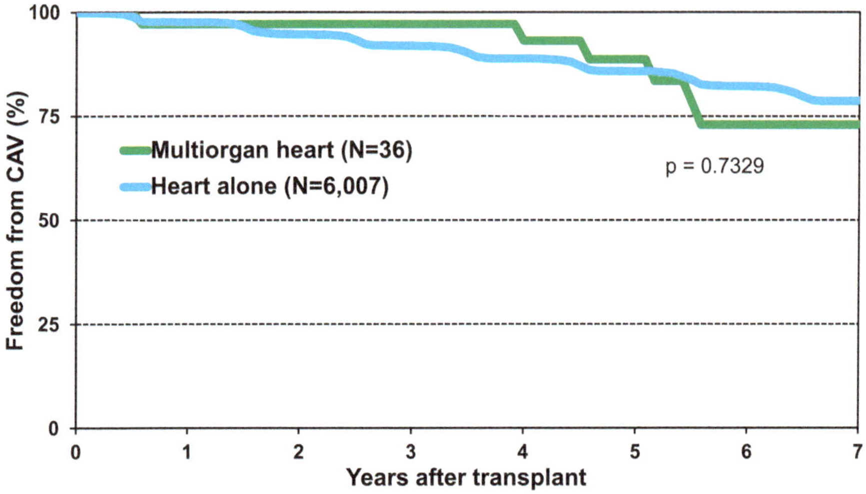

Fig. 14.4 Kaplan-Meier curve comparing time to development of cardiac allograft vasculopathy for pediatric heart-alone transplants compared to that of pediatric multiorgan transplants that involved a heart, January 1994 to June 2016, the majority of which are heart-kidney transplants. (With permission from *The Journal of Heart and Lung Transplantation* [13])

A sHKTx also offers potential advantages over kidney-after-heart transplantation, in that it avoids the potential immunologic risk from two donors and the additional induction therapy and surgical recovery. Recipients of a heart-alone transplant who develop ESRD often wait years to receive a kidney transplant and may have developed HLA antibodies related to their heart transplant, decreasing the pool of possible donors. The 25-year cohort studied by Choudhry et al. showed that 48% of heart transplant recipients on chronic dialysis had not received a kidney transplant at the time when the data were censored, and patients who remained on chronic dialysis had a significantly higher risk of death (HR 31.4, 95%CI 21–48.4, $p < 0.0001$) than those who received a kidney transplant [16].

However, sHKTx also has disadvantages for both the patient and the utility of the kidney allograft. In sHKTxs, the heart transplant is generally performed first followed by the kidney transplant [14, 20]. This results in increased cold ischemia time for the renal allograft. Heart transplant recipients may also develop vasoplegic syndrome and require ionotropic drug support, both of which compromise renal perfusion [20]. These factors likely contribute to the increased incidence of primary allograft non-function and high incidence of post-transplant dialysis (14–42%) [13, 14, 20, 21]. In the ISHLT registry, 20% of survivors of a sHKTx had severe renal dysfunction at 5 years, defined as a creatinine >2.5 g/dl or return to chronic dialysis [13]. Young children are particularly poor candidates for a simultaneous heart-kidney transplant. Heart allografts are matched to recipients based on size, but kidneys from donors less than 5 years of age have high rates of renal arterial thrombosis, delayed graft function, and early renal allograft loss [15]. Therefore, sHKTx in the smallest patients may result in worse outcomes than when kidney transplant is performed separately using an adult-sized allograft. Due to these concerns, some favor a kidney-after-heart approach, ideally using a living donor kidney [13].

Once a decision has been made to perform a sHKTx, there are several perioperative considerations. Due to the heart's relative intolerance to ischemia, the heart transplant is performed first, followed by the kidney transplant. However, it is debated whether the kidney transplant should be performed immediately, under the same anesthetic, or whether the kidney transplant should be delayed for up to 24 hours, often called a staged procedure, to allow for recovery of the newly transplanted heart and optimization of hemodynamics and volume status [20, 22]. Immediate kidney transplant minimizes renal allograft cold ischemia time, which decreases the risk of delayed graft function and worse long-term outcomes. However, it is not clear if this benefit outweighs the risks of hypotension, post-cardiopulmonary bypass inflammatory cascade, and high doses of vasoconstrictor medications [20]. Staged sHKTx also allows for reallocation of the kidney if the heart transplant procedure does not go well.

Fluid management in sHKTx is also complex. During cardiopulmonary bypass, there is often significant ultrafiltration, causing fluid shifts that can take hours to equilibrate and further impact renal allograft perfusion [20]. Renal allografts benefit from high rates of intravenous fluids, high central venous pressures (often 10–15 mm Hg), and higher mean arterial pressures. On the other hand, cardiopulmonary bypass in heart transplant is associated with acute right ventricular failure when the donor heart is unable to adapt to higher pulmonary arterial pressures in the recipient. In this state, the heart is preload dependent but sensitive to distension; high central venous pressure should be avoided [23]. Transesophageal echocardiography can be used to closely monitor the fluid balance and ventricular function, allowing maximization of central venous pressure without overwhelming the heart [20, 23]. Several measures have also been shown to improve right ventricular function including the use of inotropes to increase contractility, provision of adequate oxygenation and ventilation, and use of inhaled pulmonary vasodilators [23].

Immediately post-transplant heart recipients often have small left ventricles with decreased compliance and increased filling pressures. The denervated heart allograft also lacks the baroreceptor reflex that compensates for hypotension due to hypovolemia or systemic vasodilation. Thus, they often require ionotropic support that can decrease renal perfusion. At this time, there is no conclusive evidence to suggest that any particular ionotrope is more protective of renal perfusion after sHKTx [20].

Post-transplant, long-term management of a sHKTx requires coordinated management by both nephrology and cardiology teams. Immunosuppression protocols for both pediatric heart and kidney transplant are center-specific, and there are no guidelines for induction or maintenance immunosuppression of a sHKTx; there is also no evidence that sHKTx recipients require more or less immunosuppression than solitary organ recipients. A review of Organ Procurement and Transplant Network data on sHKTx showed improved survival with rabbit anti-thymoglobulin induction compared to no induction or interleukin-2 receptor antibody induction, though this was no longer statistically significant in an adjusted model, and pediatric patients were excluded [24]. Both organs must be monitored for rejection individually per local protocols as they can reject simultaneously or separately [25]. Blood pressure management must also be closely coordinated.

Pediatric Liver-Kidney Transplantation

Combined liver-kidney transplant (CLKT) is the most common pediatric multiorgan transplant, with 372 performed in the United States to date [1]. Nearly half of these are in children 11–17 years of age with another 30% in children 1–5 years of age; there have been only 11 CLKTs in children less than 1 year of age and none since 2015. Worldwide, only 10–30 CLKTx are performed annually [26]. Since 2000, the incidence of CLKTx in the United States has doubled from approximately 8 per year to approximately 17 per year [1]. While adult CLKT significantly increased after the introduction of MELD score, a similar increase was not seen after the introduction of the PELD score [27], possibly because the PELD score does not give priority based on renal function.

The primary indications for CLKT in children are congenital conditions that affect both the liver and kidney. A review of CLKTs between October 1987 and February 2011 showed that 37% were performed for primary hyperoxaluria and 18% for congenital hepatic fibrosis/autosomal recessive polycystic kidney disease (ARPKD) [7]. Methylmalonic acidemia, alpha-1-antitrypsin deficiency, Alagille syndrome, atypical hemolytic uremic syndrome, and glycogen storage disease 1a are other genetic diseases affecting both organ systems for which CLKT may offer benefit. CLKT in atypical hemolytic syndrome caused by genetic mutations in liver-synthesized complement factors (complement factor H, complement factor B, and C3) is less clearly indicated in the era of terminal complement inhibition medications, but it has not been entirely excluded.

Such patients should be evaluated on a case-by-case basis, including assessment of the risks of liver transplant and access to complement inhibition therapy [28]. Approximately 18% of pediatric CLKT recipients reported primary liver disease, including TPN-induced liver disease, biliary atresia, and familial and neonatal cholestasis with a second kidney disease [27]. Hepatorenal syndrome, which typically resolves with liver transplantation, is not generally considered an indication for CLKT. However, a subset of patients who require dialysis for greater than 6–8 weeks prior to liver transplantation may not recover, and CLKT has been used for adults with this indication [27].

Combined liver-kidney transplantation in children is a technically complex procedure that is mostly performed using deceased donor organs [29]. Living donation of both organs from one donor is technically possible [30] but is riskier for the donor; living donation is more commonly done as two sequential procedures. The liver is transplanted first followed by the kidney using standard surgical technique. In patients with anuric renal failure pre-transplant, such as ARPKD, fluid management during the liver transplant phase can be difficult, and continuous renal replacement therapy (CRRT) may be helpful [29]. Intraoperative CRRT can be safely performed, but its use is complicated by the patient's changing coagulation status;

systemic heparin increases the risk of bleeding, citrate anticoagulation may result in citrate excess toxicity due to impaired liver clearance, and anticoagulation-free dialysis is associated with risk of clotting [31]. In one adult cohort that largely avoided heparin or citrate anticoagulation, 40% of filters clotted during the procedure [32]. Patients with ARPKD may also require native nephrectomy to create sufficient intrabdominal space for CLKT due to the large size of the native kidneys. In this situation, the risk and benefits of performing a third procedure during the CLKT should be weighed against those of performing nephrectomy prior to transplant [26, 29].

Immediately after transplant, CLKT recipients require close monitoring for bleeding and vascular complications. Liver transplant recipients can have significant blood loss and disturbances of coagulation during transplantation, especially if intra-abdominal varices or hypersplenism was present. Overcorrection with excessive fresh frozen plasma, platelets, cryoprecipitate, and/or fibrinogen can result in vascular thrombosis after organ reperfusion. Management is therefore a matter of maintaining balance [26]. In one single-center cohort, 8 out of 18 pediatric CLKT recipients had bleeding complications [33], while another cohort reported bleeding in 6 of 12 children, half of whom required operative revision and vascular complications in two children [34]. For comparison, among pediatric liver-alone transplants, the incidence of bleeding is 5% and the incidence of vascular complications is 18% [26]. Frequent Doppler ultrasound examinations are necessary to monitor for complications.

The need for postoperative hemodialysis is also high among pediatric CLKT recipients, although these numbers are somewhat confounded by the routine use of hemodialysis after transplant in recipients with primary hyperoxaluria type 1. Harps et al. reported a cohort of 16 pediatric CLKT recipients, of whom 9 required continuous renal replacement therapy post-transplant; 8 of these had primary hyperoxaluria type 1 [35]. Similarly, Büscher et al. reported a need for dialysis in 5 of 11 children with primary hyperoxaluria type 1 and 1 of 10 patients with other indications for transplant [36]. In a review of SRTR data, Calinescu et al. reported an overall incidence of delayed graft function of only 22.4% [7], underscoring the idea that the need for dialysis is not likely related to kidney function.

Combined liver-kidney transplant may be particularly challenging in younger children due to their size. Harps et al. reported that increasing donor to recipient weight ratio and donor to recipient age ratio were strongly associated with longer intensive care unit (ICU) stay, with a receiver operating curve suggesting an age ratio of 5.34 and weight ratio of 3.4 as cutoffs for a good ICU outcome [35]. However, the use of kidneys from donors less than 5 years of age is associated with worse renal allograft outcomes due to increased vascular complications [15]. Therefore, the kidneys of young liver donors may have worse outcomes. There are reports of successful CLKTs in children under 10 kg [35, 37], but a staged procedure, with isolated liver transplant followed by kidney transplant once the patient has grown, may be necessary [36, 37]. Smaller patients also typically require split-liver transplants, which have higher rates of bleeding and thrombosis [36].

There are no guidelines regarding immunosuppression management for CLKT recipients, and induction and maintenance immunosuppression protocols are generally center-specific [29]. There are data suggesting that transplantation of a liver and kidney from the same donor is associated with a lower incidence of acute rejection and improved renal graft survival [29], and there are cases of a pre-transplant-positive lymphocytotoxic crossmatch becoming negative after liver transplant [27]. Multiple reasons for this have been theorized, including neutralization of circulating alloantibodies by soluble class I HLA antigens produced by the liver allograft, inhibition of natural killer and cytotoxic T cells by liver-produced HLA-G antigen, and liver clearance of circulating class 1 HLA antibodies [27, 29]. Adult observational studies have shown decreased kidney graft loss to chronic rejection among CLKT recipients (2%) compared to kidney-alone recipients (8%) [38]. However, a similar benefit was not seen among pediatric CLKT recipients in the European Society for Pediatric Nephrology/European Renal Association-European Dialysis and Transplant Registry [39]. In this cohort of 202 pediatric patients with ARPKD, there was no difference in 5-year death-censored kidney allograft survival between recipients of a CLKT and recipients of a kidney alone (92.1% vs 85.9%, $p = 0.4$), though age- and sex-adjusted risk for death was 6.7 times higher among the CLKT recipients [39]. Three of the four deaths within 1 month post-transplant were among the CLKT recipients; causes of death included cardiovascular disease, infection, and "other/unknown" factors [39].

A 2014 study evaluated outcomes for 152 children in the United States who had received CLKT. Patient survival for CLKT was 86.8% at 1 year, 82.1% at 5 years, and 78.9% at 10 years. A total of 12 of the 32 deaths occurred within 30 days post-operation and 17 had primary hyperoxaluria. The primary causes of death were infectious and cardiovascular complications. In comparison, patient survival after isolated liver transplant over a comparable period was 86.7% at 1 year, 81.2% at 5 years, and 77.4% at 10 years. Patient survival after isolated kidney transplant was 98.2% at 1 year, 95.4% at 5 years, and 90% at 10 years [7] (Fig. 14.5).

Liver graft survival was 81.9% at 1 year, 76.5% at 5 years, and 72.6% at 10 years. Liver graft survival was significantly worse among those with primary hyperoxaluria ($p = 0.01$), possibly due to the complications of systemic oxalosis, and the most common causes of liver graft failure were venous thrombosis (37.5%) and infection (25%). Kidney graft survival was 83.4% at 1 year, 76.5% at 5 years, and 66.8% at 10 years. Primary hyperoxaluria was significantly associated with reduced renal allograft survival ($p = 0.01$), and the most common causes of renal graft loss were chronic rejection (24%), infection (24%), and venous thrombosis (12%). Fourteen children (9.2%) had failure of both the liver and kidney, with kidney allograft failure preceding liver allograft failure in 57.1%. The time between failure of the two allografts was less than 40 days in 64.2% of children [7].

Primary Hyperoxaluria

Special consideration must be given to the question of CLKT in patients with primary hyperoxaluria. Primary hyperoxaluria type 1 is a defect in the *AXGT* gene,

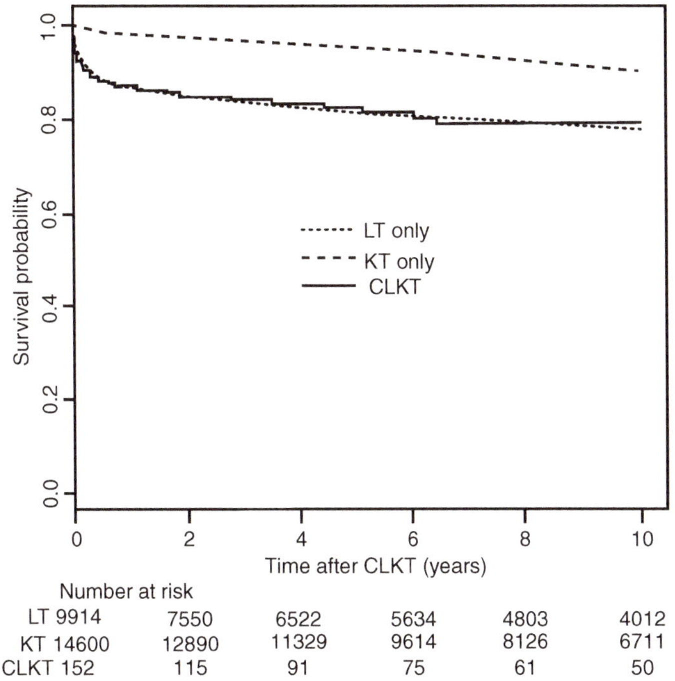

Fig. 14.5 Patient survival following pediatric combined liver-kidney transplantation (CLKT) compared to patient survival in isolated kidney transplantation (KT) and isolated liver transplantation (LT). (Reprinted with permission from *American Journal of Transplantation* [7])

resulting in defective production or trafficking of alanine-glyoxylate aminotransferase in the liver [27]. This deficiency leads to overproduction of oxalate and excessive urinary excretion of calcium oxalate that causes a decline in renal function. As the estimated glomerular filtration rate falls below 30–50 ml/min/1.73 m, renal oxalate excretion can no longer keep pace with production, and oxalate accumulates in the bones, vessels, heart, joints, and retina. Oxalate is poorly cleared by hemodialysis, with levels only decreasing by about 40% and returning to 95% of pre-dialysis levels within 48 hours; peritoneal dialysis clearance is worse. Children with primary hyperoxaluria often require daily hemodialysis with or without nightly peritoneal dialysis in order to keep pace with the continuous excess production of oxalate by the liver [40]. End-stage renal disease develops in 50% of children with primary hyperoxaluria type 1 by 15 years of age and 80% by age 30 years [27], though the course can be highly variable, even in siblings with the same genetic mutation [41].

The first step in considering CLKT for primary hyperoxaluria is genetic testing or liver biopsy to confirm alanine-glyoxylate aminotransferase deficiency [33]. Outcomes for kidney-alone transplant in primary hyperoxaluria type 1 are dismal, with a 5-year graft survival of 14% in children, primarily due to ongoing overproduction of oxalate in the liver that damages the allograft. However, the indications for liver transplantation in primary hyperoxaluria secondary to causes other than *AXGT* mutation remain unclear, with sources reporting both good outcomes and graft losses due to oxalate deposition among recipients of kidney-alone transplant in primary hyperoxaluria type 2, a milder form of the disease associated with mutations in glyoxylate reductase/hydroxypyruvate reductase and decreased risk of progression to ESRD. Another important step is determining if the patient is pyridoxine sensitive, as approximately 25–30% of patients with primary hyperoxaluria type 1 will have reduced oxalate excretion with pharmacologic doses of pyridoxine (5–10 mg/kg/dose twice a day). Soliman et al. reported that 8 of 26 patients on pyridoxine therapy were able to maintain normal renal function after 2 years of follow-up [42]. There are case reports suggesting that pyridoxine-responsive patients may have successful kidney-alone transplants, but the overall results of this practice remain unclear [33]. Similarly, there are multiple case reports of primary hyperoxaluria diagnosed only after kidney-alone transplantation; most cases resulted in early graft dysfunction (often within days to months of transplant) and early graft loss, but there also are reports of renal function stabilizing with aggressive fluid intake [43].

Among patients with confirmed primary hyperoxaluria type 1, there remains great debate about the appropriate timing of kidney transplantation [44]. After liver transplantation corrects the underlying genetic defect, systemically deposited oxalate is progressively mobilized into the blood to be filtered by, and damage, the kidneys. One management option is sequential liver and kidney transplant. The liver transplant occurs first, allowing for immediate correction of the oxalate overproduction, followed by a period of intensive dialysis to clear the mobilized systemic oxalate. Once plasma oxalate levels are lowered or normalized, the kidney transplant occurs, typically in a range of 51 days to 9 months post-liver transplant [45]. Advantages of the sequential strategy include protection of the renal allograft from systemic oxalosis and stabilization of liver function and coagulation prior to proceeding to kidney transplantation. Sequential transplant may also be more appropriate for children with the infantile form of primary hyperoxaluria type 1, for whom it is difficult to find appropriately size-matched liver and kidney allografts from the same donor. There are also multiple reports of successful sequential liver and kidney transplants using the same living donor [44, 46, 47]. However, if a patient requires a deceased donor for both organs, the wait time between liver and kidney transplants on intensive dialysis can be long [48].

In combined liver-kidney transplant, the metabolic defect and renal failure are corrected immediately, allowing earlier discontinuation of dialysis. Plasma oxalate levels drop significantly after CLKT, from >60–100 μmol/L to <20 μmol/L, but they can remain elevated for months or years as systemically deposited oxalate is mobilized [45, 49] (Fig. 14.6). Post-transplant management with high fluid intake, urine crystallization inhibitors, such as citrate, and pyridoxine (if patient is pyridoxine-responsive) is necessary to protect the renal allograft until oxalate levels are normal [33, 45]. The value of dialysis immediately after CLKT, to clear oxalate and prevent early oxalate deposition in the new renal allograft, remains unclear [33], as the anticoagulation needed for dialysis increases the risk of bleeding in a patient whose synthetic liver function is still recovering. CLKT also allows the patient to benefit from the lower rejection rates seen in CLKT [45]. In a recent case series reported by

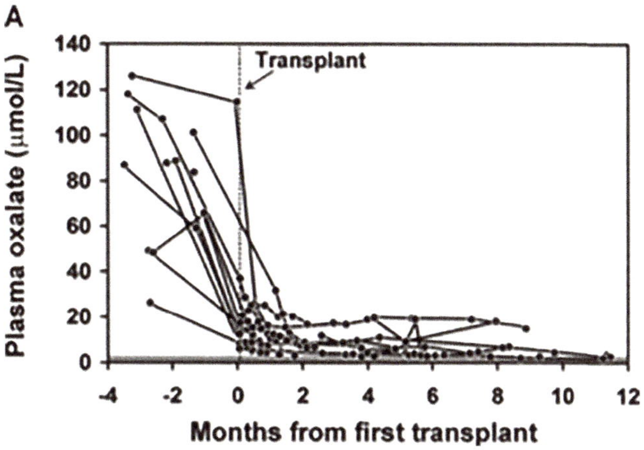

Fig. 14.6 Plasma oxalate levels declined rapidly following successful combined kidney-liver transplantation but remained above normal in most patients during the first year after transplant. The normal range for plasma oxalate levels is <1.8 µmol/L, shown in the gray-shaded area. (Reprinted with permission from *American Journal of Transplantation* [49])

Horoub et al., 24 patients with primary hyperoxaluria type 1 underwent transplantation between 2011 and 2018, 13 of whom were less than 18 years of age. Thirteen patients received sequential liver and kidney transplant and eight patients received CLKT. The authors reported no differences in mortality at 3 years, need for hemodialysis after transplant, acute cellular rejection, or estimated glomerular filtration rate between the sequential and combined transplant strategies [50].

Pre-emptive liver transplant for patients with primary hyperoxaluria type 1 remains controversial. It may be an option for patients who are diagnosed prior to significant decline in renal function, correcting the metabolic defect before systemic oxalosis develops and preventing the need for a renal transplant. "Late" pre-emptive liver transplant, in patients with a glomerular filtration rate <30 mL/min/1.73m^2, may also delay the need for kidney transplant [48]. In young children, preemptive liver transplant avoids the technical and anatomic issues of CLKT in a small abdomen [48]. However, primary hyperoxaluria has a heterogeneous course; it can present clinically in infancy with rapid progression, in adolescence with recurrent nephrolithiasis, or even in adulthood [51]. Factors predicting the onset of renal failure are unclear but may include a higher urinary oxalate level and nephrocalcinosis [52, 53]. Family history or genetic mutation is not necessarily predictive [41].

Given this uncertainty, and liver transplant graft survival outcomes of 85% at 5 years, 70% at 10 years, and 50% at 20 years [51], and the risks of immunosuppression, the difference between "preemptive" and "premature" liver transplant remains debated. There have been 24 published cases of preemptive liver transplantation for pediatric primary hyperoxaluria type 1, of which 20 patients were free of end-stage renal disease at follow-up of 0.7–16 years [48]. Ongoing research in hepatocyte transplantation [48] and the recent US Food and Drug Administration approval of lumasiran, an RNA interference-based treatment that decreases oxalate production by reducing levels of glycolate oxidase, [29] may change management of primary hyperoxaluria type 1, further complicating considerations for preemptive liver transplantation.

Pediatric Kidney-Pancreas Transplantation

Pediatric kidney-pancreas transplantation is a rare procedure, with only 69 reported cases in the US Organ Procurement and Transplantation Network [1]. The number of kidney-pancreas transplants in children has been declining in recent years, from a median of 4 per year 2006–2010 to a median of 2 per year 2016–2020. Pancreas-alone transplant is more common in children, with 703 performed since 1988. Of all pediatric kidney-pancreas transplants performed in the United States, 8 (11.5%) were in children less than 1 year old, 22 (31.9%) were in children 1–5 years old, 15 (21.7%) were in children 6–10 years old, and 22 (31.9%) were in children 11–17 years old [1].

Nearly 50 (72.4%) of the 69 pediatric kidney-pancreas recipients did not have diabetes [1]; their indications for transplant are not clearly documented in published OPTN data but may include cystic fibrosis and chronic pancreatitis [1]. Seven (10.1%) pediatric kidney-pancreas recipients reported type I diabetes, while the remainder are "unknown." Forty-three (62.3%) recipients reported "other" as their indication for renal transplant. As of writing, there were three pediatric patients waitlisted for kidney-pancreas transplant, two of whom had congenital/metabolic disorders [1].

In 1996, Bendel-Stenzel et al. published two cases of children who received simultaneous pancreas-kidney transplants. Both patients had a history of diarrhea-associated hemolytic uremic syndrome that resulted in pancreatic insufficiency requiring insulin and renal failure. One patient received a deceased donor transplant and one received a living-related simultaneous kidney and segmental pancreas transplant. Induction was with antithymocyte globulin in both patients. Both patients received tacrolimus and prednisone maintenance immunosuppression; in addition, one patient received azathioprine and one patient received mycophenolate mofetil. The need for insulin in both patients resolved within 6 hours of post-transplant; one patient continued to require pancreatic enzyme supplements. One patient had multiple episodes of rejection, while the other had none. Both patients had functioning allografts at 1-year follow-up. The authors further reported on a total of eight pediatric simultaneous kidney-pancreas transplants in the International Pancreas Transplant Registry, six of whom had function of both grafts at follow-up [54].

Due to the rarity of the procedure, published data on simultaneous kidney-pancreas transplant are largely limited to the adult population, where the primary indication is type 1 diabetes with concurrent diabetic nephropathy and patient comorbidities may be substantially different. The pancreas transplant is completed first to limit ischemic time [55]. The pancreas is transplanted heterotopically, but the exact location is a matter of surgeon and center preference. Common anastomosis sites include the pelvis, with anastomoses to the common or external iliac artery and vein, or the small bowel mesentery, with anastomoses to the iliac artery or aorta and the portal vein or superior mesenteric vein. Venous anastomosis to the systemic circulation is technically easier but carriers a higher risk of hyperinsulinemia; venous anastomosis to the portal circulation is theoretically more physiologic but has not been shown to improve graft survival [55]. The pancreas is a technically challenging organ on which to operate. Technical complications are common and include pancreatic pseudocyst and thrombosis (5–10%) [55, 56]. Abdominal infections are responsible for 9.2–15% of technical failures and remain a major cause of mortality in pancreatic transplantation [57].

As most adult simultaneous kidney-pancreas transplants are for type 1 diabetes, the patient has intact exocrine function of their native pancreas; therefore, the exocrine duct of the pancreatic allograft is typically diverted to either the bladder or jejunum. Anastomosis with the bladder was more common historically, but this can result in chronic metabolic acidosis due to loss of bicarbonate-rich fluid in the urine, infections, and damage to the urethra by pancreatic enzymes [58]. A duodenal or jejunal anastomosis of the exocrine duct is now more commonly used [55, 56], though this may result in malabsorption and diarrhea [58]. In pediatric patients with exocrine dysfunction, the location of the duct anastomosis may affect their need for pancreatic enzyme supplementation.

Post-transplant, close monitoring of blood glucose level is critical as it reflects graft function; failure to achieve normoglycemia quickly after transplant is a sign of graft dysfunction, rejection, pancreatitis, and/or an allograft that is too small for the patient [56]. Pancreatic allograft rejection in adult simultaneous kidney-pancreas recipients is concordant with kidney graft rejection in 60% of cases [55]. Elevated C-peptide and lipase are suggestive of dysfunction. Biopsy of the pancreatic graft is technically challenging and may be nondiagnostic in 12% of cases due to sampling error [55].

Data in adults suggest that simultaneous kidney-pancreas transplant has increased graft survival (>90% at 1 year) compared to isolated pancreas (80%) or pancreas-after-kidney (82%) transplantation [56]. Simultaneous kidney-pancreas recipients also have longer graft survival (72% at 8 years) than deceased donor kidney-alone recipients (55% at 8 years) [55]. However, wait times for simultaneous kidney-pancreas transplant are substantially longer than for kidney or pancreas alone. For example, between 2011 and 2014, the median wait time to receive a simultaneous kidney-pancreas transplant in the United States for an 11- to 17-year-old was 1033 days, compared to 680 days for a kidney alone and 758 days for a pancreas alone [1]. Therefore, the improved graft survival must be balanced with the longer wait time.

Liver-Kidney-Pancreas Transplant

There have been two pediatric liver-kidney-pancreas multiorgan transplants performed in the United States [1], which correspond to two case reports of such transplants for Wolcott-Rallison syndrome. Wolcott-Rallison syndrome is a rare genetic disorder that causes neonatal-onset insulin-dependent diabetes, skeletal dysplasia (mostly spondyloepiphyseal dysplasia), short stature, and hepatic dysfunction with recurrent acute liver failure [59]. The disease is autosomal recessive and is caused by mutations in *EIF2AK3*, which encodes pancreatic endoplasmic reticulum kinase (PERK). In the absence of PERK, the endoplasmic reticulum cannot respond to stress from accumulated unfolded proteins [60]. Infection, medications, or anesthesia can trigger episodic acute liver failure, often accompanied by acute renal failure [61]; the first "aggravation" is fatal in approximately 50% of cases [60].

Rivera et al. reported an 8-year-old girl with genetic-confirmed Wolcott-Rallison syndrome who presented with a dry cough, low-grade fever, and abdominal pain. She quickly developed multisystem organ failure, including a need for continuous renal replacement therapy. Nine days later, she underwent en bloc liver, pancreas, and kidney transplant from an 8-year-old ABO-compatible donor with thymoglobulin induction. Abdominal wall closure was completed on postoperative day 2; she was extubated and began eating on postoperative day 4. Post-transplant course was complicated by acute rejection of the liver and pancreas on day 45 and Enterococcus urosepsis at 6 months. She was in good health with good graft function at 18 months of follow-up [62].

Tzakis et al. reported a 6-year-old girl who presented with acute hepatic failure and was confirmed to have Wolcott-Rallison syndrome by genetic testing. She required mechanical ventilation, dialysis, and plasmapheresis for 6 weeks before recovering. Once she had been discharged, she was evaluated and listed for liver, pancreas, and kidney transplant. She received en bloc transplant with both kidneys; the native kidneys were not removed. The abdominal wall was closed on postoperative day 6. Post-transplant course was complicated by severe rejection of all three organs with acute respiratory distress syndrome, from which she recovered after 2 months of hospitalization. She was in good health with good graft function at 18 months of follow-up [60].

Kidney-Intestinal and Multivisceral Transplants

Composite visceral transplants are any transplant including the intestine and at least one other abdominal organ; multivisceral transplants are intestinal transplants that also include the stomach, duodenum, and pancreas with or without the liver and kidney [63]. Per OPTN data, 55 pediatric composite visceral transplants that include a kidney have been performed in the United States to date; 50 of these are liver-kidney-intestinal-pancreas transplants. Of the remainder, two were kidney-intestinal transplants, two were kidney-intestinal-pancreas transplants, and one was a liver-kidney- intestinal transplant. A total of 21 (42%) of the 50 transplants were performed in children aged 6–10 years. The incidence of multivisceral transplantation peaked in 2008–2010 before declining. In the past 5 years, multivisceral transplantation has been limited exclusively to liver-kidney-intestinal-pancreas transplants performed in children of ages 1–10 years at a rate of 1–3 transplants per year [1].

Intestinal and multivisceral transplant is the standard of care for patients with irreversible intestinal failure who can no longer be maintained on parental nutrition [63]. The primary causes of intestinal failure are short bowel syndrome, congenital enteropathies, and intestinal motility disorders. Primary treatment for intestinal failure is parental nutrition, with a goal of intestinal rehabilitation and return to full enteral nutrition, but maintenance of parental nutrition may be limited by severe cholestatic liver disease, recurrent catheter-related infections, and/or loss of vascular access [64]. Intestinal failure-associated liver disease (IFALD) occurs in 40–60% of children, and as many as 85% of neonates, who depend on parenteral nutrition for prolonged periods; approximately 15% of these will progress to end-stage liver disease [65]. IFALD is multifactorial and related to prematurity, recurrent infections, and parenteral lipid intake, especially the soybean oil routinely used in the United States [64, 65]. In infants with IFALD who are considered to have a high likelihood of intestinal adaptation and return to enteral nutrition, liver transplant alone may be considered, as liver disease has been shown to interfere with intestinal adaptation [65]. However, this can be difficult to predict. IFALD often recurs in the liver allograft, and the immunosuppressive medications may increase the risks of sepsis in children who still require parenteral nutrition [65]. Intestinal failure is less commonly associated with kidney disease; in the OPTN/SRTR 2016 Annual Data Report, only 3.7% of intestinal recipients required simultaneous kidney transplant [66]. Of note, many multivisceral transplant recipients do not require a pancreas transplant, but the pancreas is often included for technical reasons, as it eliminates the need for biliary reconstruction (and associated risk of bile leaks), simplifies backtable preparation, and allows for procurement of longer superior mesenteric artery and vein vessels [67].

The intestinal transplant procedure is complex and individualized to the patient, depending on the organs being transplanted and the abdominal anatomy of the patient. In the pre-transplant phase, a full assessment of upper and lower vascular patency is key as many patients will have vascular thrombosis related to their parental nutrition dependence that can complicate or even preclude the procedure. The kidney may be transplanted en bloc with the intestine or separately [63]. A recent case series by Kunzler de Oliveira Maia et al. reported using infant en bloc kidneys with a bladder segment, using the bladder patch technique in three children receiving multivisceral transplants [68]. All three patients had good vascular flow; one developed ureteral stenosis. One patient died of sepsis, while the other two were alive with graft function at 2 and 5 years of post-transplant [68]. Small patients may not have adequate abdominal domain to place an en bloc multivisceral transplant with abdominal wall closure, but abdominal wall closure at the time of surgery is preferred to decrease the risk of infection. There are several reports of using the abdominal rectus as fascia to allow tension-free abdominal closure with good results [69, 70]. Postoperatively, multivisceral transplant recipients typically continue parental nutrition with gradual, stepwise introduction of enteral feeds [63]. Acute kidney injury is common (25% incidence in adults), and is likely related to erratic intestinal absorption of tacrolimus, which can lead to markedly elevated tacrolimus levels and calcineurin inhibitor-related renal artery vasoconstriction [71].

Compared to other organs, the intestinal allograft includes significantly more lymphoid tissue and is highly antigenic; both rejection and graft versus host disease can and do occur. Acute cellular rejection has been reported in 30–60% of intestinal transplant recipients by 3 months of post-transplant [69, 71]. The rejection is typically isolated to the intestine with other transplanted organs relatively spared [71]. Intestinal rejection can present with fever, diarrhea, abdominal pain, dissension, and bacteremia due to translocation of bacteria. Tacrolimus levels may appear elevated during rejection due to impaired enterocyte tacrolimus metabolism [71]. To monitor for rejection, an ileostomy is commonly created to allow for surveillance biopsies [63] as often as twice a week immediately after transplant [71]. Depending on which other organs are transplanted, routine monitoring of hepatic enzymes, pancreatic enzymes, and serum creatinine is also necessary. Immunomodulatory strategies, including allograft radiation and bone marrow augmentation, have also been explored with some improvement in outcomes [63, 72].

Simultaneously, the patient must be monitored for graft versus host disease (GvHD), which occurs in 4–30% of recipients [71, 73]. The risk is highest in patients with an immunodeficiency (such as in familial multiple intestinal atresia or trichoheptoenteric syndrome) or who are under the age of 5 years [73, 74]. Unlike GvHD of after hematopoietic stem cell transplant, GvHD after multivisceral transplant nearly always involves the skin (often a maculopapular rash that starts on the palms and soles) [73], though intestine, lungs, and bone marrow involvement may occur concurrently [75]. The diagnosis is confirmed by the presence of donor leukocytes in the recipient's peripheral blood or organs [63]; management involves steroids and reduction in other immunosuppression. Mortality among multivisceral transplant recipients has been reported to be as high as 60–70% in one small case series [75, 76].

Intestinal transplant recipients have the highest rates of Epstein-Barr virus (EBV) infection and post-transplant lymphoproliferative disease (PTLD), with an incidence ranging from 13 to 33%, likely related to the comparatively younger age of recipients, more frequent use of T-cell depleting induction therapy, and larger amount of donor lymphoid tissue present in the intestine [77, 78]. One case series also reported two cases of intra-abdominal EBV-associated smooth muscle tumor, an overall incidence of 14% in the pediatric multivisceral population [78]. Both PTLD- and EBV-associated smooth muscle tumors are treated with reduction in immunosuppression, but case reports suggest that resection of smooth muscle tumors may improve survival [79].

Related to these complications, outcomes for multivisceral transplants remain significantly worse than other solid organ transplants. They are also worse than outcomes for individuals with intestinal failure who can be maintained on chronic parenteral nutrition [80]. Data on kidney-inclusive multivisceral transplants are not available, but current 5-year patient survival among all pediatric multivisceral transplant recipients is approximately 50–60% [69, 80, 81]. Younger age at transplant, receipt of a liver transplant from the same donor, and use of rapamycin as maintenance immunosuppression have all been associated with improved graft and patient outcomes [81]. However, Ramisch et al. reported that 93% of graft recipients were taking full enteral nutrition within 1 month of post-transplant [69], and quality of life is reportedly good after intestinal transplantation, though lower than the general population, especially in areas of school functioning [82, 83]. With improvements in intestinal rehabilitation and prevention of IFALD, the role of multivisceral transplant may be limited to that of a "final option" therapy until outcomes improve.

Future Directions

Despite growth in multiorgan transplantation over the last two decades, current information on management and outcomes, especially among pediatric patients, remains limited. Existing data supporting or refuting the role of multiorgan transplantation versus single-organ or sequential transplantation are often subject to confounding by indication and is difficult to interpret. National and international consensus on indications for multiorgan transplant is lacking. Peri- and post-operative management remains largely center-specific, driven by expert opinion rather than data. National and international registries often combine pediatric and adult data in their reporting, making it challenging to apply the results to children. Centers that frequently perform multiorgan transplants should be encouraged to publish their experience (especially in the field of pediatric kidney-pancreas transplantation), and existing registries should be encouraged to publish pediatric-specific outcomes from their databases to continue to improve the care we provide to this small but vulnerable population.

Questions

1. Which of the following statements is true regarding multiorgan allocation?
   - A. Incidence of multiorgan allocation to pediatric patients has risen over the last 5 years.
   - B. There are no policies surrounding allocation of organs for multiorgan transplantation.
   - C. Current allocation policies result in multiorgan transplant recipients receiving kidneys with a lower KDPI than kidney-alone transplant recipients.
   - D. There are simple and straightforward ways to balance equity and utility in multiorgan transplant allocation.

   C. Because multiorgan transplant takes priority over solo pediatric kidney, recipients of multiorgan transplants often receive better quality kidneys (lower KDPI) than recipients of kidney alone.
2. Outcomes among pediatric simultaneous heart-kidney transplant recipients:
   - A. Show increased rejection within the first-year post-transplant compared to heart-alone transplantation
   - B. Show increased rates of primary allograft nonfunction compared to kidney-alone transplantation
   - C. Are likely to be better for infants <10 kg than for larger children

D. Show increased mortality compared to heart-alone transplantation

B. Recipients of combined heart-kidney transplant have significantly lower mortality than heart transplant recipients who remain on dialysis but have high incidence of primary nonfunction and post-transplant dialysis, despite generally receiving higher quality (low KDPI) kidneys than kidney-alone recipients.

3. Perioperative management of combined liver-kidney transplant recipients involves:
   A. Transplanting the kidney first, followed by the liver
   B. Routine use of CRRT with heparin anticoagulation in all patients
   C. Careful balancing of bleeding and thrombosis risks
   D. Rare use of postoperative dialysis

   C. Immediately after transplant, CLKT recipients require close monitoring for bleeding and vascular complications. Liver transplant recipients can have significant blood loss and disturbances of coagulation during transplantation, especially if intra-abdominal varices or hypersplenism was present. Overcorrection with excessive fresh frozen plasma, platelets, cryoprecipitate, and/or fibrinogen can result in vascular thrombosis after organ reperfusion.

4. Compared to other solid-organ transplant recipients, multivisceral transplant recipients are at higher risk for:
   A. Graft versus host disease
   B. Rejection
   C. Post-transplant lymphoproliferative disease
   D. All of the above

   D. Multivisceral transplant recipients are at higher risk of all of the listed complications and have to be monitored carefully.

References

1. National Data - OPTN. https://optn.transplant.hrsa.gov/data/view-data-reports/national-data/#. Accessed 11 Oct 2020.
2. Cheng XS, Khush KK, Wiseman A, Teuteberg J, Tan JC. To kidney or not to kidney: applying lessons learned from the simultaneous liver-kidney transplant policy to simultaneous heart-kidney transplantation. Clin Transpl. 2020. https://doi.org/10.1111/ctr.13878.
3. OPTN/UNOS Ethics Committee. Ethical implications of multi-organ transplants. June 2019.
4. Reese PP, Veatch RM, Abt PL, Amaral S. Revisiting multi-organ transplantation in the setting of scarcity. Am J Transplant. 2014;14:21–6.
5. About the final rule - OPTN. https://optn.transplant.hrsa.gov/governance/about-the-optn/final-rule/. Accessed 11 Oct 2020.
6. Lum EL, Cárdenas A, Martin P, Bunnapradist S. Current status of simultaneous liver-kidney transplantation in the United States. Liver Transpl. 2019;25:797–806.
7. Calinescu AM, Wildhaber BE, Poncet A, Toso C, McLin VA. Outcomes of combined liver-kidney transplantation in children: analysis of the scientific registry of transplant recipients. Am J Transplant. 2014;14:2861–8.
8. Kidney-pancreas allocation system frequently asked questions - OPTN. https://optn.transplant.hrsa.gov/resources/guidance/kidney-pancreas-allocation-system-frequently-asked-questions/. Accessed 11 Oct 2020.
9. Andrews WS, Kane BJ, Hendrickson RJ. Organ allocation and utilization in pediatric transplantation. Semin Pediatr Surg. 2017;26:186–92.

10. Optn OPTN policies effective as of June 18 2020 [Eliminate the use of regions in VCA distribution].
11. Carrico R, Fridell J, Odorico J, Stewart Z. How did the new kidney and pancreas allocation systems affect pancreas utilization in the first six-months? [abstract]. Am J Transplant. 2016;16:1689–99.
12. Axelrod DA, Sung RS, Meyer KH, Wolfe RA, Kaufman DB. Systematic evaluation of pancreas allograft quality, outcomes and geographic variation in utilization. Am J Transplant. 2010;10:837–45.
13. Rossano JW, Cherikh WS, Chambers DC, et al. The International Thoracic Organ Transplant Registry of the International Society for Heart and Lung Transplantation: twenty-first pediatric heart transplantation report—2018; focus theme: multiorgan transplantation. J Heart Lung Transplant. 2018;37:1184–95.
14. Weng PL, Alejos JC, Halnon N, Zhang Q, Reed EF, Tsai Chambers E. Long-term outcomes of simultaneous heart and kidney transplantation in pediatric recipients. Pediatr Transplant. 2017. https://doi.org/10.1111/petr.13023.
15. Sahney S, Chinnock R. Management of infants and young children with combined heart and kidney failure. Pediatr Transplant. 2006;10:408–12.
16. Choudhry S, Dharnidharka VR, Castleberry CD, Goss CW, Simpson KE, Schechtman KB, Canter CE. End-stage renal disease after pediatric heart transplantation: a 25-year national cohort study. J Heart Lung Transplant. 2018;37:217–24.
17. Mosconi G, Panicali L, Persici E, Conte D, Cappuccilli ML, Cuna V, Capelli I, Todeschini P, D'Arcangelo GL, Stefoni S. Native kidney function after renal transplantation combined with other solid organs in preemptive patients. Transplant Proc. 2010;42:1017–20.
18. Madsen JC, Yamada K, Allan JS, Choo JK, Erhorn AE, Pins MR, Vesga L, Slisz JK, Sachs DH. Transplantation tolerance prevents cardiac allograft vasculopathy in major histocompatibility complex class I-disparate miniature swine. Transplantation. 1998;65:304–13.
19. Sarwal MM, Cecka JM, Millan MT, Salvatierra O. Adult-size kidneys without acute tubular necrosis provide exceedingly superior long-term graft outcomes for infants and small children. Transplantation. 2000;70:1728–36.
20. Mc Loughlin S, Bianco JC, Marenchino RG. Anesthetic and perioperative considerations for combined heart-kidney transplantation. J Cardiothorac Vasc Anesth. 2018;32:44–9.
21. Riaz A, Adebiyi O, Mishler D, Yaqub M, Taber T, Sharfuddin A. Kidney graft outcomes in combined heart-kidney transplantation: a UNOS database analysis 2000–2015 [abstract].
22. Ruzza A, Czer LSC, Trento A, Esmailian F. Combined heart and kidney transplantation: what is the appropriate surgical sequence? Interact Cardiovasc Thorac Surg. 2013;17:416–8.
23. Chacon MM, Roberts EK. Dilemmas for the cardiac anesthesiologist: managing conflicting fluid management strategies during combined heart-kidney transplantation. J Cardiothorac Vasc Anesth. 2018;32:50–2.
24. Ariyamuthu VK, Amin AA, Drazner MH, et al. Induction regimen and survival in simultaneous heart-kidney transplant recipients. J Heart Lung Transplant. 2018;37:587–95.
25. Fritzsche SD, McCabe JL, Chinnock RE. Rare combined heart and kidney transplant in a pediatric patient: a case study. J Transpl Coord. 1999;9:145–8.
26. Jalanko H, Pakarinen M. Combined liver and kidney transplantation in children. Pediatr Nephrol. 2014;29:805–14.
27. Chava SP, Singh B, Pal S, Dhawan A, Heaton ND. Indications for combined liver and kidney transplantation in children. Pediatr Transplant. 2009;13:661–9.
28. Loirat C, Fakhouri F, Ariceta G, et al. An international consensus approach to the management of atypical hemolytic uremic syndrome in children. Pediatr Nephrol. 2016;31:15–39.
29. Grenda R, Kaliciński P. Combined and sequential liver–kidney transplantation in children. Pediatr Nephrol. 2018;33:2227–37.
30. Sakamoto S, Kasahara M, Fukuda A, Tanaka H, Kakiuchi T, Karaki C, Kanazawa H, Kamei K, Ito S, Nakazawa A. Pediatric liver-kidney transplantation for hepatorenal fibrocystic disease from a living donor. Pediatr Transplant. 2012;16:99–102.
31. Matuszkiewicz-Rowińska J, Małyszko J, Wieliczko M. Renal support during liver transplantation: when to consider it? Transplant Proc. 2013;45:3157–62.

32. Townsend DR, Bagshaw SM, Jacka MJ, Bigam D, Cave D, Gibney RTN. Intraoperative renal support during liver transplantation. Liver Transpl. 2009;15:73–8.
33. Bacchetta J, Mekahli D, Rivet C, Demède D, Leclerc AL. Pediatric combined liver-kidney transplantation: a 2015 update. Curr Opin Organ Transplant. 2015;20:543–9.
34. Herden U, Kemper M, Ganschow R, Klaassen I, Grabhorn E, Brinkert F, Nashan B, Fischer L. Surgical aspects and outcome of combined liver and kidney transplantation in children. Transpl Int. 2011;24:805–11.
35. Harps E, Brinkert F, Ganschow R, Briem-Richter A, Van Husen M, Schmidtke S, Herden U, Nashan B, Fischer L, Kemper MJ. Immediate postoperative intensive care treatment of pediatric combined liver-kidney transplantation: outcome and prognostic factors. Transplantation. 2011;91:1127–31.
36. Büscher R, Büscher AK, Cetiner M, Treckmann JW, Paul A, Vester U, Hoyer PF. Combined liver and kidney transplantation and kidney after liver transplantation in children: indication, postoperative outcome, and long-term results. Pediatr Transplant. 2015;19:858–65.
37. Sutherland SM, Alexander SR, Sarwal MM, Berquist WE, Concepcion W. Combined liver-kidney transplantation in children: indications and outcome. Pediatr Transplant. 2008;12:835–46.
38. Fong TL, Bunnapradist S, Jordan SC, Selby RR, Cho YW. Analysis of the United Network for Organ Sharing database comparing renal allografts and patient survival in combined liver-kidney transplantation with the contralateral allografts in kidney alone or kidney-pancreas transplantation. Transplantation. 2003;76:348–53.
39. Mekahli D, van Stralen KJ, Bonthuis M, et al. Kidney versus combined kidney and liver transplantation in young people with autosomal recessive polycystic kidney disease: data from the European Society for Pediatric Nephrology/European Renal Association–European Dialysis and Transplant (ESPN/ERA-EDTA) registry. Am J Kidney Dis. 2016;68:782–8.
40. Nair P, Al-Otaibi T, Nampoory N, Al-Qabandi W, Said T, Halim MA, Gheith O. Combined liver and kidney transplantation in primary hyperoxaluria: a report of three cases and review of the literature. Saudi J Kidney Dis Transpl. 2013;24:969–75.
41. Eytan Mor MD, Weismann I. Editorial: current treatment for primary hyperoxaluria type 1: when should liver/kidney transplantation be considered. Pediatr Transplant. 2009;13:805–7.
42. Soliman NA, Nabhan MM, Abdelrahman SM, et al. Clinical spectrum of primary hyperoxaluria type 1: experience of a tertiary center. Nephrol Ther. 2017;13:176–82.
43. Cai R, Lin M, Chen Z, et al. Primary hyperoxaluria diagnosed after kidney transplantation failure: lesson from 3 case reports and literature review. BMC Nephrol. 2019. https://doi.org/10.1186/s12882-019-1402-2.
44. Ozer A, Aktas H, Bulum B, Emiroglu R. The experience of combined and sequential liver and kidney transplantation from a single living donor in patients with primary hyperoxaluria type 1. Pediatr Transplant. 2019. https://doi.org/10.1111/petr.13406.
45. Kemper MJ. Concurrent or sequential liver and kidney transplantation in children with primary hyperoxaluria type 1? Pediatr Transplant. 2005;9:693–6.
46. Astarcioglu I, Karademir S, Gülay H, Bora S, Astarcioglu H, Kavukcu S, Türkmen M, Soylu A. Primary hyperoxaluria: simultaneous combined liver and kidney transplantation from a living related donor. Liver Transpl. 2003;9:433–6.
47. Angelico R, Guzzo I, Pellicciaro M, et al. Same donor laparoscopic liver and kidney procurement for sequential living donor liver-kidney transplantation in primary hyperoxaluria type I. J Laparoendosc Adv Surg Tech. 2019;29:1616–22.
48. Khorsandi SE, Samyn M, Hassan A, et al. An institutional experience of pre-emptive liver transplantation for pediatric primary hyperoxaluria type 1. Pediatr Transplant. 2016;20:523–9.
49. Bergstralh EJ, Monico CG, Lieske JC, Herges RM, Langman CB, Hoppe B, Milliner DS. Transplantation outcomes in primary hyperoxaluria. Am J Transplant. 2010;10:2493–501.
50. Horoub R, Shamsaeefar A, Dehghani M, Nikoopour H, Entezari M, Moradi A, Kazemi K, Eshraghian A, Nikeghbalian S, Malek-Hosseini SA. Liver transplant for primary hyperoxaluria type 1: results of sequential, combined liver and kidney, and preemptive liver transplant. Exp Clin Transplant. 2019. https://doi.org/10.6002/ect.2019.0150.

51. Squires J, Nguyen C. Complexity of pre-emptive liver transplantation in children with primary hyperoxaluria type 1. Pediatr Transplant. 2016;20:604–6.
52. Zhao F, Bergstralh EJ, Mehta RA, Vaughan LE, Olson JB, Seide BM, Meek AM, Cogal AG, Lieske JC, Milliner DS. Predictors of incident ESRD among patients with primary hyperoxaluria presenting prior to kidney failure. Clin J Am Soc Nephrol. 2016;11:119–26.
53. Tang X, Bergstralh EJ, Mehta RA, Vrtiska TJ, Milliner DS, Lieske JC. Nephrocalcinosis is a risk factor for kidney failure in primary hyperoxaluria. Kidney Int. 2015;87:623–31.
54. Bendel-Stenzel MR, Kashtan CE, Sutherland DER, Chavers BM. Simultaneous pancreas-kidney transplant in two children with hemolytic-uremic syndrome. Pediatr Nephrol. 1997;11:485–7.
55. Samoylova ML, Borle D, Ravindra KV. Pancreas transplantation: indications, techniques, and outcomes. Surg Clin North Am. 2019;99:87–101.
56. Mittel AM, Wagener G. Anesthesia for kidney and pancreas transplantation. Anesthesiol Clin. 2017;35:439–52.
57. Haidar G, Green M. Intra-abdominal infections in solid organ transplant recipients: guidelines from the American Society of Transplantation Infectious Diseases Community of Practice. Clin Transpl. 2019. https://doi.org/10.1111/ctr.13595.
58. Bottino R, Balamurugan AN, Giannoukakis N, Trucco M. Islet/pancreas transplantation: challenges for pediatrics. Pediatr Diabetes. 2002;3:210–23.
59. Rubio-Cabezas O, Patch AM, Minton JAL, et al. Wolcott-Rallison syndrome is the most common genetic cause of permanent neonatal diabetes in consanguineous families. J Clin Endocrinol Metab. 2009;94:4162–70.
60. Tzakis AG, Nunnelley MJ, Tekin A, Buccini LD, Garcia J, Uchida K, Neville HL, Nares MA, Ruiz P, Bodamer O. Liver, pancreas and kidney transplantation for the treatment of Wolcott-Rallison syndrome. Am J Transplant. 2015;15:565–7.
61. Julier C, Nicolino M. Wolcott-Rallison syndrome. Orphanet J Rare Dis. 2010. https://doi.org/10.1186/1750-1172-5-29.
62. Rivera E, Gupta S, Chavers B, Quinones L, Berger MR, Schwarzenberg SJ, Pruett T, Verghese P, Chinnakotla S. En bloc multiorgan transplant (liver, pancreas, and kidney) for acute liver and renal failure in a patient with Wolcott-Rallison syndrome. Liver Transpl. 2016;22:371–4.
63. Costa G, Parekh N, Osman M, Armanyous S, Fujiki M, Abu-Elmagd K. Composite and multivisceral transplantation nomenclature, surgical techniques, current practice, and long-term outcome. https://doi.org/10.1016/j.suc.2018.09.010.
64. D'Antiga L, Goulet O. Intestinal failure in children: the European view. J Pediatr Gastroenterol Nutr. 2013;56:118–26.
65. Nehra D, Fallon EM, Puder M. The prevention and treatment of intestinal failure-associated liver disease in neonates and children. Surg Clin North Am. 2011;91:543–63.
66. Smith JM, Weaver T, Skeans MA, Horslen SP, Harper AM, Snyder JJ, Israni AK, Kasiske BL. OPTN/SRTR 2016 annual data report: intestine. Am J Transplant. 2018;18:254–90.
67. Mercer DF, Brady MJ, Jain G. Should the pancreas be routinely included with an intestinal graft? Curr Transplant Rep. 2015;2:159–63.
68. Kunzler de Oliveira Maia F, Tekin A, Nicolau-Raducu R, Beduschi T, Selvaggi G, Vianna R, Ammar Al Nuss M, González J, Gaynor JJ, Ciancio G. Use of pediatric donor en bloc kidneys along with bladder segment in pediatric liver-kidney and multivisceral-kidney transplantation. Pediatr Transplant. 2020. https://doi.org/10.1111/petr.13596.
69. Ramisch D, Rumbo C, Echevarria C, et al. Long-term outcomes of intestinal and multivisceral transplantation at a single center in Argentina. Transplant Proc. 2016;48:457–62.
70. Caso Maestro O, Abradelo De Usera M, Justo Alonso I, Calvo Pulido J, Manrique Municio A, Cambra Molero F, García Sesma A, Loinaz Segurola C, Moreno González E, Jiménez Romero C. Porcine acellular dermal matrix for delayed abdominal wall closure after pediatric liver transplantation. Pediatr Transplant. 2014;18:594–8.
71. Hopfner R, Tran TT, Island ER, McLaughlin GE. Nonsurgical care of intestinal and multivisceral transplant recipients: a review for the intensivist. J Intensive Care Med. 2013;28: 215–29.

72. Abu-Elmagd K, Reyes J, Bond G, et al. Clinical intestinal transplantation: a decade of experience at a single center. Ann Surg. 2001;234:404–17.
73. Rambhia PH, Hanna R, Bergfeld WF. Graft versus host disease in a pediatric multiple organ transplant recipient with trichohepatoenteric syndrome - a unique case report. Int J Dermatol. 2018;57:89–91.
74. Fischer RT, Friend B, Talmon GA, Grant WJ, Quiros-Tejeira RE, Langnas AN, Coccia PF. Intestinal transplantation in children with multiple intestinal atresias and immunodeficiency. Pediatr Transplant. 2014;18:190–6.
75. Andres AM, Santamaría ML, Ramos E, Sarriá J, Molina M, Hernandez F, Encinas JL, Larrauri J, Prieto G, Tovar JA. Graft-vs-host disease after small bowel transplantation in children. J Pediatr Surg. 2010;45:330–6.
76. Kato T, Tzakis AG, Selvaggi G, et al. Intestinal and multivisceral transplantation in children. Ann Surg. 2006;243:756–64.
77. Dharnidharka VR, Tejani AH, Ho PL, Harmon WE. Post-transplant lymphoproliferative disorder in the United States: young Caucasian males are at highest risk. Am J Transplant. 2002;2:993–8.
78. Hryhorczuk AL, Kim HB, Harris MH, Vargas SO, Zurakowski D, Lee EY. Imaging findings in children with proliferative disorders following multivisceral transplantation. Pediatr Radiol. 2015;45:1138–45.
79. Boudjemaa S, Boman F, Guigonis V, Boccon-Gibod L. Brain involvement in multicentric Epstein-Barr virus-associated smooth muscle tumours in a child after kidney transplantation. Virchows Arch. 2004;444:387–91.
80. van Stralen KJ, Borzych-Dużalka D, Hataya H, et al. Survival and clinical outcomes of children starting renal replacement therapy in the neonatal period. Kidney Int. 2014;86:168–74.
81. Grant D, Abu-Elmagd K, Mazariegos G, Vianna R, Langnas A, Mangus R, Farmer DG, Lacaille F, Iyer K, Fishbein T. Intestinal transplant registry report: global activity and trends. Am J Transplant. 2015;15:210–9.
82. Andres AM, Alameda A, Mayoral O, Hernandez F, Dominguez E, Martinez Ojinaga E, Ramos E, Prieto G, Lopez Santamaría M, Tovar JA. Health-related quality of life in pediatric intestinal transplantation. Pediatr Transplant. 2014;18:746–56.
83. Ngo KD, Farmer DG, McDiarmid SV, et al. Pediatric health-related quality of life after intestinal transplantation. Pediatr Transplant. 2011;15:849–54.

Part VI

Ethical Challenges

Ethical Challenges in Pediatric Kidney Transplantation

15

James Johnston and Aviva Goldberg

Abbreviations

ADA	Americans with Disability Act
CKiD	Chronic Kidney Disease in Children
COVID-19	coronavirus Sars-Cov-2
DSM	Diagnostic and Statistical Manual of Mental Disorders
ESKD	End-stage kidney disease
HPV	Human papillomavirus
ID	Intellectual disability
IQ	Intelligence quotient
NA	NA
OPTN	Organ Procurement and Transplant Network
QOL	Quality of life
RRT	Renal replacement therapy
SRTR	Scientific Registry of Transplant Recipients
UNOS	United Network for Organ Sharing
VPI	Vaccine preventable illness

Introduction

For a young person with end-stage kidney disease (ESKD), kidney transplant can offer freedom from the strict schedule and diet of chronic dialysis and is generally associated with improved morbidity, mortality, and self-reported quality of life

J. Johnston · A. Goldberg (✉)
Department of Pediatrics and Child Health, Max Rady College of Medicine, University of Manitoba, Winnipeg, MB, Canada
e-mail: jjohnston8@manitoba-physicians.ca; aviva.goldberg@umanitoba.ca

K. E. Twombley (ed.), *Challenges in Pediatric Kidney Transplantation*,
https://doi.org/10.1007/978-3-030-74783-1_15

(QOL) [1, 2]. Kidney transplant is not a cure for ESKD and the transplant process involves significant short-term surgical and medical risks, as well as its own invasive and intensive chronic long-term management and surveillance. Despite the burdens of post-transplant care, the benefits of kidney transplantation will usually outweigh the short- and long-term concerns, making transplant the preferred form of kidney replacement therapy for most children.

The demand for solid organ transplantation outweighs the supply of available organs. In 2018, 897 children in the United States received either a living-donor or deceased-donor kidney transplant, while an additional 966 children were newly added to the waiting list. Over the course of that year, 25 children on the active kidney transplant waiting list died while waiting [3]. Because this shortage exists, it is important to ensure not only that donation opportunities are maximized but also that those who receive organs can truly benefit from them.

When considering an individual transplant recipient, the ethical principles of beneficence, nonmaleficence, and respect for persons are paramount to determining the suitability of the transplant for that child and the optimal timing of the transplant. A transplant done too early (i.e., before the glomerular filtration rate (GFR) is low enough to require it or before the child is prepared to receive it) risks burdening the child with post-transplant complications without benefit. Delaying or denying transplant access to a child and leaving them on dialysis may rob them of the benefits that transplant can provide. Respect for persons dictates that we allow capable people to make the choices that are consistent with their personal values. While this autonomy has limits, including when individual choices harm others, just transplant policy will allow for some degree of personal choice [4].

Because the demand for organs exceeds the supply, the individual transplant candidate must be considered within the larger group of candidates, so the ethical principles of utility and equity are relevant [5, 6]. Utility describes the effort to maximize the good to individual and society with each transplanted organ. For the most part, this requires that any particular organ that is available ought to be given to the person who is likely to realize the most benefit [5]. The principle of equity requires that all potential candidates for organ transplant be given the opportunity to undergo a fair and balanced assessment of their eligibility and that allocation decisions be made on morally relevant criteria alone [5]. Transplant eligibility focuses on medical suitability for transplant and aims to disregard morally irrelevant criteria like wealth or social status. Reciprocity may play a role in just allocation as well, acknowledging that there is a duty owed to those who contribute to their communities that may elevate them in terms of transplant priority.

In addition to the principles guiding ethical transplant policy in general, ethical decision-making in children is guided by the best interest standard, at least as long as children lack capacity to make the decisions most consistent with their own values and priorities. In the best interest standard, the balance of benefits and burdens of a proposed treatment are used to determine whether a proposed treatment is permissible and ethically supportable [7]. Burdens are understood to take many forms, and they include pain, activity limitation, fear, anxiety, isolation, disruption, and medical/surgical risks and complications [8, 9]. No one combination of burdens is sufficient to deem a proposed intervention impermissible, although burdens that are significant, recurring, or enduring ought to be strongly considered before pursuing a proposed intervention. Another important standard used in pediatric decision-making is the harm principle, which sets a threshold for state intervention in parental decision-making when "there is evidence that parental actions or decisions are likely to harm a child" [10].

Organ transplant authorities, international societies, and sometimes legislatures have created standards and guidelines to guide how organ allocation decisions are made and justified. Although there is characteristically application and consideration of utility, equity, and respect for persons across these laws and policies, individual institutional protocols and society guidelines are not uniform, and certain patient factors remain controversial with respect to their suitability for receiving an organ transplant [11, 12]. There are stark inequities in access to transplantation for children of different races, intellectual capacity, and citizenship status, indicating that we need to continually interrogate our transplant policy and aim for better outcomes for all children. Throughout this chapter, we will explore various potential ethical dilemmas and challenges as they relate to kidney transplantation.

Children with Intellectual Disability and Other Co-morbidities

Intellectual disability (ID; also referred to as "intellectual development disorder" and replacing the outdated term "mental retardation") is defined by the presence of deficits in both intellectual and adaptive functioning in conceptual, social, and practical domains. ID has a prevalence of 1% among the general population, and "severe" ID has a prevalence of 0.6% [13]. The diagnosis of ID requires standardized assessment of both intelligence and adaptive function. Intelligence quotient (IQ) test scores, which formed the basis of diagnosing ID in previous editions of the Diagnostic and Statistical Manual of Mental Disorders (DSM), are now recognized to be only approximations of an individual's ability to accommodate, adapt, and perform tasks [14]. An individual's adaptive function may be above, at, or below what would be expected given their IQ test score, hence the recent de-emphasis on formal IQ testing when it comes to making a diagnosis of ID. Differences in adaptive functioning may be at least partly related to differences in social and community supports for an individual living with ID [14, 15]. The American Psychiatric Association recommends that assessment of adaptive function be based on clinical interpretation of standardized assessments and interviews and information from multiple informants [13]. There is no standardized method of assessing adaptive function that is recommended by the transplant community at present [11, 12].

The exact prevalence of ID among children with CKD/ESKD is unknown, although there are a number of conditions, including genetic syndromes and peri- and neonatal complications that can lead to both intellectual disability and chronic kidney disease (CKD). Registries like the Chronic Kidney Disease in Children (CKiD) have found that 21–40% of participants scored at least one standard deviation (SD) below the mean on measures of IQ, academic achievement, attention regulation, or executive functioning [16]. In a review of kidney allograft outcomes among all children from 2008 to 2011, 16% of all first kidney transplant recipients had definite or probable ID of some severity [17]. The United Network of Organ Sharing (UNOS) has collected data on intellectual disability in solid organ transplant recipients since 2012. Due to differences in listing criteria, transplant center-specific reports may not accurately represent the number of children and young people with ID who could be a candidate for kidney transplant but who may not have been referred or listed. As more children with complex medical conditions are surviving through advances in technology and therapeutics, and that some of these children will have both ID and CKD/ESKD as a result of their underlying condition or complications of their medical treatment, it is therefore possible that the rates of ID in children with chronic kidney disease may rise and that more of these children may present as transplant candidates.

Individuals with ID have and continue to face discrimination and limited opportunities from societies in which their disabilities are not accommodated; solid organ transplant is no exception. Individuals with ID were historically excluded from consideration for solid organ transplant with little discussion [12]. In the 1990s, the cases of Terry Urquhart and Sandra Jensen received widespread attention toward these exclusionary practices from the public at large. Mr. Urquhart and Ms. Jensen both had trisomy 21 and ID; Mr. Urquhart was considered for a lung transplant and Ms. Jensen for a combined heart-lung transplant. Both were initially denied listing on the basis of their respective listing committee's concerns that they would not have the "satisfactory intelligence" or ability to comply with complicated immunosuppressive regimens necessary to maintain a functioning allograft [12, 15]. In 2012, Amelia Rivera, a then 3-year-old girl with Wolf-Hirschhorn syndrome, ID, and ESKD, was allegedly refused a kidney transplant on the basis of her ID [18]. The public outcry from these cases was strongly in favor of approving them for transplant candidacy, and eventually all three did get access to solid organ transplants.

The transplant community has generally moved toward more acceptance of candidates with ID, but there is still no uniform consensus. A 2009 survey of pediatric centers across different organ groups found that neurodevelopmental status (including ID) was considered by 85% of transplant centers as part of their listing criteria at least some of the time, with 33% of transplant centers "always" considering neurodevelopmental delay as part of their listing criteria [11]. None of the centers that were included in the study reported having a formal method of assessing neurodevelopmental status. A recent international survey of pediatric nephrologists found that 34% of those surveyed oppose transplantation for children with ID [19]. Notably, 38% of pediatric transplant centers reported that there had been cases of an individual child who had been denied listing for organ transplant, but would have been listed if not for their neurodevelopmental status, while 40% of transplant centers reported that neurodevelopmental delay was never an absolute contraindication to listing for transplant [11].

Most major transplant society guidelines now incorporate some degree of consideration of ID into their recommended practices with many more recent documents supporting transplant candidacy. The 2020 KDIGO guidelines on transplant candidacy recommend that children "should not be excluded from kidney transplantation because of non-progressive intellectual, developmental, or cognitive disability" [20]. An American Academy of Pediatrics position statement regarding children with intellectual and developmental disabilities as organ transplant recipients states that "the notion that children with disabilities have a lower quality of life than children with typical development is both incorrect and ethically problematic in decisions regarding organ transplant" [15]. The Canadian Society of Transplantation mentions that "children who would otherwise be considered for kidney replacement therapy should not be excluded from consideration for transplantation solely on the basis of diminished cognitive or physical capacity" [21]. Others have changed their approach to ID over time. The Transplantation Society of Australia and New Zealand stated in their 2011 guidelines that ID may be considered a relative contraindication based on concern for adherence with the post-transplant regimen in the absence of a caregiver, but in their more recent guidelines, neurocognitive disability is only considered a possible contraindication "in the absence of a carer capable of facilitating adherence to therapy" [22].

The Americans with Disability Act (ADA) prohibits disability-based discrimination in any healthcare setting and specifically includes healthcare settings that are funded by Medicare, Medicaid, and organizations such as United Network for Organ Sharing (UNOS) that operate under a federal contract [17]. However, as of 2019, only 10 US states had specific state legislation that prohibited individuals with intellectual and physical disability from being disqualified from transplant assessment on the basis of their disability [23].

There are a number of established medical contraindications to transplantation that are related to the concept of reduced graft utility; these include diseases that could be expected to recur post-transplant, diseases that could be expected to be worsened by post-transplant immunosuppression, and diseases that could make transplant surgery unsafe for the patient [24]. In those cases, withholding a scarce resource from a patient with a medical contraindication is ethically permissible if there is another patient who could benefit without the increased risk for graft failure or poor patient outcome.

Arguments against providing kidney transplants for individuals with ID have included concerns about poorer allograft function in individuals with ID, concerns about the amount of benefit that is gained from providing an organ transplant to an individual with ID, and concerns that other wait-listed patients could suffer on account of transplants being offered to individuals with ID [12, 15, 16]. As a prominent physician stated in regard to the Rivera case, her transplant should have been denied "because there is a shortage of kidneys… and her impairments are too significant" [32].

However, the existing literature on graft and patient outcomes in transplant recipients with ID is that they do just as well as those of average intellect. Several studies examining patient and allograft outcomes among children with ID have observed excellent graft and patient survival [12]. Importantly, no significant difference in patient or graft outcomes was observed when pediatric kidney transplant recipients with ID were compared to pediatric kidney transplant recipients without ID [17].

This is likely due to the fact that all of these children who need a kidney transplant also need support to manage that transplant. All children with ESKD and who receive chronic kidney replacement therapies, including kidney transplantation, will require considerable social support from their caregivers and transplant teams. Some children will never reach a level of independence that permits them to entirely self-manage their chronic post-transplant regimen, including many individuals with ID, and may remain dependent on their caregivers well past the age of legal maturity. The spectrum of support needs among individuals with ID is broad, but there are resources in place to address the various and proportionate needs of people with intellectual and physical disabilities. These needs should therefore not be used as reason to deny these individuals access to transplant [15, 23].

Individuals with ID may have other conditions that are potentially life limiting, but it is important to make decisions on their transplant candidacy based on an assessment of how transplant could improve their life, not a simple weighting of how many disabilities they face. If a child's lifespan would not be significantly improved by undergoing kidney transplantation, or if their medical conditions were expected to drastically reduce the likelihood of transplant function, then it may be reasonable to not offer kidney transplantation, for the same utility-based rationale that kidney transplantations are withheld for other medical contraindications. An example of this may be co-existing and non-remediable severe heart failure. However, it is also not uncommon for individuals with ID to have multiple medical conditions that do not significantly reduce their expected life span or quality of life. For example, a child with Bardet-Biedl syndrome might have visual impairment, ID, and kidney disease. In this case, kidney transplant may improve the child's length of life and allow them the time to live well with supports for their other conditions. It would be inappropriate to withhold kidney transplantation from such a child simply because she has multiple challenges since none of them reduce the utility of the transplant itself.

Advances in medical technology have also changed our understanding of life-limiting conditions and ID, and we now understand better that children can live meaningful lives even when they have multiple disabilities. Trisomy 13 and trisomy 18, for example, were until very recently considered universally fatal in the perinatal/neonatal period. Due to changing perception of ID and the advocacy of parents of children with these conditions, changes in the approach to providing life-sustaining support for these individuals became accepted practice in some centers, and some of these children now live well into their childhoods and beyond, making interventions like heart surgery and even transplantation possible for these children [25, 26]. Conditions that were once barriers to successful intervention now have better therapies to ameliorate them. For example, tracheostomy and feeding tube placement can extend the lifespan and improve the quality of life for individuals with chronic respiratory and nutritional issues, such that medical multi-morbidity may not necessarily be a contraindication to other interventions. While the cumulative burdens of these intensive therapies needs to be considered prior to proceeding with a transplant evaluation, even a high technology intervention can be ethically considered so long as the overall benefits are expected to outweigh the burdens. This does not mean that any child or individual with ESKD, ID, and medical complexity is obligated to receive a kidney transplant, as there are situations in which the burdens will exceed the benefits [24].

Implicit and explicit biases have discriminated against individuals with ID (and other disabilities) and influenced their eligibility to be evaluated for transplantation. A 2004 survey of individuals living with disabilities and solid organ failure reported that 80% of participants faced some degree of discrimination (both physical/structural and attitudinal) during their transplant process [27]. The concept of "quality of life" is a core issue in organ transplantation. Kidneys are allocated to individuals who are felt to most benefit from them, and this is often communicated on the basis of improvement in quality of life. However, these assessments are fraught with troubling limitations. Many tests of quality of life rely on assessment of functional abilities, which are interpreted through the eyes of an individual without the disability, thus reflecting the viewpoint of the person without disability rather than the individual being assessed [28]. When individuals with disabilities have self-reported their own quality of life, it has tended to be similar to individuals without disability, whereas the physicians of those individuals tend to report their quality of life as lower [29, 30]. Such interpretations of quality of life are rooted in a social worth framework, in which "normal function" is prioritized and privileged due to a perceived ability to "contribute" to society, and disability is discounted and undervalued due to an apparent inability to contribute [28, 29]. Solid organ allocation decisions made on the basis of social value criteria therefore violate the fundamental principle of justice by incorporating morally irrelevant factors, as it fundamentally devalues the lives and societal and relational contributions of individuals with disabilities. The public at large has indicated their support for organ allocation programs that incorporate considerations beyond simply maximal outcomes, including need for transplant, and equal chances for all candidates to receive an organ [31].

While there is a strong case to be made for transplant candidacy for children with mild or moderate ID, children with severe ID and/or neurodevelopmental impairment may merit additional consideration. There may be cases in which an individual child's disabilities and impairments are so severe and significant, that the concept of burdens and benefits becomes meaningless. There is also the possibility that an individual's disabilities make it such that significant burdens cannot be sufficiently alleviated, even with a transplant, or, that an individual's disabilities make it so that substantial benefits cannot be sufficiently enjoyed [32]. For example, Kamin and colleagues argue that conditions such as persistent vegetative state may represent an absolute contraindication to transplantation due to an absolute lack of benefit on the part of the child with persistent vegetative state [33]. Ideally, an individualized assessment of an individual's specific circumstances and their ability to benefit from an organ transplant ought to be made in these cases [24, 33]. However, the ability of a severely intellectually disabled or neurodevelopmentally impaired child to benefit from a transplant may be challenging to measure or interpret. In these cases, the concept of a relational potential has been considered, referring to the presence or absence of self-consciousness and ability to form relationships. Under a relational potential standard, offering life-sustaining therapies to individuals with severe impairments but preserved relational potential would be ethically reasonable, whereas it would be permissible to withhold or withdraw such therapies from individuals who did not possess a relational potential and was therefore incapable of interacting meaningfully with another person [34]. Rather than focus on "normal function" and social worth as a marker of quality of life, relational potential places value on the ability to interact with others as a marker of a quality life. Wightman et al. discuss an expanded conceptualization of the relational potential standard, in which the presence or capacity for a caring relationship – even if one-sided – is sufficient to satisfy the relational potential standard [34]. In this conceptualization, the values and virtues of a relationship are evidence of a good, quality life, and so long as the burdens of a proposed treatment are not significant, excruciating, recurring, or enduring beyond an alleviation or an individual's capacity to reasonably bear them, proceeding with a life-sustaining treatment, such as organ transplantation, is ethically permissible [24, 34].

While the transplant and post-transplant processes may be made less straightforward by the presence of severe ID or multiple medical conditions and complexity, transplant should not be withheld if the individual's quality of life could reasonably be expected to improve with transplant and there is no other medical or relevant factor that cannot be adequately addressed. The literature demonstrates that ID is not a relevant factor to patient and graft survival, and graft success and cases of medical complexity would be best addressed by an individualized approach that seeks to optimize all modifiable factors before (or in conjunction with) deciding on the basis of the best interest standards whether a solid organ transplantation is appropriate for the individual child in front of them [12, 17, 35]. An algorithm proposed by Goldberg et al. highlights the need for comprehensive, individualized assessment characterized by multidisciplinary input and clear, transparent communication throughout the transplant evaluation [24]. In light of the inconsistent methods of psychosocial evaluation used in different transplant centers, the algorithm can serve as the foundation from which to build an equitable transplant evaluation process (Fig. 15.1).

Undocumented Children

There are over one million children in the United States who are living with undocumented status [36]. Only a small portion of these children will develop end-stage kidney disease, but those who do may not have access to kidney transplantation. While dialysis is available as emergency therapy across the United States through the federal Emergency Medical Treatment and Labor Act (EMTALA) legislation and state laws, undocumented children may not have access to the state-funded programs that finance transplant and post-transplant care. Parents and other relatives, who may lack their own health insurance, may not be able to easily volunteer as living kidney donors. Some states, like Illinois and California, have included undocumented children in their state funding for organ transplant, but many others have yet to do so [37, 38].

Access to donated organs is not restricted by residency status as UNOS allows non-citizens to receive solid organ transplants. There was previously a rule that led

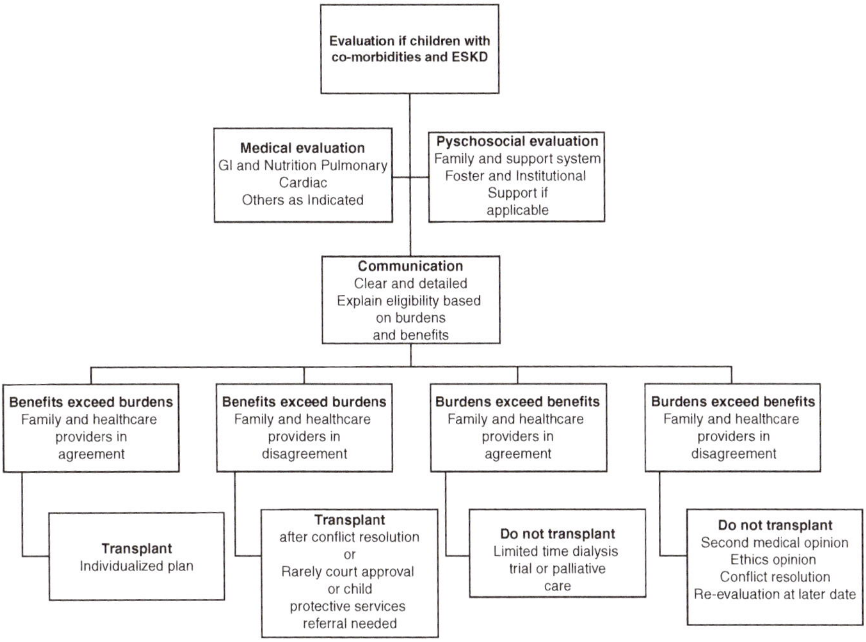

Fig. 15.1 Proposed decision tree to evaluate transplant candidacy in children with multiple comorbidities. (Reproduced from Goldberg et al. [24])

to audit if a center's non-citizen transplant rate exceeded 5% of their transplants in a year [39]. Although apparently designed to reduce transplant tourism to the United States, the policy also discouraged transplant for undocumented residents as centers feared audit if they transplanted too many non-citizen residents as well. The 5% cap has now been replaced by a policy that allows review of registrations or transplants of non-US citizens/non-US residents without a hard cap or specific punitive measures, and non-citizen/residents are now tracked separately from non-citizen/non-residents [40]. In 2018, 13 of the 1084 children under 10 years who received a solid organ transplant were non-citizen/residents [41]. Since undocumented residents are estimated to make up 3% of the US population, this low percentage indicates that undocumented residents receive transplants at a lower rate than the general American population. A 2014 paper estimated that 3.3% of donated organs came from non-citizens, so it is quite likely that undocumented residents actually donate in a larger proportion to what they receive.

Responsible stewardship of scarce resource does require drawing lines between those who are part of a funded or serviced group, and those who will not be included. These lines are often drawn based on residency status and relate to who will pay for the healthcare, even in countries where funding comes primarily from the government. In Canada, for example, health care is federally funded and provincially managed. Visitors to such countries, like tourists or international students, are required to pay for the health care they receive (either directly or through insurance) as they are outside the boundaries of the Canada Health Act [42]. Such a rule allows health care resources which are funded primarily through the tax base to be allocated toward those who contribute to that tax base and to other aspects of Canadian society through their permanent residency in the country. This is consistent with the Rawls' contractarian view of social justice, in which those who contribute to a society are entitled to the benefit of society membership [41].

Some have argued that non-residents should not be granted transplant access, or should only be granted that access after legal citizens of a country are first prioritized, based on the view that they are not members of the community [43]. Some argue that including undocumented residents in a country's publicly funded system will lead to "free riders" who take from the system but do not contribute to it [44]. Others offer utilitarian perspectives that recipients of these organs may return to their home countries which lack the resources to help them maintain their grafts and that their home countries will not develop sufficient resources if their citizens can get access to transplant in more resource-rich countries [43]. Some have argued that in the case of undocumented children, their parents have displayed a pattern of rule breaking as proven by their illegal immigration and worry that such a pattern may be a predictor of future nonadherence to post-transplant care [45]. Of course, in some jurisdictions, a center may be willing to transplant a patient, but it may be restricted from doing so because the insurance to pay for the transplant and post-transplant medications is simply not available to that child [41].

While justified in some areas of resource allocation, excluding undocumented children from receiving transplants on the basis of their community membership is not justified – they are as much a part of the community as are their legal peers. Undocumented residents contribute financially to the wealth of their resident country with their labor, contributing an estimated 11 billion dollars to state and local tax bases in the United States in 2017 [46]. As stated above, they contribute organs to the donor pool, likely more than they take from it. In one study, 60% of undocumented residents with ESKD who lacked the insurance necessary to receive a transplant had at least one potential living donor, further reducing the potential impact on the deceased donor pool if they were allowed to move forward [47].

Undocumented children and their families are part of the complex social structure of American life, and as the widespread public support for the Deferred Action for Childhood Arrivals (DACA) "Dreamers" indicates, American citizens want them to stay [48]. While it is possible that some undocumented children may be forced to return to their country of origin at some point, most will continue to live in the United States even if they lack legal status. They should be treated as the community members that they are.

Transplanting these children may improve overall utility by removing undocumented children from state-funded dialysis (although only a minority of states provide state-funded dialysis for non-documented children.) The transplant therapy that can save these children's lives costs much less than maintaining them on dialysis, thus benefiting the public purse.

Concerns that these children are somehow prone to be less adherent than their legal peers because of their parents' decision to bring them to a country of refuge without legal approval is simply unfounded, as undocumented children who received kidney transplants and can continue to pay for their transplant medication do well regardless of their immigration status. A 2015 study by McEnhill and colleagues showed that undocumented children who received a kidney transplant in California between 1998 and 2010 had graft survival at 1- and 5-year post-transplant similar to their legal status peers [16]. This is partly due to the fact that these children's transplant care is funded through the state's Medi-Cal system. When these children graduate from the program and lose funding for their immunosuppressive medications, one in five of them lost their grafts. While this could be seen as a threat to utility, it is probably better conceived as justification for extending state funding of transplant immunosuppression past childhood, so that these healthy patients can continue to take care of their healthy grafts.

Ethical allocation policy distributes organs on the basis of medical need and likelihood of benefit. An undocumented child's legal status does not affect the amount of their need nor their likelihood of benefit and they are members of the community; they should receive the same access to transplant as other American children with ESKD. As stated by Gordon and Gill, "Maintaining a just and compassionate transplant system in the increasingly protectionist US environment demands continuation of the tradition of supporting access to transplantation to persons in need regardless of their citizenship or place of residence" [49].

Non-adherent Children

While transplant is widely regarded as the treatment of choice for pediatric ESKD, it is not a cure. The long-term survival of the kidney allograft is dependent on diligent adherence to the immunosuppressive regimen, lest the graft be lost to rejection. Adherence is defined as "the extent to which a person's behavior, in terms of taking medications, following diets, or executing lifestyle changes, coincides with medical or health advice" [50]. While important in the management of all chronic illness, it is a particularly relevant topic in solid organ transplant, and even more so for adolescents since they have been consistently documented to have the highest rates of non-adherence (NA) among all kidney transplant recipients [51, 52]. Should transplant eligibility hinge on a candidate's proven or predicted non-adherence? Should the rules for a second transplant be stricter if an initial graft is lost due to non-adherence?

There is no ideal way to measure adherence and many commonly used methods have their drawbacks [53]. Self-reported NA can be easily assessed and offers an immediate opportunity to address the causes and contributors, but it can sometimes be unreliable, as individuals may be reluctant to report NA fearing they will upset their providers or face punitive consequences from the medical team or parents [54]. Random drug monitoring can root out unreported issues, but it may undermine the therapeutic relationship between patient and provider. Outcome-based assessments, such as biopsy-proven rejection and graft failure, offer limited opportunity to intervene before adverse outcomes occur. Directly administered or directly observed therapy is intrusive and difficult to sustain for patients and providers, particularly for multiple daily medications that must be taken life-long. Measurement of drug metabolite levels is possible for some anti-rejection drugs, but increased adherence in the days leading up to a clinical visit in anticipation of impending drug level testing may falsely reassure providers (aka "white coat adherence") [55]. More complex methods of measuring adherence can work well in study environments but may lack generalizability to all clinical situations [56, 57].

Acknowledging the difficulty in accurate detection, systematic review of medication NA in pediatric kidney transplant recipients has reported rates of 30% or higher [51]. Medication NA has been consistently associated with higher rates and faster progression of graft failure and loss [58, 59], mediated through the development of donor-specific antibodies (DSAs) and consequent antibody-mediated rejection. NA is more of a problem in adolescents, when rates are reported at just above 40%, compared with just over 20% of recipients <10 years old [51]. Just under 15% of all pediatric kidney allograft failures are attributed to medication NA, but amount for over 30% of all adolescent kidney allograft failures. Economic modeling has shown a significant increase in health care costs over $12,000 US dollars (USD) (which may be shouldered by the individual or the health care system or both) associated with persistently low adherence to the recommended post-transplant regimen [60]. As stewards of a scarce resource, clinicians are understandably apprehensive about the possibility of graft failure due to NA as unsuccessful transplants violate the principle of utility. Surveys have shown that a majority of transplant providers consider previous medication NA to be – or ought to be – a contraindication to transplant [61]. Approximately 5% of transplant candidates are refused on the basis of previous medication NA, and it is reasonable to assume that more potential candidates are likely not referred for evaluation on the basis of NA [62].

Explanations for increased incidence of medication NA in adolescents are manifold. Unintentional forgetfulness is by far the most commonly reported reason for missing or delaying doses of the immunosuppressive regimen but is by no means the only reason [63, 64]. Adolescence involves an interplay of physical, sexual, cognitive, and psychosocial changes as a young person forms their adult identity independent from their parents and peers. The various domains of adolescent development occur in tandem but are not uniform. Furthermore, the progress of stable, functional adolescent development can be challenged by any number of factors, including chronic illness, mental health struggles, psychosocial issues, and challenges in cognition. The experience of chronic kidney disease and exposure to chronic uremia may contribute to any one of these challenges, particularly cognitive dysfunction [16]. Developmental cognitive changes from concrete to abstract thinking and formal operations are inconsistent in early adolescence and are vulnerable to regression in times of stress [50, 65]. Persistence of concrete thinking can contribute to a sense of invulnerability in adolescents if they cannot conceptualize themselves succumbing to complications that are not experienced personally, or those that are not immediately recognizable, such as the development of DSAs or chronic rejection [50, 64, 65]. Adolescent self-concept and self-esteem can be challenged or consolidated by the experience of living with a chronic illness. Those adolescents who fail to incorporate their chronic illness into their self-conception may struggle to adhere to recommended treatments if they fail to recognize the importance of managing their condition [64, 66]. Cosmetic side effects, which can impact adherence at any age, may be particularly bothersome to adolescents [64]. Chronic illness may contribute to a sense of isolation from one's peers that in turn may lead to the adolescent rejecting the label of the chronic illness. The affected adolescent may try to hide evidence of their difference, manifesting as inconsistent adherence to medications, therapies, or appointments [50, 64]. Parents may struggle with how to transition responsibility for medications and appointments to their adolescent child, which could result in a lack of medication oversight. The adolescent's desire for independence and control over one's life may manifest as rejection of the medications or appointments that have been foisted on the adolescent by nature of having chronic organ failure [50, 64, 66]. However, it is important to recognize that adherence issues are not uniform among all adolescents. The experience of living with chronic illness can just as easily build resiliency and facilitate self-management capacity among young people as the pressures of adolescence can undermine adherence to a recommended treatment.

There is now increasing recognition that NA cannot be attributed to patient factors alone. Rather, NA should be conceptualized as a common outcome of varying, interacting, additive risk factors arising from patient-, condition-, treatment-, sociodemographic-, and health care system-related considerations [51, 56]. Figure 15.2 illustrates these contributory factors (with examples provided) in the form of a pie chart [56]. This conception highlights the equal weight that each of these factors can play in the propagation of NA.

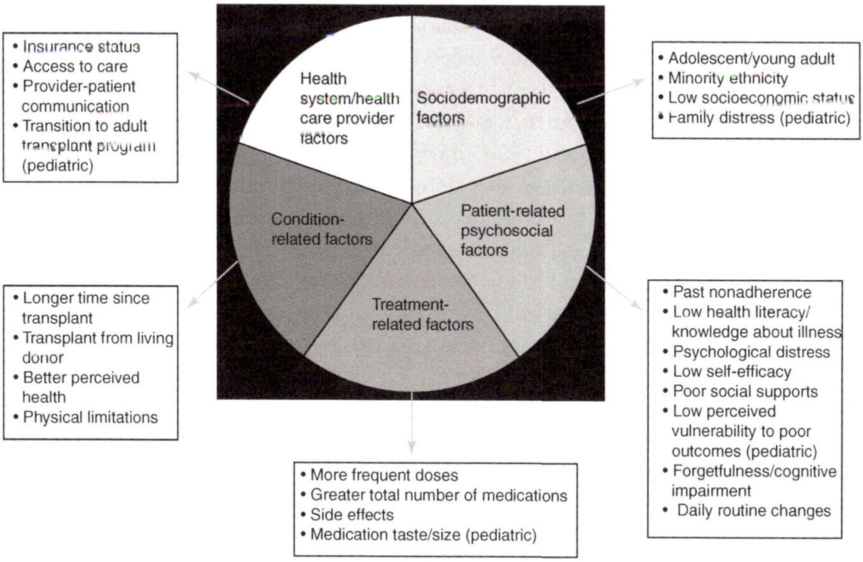

Fig. 15.2 Multifactorial contributors to NA. (Reproduced from Nevins et al. [56])

Given the significant adverse outcomes associated with NA and the desire to optimize successful utilization of a scarce resource, predictive modeling for post-transplant NA has been proposed [67, 68]. There is some evidence in support of the notion that pre-transplant medication adherence predicts post-transplant medication adherence [68] and some evidence that psychosocial stressors are associated with NA and graft failure [69]. The argument in favor of denying a kidney transplant on the basis of NA is based on the principle of utility – providing a kidney allograft to an individual who later loses their transplant due to medication NA not only harms the individual in question but also disservices the individuals on the transplant waiting list who could have benefitted from the graft that is now lost to all. However, there is no predictive pattern, model, tool, or collection of factors that can definitively predict post-transplant NA; thus, these tools are at best suggestive. It is important to recognize that the tasks involved in living on chronic dialysis and living with a kidney transplant (such as fluid intake and dietary restrictions) are significantly different, and the relief of uremic symptoms may make it easier to tolerate pills and perform cognitive tasks like remembering to take pills on time. Without the ability to conclusively predict whether someone will be non-adherent post-transplant, denying their access to a life-changing therapy on the basis of a flawed assessment cannot be ethically supported.

Predictive models and psychosocial assessments can play an important role in the peri-transplant process, but dismissive, prejudicial, or punitive use risks denying children who could benefit from a kidney transplant from receiving one. It risks labeling an individual with a marker that is difficult to shake and can color their future experiences with health care. It also risks further restricting access to marginalized groups, who in addition to experiencing barriers at all points along the transplant process are more likely to be labeled as non-adherent [70–73]. The ethical use of these models and assessments should be systematic, individualized, thoughtful, and solution-focused. We can respect the utility of the graft while also equipping our patients with the necessary tools for success. NA may still occur despite comprehensively addressing risk factors, and there are some contributory factors that are beyond the ability of an individual patient or care team to mitigate. But, as we have discussed elsewhere, denying transplantation on the basis of possible future challenges is not ethically supportable, particularly when the consequences of doing so are so significant. Medication adherence and NA can fluctuate over time, so as pediatric kidney transplant recipients continue to grow up, addressing NA must be thought of as an ongoing, essential process that requires us to be vigilant and attuned to its presence [74]. A number of different strategies are available for addressing incident, chronic, and recurrent NA. There is emerging evidence that promoting self-management can help to reduce the incidence of NA in transplant recipients [64, 66], and this may represent an effective way of preventing problems associated with medication NA, rather than dealing with the consequences.

Between 3% and 11% of the deceased donor kidney transplant waiting list is made up of those relisted after previous graft failure [75]. Although graft loss due to NA can be difficult to accurately ascertain, we know that NA is a common cause of rejection, and rejection a common cause of graft loss [59]. When NA leads to graft loss, it is reasonable to consider how much that nonadherence should factor into the decision to reactivate that patient for a second kidney transplant. There may be concerns that a second transplant may not actually benefit the recipient unless the reasons for the first graft loss have been ameliorated. Moreover, there may be a justice-based argument against re-transplantation in that patients who receive two kidney allografts are benefitting disproportionately compared to patients who have remained waiting for their first. Since most deceased donor allocation systems prioritized pediatric recipients for a transplant, it is possible that a child who lost their first transplant to nonadherence could receive a second transplant faster than an adult waiting for their first.

There is overall limited evidence on the outcomes of re-transplantation in previously non-adherent kidney transplant recipients, likely because transplant programs are apprehensive about pursuing re-transplantation in the first place. When outcomes from re-transplantation were examined using a carefully selected population, the rates of second graft loss in previously non-adherent transplant recipients are higher than that in individuals without previously documented NA (14% to 2%) [76]. However, within that same study population, the majority of previously non-adherent re-transplanted individuals were able to change their medication-taking behavior and had outcomes similar to those who were re-transplanted for graft failures not related to non-adherence [76]. Of particular note is the finding that adolescents who lost their transplant due to NA were more likely to improve their medication-taking behavior than those who were already adults when they lost their graft [76], suggesting that developmental susceptibility to NA can effectively be outgrown. The possibility for behavior change exists and should be considered. NA arises for reasons beyond just individual factors, and therefore resolutely punishing an individual who has been non-adherent by barring them from receiving another chance at a life-changing therapy would seen to go againts the fundamental principles of beneficence and non-maleficence that guide medical ethics. If we can recognize, intervene, and support individuals who are non-adherent, we can do our duty to the person, organ, and community that we serve and honor the principles of utility and justice that guide transplant decision-making.

There are well-established associations between transition to adult care and graft failure [77], and published associations between race and rates of NA [67, 78]. Acknowledging NA as a multifactorial process broadens and complicates our understanding of these associations. Easily measured patient factors are thus revealed as superficial proxies for deeper, more complex matters like access and affordability of medications, ease of appointment scheduling, family dysfunction, and beyond [51, 56]. A multifactorial-informed approach creates many potential avenues for intervention and addressing root causes of NA and can increase equity among children in need of kidney transplant. The rates of NA observed during the young adult transition period should therefore be recognized to occur not only to developmental susceptibility. There should be at least partial onus on the medical system to create a process that does not leave transitioning teenagers without adequate therapeutic supervision and oversight when they leave pediatric and enter adult medical care [77].

A discussion of NA should necessarily include a discussion of race and acknowledgement of systemic racism. Race is a social construct that nevertheless is frequently found to have a significant effect on medical outcomes, mostly due to the barriers and systemic racism that exists in healthcare, economic, and social policies. As a readily measured factor that can distinguish between individuals and groups, race is frequently reported in the medical literature, including in kidney transplant and adherence [79]. Racialized groups are more frequently identified or predicted to be non-adherent [72] than white comparators, and predicted NA has been reported as a basis from which to deny access to kidney transplant to a minority group [73, 80]. The experience of racialized groups is inherently influenced by socioeconomic and cultural factors, which are often discriminatory and inequitable. There is little doubt that the differences observed among racialized groups exist, but the relevant socioeconomic and systemic factors that propogate these differences can be overlooked when race alone is used at the reported variable in outcome data [81]. The experiences of racialized individuals cannot adequately be conveyed by reporting of skin color alone; however, ongoing systemic discrimination and marginalization persist when skin color alone is used to predict risk and restrict access. For example, the association between skin color and predicted NA has been directly cited as reason for nephrologists to restrict transplant listing among Indigenous peoples in Australia [73].

In summary, adherence is likely the most important and most modifiable factor within the patient's locus of control that contributes to good graft outcomes. Having said that, assessment and amelioration of non-adherence are rife with potential biases. An ethical approach to using non-adherence in the evaluation of pediatric kidney transplant candidates will acknowledge the potential biases and pitfalls, while working with families toward greater trust and co-management throughout their transplant journeys.

Under-Vaccinated Children

Vaccines save lives and vaccines are safe. Children with suppressed immune systems, including those with kidney transplants, are more susceptible to vaccine-preventable illnesses than are their healthy peers [82, 83]. While many vaccines can be given after kidney transplant or need to be repeated intermittently (like the influenza vaccine), there are some vaccines that are safer or more effective to give prior to transplant. Live virus vaccines are safest to give prior to solid organ transplant due to the risk for disease activation from a post-transplant inoculation [84]. Many vaccines, like the human papillomavirus (HPV) vaccine, can be given after transplant but are more immunogenic if they can be given pre-transplant [85].

Because of the benefits of pre-transplant vaccination, major pediatric and transplant associations recommend both routine and enhanced vaccination for children preparing for kidney transplantation [84]. As general vaccination rates decline, so does the degree of herd immunity, making vaccinations for individual transplant candidates even more important [82]. There is no question that vaccination should be strongly recommended as part of any transplant workup and that the kidney transplant team should strongly support vaccination. In the midst of the current coronavirus-19 (COVID-19) pandemic, vaccines are likely to become even more of a "hot topic" in the years to come. There is growing data on vaccine hesitancy in the general pediatrics population, but relatively little specific to pediatric transplant candidates.

Despite the strong support for vaccinations among transplant professionals, there may be situations in which patients or families decline vaccination with some or all of the medically recommended pre-transplant vaccines. Transplant programs are then left with a difficult decision – do they proceed with transplant listing if the vaccine schedule is not complete or do they refuse to list patients who do not complete the entire recommended schedule?

Some have argued that mandated vaccination for non-emergent transplant candidates is medically beneficial and ethically justified [86]. In the general pediatrics population, universal vaccination serves to both protect the individual child and improve herd immunity. Both beneficence and justice are served by this approach, as vaccinating one's child protects both them and their peers from vaccine preventable illnesses (VPIs). In the case of children preparing for kidney transplant, the self-protection aspect of vaccination is even higher, as immune-suppressed children are more prone to vaccine-preventable diseases and suffer greater mortality when they contract them. Likewise, the other transplant recipients who they interact with in busy waiting rooms or at transplant camps benefit from herd immunity when all transplant recipients follow the recommended vaccine schedules. Since kidney transplant is generally a non-emergent procedure, those who favor mandated vaccination accept the risk of mortality while waiting for parents to comply to be an acceptable risk given the post-transplant risk of VPIs.

There is also a potential concern that parents who refuse to vaccinate may not follow other medically sound advice post-transplant, leading to higher rates of nonadherence, rejection, and graft loss. As discussed in the section on adherence, psychosocial readiness is a critical part of the transplant work-up. A parent who is unwilling to follow basic public health advice, or who insists on following recommendations that are not based in sound science, may be suspected as a parent who is not ready for the rigors of transplant.

Some argue that restricting transplant to those who follow the pre-transplant vaccine guidelines serves a utilitarian goal. Feldman and colleagues argue that since donated organs are a limited resource, refusing transplant to those who do not vaccinate will result in allocation of organs to "those recipients who have proactively maximized the health of their new organ by getting immunized pretransplant" [82].

While it is completely reasonable to promote and strongly encourage vaccination pre-transplant, there are also potential downsides to mandating this adherence. If a program is serious about enforcing a vaccine mandate, then they must be willing to delay or deny a child access if their parents do not agree to the pre-transplant schedule. While this hardline approach may convince some reluctant parents to agree to the recommendations, in some cases, it will leave an otherwise medically suitable child languishing on dialysis. A delay in transplantation means a delay to the benefits of transplantation – the rate of post-transplant vaccine-preventable infections may well go down, but the rate of dialysis complications and related morbidity and mortality may rise. The child left waiting will be less immune compromised but still vulnerable to VPIs and could even infect other pediatric dialysis patients if they contract a VPI. The balance of benefits and burdens from extending dialysis time vs. the morbidity and mortality of VPIs may well swing in favor of moving forward with transplant.

The under-vaccinated child remains prone to VPIs while they remain on dialysis, so the goals of reducing VPIs are not attained by denying them transplant outright. While their risk of serious complications may be somewhat lower since they are not yet as immune suppressed as they will be post-transplant, they still pose a danger to themselves and others and could infect other children in the dialysis unit as easily, or even more easily, than they could infect other children in the transplant clinic.

A survey by Ladd and colleagues found that 82% of transplant centers would list a child who was incompletely vaccinated for medical reasons, but only 47% would list if the parents refused [87]. This finding suggests that the suspicion and/or anger we have toward parents who refuse recommended vaccinations would lead us to a different decision for this child over one who was unable to get a vaccine for medical reasons. While this anger against the parents is understandable, it is not fair to allow a child to suffer for the parent's poor choices or for the rising tide of anti-vaxxers worldwide. This violates the principle of equity because a child is treated differently than other children based on morally indefensible grounds – the providers' feelings toward the parents of the child. The best interest standard requires us to determine whether a transplant, even with the added risk of VPI, serves to benefit the child more than it does to harm them.

The harm principle sets a lower threshold for state intervention when parents make decisions that could truly harm their children. Given the risk of VPIs post-transplant, there is a possibility that vaccine hesitancy may cross that threshold – they are delaying their children's access to life-saving therapy but refusing a vaccine that is safe and effective. On the other hand, the decision of a transplant team to deny kidney transplant to a child based on incomplete vaccinations may also pass that threshold. As discussed above, the risk of vaccine-preventable infection morbidity needs to be balanced against the risk for morbidity from the myriad of complications that can occur when a child remains on dialysis – infection, cardiovascular events, etc. While there are of course some situations in which parents truly cannot support their child through transplant, state intervention should be reserved for only the most extreme cases. The parent's trust and collaboration with the transplant team is crucial to post-transplant success. We should work as much as is possible with parents to maintain and build upon that trust. It does not appear that the current available evidence puts children at such a high risk that vaccine hesitancy meets the threshold for state intervention even in the transplant scenario.

It may be tempting to assume that parents who refuse the medical advice to vaccinate their children may refuse other sound medical advice, like medication changes, regular checkup, and protocol biopsies. A choice to acquiesce to a parent's reluctance in this case may be seen as a "slippery slope" in which we have, as transplant professionals, ceded our expert opinion to a non-rational and non-science-based approach to care for a complex disease. However, there is currently a lack of evidence to support or refute this assumption – parents may well be adherent to medications and follow-ups even when they refuse some vaccines. It would be reasonable for the transplant team to discuss their adherence concerns with the family, and even to potentially contract to post-transplant adherence, but until such evidence exists we should not assume that vaccine behaviors are a clear indicator of post-transplant adherence.

As with adherence to transplant medications, there is not a one-size-fits-all approach to explain why some parents are hesitant to vaccinate their children. Vaccine hesitancy has multiple influences including contextual factors like history, individual and group influences, personal experiences, and issues specific to a particular parent, family, or community [88]. This will play out differently for different families. While race is an understudied area of vaccine hesitancy, the data that do exist show different reasons for under-vaccination between white and black Americans, with cost of vaccines, trust, and confidence playing a bigger role in vaccine decisions for black respondents [89]. While there is likely a subset of the population that is truly anti-science and/or irrational, there are many parents who are vaccine hesitant because they have concerns that, to them, are very valid, or may not have yet been able to process the medical advice that they are receiving. Lumping these parents in with the "anti-vaxxers" who "don't care" about others or who are acting "irrationally" oversimplifies a very complicated issue. Trust in one's healthcare team is built up over time and is affected by complex social, cultural, historical, and personal narratives [90].

Instead of enforcing a vaccine mandate and denying kidney transplant to those who do not comply, a more nuanced approach may be more appropriate. A reluctant parent should be approached with compassion and an interest in education over punishment. As suggested by the American Academy of Pediatrics in regard to vaccination in general, "The role of the physician in these situations is to provide parents with the risk and benefit information necessary to make an informed decision and to attempt to correct any misinformation or misperceptions that may exist" [91]. As with any other aspect of the transplant workup, an honest and open approach to risk communication about vaccines serves to build trust and hopefully move the vaccine hesitant to vaccine accepting. As suggested by Fahlquist, an approach that recognizes the "moral emotions" that parents bring to this decision may help move the needle. For example, asking questions such as: "what scares you about vaccines?", "what can we do that could reduce your fear?", and "can you understand why not vaccinating scares me as your child's physician?", can open the pathway to further communication and recognition of the role that emotion plays in decision-making.

While a full pre-transplant vaccination program should always be recommended and strongly encouraged, it may be reasonable to compromise on which vaccines are absolutely necessary pre-transplant and which are less time-sensitive and more negotiable. For example, a program might refuse listing until all live virus vaccines have been administered but be more flexible regarding the annual influenza vaccine or the HPV vaccine. Since parents may have concerns about one vaccine but be willing to accept others, focusing on the controversial vaccine and its benefits may serve to focus the discussion on what is the most important. Delaying some vaccines for reluctant parents while insisting on other parts of the pre-transplant preparation may help to build bridges and trust with a family dealing with a complex and frightening path toward transplant. Vaccination is not an all-or-nothing conversation, and a "no" right now does not mean that a family will always refuse vaccination. For annual vaccines, like influenza, or inactivated virus vaccines that require boosters, like tetanus, there is a chance to revisit and rediscuss the importance of vaccination post-transplant. With emerging evidence that live virus vaccines may be possible to give after transplant in epidemic situations, there may be further room to negotiate. For example, a vaccine-hesitant parent refusing the measles, mumps, rubella-varicella (MMR-V) vaccine pre-transplant might be offered post-transplant vaccination in case of a local outbreak [92]. While certainly not ideal due to the risks of post-transplant live vaccines, this just-in-time approach may be better than the alternatives of allowing a child to languish on dialysis or forcing a parent to agree to something without true informed consent.

There are strategies that may encourage vaccination even when parents are initially reluctant. A retrospective review of adult kidney transplant candidates showed that pre-transplant consultation with an infectious disease (ID) specialist was associated with a higher rate of pneumococcal and influenza vaccination. While it is not clear from this study that whether the improvement was due to better monitoring of immunization status in those who saw specialist or whether the ID specialists were able to convince reluctant individuals to get vaccines, this strategy may be one that can be employed in pediatric kidney transplant candidates as well. Transplant programs should do everything possible to promote full vaccination by reducing other barriers, such as insurance coverage for vaccines and clear communication with primary care providers around vaccine schedules, for example, well-designed digital health solutions that could better track vaccinations in these patients and connect nephrology teams to primary care providers and public health [93].

Vaccines are safe, effective, and recommended as part of a complete transplant workup. Working with vaccine-hesitant parents to complete that schedule to the greatest degree possible is a difficult and time-consuming endeavor. With a nuanced and compassionate approach that acknowledges the fear and mistrust that may be underlying this hesitancy, transplant professionals can advocate for the best possible preparation for transplant while working with reluctant families to achieve the best outcomes for their children with ESKD.

Conclusions

In this chapter, we discussed four types of children who have and continue to be questioned as worthy or optimal kidney transplant candidates. We have explained the underpinning ethical principles of a just organ allocation system, the difficulties with assessment of some of these factors, and the arguments that may justify delay or denial of transplant based on these grounds. Ultimately, we argue for an allocation system that is as inclusive as possible and that gives most children with ESKD a chance at transplant. We acknowledge that there may be significant logistical and practical barriers to achieving transplant success for these children, but it is a goal toward which we should be striving, both as individual transplant centers and as a transplant community. With better funding for transplant care and research, better evidence to support or refute our assumptions, and a continued commitment to do the very best for our patients, we are hopeful that all children for whom transplant will be of more benefit than burden will be able to access this lifesaving and life-improving technology.

Multiple Choice Questions

1. Which of the following is the best definition for the ethical principle of "equity" as it relates to kidney transplant?
   (a) All potential candidates are given an opportunity for a fair and balanced assessment, which focuses on medical suitability rather than social status, wealth, or other morally irrelevant criteria.
   (b) Renal allografts should preferentially be allocated to individuals from socio-economic groups that have historically been disadvantaged.
   (c) Potential candidates are given the opportunity to accept or decline a transplant evaluation based on their personal beliefs and values.
   (d) All potential candidates are given an opportunity for a transparent assessment, which focuses only on a specific set of predefined criteria and ignores other aspects of that individual's personal and medical history.
   (e) Renal allografts should preferentially be allocated to individuals who are likely to benefit most from the transplant.

   (a). The principle of equity requires that all potential candidates for organ transplant be given the opportunity to undergo a fair and balanced assessment of their eligibility and that allocation decisions be made on morally relevant criteria alone.
2. Compared to children without intellectual disability, renal allograft and patient survival among pediatric kidney transplant recipients with intellectual disability is:
   (a) Generally better
   (b) Generally worse
   (c) Generally similar
   (d) Dependent on the severity of the intellectual disability
   (e) Impossible to determine empirically

   (c). Children with intellectual disability generally have similar outcomes when compared to children without intellectual disability.
3. What proportion of all adolescent kidney transplant allograft failures is thought to be related to medication non-adherence?
   (a) 40%
   (b) 30%
   (c) 20%
   (d) 15%
   (e) 10%

(b). Medication NA in pediatric kidney transplant recipients has reported rates of 30% or higher. Medication NA has been consistently associated with higher rates and faster progression of graft failure and loss. NA is more of a problem in adolescents, when rates are reported at just above 40%, compared with just over 20% of recipients <10 years old. Just under 15% of all pediatric kidney allograft failures are attributed to medication NA, but amount for over 30% of all adolescent kidney allograft failures.

References

1. Wightman A, Bradford MC, Smith J. Health-related quality of life changes following renal transplantation in children. Pediatr Transplant. 2019;23(2):e13333.
2. Francis A, Didsbury MS, van Zwieten A, Chen K, James LJ, Kim S, et al. Quality of life of children and adolescents with chronic kidney disease: a cross-sectional study. Arch Dis Child. 2019;104(2):134–40.
3. Hart A, Smith JM, Skeans MA, Gustafson SK, Wilk AR, Castro S, et al. OPTN/SRTR 2018 annual data report: kidney. Am J Transplant. 2020;20(s1):20–130.
4. Council NHaMR. Ethical guidelines for organ transplantation from deceased donors. National Health and Medical Research Council: Canberra; 2016.
5. Courtney AE, Maxwell AP. The challenge of doing what is right in renal transplantation: balancing equity and utility. Nephron Clin Pract. 2009;111(1):c62–7; discussion c8.
6. Quality CfBHSa. Behavioral health trends in the United States: results from the 2014 National Survey on Drug Use and Health (HHS Publication No. SMA 15–4927, NSDUH series H-50); 2015.
7. Kopelman LM. The best-interests standard as threshold, ideal, and standard of reasonableness. J Med Philos. 1997;22(3):271–89.
8. Coughlin KW. Medical decision-making in paediatrics: infancy to adolescence. Paediatr Child Health. 2018;23(2):138–46.
9. Katz AL, Webb SA, Committee on Bioethics. Informed consent in decision-making in pediatric practice. Pediatrics. 2016;138(2):e20161485.
10. Diekema DS. Parental refusals of medical treatment: the harm principle as threshold for state intervention. Theor Med Bioeth. 2004;25(4):243–64.
11. Richards CT, Crawley LM, Magnus D. Use of neurodevelopmental delay in pediatric solid organ transplant listing decisions: inconsistencies in standards across major pediatric transplant centers. Pediatr Transplant. 2009;13(7):843–50.
12. Wightman A, Diekema D, Goldberg A. Consideration of children with intellectual disability as candidates for solid organ transplantation-a practice in evolution. Pediatr Transplant. 2018;22(1):e13091.
13. Association. AP. Neurodevelopmental disorders. In: Diagnostic and statistical manual of mental disorders. 5th ed. Arlington: American Psychiatric Association; 2013.
14. Tassé MJ, Schalock RL, Balboni G, Bersani H Jr, Borthwick-Duffy SA, Spreat S, et al. The construct of adaptive behavior: its conceptualization, measurement, and use in the field of intellectual disability. Am J Intellect Dev Disabil. 2012;117(4):291–303.
15. Statter MB, Noritz G. Children with intellectual and developmental disabilities as organ transplantation recipients. Pediatrics. 2020;145(5):e20200625.
16. Mendley SR, Matheson MB, Shinnar S, Lande MB, Gerson AC, Butler RW, et al. Duration of chronic kidney disease reduces attention and executive function in pediatric patients. Kidney Int. 2015;87(4):800–6.
17. Wightman A, Young B, Bradford M, Dick A, Healey P, McDonald R, et al. Prevalence and outcomes of renal transplantation in children with intellectual disability. Pediatr Transplant. 2014;18(7):714–9.

18. Allow the kidney transplant Amelia Rivera needs to survive: Change.org. 2012. Available from: https://www.change.org/p/children-s-hospital-of-philadelphia-allow-the-kidney-transplant-amelia-rivera-needs-to-survive.
19. Willem L, Knops N, Mekahli D, Cochat P, Edefonti A, Verrina E, et al. Renal replacement therapy in children with severe developmental disability: guiding questions for decision-making. Eur J Pediatr. 2018;177(12):1735–43.
20. Chadban SJ, Ahn C, Axelrod DA, Foster BJ, Kasiske BL, Kher V, et al. KDIGO clinical practice guideline on the evaluation and management of candidates for kidney transplantation. Transplantation. 2020;104(4S1):S11–S103.
21. Knoll G, Cockfield S, Blydt-Hansen T, Baran D, Kiberd B, Landsberg D, et al. Canadian Society of Transplantation consensus guidelines on eligibility for kidney transplantation. CMAJ Can Med Assoc J/journal de l'Association medicale canadienne. 2005;173(10):1181–4.
22. Zealand TTSoAaN. Clinical guidelines for organ transplantation from deceased donors Version 1.4; 2016.
23. Chen A, Ahmad M, Flescher A, Freeman WL, Little S, Martins PN, et al. Access to transplantation for persons with intellectual disability: strategies for nondiscrimination. Am J Transplant. 2020;20(8):2009–16.
24. Goldberg AM, Amaral S, Moudgil A. Developing a framework for evaluating kidney transplantation candidacy in children with multiple comorbidities. Pediatr Nephrol (Berlin, Germany). 2015;30(1):5–13.
25. Kett JC. Who is the next "Baby Doe?" From trisomy 21 to trisomy 13 and 18 and beyond. Pediatrics. 2020;146(Suppl 1):S9–s12.
26. Janvier A, Farlow B, Barrington K. Cardiac surgery for children with trisomies 13 and 18: where are we now? Semin Perinatol. 2016;40(4):254–60.
27. Kappel B. Lives worth saving: organ transplantation and people with disabilities Minnesota Department of Administration. 2004. Available from: https://mn.gov/mnddc/news/newsitems/transplant.html.
28. Harris J. QALYfying the value of life. J Med Ethics. 1987;13(3):117–23.
29. Waters E, Davis E, Ronen GM, Rosenbaum P, Livingston M, Saigal S. Quality of life instruments for children and adolescents with neurodisabilities: how to choose the appropriate instrument. Dev Med Child Neurol. 2009;51(8):660–9.
30. Janse AJ, Sinnema G, Uiterwaal CS, Kimpen JL, Gemke RJ. Quality of life in chronic illness: perceptions of parents and paediatricians. Arch Dis Child. 2005;90(5):486–91.
31. Ratcliffe J. Public preferences for the allocation of donor liver grafts for transplantation. Health Econ. 2000;9(2):137–48.
32. Wilkinson D. Is it in the best interests of an intellectually disabled infant to die? J Med Ethics. 2006;32(8):454–9.
33. Kamin DS, Freiberger D, Daly KP, Oliva M, Helfand L, Haynes K, et al. What is the role of developmental disability in patient selection for pediatric solid organ transplantation? Am J Transplant. 2016;16(3):767–72.
34. Wightman A, Kett J, Campelia G, Wilfond BS. The relational potential standard: rethinking the ethical justification for life-sustaining treatment for children with profound cognitive disabilities. Hastings Cent Rep. 2019;49(3):18–25.
35. Martens MA, Jones L, Reiss S. Organ transplantation, organ donation and mental retardation. Pediatr Transplant. 2006;10(6):658–64.
36. Gleeson S, Gonzales RG. When do papers matter? An institutional analysis of undocumented life in the United States. Int Migr. 2012;50(4):1–19.
37. Medicare-Medicaid Alignment Initiative (MMAI) Nursing Home Residents' Managed Care Rights Law., 305 ILCS 5/5F-1; 2014.
38. An act to amend Section 14007.8 of the Welfare and Institutions Code, relating to health care coverage., S. 709, California Senate; 2015.
39. Goldberg AM, Simmerling M, Frader JE. Why nondocumented residents should have access to kidney transplantation: arguments for lifting the federal ban on reimbursement. Transplantation. 2007;83(1):17–20.

40. Network OPaT. OPTN policy 17- International organ transplantation.
41. Charnaya O, Verghese P, Goldberg A, Ladin K, Porteny T, Lantos JD. Access to transplantation for undocumented pediatric patients. Pediatrics. 2020;146(1):e20193692.
42. Canada Health Act, RSC 1985, c C-6; 1985.
43. Hartsock JA, Ivy SS, Helft PR. Liver allocation to non-U.S. citizen non-U.S. residents: an ethical framework for a last-in-line approach. Am J Transplant. 2016;16(6):1681–7.
44. Dwyer J. Illegal immigrants, health care, and social responsibility. Hastings Cent Rep. 2004;34(1):34–41.
45. Friedman AL, Friedman EA. Illegal aliens are not entitled to federally funded organ transplants. Transplantation. 2007;83(1):21–3.
46. Gee LC, Hill MG, Weibe, ME. "Undocumented Immigrants' State & Local Tax Contributions" Washington, DC: Institute on Taxation and Economic Policy; 2017.
47. Baru JS, Lucas BR, Martinez C, Brauner D. Organ donation among undocumented hispanic immigrants: an assessment of knowledge and attitudes. J Clin Ethics. 2013;24(4):364–72.
48. Krogstad JM. Americans broadly support legal status for immigrants brought to the U.S. illegally as children: Pew Research. 2020 [cited 2020 November 1]. Available from: https://www.pewresearch.org/fact-tank/2020/06/17/americans-broadly-support-legal-status-for-immigrants-brought-to-the-u-s-illegally-as-children/.
49. Gordon EJ, Gill JS. US transplant policy should strengthen bridges, not build walls. Am J Transplant. 2016;16(6):1645–6.
50. Taddeo D, Egedy M, Frappier JY. Adherence to treatment in adolescents. Paediatr Child Health. 2008;13(1):19–24.
51. Dobbels F, Ruppar T, De Geest S, Decorte A, Van Damme-Lombaerts R, Fine RN. Adherence to the immunosuppressive regimen in pediatric kidney transplant recipients: a systematic review. Pediatr Transplant. 2010;14(5):603–13.
52. Foster BJ, Dahhou M, Zhang X, Platt RW, Samuel SM, Hanley JA. Association between age and graft failure rates in young kidney transplant recipients. Transplantation. 2011;92(11):1237–43.
53. Schäfer-Keller P, Steiger J, Bock A, Denhaerynck K, De Geest S. Diagnostic accuracy of measurement methods to assess non-adherence to immunosuppressive drugs in kidney transplant recipients. Am J Transplant. 2008;8(3):616–26.
54. Glass TR, De Geest S, Hirschel B, Battegay M, Furrer H, Covassini M, et al. Self-reported non-adherence to antiretroviral therapy repeatedly assessed by two questions predicts treatment failure in virologically suppressed patients. Antivir Ther. 2008;13(1):77–85.
55. Modi AC, Ingerski LM, Rausch JR, Glauser TA, Drotar D. White coat adherence over the first year of therapy in pediatric epilepsy. J Pediatr. 2012;161(4):695–9.e1.
56. Nevins TE, Nickerson PW, Dew MA. Understanding medication nonadherence after kidney transplant. J Am Soc Nephrol JASN. 2017;28(8):2290–301.
57. Nevins TE, Robiner WN, Thomas W. Predictive patterns of early medication adherence in renal transplantation. Transplantation. 2014;98(8):878–84.
58. Wiebe C, Gibson IW, Blydt-Hansen TD, Pochinco D, Birk PE, Ho J, et al. Rates and determinants of progression to graft failure in kidney allograft recipients with de novo donor-specific antibody. Am J Transplant. 2015;15(11):2921–30.
59. Sellarés J, de Freitas DG, Mengel M, Reeve J, Einecke G, Sis B, et al. Understanding the causes of kidney transplant failure: the dominant role of antibody-mediated rejection and nonadherence. Am J Transplant. 2012;12(2):388–99.
60. Pinsky BW, Takemoto SK, Lentine KL, Burroughs TE, Schnitzler MA, Salvalaggio PR. Transplant outcomes and economic costs associated with patient noncompliance to immunosuppression. Am J Transplant. 2009;9(11):2597–606.
61. Tong A, Jan S, Wong G, Craig JC, Irving M, Chadban S, et al. Rationing scarce organs for transplantation: healthcare provider perspectives on wait-listing and organ allocation. Clin Transpl. 2013;27(1):60–71.
62. Levenson JL, Olbrisch ME. Psychosocial evaluation of organ transplant candidates. A comparative survey of process, criteria, and outcomes in heart, liver, and kidney transplantation. Psychosomatics. 1993;34(4):314–23.

63. Siegal B, Greenstein S. Compliance and noncompliance in kidney transplant patients: cues for transplant coordinators. J Transpl Coord. 1999;9(2):104–8.
64. Jamieson NJ, Hanson CS, Josephson MA, Gordon EJ, Craig JC, Halleck F, et al. Motivations, challenges, and attitudes to self-management in kidney transplant recipients: a systematic review of qualitative studies. Am J Kidney Dis. 2016;67(3):461–78.
65. Diekema DS. Adolescent brain development and medical decision-making. Pediatrics. 2020;146(Suppl 1):S18–s24.
66. Tong A, Morton R, Howard K, Craig JC. Adolescent experiences following organ transplantation: a systematic review of qualitative studies. J Pediatr. 2009;155(4):542–9.
67. Connelly J, Pilch N, Oliver M, Jordan C, Fleming J, Meadows H, et al. Prediction of medication non-adherence and associated outcomes in pediatric kidney transplant recipients. Pediatr Transplant. 2015;19(5):555–62.
68. Dobbels F, Vanhaecke J, Dupont L, Nevens F, Verleden G, Pirenne J, et al. Pretransplant predictors of posttransplant adherence and clinical outcome: an evidence base for pretransplant psychosocial screening. Transplantation. 2009;87(10):1497–504.
69. Dew MA, Switzer GE, DiMartini AF, Matukaitis J, Fitzgerald MG, Kormos RL. Psychosocial assessments and outcomes in organ transplantation. Prog Transplant (Aliso Viejo, Calif). 2000;10(4):239–59; quiz 60-1.
70. Omoloja A, Stolfi A, Mitsnefes M. Racial differences in pediatric renal transplantation-24-year single center experience. J Natl Med Assoc. 2006;98(2):154–7.
71. Yeates KE, Cass A, Sequist TD, McDonald SP, Jardine MJ, Trpeski L, et al. Indigenous people in Australia, Canada, New Zealand and the United States are less likely to receive renal transplantation. Kidney Int. 2009;76(6):659–64.
72. van Ryn M, Burke J. The effect of patient race and socio-economic status on physicians' perceptions of patients. Soc Sci Med. 2000;50(6):813–28.
73. Anderson K, Devitt J, Cunningham J, Preece C, Jardine M, Cass A. If you can't comply with dialysis, how do you expect me to trust you with transplantation? Australian nephrologists' views on indigenous Australians' 'non-compliance' and their suitability for kidney transplantation. Int J Equity Health. 2012;11:21.
74. KDIGO clinical practice guideline for the care of kidney transplant recipients. Am J Transplant. 2009;9 Suppl 3:S1–155.
75. Dobbels F, Hames A, Aujoulat I, Heaton N, Samyn M. Should we retransplant a patient who is non-adherent? A literature review and critical reflection. Pediatr Transplant. 2012;16(1): 4–11.
76. Dunn TB, Browne BJ, Gillingham KJ, Kandaswamy R, Humar A, Payne WD, et al. Selective retransplant after graft loss to nonadherence: success with a second chance. Am J Transplant. 2009;9(6):1337–46.
77. Samuel SM, Nettel-Aguirre A, Hemmelgarn BR, Tonelli MA, Soo A, Clark C, et al. Graft failure and adaptation period to adult healthcare centers in pediatric renal transplant patients. Transplantation. 2011;91(12):1380–5.
78. Jarzembowski T, John E, Panaro F, Heiliczer J, Kraft K, Bogetti D, et al. Impact of non-compliance on outcome after pediatric kidney transplantation: an analysis in racial subgroups. Pediatr Transplant. 2004;8(4):367–71.
79. Moseley KL, Kershaw DB. African American and white disparities in pediatric kidney transplantation in the United States -- unfortunate or unjust? Camb Q Healthc Ethics. 2012;21(3):353–65.
80. Epstein AM, Ayanian JZ, Keogh JH, Noonan SJ, Armistead N, Cleary PD, et al. Racial disparities in access to renal transplantation--clinically appropriate or due to underuse or overuse? N Engl J Med. 2000;343(21):1537–44, 2 p preceding.
81. LaVeist TA. Beyond dummy variables and sample selection: what health services researchers ought to know about race as a variable. Health Serv Res. 1994;29(1):1–16.
82. Feldman AG, Hsu EK, Mack CL. The importance of prioritizing pre and posttransplant immunizations in an era of vaccine refusal and epidemic outbreaks. Transplantation. 2020;104(1):33–8.

83. Feldman AG, Beaty BL, Curtis D, Juarez-Colunga E, Kempe A. Incidence of hospitalization for vaccine-preventable infections in children following solid organ transplant and associated morbidity, mortality, and costs. JAMA Pediatr. 2019;173(3):260–8.
84. Danziger-Isakov L, Kumar D. Vaccination of solid organ transplant candidates and recipients: guidelines from the American society of transplantation infectious diseases community of practice. Clin Transplant. 2019;33:e13563.
85. Chin-Hong PV. Human papillomavirus in kidney transplant recipients. Semin Nephrol. 2016;36(5):397–404.
86. Feldman AG, Curtis DJ, Moore SL, Kempe A. Under-immunization of pediatric transplant recipients: a call to action for the pediatric community. Pediatr Res. 2020;87:277–81.
87. Ladd JM, Karkazis K, Magnus D. Parental refusal of vaccination and transplantation listing decisions: a nationwide survey. Pediatr Transplant. 2013;17(3):244–50.
88. Larson HJ, Smith DM, Paterson P, Cumming M, Eckersberger E, Freifeld CC, et al. Measuring vaccine confidence: analysis of data obtained by a media surveillance system used to analyse public concerns about vaccines. Lancet Infect Dis. 2013;13(7):606–13.
89. Quinn S, Jamison A, Musa D, Hilyard K, Freimuth V. Exploring the continuum of vaccine hesitancy between African American and white adults: results of a qualitative study. PLoS Curr. 2016;8:ecurrents.outbreaks.3e4a5ea39d8620494e2a2c874a3c4201.
90. Nihlén FJ. Vaccine hesitancy and trust. Ethical aspects of risk communication. Scand J Public Health. 2018;46(2):182–8.
91. Diekema DS. Responding to parental refusals of immunization of children. Pediatrics. 2005;115(5):1428–31.
92. Suresh S, Upton J, Green M, Pham-Huy A, Posfay-Barbe KM, Michaels MG, et al. Live vaccines after pediatric solid organ transplant: proceedings of a consensus meeting, 2018. Pediatr Transplant. 2019;23(7):e13571.
93. Feldman AG, Atkinson K, Wilson K, Kumar D. Underimmunization of the solid organ transplant population: an urgent problem with potential digital health solutions. Am J Transplant. 2020;20(1):34–9.

Index

K. E. Twombley (ed.), *Challenges in Pediatric Kidney Transplantation*, https://doi.org/10.1007/978-3-030-74783-1

D

GPSR Compliance

The European Union's (EU) General Product Safety Regulation (GPSR) is a set of rules that requires consumer products to be safe and our obligations to ensure this.

If you have any concerns about our products, you can contact us on ProductSafety@springernature.com

In case Publisher is established outside the EU, the EU authorized representative is:

Springer Nature Customer Service Center GmbH
Europaplatz 3
69115 Heidelberg, Germany

Batch number: 10726133

Printed by Printforce, the Netherlands